DEDICATION

To Tai Le, who brought us immeasurable love and joy.

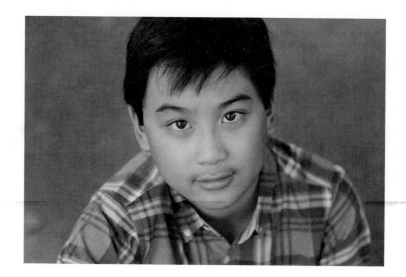

FIRST AID FOR THE® USMLE Step 2 CK

Tenth Edition

TAO LE, MD, MHS
Associate Clinical Professor
Chief, Section of Allergy and Immunology
Department of Medicine
University of Louisville School of Medicine

VIKAS BHUSHAN, MD
Boracay

MANIVER DEOL, MD
Senior Editor and Manager of Faculty Affairs
USMLE-Rx

GABRIEL REYES, MD, PhD
Resident, Department of Anesthesiology
Preoperative and Pain Medicine
Stanford University School of Medicine

Mc Graw Hill Education

New York   Chicago   San Francisco   Athens   London   Madrid   Mexico C
Milan   New Delhi   Singapore   Sydney   Toronto

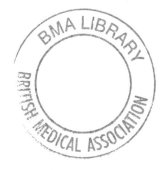

First Aid for the® USMLE Step 2 CK, Tenth Edition

Copyright © 2019, 2016, 2012, 2010, 2007, by Tao Le. Printed in the United States of America. Except as permitted under the United States Copyright Act of 1976, no part of this publication may be reproduced or distributed in any form or by any means, or stored in a data base or retrieval system, without the prior written permission of the publisher.

Previous edition copyright © 2006, 2003, 2001 by The McGraw-Hill Companies, Inc; copyright © 1999, 1996 by Appleton and Lange.

First Aid for the® is a registered trademark of McGraw-Hill Education.

1 2 3 4 5 6 7 8 9 LMN 23 22 21 20 19 18

ISBN 978-1-260-44029-4
MHID 1-260-44029-X
ISSN 1532-320X

NOTICE

Medicine is an ever-changing science. As new research and clinical experience broaden our knowledge, changes in treatment and drug therapy are required. The authors and the publisher of this work have checked with sources believed to be reliable in their efforts to provide information that is complete and generally in accord with the standards accepted at the time of publication. However, in view of the possibility of human error or changes in medical sciences, neither the authors nor the publisher nor any other party who has been involved in the preparation or publication of this work warrants that the information contained herein is in every respect accurate or complete, and they disclaim all responsibility for any errors or omissions or for the results obtained from use of the information contained in this work. Readers are encouraged to confirm the information contained herein with other sources. For example and in particular, readers are advised to check the product information sheet included in the package of each drug they plan to administer to be certain that the information contained in this work is accurate and that changes have not been made in the recommended dose or in the contraindications for administration. This recommendation is of particular importance in connection with new or infrequently used drugs.

This book was set in Electra LT Std by Graphic World.
The editors were Bob Boehringer and Christina M. Thomas.
The production supervisor was Jeffrey Herzich.
Project management was provided by Graphic World.
LSC Communications was printer and binder.

McGraw-Hill books are available at special quantity discounts to use as premiums and sales promotions, or for use in corporate training programs. To contact a representative please visit the Contact Us pages at www.mhprofessional.com.

Contents

CONTRIBUTING AUTHORS

Anup K. Bhattacharya, MD
Transitional Year Intern
Scripps Mercy Hospital San Diego

Jeff M. Cross, MD
Oakland University William Beaumont School of Medicine
Class of 2018

Linna Guan
Case Western Reserve University School of Medicine
Class of 2019

W. Preston Hewgley, MD
Resident, Department of Surgery
University of Texas Southwestern Medical Center

Blake Hollowoa, MD
Resident, Department of Otolaryngology-Head & Neck Surgery
University of Arkansas for Medical Sciences

Aamir Hussain
The University of Chicago
Pritzker School of Medicine
Harris School of Public Policy
Class of 2019

Deepika Manoharan, MD, MSc
University of Edinburgh, College of Medicine

Divya Manoharan, MD, MSc
University of Edinburgh, College of Medicine

Matthew Mui, MD
Resident, Department of Emergency Medicine
University of Florida, Jacksonville

Jun Yen Ng, MBBS
Princess Alexandra Hospital

Christopher Payette, MD
Resident, Department of Emergency Medicine
The George Washington University

Tegveer Singh Sandhu, MD
Resident, Department of Internal Medicine
BronxCare Health System

Cody Stothers
Vanderbilt University School of Medicine
Medical Scientist Training Program
Class of 2021

Visakha Suresh
Duke University School of Medicine
Class of 2019

Gefei Alex Zhu, MD
Resident, Department of Dermatology
Stanford University

FACULTY REVIEWERS

Amitha Aravapally, MD, MMM
Program Director, Department of Internal Medicine
Henry Ford Macomb Hospital

S. Ausim Azizi, MD, PhD
Professor of Neurology and Psychiatry
Mathew T. Moore Chair of Neurology
Department of Neurology
Lewis Katz School of Medicine, Temple University

Elizabeth E. Bailey, MD, MPH
Clinical Assistant Professor, Department of Dermatology
Associate Program Director, Stanford Dermatology Residency
    Program
Stanford University School of Medicine

Jeffrey Band, MD
Physician
Beaumont Hospital, Farmington Hills

Abdullah Chahin, MD
Assistant Professor, Department of Medicine
The Warren Alpert Medical School of Brown University
Associate Program Director, Internal Medicine Residency Program
Memorial Hospital of Rhode Island

Sarah K. Dotters-Katz, MD
Assistant Professor, Department of Obstetrics and Gynecology
Assistant Director, Undergraduate Medical Education
Division of Maternal Fetal Medicine
Duke University Medical Center

Andrea T. Flynn, MD
Attending Physician, Division of Oncology
Children's Hospital of Philadelphia

Germán E. Giese, MD
Physician, Department of Internal Medicine
Memorial Healthcare System

Visa S. Haran, MD
Adjunct Professor
Medical Careers Institute, College of Health Science
ECPI University

Skyler Kalady, MD
Assistant Professor, Department of Pediatrics
Cleveland Clinic
Case Western Reserve University School of Medicine

Ankur Kalra, MD
Clinical Assistant Professor of Medicine
Division of Cardiovascular Medicine, Department of Medicine
Case Western Reserve University School of Medicine
Structural Heart Interventional Cardiologist
University Hospitals Cleveland Medical Center

Jeannine Rahimian, MD, MBA
Associate Professor, Department of Obstetrics and Gynecology
David Geffen School of Medicine at UCLA

Janet Roscoe, MDCM
Associate Professor
The University of Toronto Faculty of Medicine
Nephrologist, The Scarborough and Rouge Hospital

Sherryn N. L. Roth, MD
Assistant Professor
The University of Toronto Faculty of Medicine
Cardiologist, The Scarborough and Rouge Valley Hospital

Robert A. Sasso, MD
Professor, Obstetrics and Gynecology
Director, Department of Medical Simulation
Central Michigan University College of Medicine and CMU
    Health

John P. Sharpe, MD
Assistant Professor, Department of General Surgery
Division of Trauma and Surgical Critical Care
University of Tennessee Health Science Center

Morgan I. Soffler, MD
Instructor
Harvard Medical School and Beth Israel Deaconess Medical Center

Mary Steinmann, MD
Assistant Professor, Department of Psychiatry
University of Utah School of Medicine

Amrita Sukhi, MD
Lecturer
The University of Toronto Faculty of Medicine
Physician, Trillium Health Partners

Adam Weinstein, MD
Associate Professor, Pediatric Nephrology and Medical Education
Geisel School of Medicine at Dartmouth

Preface

With the tenth edition of *First Aid for the USMLE Step 2 CK*, we continue our commitment to providing students with the most useful and up-to-date preparation guide for the USMLE Step 2 CK exam. The tenth edition represents a thorough revision in many ways and includes:

- Best initial steps in diagnosis and management.
- Vignette-style flash cards embedded in the margins to reinforce key concepts.
- Hundreds of color images and illustrations throughout the text designed for better learning.
- A revised and updated exam preparation guide for the USMLE Step 2 CK that includes updated study and test-taking strategies.
- Revisions and new material based on student experience with recent administrations of the USMLE Step 2 CK.
- Concise summaries of more than 1,000 heavily tested clinical topics written for fast, high-yield studying.
- An updated "rapid review" section that tests your knowledge of each topic for last-minute cramming.
- A completely revised, in-depth, student-to-student guide to clinical science review and sample examination resources.

The tenth edition would not have been possible without the help of the many students and faculty members who contributed their feedback and suggestions. We invite students and faculty to continue sharing their thoughts and ideas to help us improve *First Aid for the USMLE Step 2 CK*. (See How to Contribute, p. xiii.)

Tao Le
Louisville

Vikas Bhushan
Boracay

Maniver Deol
New York

Gabriel Reyes
San Francisco

Acknowledgments

This has been a collaborative project from the start. We gratefully acknowledge the thoughtful comments, corrections, and advice of the many medical students, international medical graduates, and faculty who have supported the authors in the continuing development of *First Aid for the USMLE Step 2 CK*.

For support and encouragement throughout the process, we are grateful to Thao Pham and Jinky Flang.

Thanks to our publisher, McGraw-Hill Education, for the valuable assistance of its staff, including Bob Boehringer, Christina Thomas, and Jeffrey Herzich. For outstanding editorial work, we thank Isabel Nogueira, Emma Underdown, and Catherine Johnson. We are also grateful to our medical illustrator, Hans Neuhart, and illustration manager, Susan Mazik. For administrative support we thank Louise Petersen and Jonathan Kirsch. A special thanks to Graphic World and Megan Chandler for remarkable production work.

For contributions and corrections, we thank Naief Abu Daff, Mohamad Adada, Malak Albattah, Sinan Albear, Amal Algahmi, Moatasem Al-Janabi, Chadi Allam, Gabriela Alvarez, David Anderson, Rami Arabi, Emma Bacharach, Katrina Bang, Esther Bell, Kristin Bevington, Inna Bulaevsky, Molly Cain, Stephania Cavallaro, Khalil Chahine, Anup Chalise, William Chang, Vincent Chen, Melissa Chua, Angela Chung, Spencer Church, Sara Clemens, Luis Compres, Jason Crowther, Marcin Czarniecki, Melad Dababneh, Sophia Dang, Nicole Desai, Hanah Detalla, Michael Dever, Steven Dragosljvich, Matthew Drogowski, Morgan Drucker, Sam Duddempudi, Madeleine Durand, Aslan Efendizade, Tracy El Khoury, Roberta Enes, Matthew Gao, Susan Garcia, Angela Gauthier, Joel Gieswein, Luis Fernando Gonzalez-Ciccarelli, Rachna Goswami, Indrit Greca, Morgan Gruner, Carlos Guerrero Rodríguez, Kerbi Alejandro Guevara Noriega, Camille Guzel, John Halloran, Aeman Hana, Hassan Hashm, Kamran Hassan, Joseph Heinemann, Kate Hentschel, Katrina Herbst, Daniela Hinojosa, Joyce Ho, Sylvester Homsy, Mehrzad Hosseini, Arshia Hussaini, Jay Jarodiya, Noman Javed, Molly Kaplan, David Karcnik, Aaron R. Kaufman, Maryam Khan, Yousaf Khan, Ann Kim, David Kohn, Kalyani Kumar, Matthew Lavallee, Luke Laws, Andrew Lin, Robin Lo, Alexander Mach, Anushka Magal, Amanda Maisel, Arslan Tariq Malik, Athanasios Mamarelis, Daniel Marchuk, Dylan Marshall, Otakhon Matchanov, Zachary McRae, Goran Micevic, John Mixer, Rachel Moss, Safa Moursy, Jully Munoz, Lindsay Nadkarni, Shanthi Narla, Ololade Ogunsuyi, Taofeek Olajire-Aro, Carlos Ordenana, Vasily Ovechko, Matt Parker, Brian Pham, Daria Popescu, Meryim Poursheykhi, Charleston Powell, Ryan Raffel, Jason Raina, Chumsab Rattanaruangrit, Jonathan Reeder, Kyle Richardson, Elane Rivera, Jorge Roman, Giulio Francesco Romiti, Kacie Rounds, Michellene Saegh, Apameh Salari, Jennifer Saluk, Hampton Sasser, Zachary Schoepflin, John Scholz, Charlotte Seasly, Sneha Selvaraj, Haikoo Shah, Ritu Shah, Zan Shareef, Soomin Shin, Jagoda Siembida, Jaspreet Singh, Jordan Smith, Morgan Smith, Jordan Stav, Jing Sun, Muhammad Waqas Tahir, Nitin Tandan, Vaishnavi Vaidyanathan, Luis Vargas, Lukas Voboril, Habiba Wada, Stephen Woo, Isabella Wu, Wm. Kendall Wyatt, Erwin Xia, Anastasiya Yakovenko, Tiffany Yu, Maya Zorkot, and Andy Zureick.

Tao Le
Louisville

Vikas Bhushan
Boracay

Maniver Deol
New York

Gabriel Reyes
San Francisco

How to Contribute

In our effort to continue to produce a high-yield review source for the Step 2 CK exam, we invite you to submit any suggestions or corrections. We also offer paid internships in medical education and publishing ranging from three months to one year (see below for details). Please send us your suggestions for the following:

- Study and test-taking strategies for the Step 2 CK exam
- New high-yield facts, mnemonics, diagrams, and illustrations
- Low-yield topics to remove

For each entry incorporated into the next edition, you will receive up to a $20 gift certificate to Amazon as well as personal acknowledgment in the next edition. Diagrams, tables, partial entries, updates, corrections, and study hints are also appreciated, and significant contributions will be compensated at the discretion of the authors. Also let us know about material in this edition that you feel is low yield and should be deleted.

The preferred way to submit entries, suggestions, or corrections is via our blog:

www.firstaidteam.com

We are also reachable by e-mail at firstaidteam@yahoo.com.

NOTE TO CONTRIBUTORS

All entries become property of the authors and are subject to editing and reviewing. Please verify all data and spellings carefully. If similar or duplicate entries are received, only the first entry received will be used. Include a reference to a standard textbook to facilitate verification of the fact. Please follow the style, punctuation, and format of this edition if possible.

INTERNSHIP OPPORTUNITIES

The author team is pleased to offer part-time and full-time paid internships in medical education and publishing to motivated physicians. Internships may range from three months (eg, a summer) up to a full year. Participants will have an opportunity to author, edit, and earn academic credit on a wide variety of projects, including the popular *First Aid* series. Writing/editing experience, familiarity with Microsoft Word and Google Docs, and illustration skills are highly desired. For more information, e-mail a résumé or a short description of your experience along with a cover letter to firstaidteam@yahoo.com.

How to Use This Book

We have made many improvements and added several new features to this edition of *First Aid for the USMLE Step 2 CK*. In particular, we have added more tables, charts, and images throughout the text to facilitate studying. We encourage you to read all aspects of the text to learn the material in context. We have also included comments in the margins and additional vignette questions to periodically test your knowledge of key concepts. These questions are located in the lower corner of certain pages. To prevent peeking at the answers, you'll find the answer on the back of the same page in the lower corner. These questions are not always representative of test questions.

To practice for the exam and simulate the actual test day, you can use the *USMLE-Rx Step 2 CK Qmax* question test bank (www.usmle-rx.com), which was developed by the *First Aid* author team. If you are constantly on the move, use the *USMLE-Rx Step 2 CK* app for smartphones. The question bank and this text are more than enough to allow many students to ace the exam.

Good luck!

GUIDE TO EFFICIENT EXAM PREPARATION

Introduction

The United States Medical Licensing Examination (USMLE) Step 2 allows you to pull together your clinical experience on the wards with the numerous "factoids" and classical disease presentations that you have memorized over the years. Whereas Step 1 stresses basic disease mechanisms and principles, Step 2 places more emphasis on clinical diagnosis and management, disease pathogenesis, and preventive medicine. The Step 2 examination consists of the following 2 parts:

- The Step 2 Clinical Knowledge examination (Step 2 CK).
- The Step 2 Clinical Skills examination (Step 2 CS).

The USMLE Step 2 CK is the second of three examinations that you must pass to become a licensed physician in the United States. The computerized Step 2 CK is a 1-day (9-hour) multiple-choice examination.

Students are also required to take the Step 2 CS, a 1-day live examination in which students examine 12 standardized patients. For more information on this examination, please refer to *First Aid for the USMLE Step 2 CS*. Information about the Step 2 CS format and eligibility, registration, and scoring can be found at http://www.nbme.org.

The information found in this section as well as in the remainder of the book will address only the Step 2 CK.

KEY FACT

The goal of the Step 2 CK is to apply your knowledge of medical facts to clinical scenarios that you may encounter as a resident.

USMLE Step 2 CK—Computer-Based Testing Basics

HOW WILL THE CBT BE STRUCTURED?

The Step 2 CK exam is a computer-based test (CBT) administered by Prometric, Inc. It is a 1-day examination with 318 items divided into eight 1-hour blocks that are administered during a single 9-hour testing session. The number of items in a block are displayed at the beginning of each block. This number may vary from block to block, but will not exceed 40 items.

Two question styles predominate throughout. The most common format is the **single one-best-answer** question. This is the traditional multiple-choice format in which you are tasked with selecting the "most correct" answer. **Sequential item sets** is the second question style. These are sets of multiple-choice questions that are related and must all be answered in sequence without skipping a question in the set. As you answer questions in a set, the previous answers become locked and cannot be changed. These are the only questions on the USMLE examination that are locked in such a way. There are no more than five sequential item sets within each USMLE Step 2 CK exam.

During the time allotted for each block in the USMLE Step 2 CK exam, you can answer test questions in any order and can also review responses and change your answers (except for responses within the sequential item sets described earlier). However, under no circumstances can you return to previous blocks and change your answers. Once you have finished a block, you must click on a screen icon to continue to the next block. Time not used during a testing block will be added to your overall break time, but it cannot be used to complete other testing blocks.

TESTING CONDITIONS: WHAT WILL THE CBT BE LIKE?

Even if you are familiar with CBT and the Prometric test centers, you should still access the latest practice software from the USMLE Web site (http://www.usmle.org) and try out prior to the examination. If you familiarize yourself with the USMLE testing interface ahead of time, you can skip the 15-minute tutorial offered on examination day and add those minutes to your allotted break time of 45 minutes.

For security reasons, you are not allowed to bring personal equipment (except those needed for medical reasons and soft-foam earplugs as detailed later) into the testing area—which means that writing implements, outerwear, watches (even analog), cellular telephones, and electronic paging devices are all prohibited. Food and beverages are prohibited as well. The proctor will assign you a small locker to store your belongings and any food you bring for the day. You will also be given two (8″ × 11″) laminated writing surfaces, pens, and erasers for note taking and for recording your test Candidate Identification Number (CIN). You must return these materials after the examination. Testing centers are monitored by audio and video surveillance equipment. Each time you enter the testing room, you will have to undergo a screening process to ensure that you are not bringing in personal items.

You should become familiar with a typical question screen. A window to the left displays all the questions in the block and shows you the unanswered questions (marked with an "i"). Some questions will contain figures, color illustrations, audio, or video adjacent to the question. Although the contrast and brightness of the screen can be adjusted, there are no other ways to manipulate the picture (eg, zooming or panning). Larger images are accessed with an **"exhibit"** button. You can also call up a window displaying normal **lab values.** You may **mark** questions to review at a later time by clicking the check mark at the top of the screen. The annotation feature functions like the provided dry-erase sheets and allows you to jot down notes during the examination. Play with the **highlighting/strike-out** and annotation features with the vignettes and multiple answers.

You should also do a few practice blocks to determine which tools will help you process questions more efficiently and accurately. If you find that you are not using the marking, annotation, or highlighting tools, then **keyboard shortcuts** can be quicker than using a mouse. Headphones are provided for listening to audio and blocking outside noise. Alternatively, you can bring soft earplugs to block excess noise. These earplugs must be examined by Prometric staff before you can take them into the testing area.

WHAT DOES THE CBT FORMAT MEAN FOR ME?

The CBT format is the same format as that used on the USMLE Step 1. If you are uncomfortable with this testing format, spend some time playing with a Windows-based system and pointing and clicking icons or buttons with a mouse.

KEY FACT

Expect to spend up to 9 hours at the test center.

KEY FACT

Keyboard shortcuts:
- A–E—Letter choices.
- Enter or space bar—Move to the next question.
- Esc—Exit pop-up Lab and Exhibit windows.
- Alt-T—Countdown and time-elapsed clocks for current session and overall test.

The USMLE also offers students an opportunity to take a simulated test, or practice session, at a Prometric center. The session is divided into three 1-hour blocks of up to 50 questions each. The 143 Step 2 CK sample test items that are available on the USMLE Web site (http://www.usmle.org) are the same as those used at CBT practice sessions. **No new items are presented.** The cost is about $75 for US and Canadian students but is higher for international students. Students receive a printed percent-correct score after completing the session. No explanations of questions are provided. You may register for a practice session online at http://www.usmle.org.

The National Board of Medical Examiners (NBME) provides another option for students to assess their Step 2 CK knowledge with the Comprehensive Clinical Science Self-Assessment (CCSSA) test. This test is available on the NBME Web site for $60, which will display at the end of the exam all of the questions that you answered incorrectly, without additional explanations. The content of the CCSSA items resembles that of the USMLE Step 2 CK. After you complete the CCSSA, you will be given a performance profile indicating your strengths and weaknesses. This feedback is intended for use as a study tool only and is not necessarily an indicator of Step 2 CK performance. For more information on the CCSSA examination, visit the NBME's Web site at http://www.nbme.org, and click on the link for "Students and Residents."

HOW DO I REGISTER TO TAKE THE EXAMINATION?

Information on the Step 2 CK exam's format, content, and registration requirements are found on the USMLE Web site. To register for the examination, students/graduates of accredited schools in the United States and Canada can apply online at the NBME Web site (http://www.nbme.org), whereas students/graduates of non-US/Canadian schools should apply through the Educational Commission for Foreign Medical Graduates (ECFMG) (https://iwa2.ecfmg.org). A printable version of the application is also available on these sites. The preliminary registration process for the USMLE Step 2 CK exam is as follows:

- Complete a registration form, and send your examination fees to the NBME (online).
- Select a 3-month block in which you wish to be tested (eg, June/July/August).
- Attach a passport-type photo to your completed application form.
- Complete a Certification of Identification and Authorization form. This form must be signed by an official at your medical school such as from the registrar's office (if you are a student) or a notary public (if you have graduated) to verify your identity. It is valid for 5 years, allowing you to use only your USMLE identification number for future transactions.
- Send your certified application form to the NBME for processing. (Applications may be submitted more than 6 months before the test date, but examinees will not receive their scheduling permits until 6 months prior to the eligibility period.)
- The NBME will process your application within 4–6 weeks and will send you a slip of paper that will serve as your scheduling permit.
- Once you have received your scheduling permit, decide when and where you would like to take the examination. For a list of Prometric locations nearest you, visit https://www.prometric.com.
- Call Prometric's toll-free number, or visit https://www.prometric.com to arrange a time to take the examination.

- The Step 2 CK is offered on a year-round basis except for the first 2 weeks in January. For the most up-to-date information on available testing days at your preferred testing location, refer to http://www.usmle.org.

The scheduling permit you receive from the NBME will contain the following important information:

- Your USMLE identification number.
- The eligibility period during which you may take the examination.
- Your "scheduling number," which you will need to make your examination appointment with Prometric.
- Your CIN, which you must enter at your Prometric workstation in order to access the examination.

Prometric has no access to the codes and will not be able to supply these numbers, so do not lose your permit! You will not be allowed to take the Step 2 CK unless you present your permit along with an unexpired, government-issued photo identification that contains your signature (eg, driver's license, passport). Make sure the name on your photo ID exactly matches the name that appears on your scheduling permit.

WHAT IF I NEED TO RESCHEDULE THE EXAMINATION?

You can change your date and/or center within your 3-month period by contacting Prometric if space is available. If you reschedule 31 days before your scheduled testing date, there is no fee; between 6 and 30 days before, there is a $50 fee; 5 or fewer days before, there is a larger fee (based on your testing region). If you need to reschedule outside your initial 3-month period, you can apply for a single 3-month extension (eg, April/May/June can be extended through July/August/September) after your eligibility period has begun (visit http://www.nbme.org for more information). This extension currently costs $70. For other rescheduling needs, you must submit a new application along with another application fee.

WHAT ABOUT TIME?

Time is of special interest on the CBT examination. The following is a breakdown of the examination schedule:

Tutorial	15 minutes
1-hour question blocks (44 questions per block)	8 hours
Break time (includes time for lunch)	45 minutes
Total test time	9 hours

The computer will keep track of how much time has elapsed during the examination. However, the computer will show you only how much time you have remaining in a block. Therefore, it is up to you to determine if you are pacing yourself properly.

The computer will not warn you if you are spending more than the 45 minutes allotted for break time. The break time includes not only the usual concept of a break—when you leave the testing area—but also the time it takes for you to make the transition to the next block, such as entering your CIN or

KEY FACT

Because the Step 2 CK examination is scheduled on a "first-come, first-served" basis, you should be sure to call Prometric as soon as you receive your scheduling permit.

even taking a quick stretch. **If you do exceed the 45-minute break time, the time to complete the last block of the test will be reduced.** However, you can elect not to use all of your break time, or you can gain extra break time either by skipping the tutorial or by finishing a block ahead of the allotted time.

SECURITY MEASURES

Smile! The NBME uses a check-in/check-out process that includes electronic capture of your fingerprints and photograph. These measures are intended to increase security by preventing fraud, thereby safeguarding the integrity of the examination. These procedures also decrease the amount of time needed to check in and out of the examination throughout the day, thereby maximizing your break time. However, you still need to sign out and sign in with the Test Center Log when exiting and entering the testing area.

IF I LEAVE DURING THE EXAMINATION, WHAT HAPPENS TO MY SCORE?

You are considered to have started the examination once you have entered your CIN onto the computer screen, but to receive an official score, you must finish the entire examination. This means that you must start and either finish or run out of time for each block of the examination. If you do not complete all of the question blocks, your examination will be documented on your USMLE score transcript as an incomplete attempt, but no actual score will be reported.

The examination ends when all blocks have been completed or time has expired. As you leave the testing center, you will receive a written test completion notice to document your completion of the examination.

WHAT TYPES OF QUESTIONS ARE ASKED?

The Step 2 CK is an integrated examination that tests understanding of normal conditions, disease categories, and physician tasks. Almost all questions on the examination are case based. Some questions will involve interpreting a study or drug advertisement. A substantial amount of extraneous information may be given, or a clinical scenario may be followed by a question that could be answered without actually requiring that you read the case. It is your job to determine which information is superfluous and which is pertinent to the case at hand. Content areas include internal medicine, OB/GYN, pediatrics, preventive services, psychiatry, surgery, and other areas relevant to the provision of care under supervision. Physician tasks are distributed as follows:

- Establishing a diagnosis (25–40%).
- Understanding the mechanisms of disease (20–35%).
- Applying principles of management (15–25%).
- Promoting preventive medicine and health maintenance (15–25%).

Most questions on the examination have a **single best-answer** format. The part of the vignette that actually asks the question—the **stem**—is usually found at the end of the scenario and generally relates to the physician task. From student experience, there are a few stems that are consistently addressed throughout the examination:

- What is the most likely diagnosis? (40%)
- Which of the following is the most appropriate initial step in management? (20%)

- Which of the following is the most appropriate next step in management? (20%)
- Which of the following is the most likely cause of...? (5%)
- Which of the following is the most likely pathogen...? (3%)
- Which of the following would most likely prevent...? (2%)
- Other (10%)

Additional examination tips are as follows:

- Note the age and race of the patient in each clinical scenario. When ethnicity is given, it is often relevant. Know these well (see high-yield facts), especially for more common diagnoses.
- Be able to recognize key facts that distinguish major diagnoses.
- Questions often describe clinical findings rather than naming eponyms (eg, they cite "audible hip click" instead of "positive Ortolani sign").
- Questions about acute patient management (eg, trauma) in an emergency setting are common.

The cruel reality of the Step 2 CK examination is that no matter how much you study, there will still be questions you will not be able to answer with confidence. If you recognize that a question cannot be solved in a reasonable amount of time, make an educated guess and move on; you will not be penalized for guessing. Also bear in mind that some of the USMLE questions are "experimental" and will not count toward your score.

HOW LONG WILL I HAVE TO WAIT BEFORE I GET MY SCORES?

The USMLE reports scores 3–4 weeks after the examinee's test date. During peak periods, however, as many as 6 weeks may pass before reports are scored. Official information concerning the time required for score reporting is posted on the USMLE Web site, http://www.usmle.org.

HOW ARE THE SCORES REPORTED?

Like the Step 1 score report, your Step 2 CK report includes your pass/fail status, a numeric score, and a performance profile organized by discipline and disease process (see Figures 1-1A and 1-1B). The score is a 3-digit scaled score based on a predefined proficiency standard. The current required passing score is **209**. This score requires answering 60–70% of questions correctly. Any adjustments in the required passing score will be available on the USMLE Web site.

Defining Your Goal

The first and most important thing to do in your Step 2 CK preparation is define how well you want to do on the exam, as this will ultimately determine the extent of preparation that will be necessary. Step 2CK scores are becoming increasingly used for residency selection. The amount of time spent in preparation for this examination varies widely among medical students. Possible goals include the following:

- **Simply passing.** This goal meets the requirements for becoming a licensed physician in the United States. However, if you are taking the Step 2 CK in a time frame in which residency programs will see your score, you should strive to do as well as or better than you did on Step 1.

UNITED STATES MEDICAL LICENSING EXAMINATION ®

STEP 2 CLINICAL KNOWLEDGE (CK) SCORE REPORT

This score report is provided for the use of the examinee.
Third party users of USMLE information are advised to rely solely on official USMLE transcripts.

Schmoe, Joe

USMLE ID: 1-234-567-8   Test Date: July 2018

The USMLE is a single examination program consisting of three Steps designed to assess an examinee's understanding of and ability to apply concepts and principles that are important in health and disease and that constitute the basis of safe and effective patient care. Step 2 is designed to assess whether an examinee can apply medical knowledge, skills, and understanding of clinical science essential for the provision of patient care under supervision, including emphasis on health promotion and disease prevention. The inclusion of Step 2 in the USMLE sequence is intended to ensure that due attention is devoted to principles of clinical sciences and basic patient-centered skills that provide the foundation for the safe and competent practice of medicine. There are two components to Step 2: a Clinical Knowledge (CK) examination and a Clinical Skills (CS) examination. This report represents results for the Step 2 CK examination only. Results of the examination are reported to medical licensing authorities in the United States and its territories for use in granting an initial license to practice medicine. This score[§] represents your result for the administration of Step 2 CK on the test date shown above.

PASS	This result is based on the minimum passing score recommended by USMLE for Step 2 CK. Individual licensing authorities may accept the USMLE-recommended pass/fail result or may establish a different passing score for their own jurisdictions.

240	This score is determined by your overall performance on Step 2 CK. For recent administrations, the mean and standard deviation for first-time examinees from U.S. and Canadian medical schools are approximately 238 and 19, respectively, with most scores falling between 140 and 260. A score of 209 is set by USMLE to pass Step 2 CK. The standard error of measurement (SEM)[‡] for this scale is six points.

[§]Effective April 1, 2013, test results are reported on a three-digit scale only. Test results reported as passing represent an exam score of 75 or higher on a two-digit scoring scale.

[‡]Your score is influenced both by your general understanding of clinical science and the specific set of items selected for this Step 2 CK examination. The Standard Error of Measurement (SEM) provides an index of the variation in scores that would be expected to occur if an examinee were tested repeatedly using different sets of items covering similar content.

FIGURE 1-1A.   **Sample score report—front page.**

- **Beating the mean.** This signifies an ability to integrate your clinical and factual knowledge to an extent that is superior to that of your peers (around 240 for recent examination administrations). Others redefine this goal as achieving a score 1 standard deviation above the mean (usually in the range of 245–250). Highly competitive residency programs may use your Step 1 and Step 2 scores (if available) as a screening tool or as a selection requirement (see Figure 1-2). International medical graduates should aim to beat the mean, as USMLE scores are likely to be a selection factor even for less competitive US residency programs.
- **Acing the exam.** Perhaps you are one of those individuals for whom nothing less than the best will do—and for whom excelling on standardized examinations is a source of pride and satisfaction. A high score on the Step 2 CK might also represent a way to strengthen your application and "make up" for a less-than-satisfactory score on Step 1.

INFORMATION PROVIDED FOR EXAMINEE USE ONLY

The Performance Profile below is provided solely for the benefit of the examinee.
These profiles are developed as self-assessment tools for examinees only and will not be reported or verified to any third party.

USMLE STEP 2 CK PERFORMANCE PROFILE

	Lower Performance	Borderline Performance	Higher Performance
PHYSICIAN TASK PROFILE			
Preventive Medicine & Health Maintenance			xxxxxxxxxxxxxxxxxxx
Understanding Mechanisms of Disease			xxxxxxxxxxxxxx
Diagnosis			xxxxxxxxxxx
Principles of Management			xxxxxxxxxxxxx
NORMAL CONDITIONS & DISEASE CATEGORY PROFILE			
Normal Growth & Development; Principles of Care			xxxxxxxxxxxxxxxxxx
Immunologic Disorders		xxxxxxxxxxxxxxxxxxxxxx	
Diseases of Blood & Blood Forming Organs			xxxxxxxxxxxxxxxxxxxx
Mental Disorders		xxxxxxxxxxxxxxxxxxx	
Diseases of the Nervous System & Special Senses			xxxxxxxxxxxxxxxx
Cardiovascular Disorders			xxxxxxxxxxxxxxx
Diseases of the Respiratory System			xxxxxxxxxxxxxxxxxxx
Nutritional & Digestive Disorders		xxxxxxxxxxxxxxxxxxx	
Gynecologic Disorders		xxxxxxxxxxxxxxxx	
Renal, Urinary & Male Reproductive Systems		xxxxxxxxxxxxxxxxxx	
Disorders of Pregnancy, Childbirth & Puerperium		xxxxxxxxxxxxxxxxxx	
Musculoskeletal, Skin & Connective Tissue Diseases		xxxxxxxxxxxxxxxx	
Endocrine & Metabolic Disorders			xxxxxxxxxxxxxxxxxxxx
DISCIPLINE PROFILE			
Medicine			xxxxxxxxxx
Obstetrics & Gynecology		xxxxxxxxxxxxxxxx	
Pediatrics			xxxxxxxxxxxx
Psychiatry		xxxxxxxxxxxxxxxxxx	
Surgery			xxxxxxxxxxxxx

The above Performance Profile is provided to aid in self-assessment. The shaded area defines a borderline level of performance for each content area; borderline performance is comparable to a HIGH FAIL/LOW PASS on the total test.

Performance bands indicate areas of relative strength and weakness. Some bands are wider than others. The width of a performance band reflects the precision of measurement: narrower bands indicate greater precision. The band width for a given content area is the same for all examinees. An asterisk indicates that your performance band extends beyond the displayed portion of the scale. Small differences in the location of bands should not be over interpreted. If two bands overlap, performance in the associated areas should be interpreted as similar. Because Step 2 CK is designed to be integrative, many items contribute to more than one content area. As a consequence, caution should be used when interpreting differences in performance across content areas.

This profile should not be compared to those from other Step 2 CK administrations.

Additional information concerning the topics covered in each content area can be found in the *USMLE Step 2 CK Content Description and Sample Test Materials*.

FIGURE 1-1B. **Sample score report—back page.**

- **Evaluating your clinical knowledge.** In many ways, this goal should serve as the ultimate rationale for taking the Step 2 CK, as it is technically the reason the examination was initially designed. The case-based nature of the Step 2 CK differs significantly from the more fact-based Step 1 examination in that it more thoroughly assesses your ability to recognize classic clinical presentations, deal with emergent situations, and follow the step-by-step thought processes involved in the treatment of particular diseases.
- **Preparing for internship.** Studying for the USMLE Step 2 CK is an excellent way to review and consolidate all of the information you have learned in preparation for internship.

Matching statistics, including examination scores related to various specialties, are available at the National Resident Matching Program Web site at https://www.nrmp.org under "Data and Reports."

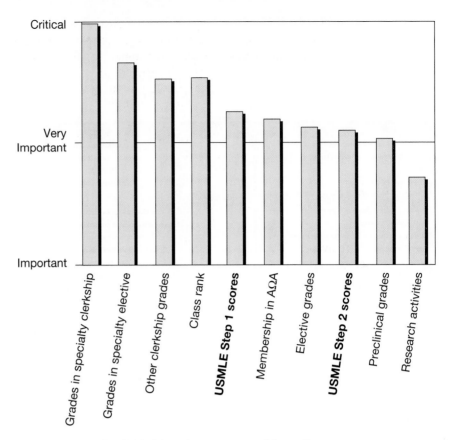

FIGURE 1-2. **Academic factors important to residency directors.**

WHEN TO TAKE THE EXAM

The second most important thing to do in your examination preparation is to decide when to take the examination. With the CBT, you now have a wide variety of options regarding when to take the Step 2 CK. Here are a few factors to consider:

- **The nature of your objectives,** as defined earlier.
- **The specialty to which you are applying.** An increasing number of residency programs are viewing the Step 2 CK as an integral part of the residency application process. Several research publications demonstrate the increasing importance placed on this examination by residency directors. Some programs are now requiring the Step 2 CK score in order to rank candidates for a residency position. It is therefore in the best interest of candidates to have this examination done in time for scores to be available for the residency application. Taking the examination in June or July ensures that scores will be available for the Match period that begins in September. Some programs, however, will accept scores after the application process starts. Check with programs in your desired specialty to determine when to take the exam.
- **Prerequisite to graduation.** If passing the USMLE Step 2 CK is a prerequisite to graduation at your medical school, you will need to take the examination in the fall or winter at the latest.
- **Proximity to clerkships.** Many students feel that the core clerkship material is fresher in their minds early in the fourth year, making a good argument for taking the Step 2 CK earlier in the fall.
- **The nature of your schedule.**
- **Considerations for MD/PhD students.** The dates of passing the Step 1, Step 2, and Step 3 examinations should occur within a 7-year period.

However, the typical pathway for MD/PhD students consists of 2–3 years of preclinical (and sometimes clinical) work in medical school, 3–4 years of graduate work with research, and finally returning to medical school for clinical work. MD/PhD students typically exceed the 7-year limit. Depending on the state in which licensure is sought, such students may need to petition their licensure body for an exception to this rule.

Study Resources

QUALITY CONSIDERATIONS

Although an ever-increasing number of USMLE Step 2 CK review books and software packages are available on the market, the quality of these materials is highly variable (see Section 3). Some common problems include the following:

- Some review books are too detailed to be reviewed in a reasonable amount of time or cover subtopics that are not emphasized on the examination (eg, a 400-page anesthesiology book).
- Many sample question books have not been updated to reflect current trends on the Step 2 CK.
- Many sample question books use poorly written questions, contain factual errors in their explanations, give overly detailed explanations, or offer no explanations at all.
- Software for boards review is of highly variable quality, may be difficult to install, and may be fraught with bugs.

CLINICAL REVIEW BOOKS

Many review books are available, so you must decide which ones to buy by carefully evaluating their relative merits. Toward this goal, you should compare differing opinions from other medical students; read the reviews and ratings in Section 3 of this guide, and examine the various books closely in the bookstore. Do not worry about finding the "perfect" book, as many subjects simply do not have one.

There are two types of review books: those that are stand-alone titles and those that are part of a series. Books in a series generally have the same style, and you must decide if that style is helpful for you and optimal for a given subject.

TEST BANKS

A test bank can serve multiple functions, including the following:

- Provide information about strengths and weaknesses in your fund of knowledge.
- Add variety to your study schedule.
- Serve as the main form of study.
- Improve test-taking skills.
- Familiarize examinees with the style of the USMLE Step 2 CK examination.

Students report that some test banks have questions that are, on average, shorter and less clinically oriented than those on the current Step 2 CK exam. Step 2 CK questions demand fast reading skills and the application of clinical facts in a problem-solving format. Approach sample examinations critically, and do not waste time with low-quality questions until you have exhausted better sources.

After you have taken a practice test, try to identify concepts and areas of weakness, not just the facts that you missed. Use this experience to motivate your study and to prioritize the areas in which you need the most work. Analyze the pattern of your responses to questions to determine if you have made systematic errors in answering questions. Common mistakes include reading too much into the question, second-guessing your initial impression, and misinterpreting the question.

TEXTS AND NOTES

Most textbooks are too detailed for high-yield boards review and should be avoided. When using texts or notes, engage in active learning by making tables, diagrams, new mnemonics, and conceptual associations whenever possible. If you already have your own mnemonics, do not bother trying to memorize someone else's. Textbooks are useful, however, to supplement incomplete or unclear material.

COMMERCIAL COURSES

Commercial preparation courses can be helpful for some students, as they offer an effective way to organize study material. However, multiweek courses are costly and require significant time commitment, leaving limited time for independent study. Also note that some commercial courses are designed for first-time test takers, students who are repeating the examination, or international medical graduates.

NBME/USMLE PUBLICATIONS

We strongly encourage students to use the free materials provided by the testing agencies and to study the following NBME publications:

- ■ **USMLE Step 2 Clinical Knowledge (CK): Content Description and General Information.** This publication provides you with nuts-and-bolts details about the examination (included on the Web site http://www.usmle.org; free to all examinees).
- ■ **USMLE Step 2 Clinical Knowledge (CK): Sample Test Questions.** This is a PDF version of the test questions and test content also found at http://www.usmle.org.
- ■ **USMLE Web site** (http://www.usmle.org). In addition to allowing you to become familiar with the CBT format, the sample items on the USMLE Web site provide the only questions that are available directly from the test makers. Student feedback varies as to the similarity of these questions to those on the actual exam, but they are nonetheless worthwhile to know.

Test-Day Checklist

THINGS TO BRING WITH YOU TO THE EXAM

- ■ Be sure to bring your scheduling permit and a photo ID with signature. (You will not be admitted to the examination if you fail to bring your permit, and Prometric will charge a rescheduling fee.)

- Remember to bring lunch, snacks (for a little "sugar rush" on breaks), and fluids (including a caffeine-containing drink if needed).
- Bring clothes to layer to accommodate temperature variations at the testing center.
- Earplugs will be provided at the Prometric center.
- Remove all jewelry (eg, earrings, necklaces) before entering the testing center.
- Bring acetaminophen/ibuprofen, in case you develop a headache during the exam.
- Check the USMLE Web site (http://www.usmle.org/test-accommodations/PIEs.html) for the personal item exception list to see if a medical device or personal item that you need is allowed into the testing facility without submitting a special request.
- If you have a medical condition that requires use of an item NOT on the above list, contact the NBME personal item exception (PIE) coordinator at pie@nbme.org or (215) 590-9700 for additional information on how to request a personal item exception.

Testing Agencies

National Board of Medical Examiners (NBME)
Department of Licensing Examination Services
3750 Market Street
Philadelphia, PA 19104-3102
(215) 590-9700
Fax: (215) 590-9460
http://www.nbme.org/contact/
e-mail: webmail@nbme.org

USMLE Secretariat
3750 Market Street
Philadelphia, PA 19104-3190
(215) 590-9700
Fax: (215) 590-9460
http://www.usmle.org
e-mail: webmail@nbme.org

Educational Commission for Foreign Medical Graduates (ECFMG)
3624 Market Street
Philadelphia, PA 19104-2685
(215) 386-5900
Fax: (215) 386-9196
http://www.ecfmg.org/contact.html
e-mail: info@ecfmg.org

Federation of State Medical Boards (FSMB)
400 Fuller Wiser Road, Suite 300
Euless, TX 76039
(817) 868-4041
Fax: (817) 868-4098
http://www.fsmb.org/contact-us
e-mail: usmle@fsmb.org

NOTES

DATABASE OF HIGH-YIELD FACTS

How to Use the Database

The tenth edition of *First Aid for the USMLE Step 2 CK* contains a revised and expanded database of clinical material that student authors and faculty have identified as high yield for boards review. The facts are organized according to subject matter, whether medical specialty (eg, Cardiovascular, Renal) or high-yield topic (eg, Ethics). Each subject is then divided into smaller subsections of related facts.

Individual facts are generally presented in a logical fashion, from basic definitions and epidemiology to History/Physical Exam, Diagnosis, and Treatment. Lists, mnemonics, pull quotes, vignette flash cards, and tables are used when they can help the reader form key associations. In addition, color and black-and-white images are interspersed throughout the text. At the end of Section 2, we also feature a Rapid Review chapter consisting of key facts and classic associations that can be studied a day or two before the exam.

The content contained herein is useful primarily for the purpose of reviewing material already learned. The information presented is not ideal for learning complex or highly conceptual material for the first time.

The Database of High-Yield Facts is not meant to be comprehensive. Use it to complement your core study material, not as your primary study source. The facts and notes have been condensed and edited to emphasize essential material. Work with the material, add your own notes and mnemonics, and recognize that not all memory techniques work for all students.

We update Section 2 biannually to keep current with new trends in boards content as well as to expand our database of high-yield information. However, we must note that inevitably many other high-yield entries and topics are not yet included in our database.

We actively encourage medical students and faculty to submit entries and mnemonics so that we may enhance the database for future students. We also solicit recommendations of additional study tools that may be useful in preparing for the exam, such as diagrams, charts, and computer-based tutorials (see How to Contribute, p. xiii).

DISCLAIMER

The entries in this section reflect student opinions of what is high yield. Owing to the diverse sources of material, no attempt has been made to trace or reference the origins of entries individually. We have regarded mnemonics as essentially in the public domain. All errors and omissions will gladly be corrected if brought to the attention of the authors, either through the publisher or directly by e-mail.

CARDIOVASCULAR

At usual speed (25 = mm/s), each large square = 200 msec, and each small square = 40 msec.

Heart rate = 300/number of large boxes between two consecutive QRS complexes.

Axis deviation—

RAD RALPH, the LAD from VILLA hates WOLVES

Right **A**xis **D**eviation
  Right ventricular hypertrophy
  Anterolateral MI
  Left **P**osterior **H**emiblock
    (also consider PE)
Left **A**xis **D**eviation
  Ventricular tachycardia
  Inferior myocardial infarction
  Left ventricular hypertrophy
  Left **A**nterior hemiblock
WOLVES – Wolf-Parkinson-White
  syndrome can cause BOTH

Electrocardiogram

Assesses the ECG for rate, rhythm, axis, intervals, ischemia, and chamber enlargement (see Figure 2.1-1).

Rate

Normal adult HR is 60–100 bpm. HR < 60 bpm is bradycardia. HR > 100 bpm is tachycardia. Common causes of sinus bradycardia are physical fitness, sick sinus syndrome, drugs, vasovagal attacks, acute MI, ↑ intracranial pressure. Common causes of sinus tachycardia are anxiety, anemia, pain, fever, sepsis, CHF, PE, hypovolemia, thyrotoxicosis, CO_2 retention, and sympathomimetics.

Rhythm

Sinus rhythm: Normal rhythm that originates from sinus node. It is characterized by a P wave (upright in II, III, and aVF; inverted in aVR) preceding every QRS complex and a QRS complex following every P wave. Sinus arrhythmia is common in young adults.

Axis

Can be determined by examining the QRS in leads I, II, and aVF (see Table 2.1-1 and Figure 2.1-2).

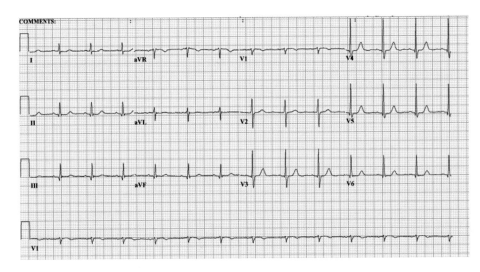

FIGURE 2.1-1. **Normal electrocardiogram from a healthy subject.** (Reproduced with permission from USMLE-Rx.com.)

TABLE 2.1-1. **Axis Deviation by ECG Findings**

	LEAD I	**LEAD II**	**LEAD aVF**	**DEGREES**
Normal axis	↑	↑	↑	⊖30–⊕90
Left axis deviation	↑	↓	↓	⊖30–⊖90
Right axis deviation	↓	↑	↑	⊕90–⊕180
Extreme axis	↓	↓	↓	⊖90–⊖180

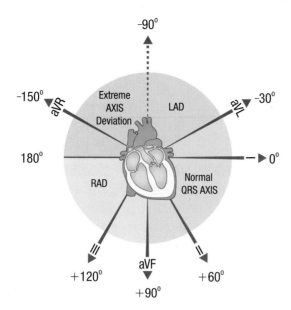

FIGURE 2.1-2. **ECG axis interpretation.** QRS axis and frontal leads. (Reproduced with permission from USMLE-Rx.com.)

Intervals

- **PR interval:** Normally 120–200 msec (3–5 small boxes).
  - Prolonged = delayed AV conduction (eg, first-degree heart block).
  - Short = fast AV conduction down accessory pathway (eg, WPW syndrome).
- **QRS interval:** Normally < 120 msec. A normal Q wave is < 40 msec wide and < 2mm deep. Ventricular conduction defects can cause a widened QRS complex (> 120 msec):
  - **Left bundle branch block (LBBB):** Deep S wave and no R wave in V_1 ("W"-shaped); wide, tall and broad, or notched ("M"-shaped) R waves in I, V_5, and V_6 (see Figure 2.1-3). A new LBBB is pathologic and may be a sign of acute MI.
  - **Right bundle branch block (RBBB):** RSR′ complex ("rabbit ears;" "M"-shaped); qR or R morphology with a wide R wave in V_1; QRS pattern with a wide S wave in I, V_5, and V_6 (see Figure 2.1-4).
- **QT interval:** Normally QTc (the QT interval corrected for extremes in heart rate) is 380–440 msec (QTc = QT/√RR). Long QT syndrome (QTc > 440 msec) is an underdiagnosed congenital disorder that predisposes to ventricular tachyarrhythmias. Other common causes of prolonged QTc: acute MI, bradycardia, myocarditis, ↓ K^+, ↓ Ca^{2+}, ↓ Mg^{2+}, congenital syndromes, head injury, drugs.
- **Jervell and Lange-Nielsen syndrome:** Long QT syndrome due to a defect in K^+ channel conduction. Associated with sensorineural deafness. Treat with β-blockers and pacemaker.

Ischemia/Infarction

Acute ischemia:

- Within hours, peaked T-waves and ST-segment changes (either depression or elevation).
- Within 24 hours, T-wave inversion and ST-segment resolution.
- Within a few days, pathologic Q waves (> 40 msec or more than one-third of the QRS amplitude). Q waves usually persist, but may resolve in 10% of patients. Because of this, Q waves signify either acute or prior ischemic events.

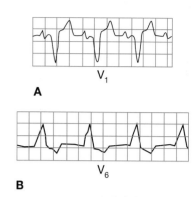

FIGURE 2.1-3. **Left bundle branch block.** Characteristic ECG findings are seen in leads V_1 (**A**) and V_6 (**B**). (Modified with permission from USMLE-Rx.com.)

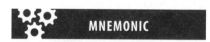

MNEMONIC

Left bundle branch block—

WiLLiaM

V1 = **W** QRS pattern
V6 = **M** QRS pattern

Right bundle branch block—

MaRRoW

V1 = **M** QRS pattern
V6 = **W** QRS pattern

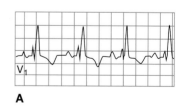

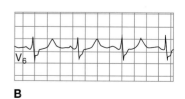

FIGURE 2.1-4. **Right bundle branch block.** Characteristic ECG findings are seen in leads V_1 (**A**) and V_6 (**B**). (Modified with permission from USMLE-Rx.com.)

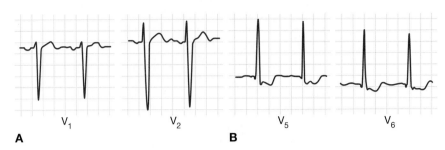

FIGURE 2.1-5. **Left ventricular hypertrophy.** Shown are leads V_1, V_2, V_5, and V_6. → S wave in V_1 + R wave in V_5 = 45 mm. Note ST changes and T-wave inversion in V_5 and V_6, suggesting strain. (Reproduced with permission from USMLE-Rx.com.)

- Non–Q-wave infarcts (also known as subendocardial infarcts) have ST and T changes without Q waves.
- In a normal ECG, R waves increase in size compared to the S wave between leads V_1 and V_5. Poor R-wave progression refers to diminished R waves in these precordial leads, and can be a sign of infarction, although it is not specific.

Chamber Enlargement

- **Atrial enlargement:**
  - **Right atrial abnormality (P pulmonale):** The P-wave amplitude in lead II is > 2.5 mm.
  - **Left atrial abnormality (P mitrale):** The P-wave width in lead II is > 120 msec, or terminal ⊖ deflection in V_1 is > 1 mm in amplitude and > 40 msec in duration. Notched P waves can frequently be seen in lead II.
- **Left ventricular hypertrophy** (LVH; see Figure 2.1-5):
  - **Amplitude of S in V_1 + R in V_5 or V_6 is > 35 mm.**
  - **Alternative criteria:** The amplitude of R in aVL + S in V_3 is > 28 mm in men or > 20 mm in women.
  - Usually associated with ST depression and T-wave changes.

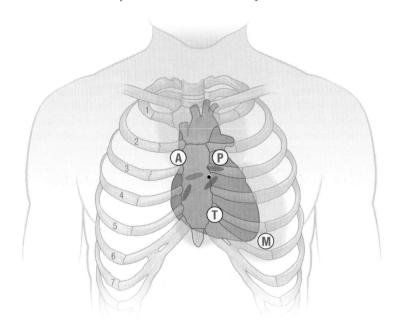

Aortic
Pulmonic
Tricuspid
Mitral

FIGURE 2.1-6. **Auscultation locations.** Auscultation sites are shown with associated valves. A, aortic valve; M, mitral valve; P, pulmonic valve; T, tricuspid valve. (Modified with permission from USMLE-Rx.com.)

- **Right ventricular hypertrophy (RVH):**
  - Right-axis deviation and an R wave in $V_1 > 7$ mm.

Cardiac Physical Exam

Key exam findings that can narrow the differential include the following:

- **Jugular venous distention** (JVD > 4 cm above the sternal angle): Most typically from volume overload, stemming from conditions such as right heart failure or pulmonary hypertension.
- **Hepatojugular reflux** (distention of neck veins upon applying pressure to the liver): Seen in same conditions as JVD.
- **Kussmaul sign** (↑ in jugular venous pressure [JVP] with inspiration): Often seen in constrictive pericarditis.
- **Systolic murmurs** (see Table 2.1-2 and Figures 2.1-6 and 2.1-7):
  - **Aortic stenosis:** A harsh systolic ejection murmur that radiates to the carotids.
  - **Mitral regurgitation:** A holosystolic murmur that radiates to the axilla.
  - **Mitral valve prolapse:** A midsystolic or late systolic murmur with a preceding click.
  - **Flow murmur:** Usually a soft murmur that is position-dependent (very common and does not imply cardiac disease).
- **Diastolic murmurs** (see Table 2.1-2 and Figures 2.1-6 and 2.1-7): Always abnormal.
  - **Aortic regurgitation:** An early decrescendo murmur.
  - **Mitral stenosis:** A mid to late low-pitched murmur.
- **Gallops:**
  - **S3 gallop:** A sign of fluid overload (ie, heart failure, mitral valve disease); often normal in younger patients and in high-output states (eg, pregnancy).
  - **S4 gallop:** A sign of decreased compliance (ie, hypertension, aortic stenosis, diastolic dysfunction); usually pathologic but can be normal in younger patients and in athletes.
- **Edema:**
  - **Pulmonary:** Left heart failure (fluid "backs up" into the lungs).
  - **Peripheral:** Right heart failure and biventricular failure (fluid "backs up" into the periphery), nephrotic syndrome, hepatic disease, lymphedema, hypoalbuminemia, and drugs.
- **Hands:**
  - **Finger clubbing:** Congenital cyanotic heart disease; endocarditis.
  - **Infective endocarditis:** Splinter hemorrhages; Osler nodes, Janeway lesions.

KEY FACT

Axis deviation can be a sign of ventricular enlargement.

KEY FACT

Right-sided murmurs increase with inspiration. Left-sided murmurs increase with expiration.

TABLE 2.1-2. Cardiac Murmurs

Systolic Murmurs	Diastolic Murmurs
Aortic stenosis	Aortic regurgitation
Mitral regurgitation	Mitral stenosis
Mitral valve prolapse	
Tricuspid regurgitation	

A college-age man passed out while playing basketball and had no prodromal symptoms or signs of seizure. His cardiac exam is unremarkable, and an ECG shows a slurred upstroke of the QRS. What are the next best steps?

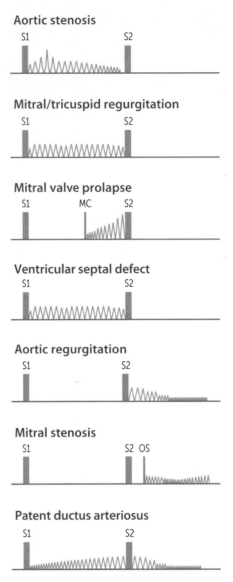

FIGURE 2.1-7. Heart murmurs. Visual representations of common heart murmurs are shown in relation to S1 and S2. MC, midsystolic click; OS, opening snap. (Reproduced with permission from USMLE-Rx.com.)

KEY FACT

An atrial myxoma is a benign tumor of the heart, commonly found within the left and right atria on the interatrial septum that can present with atrial fibrillation or mimic infective endocarditis. On auscultation, you will often hear a tumor "Plop" or see a tumor on echocardiography. Patients may develop systemic embolization from breakoff of tumor, leading to stroke. Resection of the tumor is the only treatment.

A

This is Wolff-Parkinson-White syndrome (WPW). Advise against vigorous physical activity, use procainamide for arrhythmias, and refer for an electrophysiology study. Calcium channel blockers are contraindicated.

- **Peripheral pulses:**
  - **Increased:** Compensated aortic regurgitation (bounding pulses); coarctation (greater in arms than in legs); patent ductus arteriosus.
  - **Decreased:** Peripheral arterial disease; late-stage heart failure.
  - **Collapsing** ("waterhammer"): Aortic incompetence; AV malformations; patent ductus arteriosus; thyrotoxicosis, severe anemia.
  - **Pulsus paradoxus** (↓ systolic BP > 10 mm Hg with inspiration): Cardiac tamponade; pericardial constriction; also seen in obstructive lung diseases (eg, severe asthma), tension pneumothorax, and foreign body in airway.
  - **Pulsus alternans** (alternating weak and strong pulses): Cardiomyopathy; impaired left ventricular systolic function (LVF). Poor prognosis.
  - **Pulsus parvus et tardus** (weak and delayed pulse): Aortic stenosis.
  - **Jerky:** hypertrophic obstructive cardiomyopathy (HOCM).
  - **Pulsus bisferiens** (bifid pulse/"twice beating"): Aortic regurgitation; combined aortic stenosis and aortic regurgitation, HOCM.

Arrhythmias

BRADYARRHYTHMIAS AND CONDUCTION ABNORMALITIES

Table 2.1-3 outlines the etiologies, clinical presentation, and treatment of common bradyarrhythmias and conduction abnormalities.

MNEMONIC

Management options for atrial fibrillation—

ABCD

Anticoagulate
β-blockers to control rate
Cardiovert/**C**alcium channel blockers
Digoxin (in refractory cases)

TABLE 2.1-3. Bradyarrhythmias and Conduction Abnormalities

Type	Etiology	Signs/Symptoms	ECG Findings	Treatment
Sinus bradycardia	Normal response to cardiovascular conditioning. Can also result from sinus node dysfunction, β-blocker or CCB excess; therefore, it is important to review medications	May be asymptomatic, but may also present with light-headedness, syncope, chest pain, or hypotension	Sinus rhythm. Ventricular rate < 60 bpm	None if asymptomatic and rate > 40 bpm; atropine may be used to ↑ heart rate. Pacemaker implant is the definitive treatment in severe cases
First-degree AV block	Can occur in normal individuals; associated with ↑ vagal tone, β-blocker or CCB use	Asymptomatic	PR interval > 200 msec	None necessary
Second-degree AV block (Mobitz type I/ Wenckebach)	Drug effects (digoxin, β-blockers, CCBs) or ↑ vagal tone; right coronary ischemia or infarction	Usually asymptomatic	Progressive PR lengthening until a dropped beat occurs; the PR interval then resets	None if asymptomatic. Stop the offending drug. Atropine as clinically indicated
Second-degree AV block (Mobitz type II)	Results from fibrotic disease of the conduction system or from acute, subacute, or prior MI	Occasionally syncope; frequent progression to third-degree AV block	Unexpected dropped beat(s) without a change in PR interval	Pacemaker placement (even if asymptomatic)
Third-degree AV block (complete)	No electrical communication between the atria and ventricles	Syncope, dizziness, acute heart failure, hypotension, cannon A waves	No relationship between P waves and QRS complexes	Pacemaker placement
Sick sinus syndrome/ tachycardia-bradycardia syndrome	Heterogeneous disorder that leads to intermittent supraventricular tachyarrhythmias and bradyarrhythmias	2° to tachycardia or bradycardia; AF and thromboembolism may occur → syncope, palpitations, dyspnea, chest pain, TIA, and/or stroke		Most common indication for pacemaker placement. Anticoagulate in atrial fibrillation/flutter to prevent systemic emboli

TACHYARRHYTHMIAS

Tables 2.1-4 and 2.1-5 outline the etiologies, clinical presentation, and treatment of common supraventricular and ventricular tachyarrhythmias.

TABLE 2.1-4. Supraventricular Tachyarrhythmias

TYPE	ETIOLOGY	SIGNS/SYMPTOMS	ECG FINDINGS	TREATMENT
ATRIAL				
Sinus tachycardia	Normal physiologic response to fear, pain, and exercise Can also be 2° to hyperthyroidism, volume contraction, infection, or PE	Palpitations, shortness of breath	Sinus rhythm Ventricular rate > 100 bpm	Treat the underlying cause
Atrial fibrillation (AF)	Acute AF—**PIRATES:** **P**ulmonary disease **I**schemia **R**heumatic heart disease **A**nemia/**A**trial myxoma **T**hyrotoxicosis **E**thanol **S**epsis Chronic AF—HTN, CHF Most often caused by ectopic foci within the pulmonary veins	Often asymptomatic and incidental but can present with shortness of breath, chest pain, dizziness, fatigue, or palpitations. May present with congestive heart failure, cardiogenic shock, or devastating cerebrovascular accident Physical exam reveals an irregular pulse	No discernible P waves, with variable and irregular QRS response	For chronic AF, initial therapy: Rate control with β-blockers, CCBs, or digoxin Anticoagulate with warfarin or novel oral anticoagulant (NOAC) for patients with CHA_2DS_2-VASc score ≥ 2 For unstable AF, or new-onset AF (of < 2 days) cardiovert If > 2 days or unclear duration, must get TEE to rule out atrial clot
Atrial flutter	Circular movement of electrical activity around the atrium at a rate of approximately 300 times per minute	Usually asymptomatic but can present with palpitations, syncope, and lightheadedness	Regular rhythm; "saw-tooth" appearance of P waves can be seen The atrial rate is usually 240–320 bpm, and the ventricular rate is ~150 bpm	Anticoagulation, rate control, and cardiover-sion guidelines as in AF above
Multifocal atrial tachycardia	Multiple atrial pace-makers or reentrant pathways; associated with COPD, hypoxemia	May be asymptomatic. At least three different P-wave morphologies	Three or more unique P-wave morphologies; rate > 100 bpm	Treat as AF but avoid β-blockers because of chronic lung disease (if present)

(continues)

TABLE 2.1-4.   Supraventricular Tachyarrhythmias *(continued)*

TYPE	ETIOLOGY	SIGNS/SYMPTOMS	ECG FINDINGS	TREATMENT
ATRIOVENTRICULAR JUNCTION				
Atrioventricular nodal reentry tachycardia (AVNRT)	A reentry circuit in the AV node depolarizes the atrium and ventricle nearly simultaneously	Palpitations, shortness of breath, angina, syncope, lightheadedness	Rate 150–250 bpm; P wave is often buried in QRS or shortly after	Cardiovert if hemodynamically unstable. Vagal maneuvers (eg, carotid massage, Valsalva, ice immersion (dive reflex). Adenosine if vagal maneuver fails
Atrioventricular reentrant tachycardia (AVRT)	An ectopic connection between the atrium and ventricle that causes a reentry circuit Seen in WPW	Palpitations, shortness of breath, angina, syncope, lightheadedness	A retrograde P wave is often seen after a normal QRS A reexcitation delta wave is characteristically seen in WPW	Except for WPW, same as that for AVNRT WPW listed separately below
Wolff-Parkinson-White (WPW) syndrome	Abnormal fast accessory conduction pathway from atria to ventricle (Bundle of Kent)	Palpitations, dyspnea, dizziness, and rarely cardiac death	Characteristic delta wave with widened QRS complex and shortened PR interval (see Figure 2.1-8)	Observation for asymptomatics Acute therapy is procainamide or amiodarone SVT gets worse after CCBs or digoxin (dangerous in WPW). Radiofrequency catheter ablation is curative
Paroxysmal atrial tachycardia	Rapid ectopic pacemaker in the atrium (not sinus node)	Palpitations, shortness of breath, angina, syncope, lightheadedness	Rate > 100 bpm; P wave with an unusual axis before each normal QRS	Adenosine can be used to unmask underlying atrial activity by slowing down the rate

Congestive Heart Failure

A clinical syndrome caused by inability of the heart to pump enough blood to maintain fluid and metabolic homeostasis. Risk factors include the following:

- Coronary heart disease.
- Hypertension.
- Cardiomyopathy.
- Valvular heart disease.
- Diabetes.
- COPD (cor pulmonale).

The American Heart Association/American College of Cardiology guidelines classify heart failure according to clinical syndromes, but alternative classification systems, including that of the New York Heart Association (NYHA), include functional severity, left-sided vs right-sided failure, and systolic vs nonsystolic failure (see Tables 2.1-6–2.1-8).

KEY FACT

Use the **CHA₂DS₂-VASc** scoring system to estimate stroke risk in atrial fibrillation, and anticoagulate with NOAC (eg, dabigatran, rivaroxaban, apixaban, and edoxaban) or warfarin (used with metal valves or mitral stenosis) for a score of 2 or more:

- **C**HF (1 point).
- **H**TN (1 point).
- **A**ge ≥ 75 (2 points).
- **D**iabetes (1 point).
- **S**troke or TIA history (2 points).
- **V**ascular disease (1 point).
- **A**ge 65–74 (1 point).
- **S**ex **c**ategory (female) (1 point).

TABLE 2.1-5. **Ventricular Tachyarrhythmias**

Type	Etiology	Signs/Symptoms	ECG Findings	Treatment
Premature ventricular contraction (PVC)	Ectopic beats arise from ventricular foci. Associated with hypoxia, fibrosis, ↓ LV function, electrolyte abnormalities, and hyperthyroidism	Usually asymptomatic but may lead to palpitations	Early, wide QRS not preceded by a P wave PVCs are usually followed by a compensatory pause	Treat the underlying cause If symptomatic, give β-blockers or, occasionally, other antiarrhythmics
Ventricular tachycardia (VT)	Can be associated with CAD, MI, and structural heart disease	Nonsustained VT (lasts < 30 seconds) is often asymptomatic; sustained VT (lasts > 30 seconds) can lead to palpitations, hypotension, angina, and syncope Can progress to VF and death	Three or more consecutive PVCs; wide QRS complexes in a regular rapid rhythm; may see AV dissociation	Cardioversion if unstable. Antiarrhythmics (eg, amiodarone, lidocaine, procainamide) if stable
Ventricular fibrillation (VF)	Associated with CAD and structural heart disease Also associated with cardiac arrest (together with asystole)	Syncope, absence of BP, no pulse	Totally erratic wide-complex tracing	Immediate electrical defibrillation and ACLS protocol
Torsades de pointes	Associated with long QT syndrome, proarrhythmic response to medications, hypokalemia, congenital deafness, and alcoholism	Can present with sudden cardiac death; typically associated with palpitations, dizziness, and syncope	Polymorphous QRS; VT with rates between 150 and 250 bpm	Give magnesium initially and cardiovert if unstable Correct hypokalemia; withdraw offending drugs

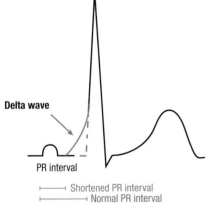

FIGURE 2.1-8. **Ventricular tachyarrhythmias.** Characteristic delta wave with widened QRS complex and shortened PR interval in WPW. (Reproduced with permission from USMLE-Rx.com.)

TABLE 2.1-6. **NYHA Functional Classification of CHF**

Class	Description
I	No limitation of activity; no symptoms (palpitations, dyspnea, and fatigue) with normal activity
II	Slight limitation of activity. Comfortable at rest or with mild exertion
III	Marked limitation of activity; comfortable only at rest
IV	Any physical activity brings on discomfort; symptoms (palpitations, dyspnea, and fatigue) present at rest

TABLE 2.1-7.   Comparison of Systolic and Diastolic Dysfunction

Variable	Systolic Dysfunction/Heart Failure with Reduced Ejection Fraction (HFrEF)	Diastolic Dysfunction/Heart Failure with Preserved Ejection Fraction (HFpEF)
Patient age	Often < 65 years of age	Often > 65 years of age
Comorbidities	Dilated cardiomyopathy, valvular heart disease, myocardial infarction	Restrictive or hypertrophic cardiomyopathy; renal disease or HTN
Physical exam	Displaced PMI, S3 gallop ("KEN"-tuc-ky)	Sustained PMI, S4 gallop ("Tenn"-es-SEE)
CXR	Pulmonary congestion, cardiomegaly	Pulmonary congestion
ECG/echocardiography	Q waves, ↓ EF (< 40%), dilation of the heart	LVH, normal/preserved EF (> 55%), abnormal LV diastolic indices

SYSTOLIC DYSFUNCTION/HEART FAILURE WITH REDUCED EJECTION FRACTION

A ↓ EF (< 40%) and ↑ left ventricular end-diastolic volumes. It is caused by inadequate left ventricular contractility or ↑ afterload. The heart compensates for ↓ EF and ↑ preload through hypertrophy and ventricular dilation (Frank-Starling law), but the compensation ultimately fails, leading to ↑ myocardial work and worsening systolic function.

HISTORY/PE

- Exertional dyspnea that progresses to orthopnea, paroxysmal nocturnal dyspnea (PND), and finally dyspnea at rest.
- Chronic cough, fatigue, and peripheral edema may be reported.
- Exam: parasternal lift, an elevated and sustained left ventricular impulse, an S3/S4 gallop, JVD, rales on lung exam, and peripheral edema.
- Look for signs to distinguish left- from right-sided failure (see Table 2.1-8).

DIAGNOSIS

- CHF is a clinical syndrome whose diagnosis is based on signs and symptoms.
- Diagnostic studies that may support diagnosis include the following:
  - **Best initial test:** Echocardiogram (transthoracic echocardiogram). ↓ EF and ventricular dilation may help pinpoint underlying cause (ie, AF, old MI, or LVH).
  - **ECG:** May show MI, heart block, arrhythmia.

KEY FACT

The most common cause of right-sided heart failure is left-sided heart failure.

KEY FACT

Hyponatremia parallels severity of heart failure and is an independent predictor of mortality in these patients.

MNEMONIC

CXR findings in CHF diagnosis—

ABCDE

Alveolar edema ("Bat's wings")
Kerley **B** lines (interstitial edema)
Cardiomegaly
Dilated prominent upper lobe vessels
Effusion (pleural)

TABLE 2.1-8.   Left-Sided vs Right-Sided Heart Failure

Left-Sided CHF Symptoms	Right-Sided CHF Symptoms
Dyspnea predominates	Fluid retention predominates
Left-sided S3/S4 gallop	Right-sided S3/S4 gallop
Bilateral basilar rales	JVD
Pleural effusions	Hepatojugular reflux
Pulmonary edema	Peripheral edema
Orthopnea, paroxysmal nocturnal dyspnea	Hepatomegaly, ascites

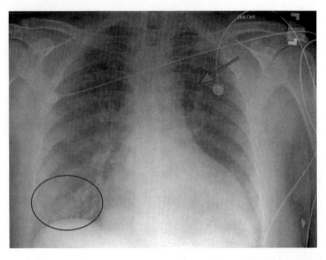

FIGURE 2.1-9. **Chest x-ray (CXR) with evidence of congestive heart failure.** Frontal CXR demonstrates marked cardiomegaly, cephalization of vessels *(arrow)*, interstitial edema *(circle)*, and left-sided pleural effusion that raise concern for CHF. (Reproduced with permission from Tintinalli JE et al. *Tintinalli's Emergency Medicine: A Comprehensive Study Guide,* 7th ed. New York, NY: McGraw-Hill; 2011.)

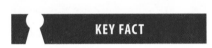

KEY FACT

Atrial tachycardia with AV block occurs 2° to digoxin toxicity.

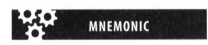

MNEMONIC

Acute CHF management—

LMNOP

Lasix (furosemide)
Morphine
Nitrates
Oxygen
Position (sit upright)

- **CXR:** May show cardiomegaly, cephalization of pulmonary vessels, pleural effusions, vascular congestion, pulmonary edema, and prominent hila (see Figure 2.1-9).
- **Lab abnormalities:** Brain natriuretic peptide > 500 pg/mL, ↓ CBC (anemia), ↑ creatinine (sometimes), ↓ sodium in later stages, ↑ or ↓ TSH/T4 levels.

TREATMENT

Acute:
- **Pharmacologic therapy** (see Table 2.1-9):
  - Loop diuretics (most commonly) for aggressive diuresis.
  - ACEIs or ARB in combination with loop diuretics.
  - β-blockers should be avoided during decompensated CHF but should be restarted once patient is euvolemic.
- Correct underlying causes such as arrhythmias, myocardial ischemia, and drugs (eg, CCBs, antiarrhythmics, NSAIDs, alcohol, anemia, thyroid and valvular disease, high-output states).

TABLE 2.1-9. **Types of Diuretics**

CLASS	EXAMPLES	SIDE EFFECTS
Loop diuretics	Furosemide, ethacrynic acid, bumetanide, torsemide	Ototoxicity, hypokalemia, hypocalcemia, hyperuricemia, dehydration, gout
Thiazide diuretics	Hydrochlorothiazide, chlorothiazide, chlorthalidone	Hypokalemic metabolic alkalosis, hyponatremia, and hyper**GLUC** (hyper**G**lycemia, hyper**L**ipidemia, hyper**U**ricemia, hyper**C**alcemia)
K⁺-sparing agents	Spironolactone, eplerenone, triamterene, amiloride	Hyperkalemia, gynecomastia, sexual dysfunction. Eplerenone does not have antiandrogenic effects that lead to gynecomastia
Carbonic anhydrase inhibitors	Acetazolamide	Hyperchloremic metabolic acidosis, neuropathy, NH_3 toxicity, sulfa allergy
Osmotic agents	Mannitol	Pulmonary edema, dehydration. Contraindicated in anuria and CHF

- Treat acute pulmonary congestion with LMNOP (see Acute CHF management mnemonic).
- **Acute decompensated heart failure:** Inotropic agents (eg, dobutamine) reduce left ventricular end-systolic volume for symptomatic improvement.

Chronic:
- **Lifestyle:** Control comorbid conditions, and limit dietary sodium and fluid intake.
- **Pharmacologic therapy:**
  - **β-blockers and ACEIs/ARBs:** Help prevent remodeling of the heart and ↓ mortality for NYHA class II–IV patients. Avoid CCBs (can worsen edema).
  - **Low-dose spironolactone:** Shown to ↓ mortality risk in patients with NYHA class III–IV heart failure.
  - **Diuretics** (most commonly loop diuretics): Prevent volume overload.
  - **Digoxin:** Symptomatic control of dyspnea and ↓ frequency of hospitalizations.
  - Daily ASA and a statin are recommended if the underlying cause is a prior MI.
- **Advanced pharmacologic therapy:**
  - **Sacubitril/valsartan:** angiotensin receptor-neprilysin inhibitor (ARNI) is a new drug class used in patients who continue to be dyspneic despite using the initial pharmacologic regimen. Provides mortality benefit for systolic dysfunction.
  - **Ivabradine:** Reduces heart rate through SA nodal inhibition of the "funny channels." Indicated in patients with systolic dysfunction if pulse is > 70 bpm or β-blockers are contraindicated.

Advanced treatments:
- Implantable cardiac defibrillator (ICD) in patients with an EF < 35%. Shown to ↓ mortality risk.
- Biventricular pacemaker in patient with an EF < 35%, dilated cardiomyopathy, and widened QRS complex with persistent symptoms.
- Left ventricular assist device (LVAD) or cardiac transplantation may be necessary in patients who are unresponsive to maximal medical therapy and biventricular pacemaker failure.

NONSYSTOLIC DYSFUNCTION/HEART FAILURE WITH PRESERVED EJECTION FRACTION

Defined by ↓ ventricular compliance with normal systolic function. The ventricle has either impaired active relaxation (2° to hypertension, ischemia, aging, and/or hypertrophy) or impaired passive filling (scarring from prior MI; restrictive cardiomyopathy). Left ventricular end-diastolic pressure ↑, cardiac output remains essentially normal, and EF is normal or ↑.

HISTORY/PE

Associated with stable and unstable angina, shortness of breath, dyspnea on exertion, arrhythmias, MI, heart failure, and sudden death.

TREATMENT

- **Best initial treatment:** Diuretics (see Table 2.1-9).
- Maintain rate and BP control via β-blockers (first-line), ACEIs, ARBs, or CCBs.
- Digoxin and spironolactone are not beneficial in these patients.

KEY FACT

ACEIs/ARBs, ARNI, β-blockers, spironolactone or eplerenone, hydralazine/nitrates, and implantable defibrillator have mortality benefit in systolic dysfunction. Diuretics and digoxin (as well as other positive inotropic agents) are for symptomatic relief only and confer no mortality benefit. CCBs may ↑ mortality.

KEY FACT

Loops lose calcium; thiazides take it in. Both cause hypokalemia and hyperuricemia.

Q   **1**

A man was admitted for a CHF exacerbation with low EF. The patient is now ready for discharge, and his medications include furosemide and metoprolol. Assuming no contraindications, what medication would be appropriate to add to his treatment regimen?

Q   **2**

A woman with HTN and prior MI has an exam notable for a displaced PMI, an S3, a nonelevated JVP, and bibasilar rales. What is the next best step in diagnosis?

Cardiomyopathy

Myocardial disease; categorized as dilated, hypertrophic, or restrictive (see Table 2.1-10 and Figure 2.1-10).

DILATED CARDIOMYOPATHY

The most common cardiomyopathy. Left ventricular dilation and ↓ EF must be present for diagnosis. Most cases are idiopathic, but known 2° causes include alcohol, postviral myocarditis, postpartum status, drugs (doxorubicin, AZT, cocaine), radiation, endocrinopathies (thyrotoxicosis, acromegaly, pheochromocytoma), infection (coxsackievirus, HIV, Chagas disease, parasites), genetic factors, and nutritional disorders (wet beriberi). The most common causes of 2° dilated cardiomyopathy are ischemia and long-standing hypertension.

HISTORY/PE

- Often presents with gradual development of CHF symptoms such as dyspnea on exertion, and diffuse edema of the ankles, feet, legs, and abdomen.
- Exam often reveals displacement of the left ventricular impulse, JVD, rales, an S3/S4 gallop, or mitral/tricuspid regurgitation.

DIAGNOSIS

- Echocardiography is diagnostic.
- CXR shows an enlarged, "balloon-like" heart and pulmonary congestion.

TREATMENT

- Address the underlying etiology (eg, alcohol use, endocrine disorders, infection).
- Treat CHF as noted in above section with lifestyle changes, and pharmacologic and advanced treatments.

KEY FACT

An S3 gallop signifies rapid ventricular filling in the setting of fluid overload and is associated with dilated cardiomyopathy. A S3 gallop sounds similar to the word "KEN-tuc-ky."

KEY FACT

An S4 gallop signifies a stiff, noncompliant ventricle and ↑ "atrial kick," and may be associated with hypertrophic cardiomyopathy. A S4 gallop sounds similar to the word "Tenn-es-SEE."

1 **A**

Add an angiotensin-converting enzyme inhibitor (ACEI) to this patient's current regimen. ACEIs have been shown to have a ⊕ mortality benefit when used with β-blockers in NYHA class II–IV heart failure patients.

2 **A**

This patient has evidence of dilated cardiomyopathy. An echocardiogram would be the next best diagnostic step.

TABLE 2.1-10. **Differential Diagnosis of Cardiomyopathies**

	TYPE		
VARIABLE	**DILATED**	**HYPERTROPHIC**	**RESTRICTIVE**
Major abnormality	Impaired contractility	Impaired relaxation	Impaired elasticity
Left ventricular cavity size (end diastole)	↑↑	↓	↓
Left ventricular cavity size (end systole)	↑↑	↓↓	↓
EF	↓↓	↑ (or normal)	Normal
Wall thickness	Usually ↓	↑↑	Usually ↑

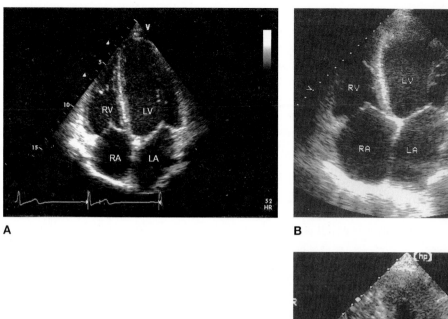

A

B

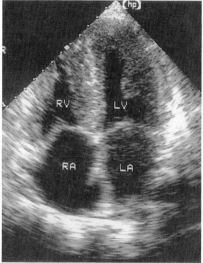

C

FIGURE 2.1-10. **Cardiomyopathies.** Echocardiogram four-chamber views of (**A**) a normal heart, (**B**) dilated cardiomyopathy, and (**C**) hypertrophic cardiomyopathy. (Reproduced with permission from Fuster V et al. *Hurst's The Heart,* 12th ed. New York, NY: McGraw-Hill; 2008.)

HYPERTROPHIC CARDIOMYOPATHY

Impaired left ventricular relaxation and filling (diastolic dysfunction) due to thickened ventricular walls secondary to stressors on the myocardium, such as HTN (most common cause) and aortic stenosis. Hypertrophy may also involve the interventricular septum, leading to left ventricular outflow tract obstruction and impaired ejection of blood due to asymmetric septal hypertrophy. The congenital form, hypertrophic obstructive cardiomyopathy (HOCM), is inherited as an autosomal dominant trait in 50% of HOCM patients and is the most common cause of sudden death in young, healthy athletes in the United States.

HISTORY/PE

- Patients are often asymptomatic but may also present with syncope, light-headedness, dyspnea, palpitations, angina, or sudden cardiac death.
- Key finding is a harsh systolic ejection crescendo-decrescendo murmur in the lower left sternal edge that ↑ with ↓ preload (eg, Valsalva maneuver, standing) and ↓ with ↑ preload (eg, passive leg raise).
- Symptoms worsen with exercise, diuretics, dehydration, ACEIs/ARBs, digoxin, and hydralazine.

KEY FACT

HOCM is the most common cause of sudden death in young, healthy athletes in the United States.

- Exam also often reveals a sustained apical impulse, an S4 gallop, paradoxical S2, and an abnormal bifid or bisferiens pulse (sudden quick rise followed by a slower longer rise due to LV outflow tract obstruction).

DIAGNOSIS

- **Best initial test:** Echocardiography is diagnostic and shows an asymmetrically hypertrophied interventricular septum and dynamic obstruction of blood flow (due to systolic anterior motion of the mitral valve against hypertrophied septum).
- ECG may be normal or show signs of LVH and nonspecific ST- and T-wave changes. Septal Q waves are common in HOCM (inferior and lateral leads).
- CXR may reveal left atrial enlargement (LAE) 2° to mitral regurgitation.

TREATMENT

- **Best initial treatment:** β-blockers are the best initial therapy for symptomatic relief in both HCM and HOCM; non-dihydropyridine CCBs (negative inotropic effect) and ventricular pacemakers are second-line agents.
- Digoxin and spironolactone are contraindicated. Diuretics may help in HCM but are contraindicated in HOCM.
- Implantable defibrillators should be used in symptomatic HOCM patients.
- Patients should avoid intense athletic competition and training.
- Surgical options for HOCM with persistent symptoms include partial excision or alcohol ablation of the myocardial septum.
- Surgical septal myomectomy is reserved for patients when medical and catheter procedures fail.

RESTRICTIVE CARDIOMYOPATHY

Decreased elasticity of myocardium leading to impaired diastolic filling without significant systolic dysfunction (a normal or near-normal EF). It is caused by infiltrative disease (eg, amyloidosis, sarcoidosis, hemochromatosis), scleroderma, Loeffler eosinophilic endocarditis, endomyocardial fibrosis, or by scarring and fibrosis (2° to radiation).

HISTORY/PE

Signs and symptoms of right-sided heart failure (JVD, peripheral edema, ascites, hepatomegaly) often predominate over left-sided failure, but dyspnea is the most common complaint.

DIAGNOSIS

- Echocardiography is key for diagnosis, with rapid early filling and a near-normal or elevated EF. CXR, MRI, and cardiac catheterization are helpful for characterization (eg, sarcoid, amyloidosis).
- Cardiac biopsy may reveal fibrosis or evidence of infiltration.
- ECG frequently shows LBBB; low voltages are seen in amyloidosis.

TREATMENT

Treat the underlying cause. Therapeutic options are limited and are generally palliative only. Medical treatment includes cautious use of diuretics for fluid overload and vasodilators to ↓ filling pressure.

Coronary Artery Disease

Also known as ischemic heart disease (IHD) or atherosclerotic heart disease. Clinical manifestations include stable and unstable angina, shortness of breath, dyspnea on exertion, arrhythmias, MI, heart failure, and sudden death.

Risk factors include the following:

- Diabetes mellitus (DM).
- Family history of premature CAD (men age < 55 years, women age < 65 years).
- Smoking.
- Hyperlipidemia.
- Abdominal obesity.
- HTN.
- Age (men age > 45 years, women age > 55 years).
- Male gender.
- CAD risk equivalents include DM, symptomatic carotid artery disease, peripheral arterial disease, and abdominal aortic aneurysm (AAA).

KEY FACT

Major risk factors for CAD include advanced age, male gender, $\uparrow$ LDL, $\downarrow$ HDL, HTN, a family history, and smoking. MI in menstruating women is rare.

ANGINA PECTORIS

Substernal chest pain 2° to myocardial ischemia (O_2 supply-and-demand mismatch). Mostly caused by atheroma. Less frequently caused by anemia, aortic stenosis, tachyarrhythmias, hypertrophic cardiomyopathy, and small vessel disease.

HISTORY/PE

- The classic triad consists of substernal chest pain that is usually precipitated by stress or exertion and is relieved by rest or nitrates (stable angina).
- The duration of stable angina is usually from 2–10 minutes (acute coronary syndrome is normally 10–30 minutes in duration).
- Pain can radiate to the neck or arm and may be associated with shortness of breath, nausea/vomiting, diaphoresis, dizziness, or lightheadedness.
- Pain is usually described as dull, squeezing, tightness, or pressure-like.
- Ischemic pain is not tender, positional, or pleuritic.

KEY FACT

Pain that is sharp or stabbing, or that changes with position, breathing, or touch, is less likely to be ischemic.

DIAGNOSIS

- **Best initial test:** ECG for any type of chest pain. Usually normal in angina pectoris, but may show ST-depression, flat or inverted T waves, or signs of past MI.
- **Cardiac enzymes (CK-MB/troponin):** Normal. May be required to be done in emergency setting after an ECG.
- **Stress testing:** ST-segment or wall-motion changes (using echo) with exercise or pharmacologic stress (dobutamine echo or dipyridamole thallium) are diagnostic of CAD. ECG stress test is not helpful without imaging for patients with abnormal baseline ECGs. (*Note:* Do not perform stress tests on asymptomatic patients with low pretest probability of disease.) Hold β-blockers, CCBs, and nitrates for 48 hours prior to stress test. Pharmacologic stress testing works due to coronary steal (diseased vessels are already maximally dilated while nondiseased vessels dilate in response to drugs, such as dipyridamole, leading to detectable ischemia).
- **Coronary angiography or CT coronary angiogram:** Coronary angiography, or a less invasive diagnostic test, CT coronary angiogram (availability

varies among centers), may be used as a last resort if ECG or stress testing is equivocal.
- Rule out pulmonary, GI, or other cardiac causes of chest pain.

Noncardiac Differential Diagnosis

- **GERD:** History described as hoarseness, bad taste, and cough; relief of symptoms with proton pump inhibitors confirms diagnosis.
- **Musculoskeletal/costochondritis:** Pain is described as tender to palpation and movement.
- **Pneumonia/pleuritis:** Pain is described as worsening with breathing (pleuritic) and is often accompanied by fever and productive cough.
- **Anxiety:** Patients may have history of panic disorder or anxiety attacks.

Treatment

- **Chronic stable angina:** ASA, β-blockers, and nitroglycerin.
  - Nitroglycerin relieves pain due to ↓ in left ventricular end-diastolic pressure and wall stress.
- Initiate risk-factor reduction (eg, smoking, cholesterol, HTN) through the initiation of ACEIs/ARBs, lipid-lowering therapies (ie, statins), and smoking cessation. Hormone replacement therapy is not protective in postmenopausal women.

PRINZMETAL (VARIANT) ANGINA

- Mimics angina pectoris but is caused by vasospasm of coronary vessels. It classically affects young women at rest (rather than during activity) in the early morning and is associated with ST-segment elevation. It is also associated with illicit drug use, especially cocaine.
- Patients usually do not have the standard risk factors for atherosclerosis.
- **Tx:** CCBs with or without long-acting nitrates. Aspirin is avoided as it can aggravate the ischemic attacks. β-blockers are contraindicated as they can ↑ vasospasm.

CAROTID ARTERY STENOSIS

Atherosclerotic lesion of either (or both) carotid arteries. Accounts for 20% of transient ischemic attacks and embolic strokes.

History/PE

- Often asymptomatic.
- Symptomatic disease is characterized by sudden-onset focal neurologic defect in the past six months (ie, TIA or stroke).
- PE may reveal carotid artery bruit.
- **Risk factors:** Advanced age, smoking, HTN, hyperlipidemia, diabetes, obesity, and family history of CAD and/or carotid artery disease.

Diagnosis

Duplex ultrasonography can determine percent occlusion.

Treatment

- **Definitive treatment:** Carotid endarterectomy (CEA).
  - Men with ≥ 60% (≥ 50% if symptomatic) stenosis or women with ≥ 70% stenosis benefit from CEA.
- Smaller lesions are monitored with serial duplex ultrasonography.

Acute Coronary Syndromes

A spectrum of clinical syndromes caused by plaque disruption or vasospasm that leads to acute myocardial ischemia.

UNSTABLE ANGINA/NON–ST-SEGMENT ELEVATION MYOCARDIAL INFARCTION

Chest pain that is (1) new onset, (2) accelerating (ie, occurs with less exertion, lasts longer, or is less responsive to medications), or (3) occurs at rest. Patient history distinguishes unstable angina from stable angina pectoris. Both stable and unstable angina have no elevated cardiac biomarkers. It signals the presence of possible impending infarction based on plaque instability. In contrast, NSTEMI indicates myocardial necrosis marked by elevations in troponin I and creatine kinase–MB isoenzyme (CK-MB) without ST-segment elevations seen on ECG.

DIAGNOSIS

- Patients should be risk stratified according to the Thrombolysis in Myocardial Infarction (TIMI) study criteria (see Table 2.1-11).
- **ECG:** Unstable angina and NSTEMI are not associated with ST elevation, but ST changes (eg, ST depression, T-wave inversion, nonspecific changes) may be seen on ECG.
- **Cardiac markers (CK-MB /troponin):** Unstable angina is not associated with elevated cardiac markers. NSTEMI is associated with elevations in cardiac markers.
- NSTEMI is diagnosed by serial cardiac enzymes and ECG.

TREATMENT

Best initial treatment:
- Admit to CCU, and monitor closely.
- If $SaO_2 < 90\%$ or breathless, administer O_2.

KEY FACT

Acute coronary syndrome:
- Unstable angina: ECG—no ST elevation; cardiac biomarkers ⊖.
- NSTEMI: ECG—no ST elevation; cardiac biomarkers ⊕.
- STEMI: ECG—ST elevation; cardiac biomarkers ⊕.

TABLE 2.1-11.   TIMI Risk Score for Unstable Angina/NSTEMI

CHARACTERISTICS	POINT
History	
Age ≥ 65 years	1
Three or more CAD risk factors (premature family history, DM, smoking, HTN, ↑ cholesterol, PAD, abdominal aortic aneurysm)	1
Known CAD (stenosis > 50%)	1
ASA use in past 7 days	1
Presentation	
Severe angina (two or more episodes within 24 hours)	1
ST deviation ≥ 0.5 mm	1
+ cardiac marker	1
Risk score—total points[a]	(0–7)

[a]Patients at higher risk (risk score ≥ 3) benefit more from enoxaparin (vs unfractionated heparin), glycoprotein IIb/IIIa inhibitors, and early angiography.

- **Analgesia:** IV morphine with IV metoclopramide.
- **Nitrates:** IV, GTN, or sublingual.
- **Antiplatelet therapy:** ASA (↓ mortality in ACS) in combination with a second agent (ie, clopidogrel, prasugrel, or ticagrelor), unless contraindicated.
- Consider β-blockers as hemodynamics allow (if hypertensive/tachycardic/ LV function < 40%).
- Low-molecular-weight heparin (eg, enoxaparin) to prevent clot formation in the coronary arteries.

Interventions:

- Assess mortality risk (eg, TIMI score, GRACE score).
- Heparin is recommended for non-ST elevation MI. Thrombolytics are only recommended in STEMI if percutaneous coronary intervention (PCI) is not available within 2 hours.
- Patients with chest pain refractory to medical therapy, a TIMI score of ≥ 3, a troponin elevation, or ST changes > 1 mm should be given GPIIb/IIIa inhibitors (abciximab, tirofiban, eptifibatide) and scheduled for angiography and possible revascularization within 72 hours (percutaneous coronary intervention [PCI] or coronary artery bypass graft [CABG]).
- Dual antiplatelet therapy with aspirin and prasugrel or ticagrelor (also $P2Y_{12}$ inhibitors but superior to clopidogrel) should be considered for up to 12 months after angioplasty and stenting to prevent restenosis of stenting.
- Ensure patient is on long-term β-blockers (if depressed LV function), ACEIs/ARBs, and statin.
- Address modifiable risk factors (ie, smoking, hypertension, hyperlipidemia, diabetes).

ST-SEGMENT ELEVATION MYOCARDIAL INFARCTION

ST-segment elevations and cardiac enzyme release 2° to prolonged cardiac ischemia and necrosis. STEMI is a common medical emergency, and prompt treatment is absolutely necessary.

HISTORY/PE

- **Presentation:** Acute-onset substernal chest pain (> 10–30 min), commonly described as a pressure, tightness, or heaviness that can radiate to the left arm, shoulders, neck, or jaw. May present without chest pain ("silent" infarct).
- **Associated symptoms:** Diaphoresis, shortness of breath, lightheadedness, anxiety, nausea/vomiting, epigastric pain (more common in women), and syncope.
- **PE:** May reveal arrhythmias, hypotension (cardiogenic shock), new S4, pansystolic murmur, and evidence of new CHF. Clear lung fields are seen in right ventricular MI (inferior MI). In a young, otherwise healthy person, consider cocaine use as the etiology.
- The best predictor of survival is left ventricular EF.
- **Differential diagnosis:** Angina, myocarditis, pericarditis, aortic dissection, pulmonary embolism, esophageal reflux/spasm.

DIAGNOSIS

- **ECG:** ST-segment elevations, hyperacute (tall) T waves, or new LBBB within hours. ST-segment depressions and dominant R waves in leads V_1–V_2 can also be reciprocal change indicating posterior wall infarct. T-wave inversion and pathologic Q waves develop within hours to days.
  - **Sequence of ECG changes:** Peaked T waves → ST-segment elevation → Q waves → T-wave inversion → ST-segment normalization → T-wave normalization over several hours to days.

MNEMONIC

Treatment for MI—

Patient is MOANing Big from MI

Morphine
Oxygen (to maintain saturations)
ASA + **A**dditional second antiplatelet agent (NSTEMI)
Nitrates
β-blockers

KEY FACT

It is important to check for aortic dissection clinically prior to administering anticoagulants or thrombolytics.

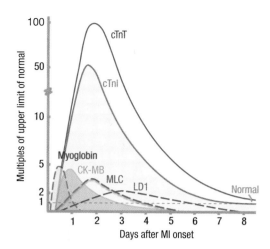

FIGURE 2.1-11. **Typical pattern of serum marker elevation after an acute myocardial infarction.** CK-MB, creatine kinase MB isoenzyme; cTnI, cardiac troponin I; cTnT, cardiac troponin T; LD1, lactate dehydrogenase isoenzyme 1; MLC, myosin light chain. (Reproduced with permission from USMLE-Rx.com.)

- ◼ Cardiac enzymes:
    - ◼ Troponin (T and I) is the most sensitive and specific cardiac marker.
    - ◼ CK-MB and the CK-MB/total CK ratio (CK index) are also regularly checked.
    - ◼ Both troponin and CK-MB can take up to 3–12 hours to rise following the onset of chest pain. Troponin peaks at 24–48 hours, and CK-MB peaks within 24 hours (see Figure 2.1-11).
- ◼ ST-segment abnormalities:
    - ◼ **Inferior MI (involving the RCA/PDA):** ST-segment elevation in leads II, III, and aVF (see Figure 2.1-12). Obtain a right-sided ECG to look for ST elevations in the right ventricle.
    - ◼ **Anterior MI (involving LAD and diagonal branches):** ST-segment elevation in leads V_1–V_4 (see Figure 2.1-13).

KEY FACT

Women, diabetics, the elderly, and post–heart transplant patients may have atypical or clinically silent MIs.

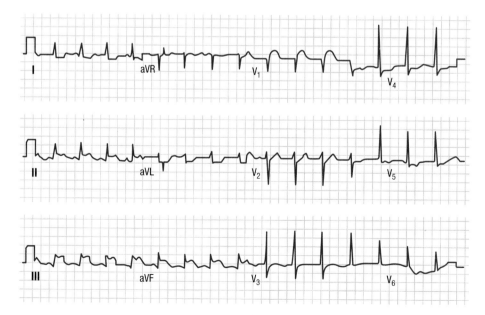

FIGURE 2.1-12. **Inferior wall myocardial infarction.** In this patient with acute chest pain, the ECG demonstrated acute ST-segment elevation in leads II, III, and aVF with reciprocal ST-segment depression and T-wave flattening in leads I, aVL, and V_4–V_6. (Reproduced with permission from USMLE-Rx.com.)

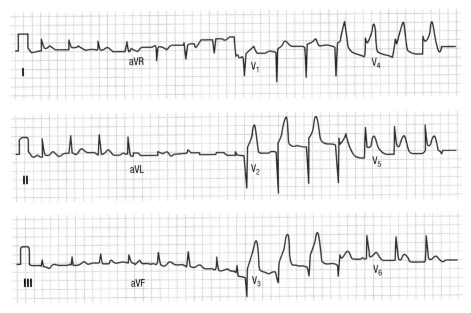

FIGURE 2.1-13. **Anterior wall myocardial infarction.** This patient presented with acute chest pain. The ECG showed acute ST-segment elevation in leads V_1–V_6 and hyperacute T waves. (Reproduced with permission from USMLE-Rx.com.)

- **Lateral MI (involving LCA):** ST-segment elevation in leads I, aVL, and V_5–V_6.
- **Posterior MI:** ST-segment depression in leads V_1–V_2 (anterior leads) can be indicative. Obtain posterior ECG leads V_7–V_9 (15-lead) to assess for ST-segment elevations.

TREATMENT

Best initial treatment:
- **First line:** Antiplatelet therapy; ASA (↓ mortality in ACS). Add prasugrel or ticagrelor (both superior to clopidogrel), or clopidogrel as second antiplatelet agent with aspirin only for patients undergoing angioplasty or stenting.
- **Analgesia:** IV morphine with IV metoclopramide.
- **Nitrates:** IV, GTN, or sublingual.
- If $SaO_2 < 95\%$, breathless, or in acute LVF, administer O_2.
- Consider β-blockers as hemodynamics allow (if hypertensive/tachycardic/LV function < 40%).
- If the patient is in heart failure or in cardiogenic shock, do not give β-blockers; instead, give ACEIs provided that the patient is not hypotensive.
- In inferior wall MI (ie, right ventricular infarction), avoid nitrates and diuretics due to risk for severe hypotension (preload dependent).

Interventions:
- Emergent angiography and PCI should be performed if possible (superior to thrombolysis).
- If PCI cannot be performed < 120 minutes (door-to-balloon time should ideally be < 90 minutes), and there are no contraindications to thrombolysis, and the patient presents within 3 hours of chest pain onset, thrombolysis with tPA, reteplase, or streptokinase should be performed instead of PCI.
- Thrombolysis target time (door-to-needle time) is < 30 minutes and is contraindicated if > 24 hours. Thrombolytics can be used up to 12 hours from the onset of symptoms (mortality benefit extends to 12 hours).
- Long-term management (for all patients) includes ASA, ACEIs, β-blockers, nitrates, and high-dose statins.

KEY FACT

Contraindications to thrombolysis:
- Previous intracranial hemorrhage or major GI bleed.
- Recent major trauma/surgery/head injury.
- Ischemic stroke within the last 6 months.
- Severe hypertension (> 180/110 mmHg).
- Known bleeding disorder.

- If PCI was performed, add clopidogrel, prasugrel, or ticagrelor (dual anti-platelet therapy).
- Address modifiable risk factors (ie, smoking, hypertension, hyperlipidemia, diabetes).

COMPLICATIONS

- **Arrhythmia:** VF and VT are the most common complications and the most common causes of sudden death following acute MI. Sinus bradycardia and third-degree (complete) heart block are also very common.
- Less common complications include reinfarction, left ventricular wall rupture, VSD, pericarditis, papillary muscle rupture (with mitral regurgitation), left ventricular aneurysm or pseudoaneurysm, and mural thrombi (with subsequent acute limb ischemia, TIA, or stroke).
- **A timeline of common post-MI complications:**
  - **First day:** Heart failure.
  - **2–4 days:** Arrhythmia, pericarditis.
  - **5–10 days:** Left ventricular wall rupture (acute pericardial tamponade causing electrical alternans, pulseless electrical activity, and JVD), papillary muscle rupture (severe mitral regurgitation, pulmonary edema), septal rupture (lower left sternal border murmur, increase in O_2 saturation in the right ventricle).
  - **Weeks to months:** Ventricular aneurysm (CHF, arrhythmia, persistent ST-segment elevation, mitral regurgitation, thrombus formation).
- Dressler syndrome, an autoimmune process occurring 2–10 weeks post-MI, presents with fever, pericarditis, pleural effusion, leukocytosis, and ↑ ESR.
- **Right ventricular infarction:** Caused by the occlusion of the RCA. Presents with hypotension, JVD, and clear lungs. Treat with high-volume fluid replacement (preload dependent), and avoid nitrates and diuretics.

Dyslipidemia

Total cholesterol level > 200 mg/dL, LDL > 130 mg/dL, triglycerides > 150 mg/dL, and HDL < 40 mg/dL, all of which are risk factors for CAD. Etiologies include obesity, DM, alcoholism, hypothyroidism, nephrotic syndrome, hepatic disease, Cushing syndrome, OCP use, high-dose diuretic use, and familial hypercholesterolemia.

HISTORY/PE

- Most patients have no specific signs or symptoms.
- Patients with extremely high triglyceride or LDL levels may have xanthomata (eruptive itchy nodules, orange streaks in palmar creases, or tuberous plaques on the elbows and knees); xanthelasma (yellow fatty deposits in the skin around the lids just below the eyes); lipemia retinalis (creamy appearance of retinal vessels); corneal arcus (deposition of lipid in the corneal stroma).
- Patients may have a history of familial primary hyperlipidemias.

DIAGNOSIS

- **Fasting lipid profile:** Total cholesterol, LDL, HDL, and triglycerides.
- Conduct a fasting lipid profile for patients > 35 years of age or in those ≥ 20 years of age with CAD risk factors, and repeat every 5 years or sooner if lipid levels are elevated.
- Total serum cholesterol > 200 mg/dL on two different occasions is diagnostic of hypercholesterolemia.
- LDL > 130 mg/dL or HDL < 40 mg/dL is diagnostic of dyslipidemia (not optimal levels), even if total serum cholesterol is < 200 mg/dL.
- Individuals with LDL > 190 mg/dL or triglycerides ≥ 500 mg/dL should be evaluated for secondary causes of hyperlipidemia.

KEY FACT

Indications for CABG:
- Left main coronary artery disease.
- Triple-vessel disease with ≥ 70% in each vessel.
- Two-vessel disease in diabetic patient.
- Symptomatic patient despite maximal medical therapy.

MNEMONIC

Complication of MI—

DARTH VADER

Death
Arrhythmia
Rupture (ventricular wall, septum, or papillary muscle)
Tamponade
Heart failure
Valvular disease
Aneurysm of ventricle
Dressler's syndrome
Emboli (mural thrombosis)
Recurrence/**R**einfarction/**R**egurgitation (mitral)

KEY FACT

Right ventricular MI is caused by the occlusion of the RCA. Nitrates and diuretics must be avoided, and the condition is treated with IV fluids.

KEY FACT

Secondary hyperlipidemia causes include Cushing syndrome, hypothyroidism, nephrotic syndrome, or cholestasis.

KEY FACT

As you cannot calculate the patient's ASCVD risk on the USMLE, focus on obvious signs of ↑ risk (smoking, diabetes) or ↓ risk (young, healthy) when deciding if statin therapy is appropriate.

TABLE 2.1-12. American College of Cardiology/American Heart Association Treatment Guidelines

PATIENT AGE	CRITERIA	TREATMENT
≥ 21 years	Atherosclerotic cardiovascular disease (ASCVD) (eg, CAD, CVA, or PAD)	High-intensity statin
≥ 21 years	LDL ≥ 190 mg/dL	High-intensity statin
40–75 years	LDL 70–189 mg/dL without ASCVD or diabetes	≥ 7.5% 10-year risk → high-intensity statin 5–7.5% 10-year risk → moderate-intensity statin ≤ 5% 10-year risk → no statin
40–75 years	LDL 70–189 mg/dL with diabetes	≥ 7.5% 10-year risk → high-intensity statin ≤ 7.5% 10-year risk → moderate-intensity statin
≤ 75 years	ASCVD	High-intensity statin

TREATMENT

- Based on risk stratification using one of many cardiovascular risk calculators.
- The American College of Cardiology/American Heart Association recommendations are listed in Table 2.1-12.
- **High-intensity therapy:** Goal reduction in LDL of > 50%, moderate-intensity as lowering by 30–50% or by specific medication and dosing guidelines (ie, atorvastatin 80 mg).
- **Smokers of all ages:** Screen for dyslipidemias due to their ↑ risk.
- **First intervention:** 12-week trial of diet and exercise in a patient with no known ASCVD. Commonly used lipid-lowering agents are listed in Table 2.1-13.
- **Secondary hyperlipidemia:** Treat underlying cause.

KEY FACT

Dyslipidemia:
- LDL > 130 mg/dL or
- HDL < 40 mg/dL.

TABLE 2.1-13. Lipid-Lowering Agents

CLASS	EXAMPLES	EFFECT ON LIPID PROFILE	SIDE EFFECTS
HMG-CoA reductase inhibitors (statins)	Atorvastatin, simvastatin, lovastatin, pravastatin, rosuvastatin	↓ LDL, ↓ triglycerides	↑ LFTs, myositis, warfarin potentiation
Lipoprotein lipase stimulators (fibrates)	Gemfibrozil	↓ Triglycerides, ↑ HDL	GI upset, cholelithiasis, myositis (especially in combination with statins), ↑ LFTs, pancreatitis
Cholesterol absorption inhibitors	Ezetimibe	↓ LDL	Diarrhea, abdominal pain. Can cause angioedema
Niacin	Niaspan	↑ HDL, ↓ LDL	Skin flushing (can be prevented with ASA, due to ↑ prostaglandins), paresthesias, pruritus, GI upset, ↑ LFTs
Bile acid resins	Cholestyramine, colestipol, colesevelam	↓ LDL	Constipation, GI upset, LFT abnormalities, myalgias. Can ↓ absorption of other drugs from the small intestine
Proprotein convertase subtilisin/kexin type 9 (PCSK9) inhibitors	Evolocumab, alirocumab (injectable medications taken every 2–4 weeks)	↓↓ LDL	Injection-site swelling, rash, muscle/limb pain, backache

TABLE 2.1-14. American College of Cardiology/American Heart Association BP Guidelines[a]

BP CATEGORY	BP	TREAT OR FOLLOW-UP
Normal	SBP < 120 mm Hg and DBP < 80 mm Hg	Yearly evaluation Lifestyle modifications to maintain normal BP
Elevated	SBP 120–129 mm Hg and DBP < 80 mm Hg	Recommend healthy lifestyle changes Reassess in 3–6 months
Hypertension: stage 1	SBP ≥ 130–139 mm Hg or DBP ≥ 80–89 mm Hg	Assess 10-year risk for heart disease and stroke (ASCVD) ■ < 10% 10-year risk: 　■ Lifestyle recommendations 　■ Reassess in 3–6 months ■ > 10% 10-year risk or the patient has known CVD, diabetes mellitus, or CKD, lifestyle changes, and BP-lowering medication: 　■ Reassess in 1 month for effectiveness of medication therapy 　■ If goal is met after 1 month, reassess in 3–6 months 　■ If goal is not met after 1 month, consider different medication or titration; continue monthly follow-up until control is achieved
Hypertension: stage 2	SBP ≥ 140 mm Hg or DBP ≥ 90 mm Hg	Recommend healthy lifestyle changes and BP-lowering medication (two medications of different classes) ■ Reassess in 1 month for effectiveness: 　■ If goal is met after 1 month, reassess in 3–6 months 　■ If goal is not met after 1 month, consider different medications or titration ■ Continue monthly follow-up until control is achieved

[a] Based on 2017 report of the American College of Cardiology/American Heart Association Task Force on Clinical Practice Guidelines.

Hypertension

A major risk factor for stroke and MI. Defined as systolic BP ≥ 140 mm Hg and/or diastolic BP ≥ 90 mm Hg based on three measurements separated in time in adults (see Table 2.1-14). Classified as 1° or 2°.

1° (ESSENTIAL) HYPERTENSION

Hypertension with no identifiable cause. Represents 95% of cases of HTN. Risk factors include a family history of HTN or heart disease, a high-sodium diet, smoking, obesity, ethnicity (African-Americans > whites), and advanced age.

HISTORY/PE

- HTN is usually asymptomatic until complications develop.
- Patients should be evaluated for end-organ damage to the brain (stroke, dementia), eye (cotton-wool exudates, hemorrhage, retinopathy), heart (LVH), and kidney (proteinuria, CKD). Renal bruits may signify renal artery stenosis as the cause of HTN.

KEY FACT

PCSK9 inhibitors are a new class of LDL-lowering drugs. They significantly increase hepatic clearance of LDL. Indicated in familial hypercholesterolemia and statin-resistant or -intolerant patients with severe hyperlipidemia.

Q

A woman is found with pulseless electrical activity on hospital day 7 after suffering a lateral wall STEMI. The ACLS protocol is initiated. What is the next best step?

DIAGNOSIS

- **Quantify overall risk:** Fasting glucose, HBA1c, lipid profile.
- **Assess end-organ damage:** ECG to check for LVH or past MI, urinalysis for proteinuria or hematuria; BUN/creatinine.
- **Exclude secondary causes (as required):** U&Es, Ca^{2+}, renal ultrasound, 24-hour urine metanephrine, renin, aldosterone, urinary cortisol.
- 24-hour ambulatory BP monitoring (ABPM) may be useful sometimes (ie, "white coat" or borderline hypertension).

TREATMENT

- Begin with lifestyle modifications (weight loss, exercise, smoking cessation, diet improvement, limit alcohol and salt intake).
- BP goals vary by category and ASCVD (see Table 2.1-14).
- Diuretics, CCBs, ACEIs, and β-blockers have been shown to ↓ mortality in uncomplicated HTN. They are first-line agents unless a comorbid condition requires another medication (see Table 2.1-15).
- For patients who are not African-American, including those with diabetes, → ACEI/ARB (nephroprotective), thiazide, CCB.
- For African American patients, including those with diabetes, → thiazide, CCB.
- For patients ≥ 18 years of age with CKD → ACEI/ARB (nephroprotective).
- If BP goal is not reached within 1 month of commencing treatment, ↑ dose of initial drug or add a second drug, and if goal BP cannot be reached with two drugs, add and titrate a third drug. Poorer outcomes are seen if ACEIs and ARBs are used together.
- Periodically test for end-organ complications, including renal complications (BUN, creatinine, urine protein-to-creatinine ratio), hypertensive retinopathy (eye exam), and cardiac complications (ECG evidence of LVH).

2° HYPERTENSION

Hypertension 2° to an identifiable organic cause (~5% of cases). See Table 2.1-16 for the diagnosis and treatment of common causes.

MNEMONIC

Treatment of HTN—

ABCD

ACEIs/ARBs
β-blockers
CCBs
Diuretics (typically thiazide diuretics)

MNEMONIC

Causes of 2° hypertension—

CHAPS

Cushing syndrome
Hyperaldosteronism (Conn syndrome)
Aortic coarctation
Pheochromocytoma
Stenosis of renal arteries

RECENT

Renal causes (renal artery stenosis, PKD)
Endocrine (Conn syndrome, Cushing syndrome, hyperparathyroidism, pheochromocytoma)
Coarctation of the aorta
Estrogen (OCP)
Neurologic (ICP)
Thyroid disorder

A

This patient has probably suffered a left ventricular free-wall rupture with acute cardiac tamponade. Emergent pericardiocentesis is the next best therapeutic and diagnostic step.

TABLE 2.1-15. Treatment of 1° Hypertension in Specific Populations

POPULATION	AGENTS
Uncomplicated	Diuretics, CCBs, ACEIs
CHF	Diuretics, β-blockers, ACEIs, ARBs, aldosterone antagonists
Diabetes	Diuretics, ACEIs, ARBs, CCBs
Post-MI	β-blockers, ACEIs, ARBs, aldosterone antagonists
Chronic kidney disease	ACEIs, ARBs
BPH	Diuretics, α_1-adrenergic blockers
Isolated systolic HTN	Diuretics, ACEIs, CCBs (dihydropyridines)
Pregnancy	Methyldopa, β-blockers (typically labetalol), hydralazine

TABLE 2.1-16. **Common Causes of 2° Hypertension**

ETIOLOGY	DESCRIPTION	MANAGEMENT
1° Renal disease	Often unilateral renal parenchymal disease	Treat with ACEIs, which slow the progression of renal disease
Renal artery stenosis	Especially common in patients < 25 and > 50 years of age with recent-onset HTN Etiologies include fibromuscular dysplasia (younger patients) and atherosclerosis (older patients) Often present with headaches and bruits in abdomen/neck	Diagnose with MRA, CT angiography, or renal artery Doppler ultrasound May be treated with angioplasty or stenting. Consider ACEIs in unilateral disease. (In bilateral disease, ACEIs can accelerate kidney failure by preferential vasodilation of the efferent arteriole.) Open surgery is a second option if angioplasty is not effective or feasible
OCP use	Common in women > 35 years of age, obese women, and those with long-standing use	Discontinue OCPs (effect may be delayed)
Pheochromocytoma	An adrenal gland tumor that secretes epinephrine and nor-epinephrine, leading to episodic headache, sweating, and tachycardia	Diagnose with urinary metanephrines and catechol-amine levels or plasma metanephrine Surgical removal of tumor after treatment with α-blockers followed by β-blockers
Conn syndrome (hyperaldosteronism)	Most often 2° to an aldosterone-producing adrenal adenoma Causes the triad of HTN, unexplained hypokalemia, and metabolic alkalosis	Metabolic workup with plasma aldosterone and renin level; ↑ aldosterone and ↓ renin levels suggest 1° hyperaldosteronism. Surgical removal of tumor
Cushing syndrome	Due to an ACTH-producing pituitary tumor, an ectopic ACTH-secreting tumor, or cortisol secretion by an adrenal adenoma or carcinoma. Also due to exogenous steroid exposure. (See the Endocrinology chapter for more details)	Surgical removal of tumor; removal of exogenous steroids
Coarctation of the aorta	See the Pediatrics chapter	Surgical correction
Hyperparathyroidism	Either alone or as part of MEN type 2 (with pheochromocytoma) Look for ↑ calcium and vascular/valvular calcification	Treat underlying hyperparathyroidism

HYPERTENSIVE CRISES

A spectrum of clinical presentations in which there is a severe increase in BP (usually > 180/120 mm Hg) that can lead to end-organ damage.

HISTORY/PE

Present with end-organ damage revealed by acute kidney injury, severe chest pain (ischemia, MI), back pain (aortic dissection), stroke, severe headache with changes in mental status (hypertensive encephalopathy), and blurred vision. Other symptoms include nausea and vomiting, seizures, shortness of breath, and severe anxiety.

Q

A 40-year-old man presents for a routine exam. His exam is significant for a BP of 145/75 mm Hg but is otherwise unremarkable, as are his lab results. What is the next best step?

TABLE 2.1-17. **Major Classes of Antihypertensive Agents**

CLASS	AGENTS	MECHANISM OF ACTION	SIDE EFFECTS
Diuretics	Thiazide, loop, K$^+$ sparing Ethacrynic acid is the only nonsulfa loop diuretic that can be used in severe sulfa allergy patients	↓ Extracellular fluid volume and thereby ↓ vascular resistance	Hypokalemia (not with K$^+$ sparing), hyperglycemia, hyperlipidemia, hyper-uricemia, azotemia
β-blockers	Propranolol, metoprolol, nadolol, atenolol, timolol, carvedilol, labetalol	↓ Cardiac contractility and renin release	Bronchospasm (in severe active asthma), bradycardia, CHF exacerbation, impotence, fatigue, depression
ACEIs	Captopril, enalapril, fosinopril, bena-zepril, lisinopril	Blocks the conversion of angio-tensin I to angiotensin II, reducing peripheral resistance and salt/water retention. Bradykinin ↑ due to the ↓ activation of ACE	Cough and angioedema (due to ↑ brady-kinin build-up), rashes, leukopenia, hyperkalemia
ARBs	Losartan, valsartan, irbesartan	Blocks the activation of angiotensin II receptor, reducing periph-eral resistance and salt/water retention	Rashes, leukopenia, and hyperkalemia but no cough
CCBs	Dihydro pyridines (nifedipine, felodipine, amlodipine), nondihy-dropyridines (diltiazem, verapamil)	↓ Smooth muscle tone and cause vasodilation; may also ↓ cardiac output	Dihydropyridines: headache, flushing, peripheral edema Nondihydropyridines: ↓ Contractility
Vasodilators	Hydralazine, minoxidil	↓ Peripheral resistance by dilating arteries/arterioles	Hydralazine: headache, lupus-like syndrome Minoxidil: orthostasis, hirsutism
α$_1$-adrenergic blockers	Prazosin, terazosin, phenoxybenzamine	Cause vasodilation by blocking actions of norepinephrine on vascular smooth muscle	Orthostatic hypotension
Centrally acting adrenergic agonists	Methyldopa, clonidine	Inhibit the sympathetic nervous system via central α$_2$-adrenergic receptors	Somnolence, orthostatic hypotension, impotence, rebound HTN

KEY FACT

Hypertensive emergencies are diagnosed on the basis of the extent of end-organ damage, not BP measurement.

With a single BP recording and no evidence of end-organ damage, the next best step should consist of a repeat BP measurement at the end of the exam with a return visit if BP is still high.

DIAGNOSIS

- **Hypertensive urgency:** ↑ BP with mild to moderate symptoms (headache, chest pain, nausea and vomiting) without end-organ damage.
- **Hypertensive emergency:** ↑ BP with signs or symptoms of impending end-organ damage such as acute kidney injury, intracranial or retinal hemorrhage, papilledema, stroke, or ECG changes suggestive of ischemia, MI, or pulmonary edema.

TREATMENT

- **Hypertensive urgency:** BP can be reduced gradually over 24–48 hours with oral antihypertensives (eg, β-blockers, clonidine, ACEIs) (see Table 2.1-17).
- **Hypertensive emergency:** BP must be reduced immediately to prevent imminent organ damage. Treat with IV medications (labetalol, nitroprus-side, nicardipine) with the goal of lowering mean arterial pressure by no more than 25% over the first 2 hours to prevent cerebral hypoperfusion or coronary insufficiency.

Pericardial Disease

Consists of pericarditis, constrictive pericarditis, and pericardial tamponade. Results from acute or chronic pericardial insults; may lead to pericardial effusion.

PERICARDITIS

Inflammation of the pericardial sac. It can compromise cardiac output via tamponade (extravasation of large amounts of fluid secondary to pericarditis) or constrictive pericarditis (chronic pericarditis). Most commonly idiopathic, although known etiologies include viral infection (most common infection, likely etiology Coxsackie B virus), *Staphylococcus, Streptococcus*, tuberculosis (TB), systemic lupus erythematosus (SLE), uremia, drugs, radiation, connective tissue disorder (ie, rheumatoid arthritis, Goodpasture syndrome), and neoplasms. May also occur after MI (either within days after MI or as a delayed phenomenon; ie, Dressler syndrome) or open-heart surgery (see Figure 2.1-14).

HISTORY/PE

- **Presentation:** Sharp pleuritic chest pain, dyspnea, cough, and fever.
- **Key feature:** Chest pain tends to worsen in the supine position and with inspiration. Classically, patient is seen sitting up (pain improves in prone position) and bending forward.
- **Exam:** May reveal a pericardial friction rub. Elevated JVP, tachycardia, muffled S_1 and S_2, and pulsus paradoxus (a ↓ in systolic BP >10 mm Hg on inspiration) can be present with pericardial tamponade. Kussmaul sign can be present with constrictive pericarditis.

DIAGNOSIS

- **ECG:** Include diffuse ST-segment elevation and PR-segment depressions followed by T-wave inversions (see Figure 2.1-15). Classically shows concave (saddle-shaped) ST segment elevation.

KEY FACT

Pericardial calcification seen on chest x-ray (CXR) strongly suggest constrictive pericarditis due to chronic fibrosis and calcification of the pericardium.

MNEMONIC

Causes of pericarditis—

CARDIAC RINDS

Collagen vascular disease
Aortic dissection
Radiation
Drugs
Infections
Acute renal failure
Cardiac (MI) and **C**onnective tissue disease
Rheumatic fever
Injury
Neoplasms
Dressler syndrome
Surgery (postpericardiotomy syndrome)

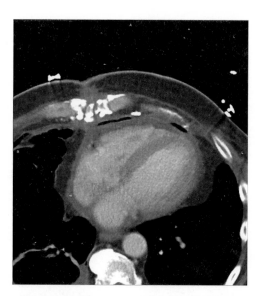

FIGURE 2.1-14. Radiographic findings in pericarditis. Contrast-enhanced CT at the level of the interventricular septum demonstrates a small pericardial effusion, with thickening and increased enhancement of the pericardium consistent with infection in this postsurgical patient. The air outlining the pericardium anteriorly is the result of dehiscence of the median sternotomy. (Reproduced with permission from USMLE-Rx.com.)

- **CXR:** Cardiomegaly may indicate a pericardial effusion.
- **Blood tests:** FBC, ESR, U&Es, cardiac enzymes (troponin may be raised), viral serology, and if indicated, autoantibodies, fungal precipitins, and TFTs.
- **Echo:** Pericardial thickening or effusion may be evident.

TREATMENT

- Treat the underlying cause (eg, corticosteroids/immunosuppressants for SLE, dialysis for uremia) or symptoms (eg, ASA for post-MI pericarditis, ASA/NSAIDs for viral pericarditis or Dressler syndrome). Avoid corticosteroids within a few days after MI, as they can predispose to ventricular wall rupture.
- Treat idiopathic cases with NSAIDs such as ibuprofen, naproxen, or indomethacin. Consider colchicine for relapse or persistent symptoms.
- Pericardial effusions without symptoms can be monitored, but evidence of tamponade requires pericardiocentesis with continuous drainage as needed.

CARDIAC TAMPONADE

Excess fluid in the pericardial sac ↑ the intrapericardial pressure, leading to compromised ventricular filling and ↓ cardiac output. The rate of fluid formation is more important than the size of the effusion. Risk factors include pericarditis, malignancy, SLE, TB, and trauma (commonly stab wounds medial to the left nipple).

HISTORY/PE

- Presents with fatigue, dyspnea, anxiety, tachycardia, and tachypnea that can rapidly progress to shock and death.
- Exam of a patient with acute tamponade may reveal Beck triad (hypotension, distant or muffled S_1 and S_2 heart sounds, and JVD), a narrow pulse pressure, and pulsus paradoxus.
- Lung fields are clear on exam.

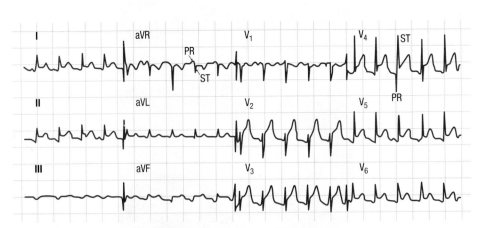

FIGURE 2.1-15. **Acute pericarditis.** Diffuse ST-segment elevations in multiple leads not consistent with any discrete coronary vascular territory and PR-segment depressions. (Reproduced with permission from USMLE-Rx.com.)

DIAGNOSIS

- Echo is diagnostic and shows right atrial and right ventricular diastolic collapse and echo-free zone around the heart.
- CXR may show an enlarged, globular, water-bottle-shaped heart with a large effusion (see Figure 2.1-16).
- If present on ECG, electrical alternans is diagnostic of a large pericardial effusion.

TREATMENT

- Aggressive volume expansion with IV fluids.
- Urgent pericardiocentesis (aspirate will be non-clotting blood). Send fluid to lab analysis to determine etiology.
- Decompensation or recurrent cases may warrant pericardial window.

Valvular Heart Disease

Until recently, rheumatic fever (which affects the mitral valve more often than the aortic valve) was the most common cause of valvular heart disease in US adults; the leading cause is now mechanical degeneration. Subtypes are listed in Table 2.1-18 along with their etiologies, presentation, diagnosis, and treatment.

Vascular Diseases

AORTIC ANEURYSM

Greater than 50% dilation of all three layers of the aortic wall. Aortic aneurysms are most commonly associated with atherosclerosis. Most are abdominal, and > 90% originate below the renal arteries.

- Ascending aortic aneurysm—think cystic medial necrosis or connective tissue disease.
- Descending aortic aneurysm—think atherosclerosis.
- **Complications:** Rupture, thrombosis, embolism, fistulae, pressure on surrounding structures.

HISTORY/PE

- Usually asymptomatic and discovered incidentally on exam or radiologic study. It may cause mild abdominal or back pain.
- Exam demonstrates a pulsatile abdominal mass or abdominal bruits.
- Risk factors include HTN, high cholesterol, other vascular disease, a ⊕ family history, smoking (strongest predictor of rupture), gender (males > females), and age.
- Ruptured aneurysm leads to hypotension and severe, tearing abdominal pain that radiates to the back, iliac fossae, or groin, and syncope.

DIAGNOSIS

- **Screening:** All men 65–75 years of age with a history of smoking are recommended for a one-time screening by ultrasound for AAA (see Figure 2.1-17).
- Abdominal ultrasound is used for diagnosis or to follow the course of an aneurysm over time.
- CT with contrast or MRA may be useful to determine the precise anatomy.

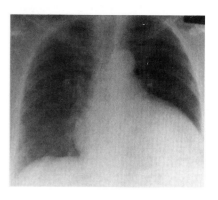

FIGURE 2.1-16. Pericardial effusion. Water-bottle-shaped heart seen on CXR with pericardial effusion. (Reproduced with permission from Chen MY et al. *Basic Radiology,* 2nd ed. New York, NY: McGraw-Hill; 2011.)

> **KEY FACT**

Beck triad can diagnose acute cardiac tamponade:
- JVD.
- Hypotension.
- Distant S_1 and S_2 heart sounds.

> **KEY FACT**

Size of AAA determines treatment:
- < 5 cm → monitoring.
- > 5 cm → surgical correction.

Q

A 20-year-old man presents with an initial BP of 150/85 mm Hg, and repeat measurement yields 147/85 mm Hg. The patient's potassium level is 3.2 mg/dL. What is the next appropriate diagnostic step?

TABLE 2.1-18. **Types of Valvular Heart Disease**

TYPE	ETIOLOGY	HISTORY	EXAM/DIAGNOSIS	TREATMENT
Aortic stenosis	Most often seen in the elderly (senile calcific aortic stenosis) Unicuspid in childhood and adolescence. Rheumatic heart disease can predispose to AS	May be asymptomatic for years despite significant stenosis Once symptomatic, usually progresses from angina to syncope to CHF to death within 2 years Sx (also indications for valve replacements): **ACS—A**ngina, **C**HF, **S**yncope	PE: Pulsus parvus et tardus (weak, delayed carotid upstroke) and a single or paradoxically split S2 sound; systolic crescendo-decrescendo murmur at the right second intercostal space radiating to the carotids Severe AS characterized by soft and single S2 Dx: Echocardiography	Aortic valve replacement (surgical or transcatheter methods)
Aortic regurgitation	Acute: Infective endocarditis, aortic dissection, chest trauma, MI Chronic: Valve malformations, rheumatic fever, connective tissue disorders (ie, Marfan syndrome), syphilis, inflammatory disorders	Acute: Rapid onset of pulmonary congestion, cardiogenic shock, and severe dyspnea Chronic: Slowly progressive onset of dyspnea on exertion, orthopnea, and PND. Uncomfortable heart pounding when lying on left side	PE: Early blowing diastolic murmur at the left sternal border, mid-diastolic rumble (Austin Flint murmur), and midsystolic apical murmur Widened pulse pressure causes de Musset sign (head bob with heartbeat), Corrigan sign (water-hammer pulse; wide and bounding), and Duroziez sign (femoral bruit) Dx: Echocardiography	Vasodilator therapy (dihydropyridines or ACEIs) for isolated aortic regurgitation until symptoms become severe enough to warrant valve replacement. Digoxin and diuretics have little benefit Monitor LV function and size
Mitral valve stenosis	The most common etiology continues to be rheumatic fever Uncommon in the US	Sx: Include dyspnea, orthopnea, PND, and hemoptysis. Unique features secondary to LAE include AF, dysphagia, and hoarseness	PE: Opening snap and mid-diastolic murmur at the apex; pulmonary edema Dx: Echocardiography	Antiarrhythmics (β-blockers, digoxin, or CCBs) and warfarin for AF. Mitral balloon valvotomy and valve replacement are effective for severe cases
Mitral valve regurgitation	Primarily 2° to rheumatic fever or chordae tendineae rupture after MI Myxomatous degeneration due to mitral valve prolapse Infective endocarditis	Patients present with dyspnea, orthopnea, PND, and fatigue	PE: Holosystolic/pansystolic murmur radiating to the axilla Dx: Echocardiography will demonstrate regurgitant flow; angiography can assess the severity of disease	ACEIs or ARBs to vasodilate and ↓ rate of progression. Antiarrhythmics if necessary (AF is common with LAE). Digoxin and diuretics may be needed in CHF Valve repair or replacement for severe cases

A hyperaldosteronism workup with serum aldosterone and renin levels is an appropriate next diagnostic step.

A

TREATMENT

- In asymptomatic patients, monitoring is appropriate for lesions < 5 cm.
- Surgical correction is indicated if the lesion is ≥ 5.5 cm (abdominal), > 6 cm (thoracic), or smaller but rapidly enlarging (watch for bowel ischemia and infarction).
- Emergent surgery for symptomatic or ruptured aneurysms.

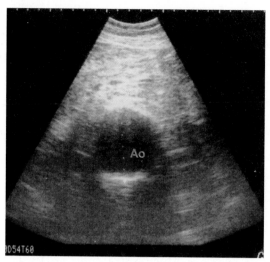
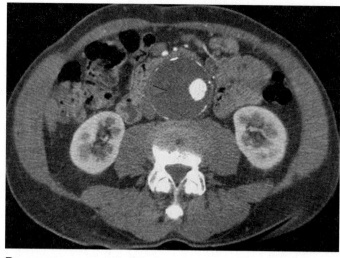

A   **B**

FIGURE 2.1-17.   Abdominal aortic aneurysm. (A) Ultrasound image of an AAA (Ao, aorta). **(B)** Transaxial image from a contrast-enhanced CT showing an aneurysm with extensive mural thrombus (*arrowhead*). (Image A reproduced with permission from Tintinalli JE et al. *Tintinalli's Emergency Medicine: A Comprehensive Study Guide,* 6th ed. New York, NY: McGraw-Hill; 2004. Image B reproduced with permission from Doherty GM. *Current Diagnosis & Treatment: Surgery,* 13th ed. New York, NY: McGraw-Hill; 2010.)

AORTIC DISSECTION

A transverse tear in the intima of a vessel that results in blood entering the media, creating a false lumen and leading to a hematoma that propagates longitudinally. Most commonly 2° to HTN, but also due to blunt chest trauma. The most common sites of origin are above the aortic valve and distal to the left subclavian artery. Most often occurs at 40–60 years of age, with a greater frequency in males than in females.

HISTORY/PE

- **Hx:** HTN, Marfan syndrome, mitral valve prolapse, trauma.
- **Presentation:** Sudden tearing/ripping pain in the anterior chest (ascending) with or without radiation to the back (descending), typically between the scapulae.
- **Exam:**
  - Patients are typically hypertensive. If hypotensive, consider pericardial tamponade, hypovolemia from blood loss, or other cardiopulmonary etiologies.
  - Asymmetric pulses and BP measurements or acute limb ischemia.
  - A murmur of aortic regurgitation may be heard if the aortic valve is involved with a proximal dissection.
  - Neurologic deficits, such as paraplegia, may be seen if the aortic arch or spinal arteries are involved.
  - Anuria may be seen if renal arteries are involved.
  - Signs of pericarditis or pericardial tamponade may be seen.

DIAGNOSIS

- **Best initial test for hemodynamically stable patients:** CT angiography. MRA can be used if contrast CT is contraindicated.
- **Best initial test for hemodynamically unstable patients:** TEE. It may also be used to visualize details of the proximal aorta and coronary vessels and can also evaluate for pericardial effusion.

> **KEY FACT**
>
> Aortic aneurysm is most often associated with atherosclerosis, whereas aortic dissection is commonly linked to HTN.

Q

A 70-year-old man with HTN presents for a routine appointment. He quit smoking 20 years ago but has a 20-pack-year history. What screening, if any, is indicated?

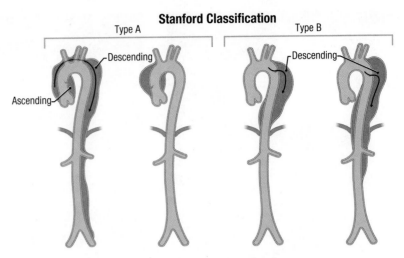

FIGURE 2.1-18. **Stanford classification of aortic dissection.** Type A involves the ascending aorta and may progress to involve the arch and thoracoabdominal aorta. Type B involves the descending thoracic or thoracoabdominal aorta distal to the left subclavian artery without involvement of the ascending aorta. (Reproduced with permission from USMLE-Rx.com.)

- The Stanford system classifies any dissection proximal to the left subclavian artery as type A and all others as type B (see Figure 2.1-18).
- Type A (~70%) is the most common and involves the ascending aorta, irrespective of the site of the tear. Type B does not involve the ascending aorta.

TREATMENT

- **BP control:** Important to monitor and medically manage BP and heart rate as necessary. Avoid thrombolytics. Begin intravenous β-blockers (eg, IV labetalol) before starting vasodilators (nitroprusside) to prevent reflex tachycardia.
- All patients with type A thoracic dissection (ascending dissections) should have surgery.
- Patients with type B thoracic dissection (descending dissections) may be managed medically with BP and heart rate control; surgery is reserved if there is a leakage, rupture, or compromised organs.

DEEP VENOUS THROMBOSIS

Clot formation in the large veins of the extremities or pelvis. The classic Virchow triad of risk factors includes venous stasis (eg, from long-haul flights, prolonged bed rest, obesity, immobility, or incompetent venous valves in the lower extremities), endothelial trauma (eg, surgery, injury to the lower extremities, trauma), and hypercoagulable states (eg, thrombophilia, malignancy, pregnancy, OCP use).

HISTORY/PE

- Presents with unilateral lower extremity pain and swelling. Calf warmth, tenderness, and erythema may be present.
- Homans sign is calf tenderness with passive foot dorsiflexion (poor sensitivity and specificity for DVT).
- Use pretest clinical probability scoring for DVT, the Wells score.

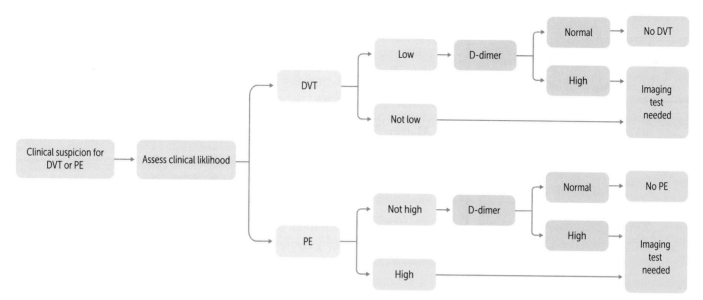

FIGURE 2.1-19. Algorithm for diagnostic imaging of deep vein thrombosis and pulmonary embolism. (Reproduced with permission from USMLE-Rx.com)

DIAGNOSIS

- D-dimer test should be ordered (sensitive but not specific) and is elevated in DVT. Also elevated in infections, malignancy, pregnancy, and postoperatively. A negative result, combined with a low clinical probability is sufficient to exclude a DVT.
- If D-dimer is elevated and the patient has a high-to-intermediate clinical probability, Doppler ultrasound is done.
- A spiral CT or V/Q scan may be used to evaluate for PE (see Figure 2.1-19).

TREATMENT

- Anticoagulate with subcutaneous low-molecular-weight heparin (LMWH) or IV unfractionated heparin followed by PO warfarin or NOACs for a total of 3–6 months.
- In patients with contraindications for anticoagulation, inferior vena cava filters should be placed.
- Hospitalized patients should receive DVT prophylaxis consisting of exercise as tolerated, antithromboembolic stockings, and subcutaneous LMWH or unfractionated heparin.

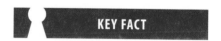

KEY FACT

A ⊖ D-dimer test can be used to rule out the possibility of PE in low-risk patients.

PERIPHERAL ARTERIAL DISEASE

Defined as a restriction of the blood supply to the extremities by atherosclerotic plaque. The lower extremities are most commonly affected. Clinical manifestations depend on the vessels involved, the extent and rate of obstruction, and the presence of collateral blood flow.

HISTORY/PE

- Presents with intermittent claudication; reproducible cramping pain in the calf, thigh, or buttock after walking for a certain distance (claudication distance) and is relieved with rest.
- As the disease progresses, it causes critical limb ischemia. Pain occurs at rest and affects the distal extremities. Dorsal foot ulcerations may develop 2° to poor perfusion. A painful, cold, numb foot is characteristic of critical limb ischemia.

The 6 P's of acute ischemia—

Pain
Pallor
Paralysis
Pulse deficit
Paresthesias
Poikilothermia

KEY FACT

$ABI = P_{leg}/P_{arm}$
Rest pain seen with an ABI < 0.4.
  (normal ABI: 1.0–1.2)

KEY FACT

Calf claudication = femoral disease
Buttock claudication = iliac disease
Buttock claudication + impotence =
  Leriche syndrome (aortoiliac occlusive
  disease)

KEY FACT

The major cause of mortality in patients with PAD is cardiovascular disease (MI, stroke); there is a 20–30% risk for these complications. There is only a 1–2% risk for developing limb ischemia.

- For more proximal lesions, there will be claudication and weak pulses below the area of occlusion (ie, aortoiliac disease; [Leriche syndrome] is characterized by the triad of hip, thigh, and buttock claudication, impotence, and symmetric atrophy of bilateral lower extremities).
- A Buerger angle of < 20 degrees and capillary filling of > 15 seconds are seen in severe ischemia.
- **Acute ischemia:**
    - May be due to thrombosis in situ (~40), emboli usually of cardiac origin (~38%), graft/angioplasty occlusion (~15%), or trauma. Acute occlusions commonly occur at bifurcations distal to the last palpable pulse (see mnemonic for signs and symptoms).
    - May also be 2° to cholesterol atheroembolism ("blue toe syndrome"), which is characterized by blue toes, livedo reticularis, renal failure (often 2° to catheterization).
- **Chronic ischemia:** Lack of blood perfusion leads to muscle atrophy, pallor, loss of sweat and sebaceous glands, cyanosis, hair loss, and gangrene/necrosis.

DIAGNOSIS

- Identify cardiovascular risk factors, especially smoking, diabetes, hypertension, and hyperlipidemia.
- **Best initial test:** Ankle-brachial index test; can provide objective evidence of atherosclerosis (rest pain usually occurs with an ABI < 0.4). A very high ABI can indicate calcification of the arteries.
- **Doppler ultrasound:** Identifies stenosis and occlusion. Normal ankle Doppler readings are > 90% of brachial readings.
- **Most accurate test:** Angiography; often not necessary unless revascularization is indicated.

TREATMENT

- Treat acute symptomatic ischemia with heparin and prompt revascularization.
- **Address modifiable risk factors:** Smoking (vital), hypertension, hyperlipidemia, and diabetes.
- Educate regarding careful hygiene and foot care. Exercise helps develop collateral circulation.
- Antiplatelet agents (ASA or vorapaxar) do not consistently reduce symptoms, but ↓ the risk for associated cardiovascular mortality.
- Cilostazol is effective medication in intermittent claudication.
- Surgery (arterial bypass), percutaneous transluminal angioplasty, and stenting, or amputation can be employed when conservative treatment fails or in acute limb ischemia.

LYMPHEDEMA

A disruption of the lymphatic circulation that results in peripheral edema and chronic infection of the extremities. Primary (or congenital) lymphedema is rare. Most often caused secondarily by surgeries involving lymph node dissection or, in developing countries, parasitic infections.

HISTORY/PE

History will differ by cause. Examples include the following:

- Postmastectomy patients present with unexplained swelling of the upper extremity (secondary to surgery).

- Patients originating from developing countries present with progressive swelling of the lower extremities bilaterally with no cardiac abnormalities (ie, filariasis infection).
- Children present with progressive, bilateral swelling of the extremities (1°).
- Patients with Turner syndrome will have lymphatic edema.

DIAGNOSIS

Diagnosis is clinical. Rule out other causes of edema, such as cardiac and metabolic disorders.

TREATMENT

- Directed at symptom management, including exercise, massage therapy, and pressure garments to mobilize and limit fluid accumulation.
- Diuretics are ineffective and relatively contraindicated.
- Maintain vigilance for cellulitis with prompt gram-⊕ antibiotic coverage for infection.

Syncope

A sudden, temporary loss of consciousness and postural tone 2° to cerebral hypoperfusion. Etiologies can be cardiac, neurologic, or other.

- **Cardiac:** Valvular lesions (aortic stenosis), arrhythmias, PE, cardiac tamponade, aortic dissection.
- **Neurologic:** Subarachnoid hemorrhage.
- **Other:** Orthostatic/hypovolemic hypotension, metabolic abnormalities, neurocardiogenic syndromes (eg, vasovagal/micturition syncope), psychiatric, medications.

HISTORY/PE

- Age, triggers, prodromal symptoms, and associated symptoms should be investigated.
- Syncope can be confused with seizures. Unlike syncope, seizures may be characterized by a preceding aura, tonic-clonic activity, tongue-biting, bladder and bowel incontinence, and a postictal phase.
- Cardiac causes of syncope are typically associated with very brief or absent prodromal symptoms, a history of exertion, lack of association with changes in position, and/or a history of cardiac disease.
- Neurocardiogenic syndrome is common in younger patients and older patients with difficulty voiding.

DIAGNOSIS

Depending on the suspected etiology:

- **Cardiac:** ECG, Holter monitors or 2-week event recorders (arrhythmias), echocardiograms (structural abnormalities), stress tests (ischemia).
- **Neurologic:** CT of head (ischemia or hemorrhage) and EEG (seizure).
- **Other:** Orthostatic BP readings (hypovolemia, autonomic dysfunction), glucose (hypoglycemia), and tilt-table testing (neurally mediated syncope).

TREATMENT

Tailored to the etiology.

KEY FACT

Cardiac syncope is associated with 1-year sudden cardiac death rates of up to 40%.

NOTES

DERMATOLOGY

Layers of the Skin

The skin is the largest organ in the human body. It provides a barrier and immunologic protection against the environment, regulates body temperature, fluids, and electrolytes, and allows for touch and sensation. Figures 2.2-1 and 2.2-2 and Table 2.2-1 outline the skin layers, cell junctions, and common terminology related to the skin.

TABLE 2.2-1.   Dermatologic Macroscopic Terms

LESION	CHARACTERISTICS	EXAMPLES
Macule	Flat lesion < 1 cm	Freckle, labial macule (see Image A)
Patch	Flat lesion > 1 cm	Birthmark (congenital nevus) (see Image B)
Papule	Elevated solid lesion < 1 cm	Mole (nevus) (see Image C), acne
Plaque	Elevated lesion > 1 cm	Psoriasis (see Image D)
Vesicle	Small fluid-containing blister < 1 cm	Chickenpox (varicella), shingles (zoster) (see Image E)
Bulla	Large fluid-containing blister > 1 cm	Bullous pemphigoid (see Image F)
Cyst	Epithelium-lined sac containing material or fluid	Pilar cyst (follicular cyst on scalp)
Pustule	Vesicle containing pus	Pustular psoriasis (see Image G)
Wheal	Transient edematous papule or plaque	Hives (urticarial) (see Image H)
Scale	Flaking off of stratum corneum	Eczema, psoriasis, SCC (see Image I)
Crust	Exudate of dried serum, blood, and/or pus	Impetigo (see Image J)
Ulcer	Defect extending through the epidermis and upper dermis	Diabetic foot ulcer
Lichenification	Hypertrophy and thickening of the epidermis with accentuation of normal skin markings	Chronic scratching (pruritic scabies, eczema)

A   B   C   D   E

F   G   H   I   J

Images reproduced with permission from Dr. Richard Usatine.

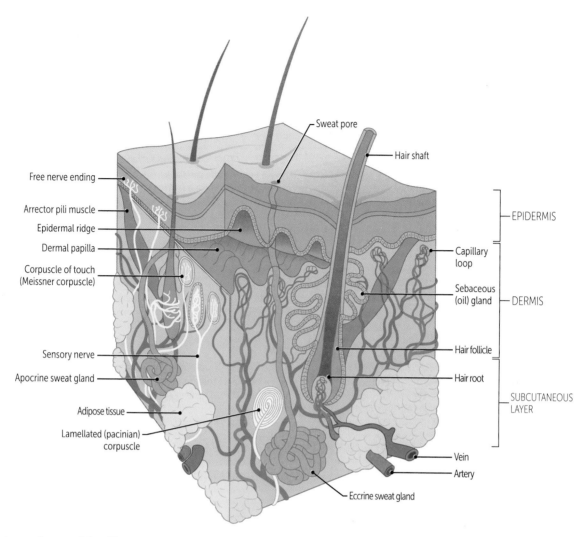

FIGURE 2.2-1.   Layers of the skin. (Reproduced with permission from USMLE-Rx-com.)

Allergic and Immune-Mediated Skin Disorders

HYPERSENSITIVITY REACTIONS

Table 2.2-2 outlines the types and mechanisms of hypersensitivity reactions.

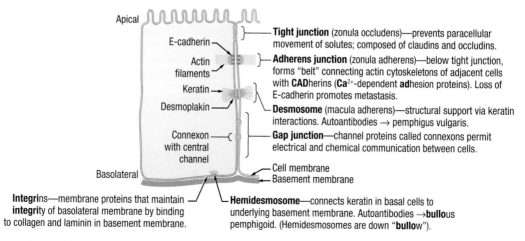

FIGURE 2.2-2.   Epithelial cell junctions. (Reproduced with permission from USMLE-Rx.com.)

TABLE 2.2-2. Types and Mechanisms of Hypersensitivity Reactions

DESCRIPTION	MECHANISM	COMMENTS	EXAMPLES
TYPE I			
Anaphylactic and atopic Mast cell or basophil — Fc receptor — IgE — Ag	Antigen cross-links preformed surface-bound IgE on mast cells and basophils, triggering the release of vasoactive amines like histamine. Reaction develops rapidly as a result of preformed antibody	**F**irst and **F**ast (like anaphylaxis) Types I, II, and III are all antibody mediated	Anaphylaxis (bee sting, food allergy), asthma, urticaria, urticarial drug reactions, local wheal and flare
TYPE II			
Cytotoxic IgG — Cell — IgG — ⓒ = complement	IgM and IgG bind to antigen on an "enemy" cell, leading to lysis by complement or phagocytosis	Cy-2-toxic Antibody and complement lead to formation of the membrane attack complex (MAC)	Autoimmune hemolytic anemia, erythroblastosis fetalis, Goodpasture syndrome, rheumatic fever
TYPE III			
Immune complex Ag — ⓒ — Ag	Antigen-antibody complexes fix complement, which attracts PMNs; PMNs release lysosomal enzymes	Imagine an immune complex as three things stuck together: antigen-antibody-complement Includes many glomerulonephritides and vasculitides	Polyarteritis nodosa, immune complex glomerulonephritis, SLE, rheumatoid arthritis
TYPE IV			
Delayed (cell-mediated) type APC — Th cells	Sensitized T lymphocytes encounter antigen and then release lymphokines (leading to macrophage activation)	Fourth and final (last)—delayed Cell mediated, not antibody mediated; therefore, it is not transferable by serum	TB skin tests, transplant rejection, contact dermatitis

Modified with permission from Le T et al. *First Aid for the USMLE Step 1 2016*. New York, NY: McGraw-Hill Education; 2016.

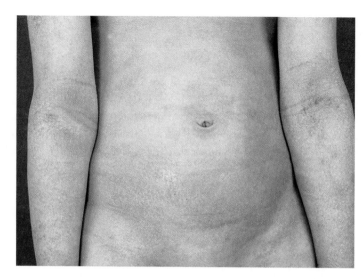

FIGURE 2.2-3.   Atopic dermatitis. Lichenification, excoriations, and ill-defined, scaly erythematous plaques are characteristic. (Reproduced with permission from Tintinalli JE et al. *Tintinalli's Emergency Medicine: A Comprehensive Study Guide,* 7th ed. New York, NY: McGraw-Hill; 2011.)

ATOPIC DERMATITIS (ECZEMA)

A chronic inflammatory dermatitis that classically manifests in infancy and persists into adulthood. It is characterized by a defective epidermal barrier, causing sensitization, inflammation, pruritus, and ultimately lichenification (see Figure 2.2-3).

HISTORY/PE

- Look for a strong family history of asthma, eczema, and allergic rhinitis ("atopic triad") as well as food allergies.
- Patients are at ↑ risk for 2° bacterial (*Staphylococcus aureus* or *Streptococcus pyogenes*) and viral (HSV or molluscum) infection due to constant waxing and waning cycles of pruritus and excoriation.
- Triggers include climate, food, skin irritants, allergens, and emotional factors.
- **Manifestations by age group:**
    - **Infants:** Erythematous, edematous, weeping, pruritic vesicles, papules, and plaques on the face, scalp, and extensor surfaces of the extremities. The diaper area is often spared.
    - **Children:** Dry, scaly, pruritic, excoriated vesicles, papules, and plaques in the flexural areas and neck.
    - **Adults:** Lichenification and dry, fissured skin in a flexural distribution. Often, there is hand or eyelid involvement.

DIAGNOSIS

Characteristic exam findings and history are sufficient. Excluding contact dermatitis by history and anatomic distribution is important. KOH prep can help distinguish chronic eczema from tinea. Mild peripheral eosinophilia and ↑ IgE may be seen but have no diagnostic value.

KEY FACT

Long-term use of immunomodulating medications may ↑ the risk for developing lymphoma.

KEY FACT

Erythema toxicum neonatorum typically begins 1–3 days after delivery and presents with red papules, pustules, and/or vesicles with surrounding erythematous halos. ↑ Eosinophils are present in the pustules or vesicles. This benign eruption usually resolves in 1–2 weeks with no treatment.

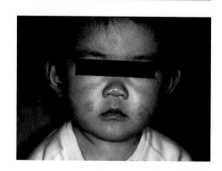

FIGURE 2.2-4.   (Reproduced with permission from Dr. Richard Usatine).

An infant with a history of eczema treated with corticosteroids is brought in with a new-onset rash and fever. Physical exam reveals grouped monomorphic vesicles involving eczematous areas of the infant's extremities and face (see Figure 2.2-4). What is the appropriate therapy?

TREATMENT

- The primary goal of therapy is to break the itch-scratch cycle with agents targeted at inflammation, pruritus, and xerosis (dry skin).
- Topical corticosteroids are first-line therapy for flares, but watch out for atrophy, telangiectasias, and rebound flares with prolonged use. Topical calcineurin inhibitors (eg, tacrolimus) are useful as steroid-sparing agents for moderate to severe eczema for patients > 2 years of age.
- H₁-blockers may be used for relief of pruritus. Choose a first-generation H₁-blocker (eg, hydroxyzine) for nighttime use.
- Aggressive use of emollients, avoidance of harsh soaps, and limiting hot showers after resolution of acute flares will prevent future episodes.

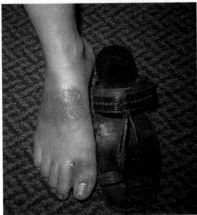

FIGURE 2.2-5. Contact dermatitis. Shown are erythematous papules and vesicles with serous weeping localized to areas of contact with the offending agent. (Reproduced with permission from Hurwitz RM. *Pathology of the Skin: Atlas of Clinical-Pathological Correlation*, 2nd ed. Stamford, CT: Appleton & Lange; 1998.)

KEY FACT

Remember that patch testing results are affected by topical steroids and calcineurin inhibitors but not antihistamines, since type IV hypersensitivity reactions are not histamine-mediated.

CONTACT DERMATITIS

A type IV hypersensitivity reaction that results from contact with an allergen to which the patient has previously been exposed and sensitized such as nickel, poison ivy, perfumes/deodorants, and neomycin. More common in adults.

HISTORY/PE

- Presents with pruritus and an eczematous rash, with the distribution of the rash often mimicking the contact event (see Figure 2.2-5). Characteristic distributions are seen where makeup, clothing, perfume, nickel jewelry, and plants come into contact with the skin.
- Often described as a "linear" or "angular" rash. It can spread over the body via transfer of allergen by the hands or via circulating T-lymphocytes.
- **Frequently implicated allergens:** Poison ivy, poison oak, nickel, topical antibiotics, cosmetics, and latex.

DIAGNOSIS

Characteristic exam findings and history are sufficient. Excluding atopic dermatitis (eczema) is important. Patch testing can be used to establish the causative allergen after the acute-phase eruption has been treated.

TREATMENT

The best initial treatment is topical corticosteroids and allergen avoidance. In severe cases, a systemic corticosteroid may be needed.

SEBORRHEIC DERMATITIS

A common chronic inflammatory skin disease that may be caused by a reaction to *Malassezia furfur*, a generally harmless yeast found in sebum and hair follicles. It has a predilection for areas with sebaceous glands.

HISTORY/PE

- **Rash presentation varies with age:**
  - **Infants:** Severe, red diaper rash with yellow scale, erosions, and blisters. Scaling and crusting ("cradle cap") may be seen on the scalp (see Figure 2.2-6A).
  - **Children/adults:** Ill-defined red, scaly thin plaques are seen around the ears, eyebrows, nasolabial fold, midchest, and scalp (see Figure 2.2-6B).
- Patients with HIV/AIDS, psychotic disorders, and Parkinson disease can develop severe, widespread seborrheic dermatitis.

This infant has eczema herpeticum, a medical emergency that is due to the propensity for HSV infection to spread systemically, potentially affecting the brain. IV acyclovir must be started immediately!

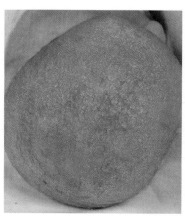 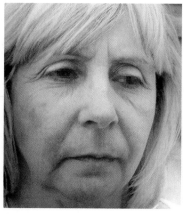

A **B**

FIGURE 2.2-6. **Seborrheic dermatitis.** (**A**) Seborrheic dermatitis (cradle cap) in an infant. Note the yellow, scaly crust present on the infant's scalp with an area of erosion. (**B**) Photo-exacerbated seborrheic dermatitis, affecting the face only at sites of predilection for the seborrheic eruption. (Image A reproduced with permission from Tintinalli JE et al. *Tintinalli's Emergency Medicine: A Comprehensive Study Guide,* 7th ed. New York, NY: McGraw-Hill; 2011. Image B reproduced with permission from Goldsmith LA et al. *Fitzpatrick's Dermatology in General Medicine,* 8th ed. New York, NY: McGraw-Hill; 2012.)

DIAGNOSIS

Characteristic exam findings and history are sufficient. Can be confused with atopic dermatitis, contact dermatitis, tinea, or psoriasis.

TREATMENT

Treat adults with ketoconazole, selenium sulfide or zinc pyrithione shampoos for the scalp, and topical antifungals (ketoconazole cream) and/or topical corticosteroids for other areas. Cradle cap often resolves with routine bathing and application of emollients in infants.

STASIS DERMATITIS

Lower extremity dermatitis due to venous hypertension forcing blood from the deep to the superficial venous system. Venous hypertension is often a result of venous valve incompetence or flow obstruction. It commonly involves the medial ankle in patients with deep vein thrombosis (DVT) history, chronic edema, and long periods of standing. If untreated, the area can become inflamed, exudative, and hyperpigmented from hemosiderin deposition (see Figure 2.2-7). Stasis ulcers may develop. Treat early with leg elevation, compression stockings, emollients, and topical steroids.

PSORIASIS

A T-cell–mediated inflammatory dermatosis characterized by well-demarcated, erythematous plaques with silvery scales (see Figure 2.2-8A) due to dermal inflammation and epidermal hyperplasia. Psoriasis can begin at any age.

HISTORY/PE

■ Lesions are classically found on the extensor surfaces, including the elbows and knees. Scalp and lumbosacral regions are often involved. Nails are frequently affected with pitting, "oil spots," and onycholysis (lifting of the nail plate, see Figure 2.2-8B).

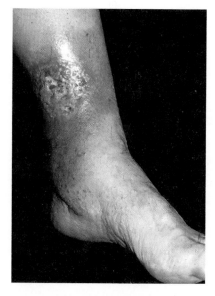

FIGURE 2.2-7. **Stasis dermatitis.** Venous ulceration with stasis dermatitis, edema, and varicosities. (Reproduced with permission from Goldsmith LA et al. *Fitzpatrick's Dermatology in General Medicine,* 8th ed. New York, NY: McGraw-Hill; 2012.)

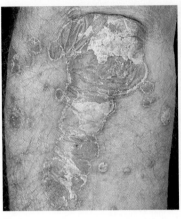
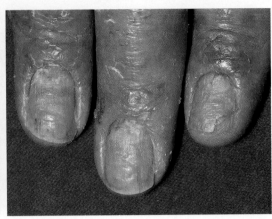

A   **B**

FIGURE 2.2-8. **Psoriasis. (A)** Skin changes. The classic sharply demarcated plaques with silvery scales are commonly located on the extensor surfaces (eg, elbows, knees). **(B)** Nail changes. Note the pitting, onycholysis, and "oil spots." (Image A reproduced with permission from Wolff K et al. *Fitzpatrick's Color Atlas and Synopsis of Clinical Dermatology,* 7th ed. New York, NY: McGraw-Hill; 2013. Image B reproduced with permission from Hurwitz RM. *Pathology of the Skin: Atlas of Clinical-Pathological Correlation,* 2nd ed. Stamford, CT: Appleton & Lange; 1998.)

- Lesions initially appear small but may become confluent and can be provoked by local irritation or trauma (Koebner phenomenon). Some medications such as β-blockers, lithium, and ACE inhibitors (ACEIs), can worsen psoriatic lesions.
- Up to 30% develop psoriatic arthritis (affecting small joints of the hands and feet).

DIAGNOSIS

- Characteristic exam findings and history are sufficient. Classical presentation: Auspitz sign (pinpoint bleeding when scale is scraped) overlying well-demarcated, erythematous plaques with silvery "micaceous" scale.
- Perform a biopsy if diagnosis is uncertain. Histology shows a thickened epidermis, elongated rete ridges, an absent granular cell layer, preservation of nuclei in the stratum corneum (parakeratosis), and a sterile neutrophilic infiltrate in the stratum corneum (Munro microabscesses).

TREATMENT

- **Local disease:** Manage with topical steroids, calcipotriene (vitamin D derivative), and retinoids such as tazarotene or acitretin (vitamin A derivative).
- **Severe disease or presence of psoriatic arthritis:** Methotrexate or anti–tumour necrosis factor (TNF) biologics (etanercept, infliximab, adalimumab). Newer agents such as ustekinumab (anti-interleukin [IL]-12/23), secukinumab (anti-IL17), and UV light therapy can be used for extensive skin involvement (except in immunosuppressed patients who can develop skin cancer from UV light).
- Before starting methotrexate or anti-TNF biologics, patients should at a minimum get a complete blood count (CBC), comprehensive metabolic panel (CMP), hepatitis panel, and a purified protein derivative (PPD).

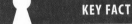

KEY FACT

If a rash involves the extensor surfaces, think psoriasis. If a rash involves the flexor surfaces, think atopic dermatitis.

KEY FACT

"Sausage digits" and pencil-in-cup x-ray findings are suggestive of psoriatic arthritis.

URTICARIA (HIVES)

Results from the release of histamine and prostaglandins from mast cells in a type I hypersensitivity response. Sharply demarcated edematous plaques with

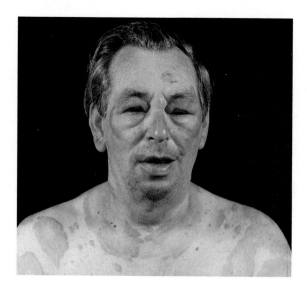

FIGURE 2.2-9. **Urticaria (hives) and angioedema.** This patient has urticaria occurring on the face, neck, and shoulders with orbital angioedema. (Reproduced with permission from Goldsmith LA et al. *Fitzpatrick's Dermatology in General Medicine,* 8th ed. New York, NY: McGraw-Hill; 2012.)

surrounding erythema ("wheal and flare") are seen, with each lesion lasting < 24 hours. Can be acute or chronic (lasting > 6 weeks).

HISTORY/PE

- Urticaria lesions (wheals) are reddish or white transient papules or plaques representing dermal edema. Lesions may be widespread and last a few hours.
- In severe allergic reactions, extracutaneous manifestations can include tongue swelling, angioedema (deep, diffuse swelling often around the eyes and mouth; see Figure 2.2-9), asthma, GI symptoms, joint swelling, and fever.
- Acute urticaria is a response to some often-unidentified trigger: food, drug, virus, insect bite, or physical stimulus (cold, heat, sun). Chronic urticaria is usually idiopathic.

DIAGNOSIS

Characteristic exam findings and history are sufficient. Positive dermatographism (formation of wheals where the skin is stroked) may help. If in doubt, drawing a serum tryptase (coreleased with histamine from mast cells) can help clinch the diagnosis. It can often be difficult to determine the cause of urticaria.

TREATMENT

Treat urticaria with systemic antihistamines. Anaphylaxis (rare) requires intramuscular epinephrine, antihistamines, IV fluids, and airway support.

DRUG ERUPTION

Drug eruptions can range from a mild morbilliform rash (most common, see Figure 2.2-10) to the rare but life-threatening toxic epidermal necrolysis (TEN). Maintain a high suspicion for a cutaneous drug reaction in patients who are hospitalized and develop rashes. Drugs can cause all four types of hypersensitivity reactions, and the same drug may cause different types of reactions in different persons.

Q

A 23-year-old woman is seen for an itchy, linear rash on her right leg. She returned from a camping trip 4 days ago and denies using any new makeup, clothing, or jewelry. What features of this presentation favor a contact dermatitis?

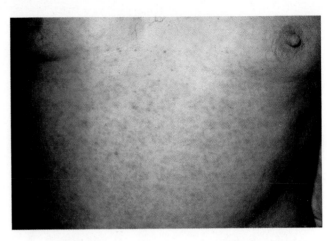

FIGURE 2.2-10. **Morbilliform rash.** Morbilliform rash following drug administration. (Reproduced with permission from Longo DL et al. *Harrison's Principles of Internal Medicine,* 18th ed. New York, NY: McGraw-Hill; 2011.)

HISTORY/PE

- Non-anaphylactoid eruptions usually occur 7–14 days after exposure: If a patient reacts within 1–2 days of starting a new drug, it is probably not the causative agent.
- Eruptions are generally widespread, relatively symmetric, and pruritic.
- Most disappear within 1–2 weeks following removal of the offending agent.
- Extreme complications of drug eruptions include erythroderma, drug reaction with eosinophilia, and systemic symptoms (DRESS), Stevens-Johnson syndrome (SJS), and TEN.

DIAGNOSIS

Characteristic exam findings and history are sufficient. Excluding other causes are important, including viral exanthema, graft-versus-host disease, and autoimmune dermatoses. A skin biopsy may be helpful if the diagnosis is not clear.

TREATMENT

Discontinue the offending agent; treat symptoms with antihistamines and topical steroids to relieve pruritus. In severe cases, systemic steroids and/or intravenous immunoglobulin may be used.

ERYTHEMA MULTIFORME

A cutaneous reaction pattern with classic targetoid lesions (see Figure 2.2-11) that has many triggers and is often recurrent.

HISTORY/PE

- Typically, lesions start as erythematous, dusky macules that become centrally clear (classic targets have three different color zones) and then develop a blister. The palms and soles are often affected.
- In its minor form, the disease is uncomplicated and localized to the skin.
- Erythema multiform (EM) major involves mucous membranes. It is a distinct entity from SJS, and there is no risk for progression to TEN.
- May have systemic symptoms, including fever, myalgias, arthralgias, and headache.

DIAGNOSIS

Characteristic exam findings and history are sufficient. As opposed to SJS or TEN, in EM the Nikolsky sign is ⊖.

The asymmetric involvement of the rash, its linear arrangement (possibly from contact with a plant during the camping trip), and the time from exposure to rash presentation all point to contact dermatitis.

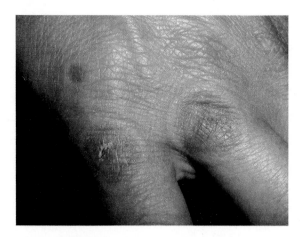

FIGURE 2.2-11. Erythema multiforme. (Reproduced with permission from Dr. Richard Usatine.)

TREATMENT

- Symptomatic treatment is all that is necessary; systemic corticosteroids are of no benefit.
- Minor cases can be managed supportively; major cases should be treated as burns.

STEVENS-JOHNSON SYNDROME/TOXIC EPIDERMAL NECROLYSIS

SJS and TEN constitute two different points on the spectrum of life-threatening exfoliative mucocutaneous diseases that are often caused by a drug-induced immunologic reaction. The epidermal separation of SJS involves < 10% of body surface area (BSA), whereas TEN involves > 30% of BSA. Mucosal involvement is present in > 90% of cases of SJS/TEN.

HISTORY/PE

- Exam reveals severe mucosal erosions with widespread erythematous, dusky red or purpuric macules, or atypical targetoid lesions (see Figure 2.2-12). The epidermal lesions often become confluent and show a ⊕ Nikolsky sign (separation of the superficial skin layers with slight rubbing) and epidermal detachment.
- Mucous membranes (eyes, mouth, and genitals) often become eroded and hemorrhagic.
- Associated with first-time exposure to drugs: sulfonamides, penicillin, seizure medications (phenytoin, carbamazepine), quinolones, cephalosporins, steroids, nonsteroidal anti-inflammatory drugs (NSAIDs).

DIAGNOSIS

- **SJS/TEN:** Biopsy shows full-thickness eosinophilic epidermal necrosis.
- Include staphylococcal scalded-skin syndrome (SSSS), graft-vs-host reaction (usually after bone marrow transplant), radiation therapy, and burns on the differential diagnosis.

TREATMENT

- High risk for mortality. Early diagnosis and discontinuation of offending agent are critical in improving survival.
- Patients have the same complications as burn victims—thermoregulatory and electrolyte disturbances and 2° infections, so cover the skin and manage fluids and electrolytes.

KEY FACT

Always include SJS and TEN in your differential diagnosis if a ⊕ Nikolsky sign is present.

KEY FACT

Do not confuse SJS and TEN with SSSS. SSSS is usually seen in children < 6 years of age and does not present with targetoid lesions. SJS/TEN is generally seen in adults and is usually caused by a drug reaction.

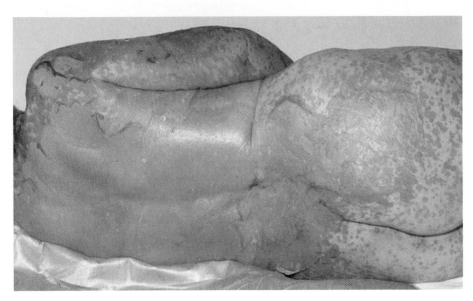

FIGURE 2.2-12. Toxic epidermal necrolysis. Note the diffuse erythematous bullae and areas of sloughing 2° to the full-thickness necrosis of the epidermis. (Reproduced with permission from Tintinalli JE et al. *Tintinalli's Emergency Medicine: A Comprehensive Study Guide,* 7th ed. New York, NY: McGraw-Hill; 2011.)

MNEMONIC

Causes of erythema nodosum—

NODOSUM

NO cause (60% idiopathic)
Drugs: sulfa, NSAIDs, iodides
Oral contraceptives
Sarcoidosis
Ulcerative colitis/Crohn disease
Microbiology (TB, leprosy, histoplasmosis, chronic infection)

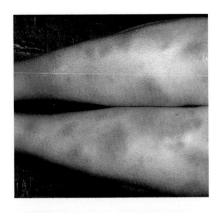

FIGURE 2.2-13. Erythema nodosum. Erythematous plaques and nodules are commonly located on pretibial areas. Lesions are painful and indurated but heal spontaneously without ulceration. (Reproduced with permission from Hurwitz RM. *Pathology of the Skin: Atlas of Clinical-Pathological Correlation,* 2nd ed. Stamford, CT: Appleton & Lange; 1998.)

- Data on pharmacologic therapy with steroids, cyclosporine, and IVIG is mixed.

ERYTHEMA NODOSUM

A panniculitis (inflammatory process of the subcutaneous adipose tissue) triggered by infection (*Streptococcus, Coccidioides, Yersinia,* TB), drugs (sulfonamides, antibiotics, oral contraceptive pills [OCPs]), and chronic inflammatory diseases (sarcoidosis, Crohn disease, ulcerative colitis, Behçet disease).

HISTORY/PE

- Painful, erythematous nodules appear on the patient's anterior shins (see Figure 2.2-13) and slowly spread, turning brown or purple. Patients may present with fever and joint pain.
- Patients with erythema nodosum may have a false-⊕ venereal disease research laboratory (as in systemic lupus erythematosus).

DIAGNOSIS

Characteristic exam findings and history are sufficient. A biopsy may help establish the diagnosis. Workup with an ASO titer, PPD in high-risk patients, an chest x-ray (CXR) to rule out sarcoidosis, or inflammatory bowel disease workup based on the patient's complaints.

TREATMENT

Investigate and treat the underlying disease. Cool compresses, bed rest, and NSAIDs are helpful. Potassium iodide may be considered for persistent cases.

BULLOUS PEMPHIGOID/PEMPHIGUS VULGARIS

Table 2.2-3 contrasts the clinical features of bullous pemphigoid with those of pemphigus vulgaris. Figure 2.2-2 shows the location of antibodies.

TABLE 2.2-3. **Acquired, Autoimmune Blistering Dermatoses**

Variable	Bullous Pemphigoid	Pemphigus Vulgaris
Location of blisters	Basement membrane zone	Intraepidermal
Autoantibodies	Against hemidesmosomal proteins	Anti-desmoglein; desmoglein is responsible for keratinocyte adhesion
Blister appearance	Firm, stable blisters (see Image A); may be preceded by urticaria	Erosions are more common than intact blisters (see Image B) because of the lack of keratinocyte adherence
Nikolsky sign	⊖	⊕
Mucosal involvement	Rare	Common
Patient age	Usually > 60 years of age	Usually 40–60 years of age
Associated medication triggers	Generally idiopathic	ACEIs, penicillamine, phenobarbital, penicillin
Mortality	Rare and milder course	Possible
Diagnosis	Look for tense bullae on the trunk. **Most accurate test:** skin biopsy with direct immunofluorescence, and/or ELISA	Look for flaccid/unroofed bullae and erosions on the extremities and mucous membranes
Treatment	Topical steroids can be sufficient	High-dose steroids (prednisone) + immunomodulatory therapy (azathioprine, mycophenolate mofetil, IVIG, rituximab)

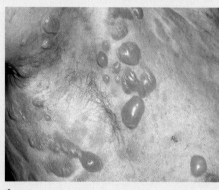
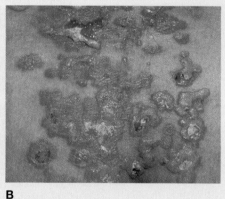

A　　　　B

Images reproduced with permission from Wolff K, Johnson RA. *Fitzpatrick's Color Atlas & Synopsis of Clinical Dermatology,* 6th ed. New York, NY: McGraw-Hill; 2009.

Infectious Disease Manifestations of the Skin

VIRAL DISEASES

Herpes Simplex

Painful, recurrent vesicular eruption of the mucocutaneous surfaces due to infection with HSV. HSV-1 usually produces oral-labial lesions, whereas HSV-2 usually causes genital lesions. The virus spreads through epidermal cells, fusing them into giant cells. The local host inflammatory response causes erythema and swelling.

KEY FACT

Dermatitis herpetiformis (DH) has vesicles and erosions like herpes but is caused by HSV. DH consists of pruritic papules, vesicles, bullae, and erosions on the elbows (see Figure 2.2-14), knees, buttocks, neck, and scalp, and it is associated with celiac disease (15–25%). Treat with dapsone and a gluten-free diet.

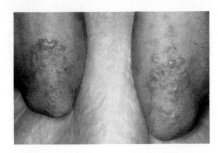

FIGURE 2.2-14. Dermatitis herpetiformis. This disorder typically displays pruritic, grouped papulovesicles on elbows, knees, buttocks, and posterior scalp. Vesicles are often excoriated due to associated pruritus. (Reproduced with permission from Longo DL et al. *Harrison's Principles of Internal Medicine,* 18th ed. New York, NY: McGraw-Hill; 2011.)

KEY FACT

No multinucleated giant cells on Tzanck smear? Tzanck goodness it's not herpes!

HISTORY/PE

- The initial infection is by direct contact, after which the herpesvirus remains dormant in local nerve ganglia. 1° Episodes are generally longer and more severe than recurrences.
- Onset is preceded by prodromal tingling, burning, or pain but can also present with lymphadenopathy, fever, discomfort, malaise, and edema of involved tissue.
- Recurrences are limited to mucocutaneous areas innervated by the involved nerve.
    - **Recurrent oral herpes (HSV-1):** The common "cold sore," or herpes labialis, which presents as a cluster of crusted vesicles on an erythematous base (see Figure 2.2-15A). Often triggered by sun and fever.
    - **Recurrent genital herpes (HSV-2):** Unilateral and characterized by a cluster of blisters on an erythematous base, but with less pain and systemic involvement than the 1° infection.

DIAGNOSIS

- Clinical diagnosis.
- **Most accurate test:** Viral culture or polymerase chain reaction (PCR) test of lesion. Direct fluorescent antigen is the most rapid test.
- Classic multinucleated giant cells on Tzanck smear (Figure 2.2-15B) support the diagnosis.

TREATMENT

- **First episode:** Immunocompetent patients with small lesions only need supportive therapy, but acyclovir, famciclovir, or valacyclovir may be given to speed healing and reduce shedding.
    - Immunocompromised patients or those with a severe painful outbreak should receive an antiviral drug within 72 hours of the start of the outbreak.
- **Recurrent episodes:** Minor lesions can be managed supportively. Acyclovir, famciclovir, or valacyclovir can be given during the episode to reduce healing time by ~ 2 days.
- **Severe frequent recurrences (> 6 outbreaks per year):** Daily prophylaxis with acyclovir, famciclovir, or valacyclovir.
- In AIDS patients, HSV can persist, with ulcers remaining resistant to antiviral therapy. Symptomatic HSV infection lasting > 1 month can be considered an AIDS-defining illness.

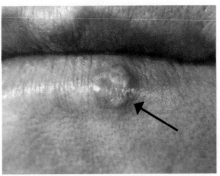

A

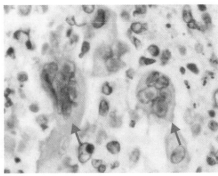

B

FIGURE 2.2-15. Herpes simplex. **(A)** Herpes labialis. **(B)** Positive Tzanck smear in genital herpes (HSV-2). Note multinucleated giant cells *(arrows).* (Image A reproduced with permission from the US Department of Health and Human Services and Dr. Herrmann. Image B reproduced with permission from Yale Rosen.)

Varicella-Zoster Virus

Varicella-zoster virus (VZV) causes two different diseases, varicella and herpes zoster—with transmission occurring via respiratory droplet or by direct contact. VZV has an incubation period of 10–20 days, with contagion beginning 24 hours before the eruption appears and lasting until lesions have crusted.

History/PE

- **Varicella:**
  - A prodrome of malaise, fever, headache, and myalgia occurs 24 hours before the rash.
  - Pruritic lesions appear in crops over 2–3 days, evolving from red macules to vesicles that then crust over.
  - At any given time, patients may have all stages of lesions present. The trunk, face, scalp, and mucous membranes are involved.
  - In adults, chickenpox is often more severe, with systemic complications such as pneumonia and encephalitis.
- **Zoster:**
  - Herpes zoster (shingles) represents the recurrence of VZV in a specific nerve, with lesions cropping up along the nerve's dermatomal distribution. Outbreaks are usually preceded by intense local pain followed by grouped blisters on an erythematous base (see Figure 2.2-16). Zoster can become disseminated in immunocompromised persons.
  - Older patients with zoster can develop postherpetic neuralgia (severe nerve pain that persists for months at the infection site).

Diagnosis

Characteristic exam findings and history are sufficient.

Treatment

- Varicella is self-limited in healthy children. A vaccine is available.
- Adults should be treated with systemic acyclovir to treat symptoms and prevent complications. Pain control with neuropathic agents (gabapentin, tricyclic antidepressants).
- Postexposure prophylaxis is rarely needed, as most patients in the United States have been vaccinated or had childhood varicella. If needed, immunocompromised individuals, pregnant women, and newborns should receive varicella-zoster immune globulin within 10 days of exposure. Immunocompetent adults should receive a varicella vaccine within 5 days of exposure.

Molluscum Contagiosum

A poxvirus infection that is most common in young children and in AIDS patients. It is spread by direct skin-to-skin contact (sports, sex) or sharing infected clothing or towels.

History/PE

- Presents as tiny flesh-colored dome-shaped waxy papules, frequently with central umbilication. In children, lesions are found on the trunk, extremities, or face (see Figure 2.2-17). In adults, they are commonly found on the genitalia and in the perineal region. Typically spares palms and soles.
- Lesions are asymptomatic unless they become inflamed or irritated.

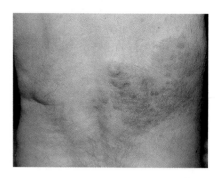

FIGURE 2.2-16. Varicella zoster. The unilateral dermatomal distribution of the grouped vesicles on an erythematous base is characteristic. (Reproduced with permission from Wolff K et al. *Fitzpatrick's Color Atlas & Synopsis of Clinical Dermatology,* 5th ed. New York, NY: McGraw-Hill; 2005.)

KEY FACT

Immunocompromised patients, cancer patients (especially those undergoing chemotherapy), the elderly, and severely stressed individuals are more susceptible to zoster infection.

KEY FACT

If you see giant molluscum contagiosum, think HIV or ↓ cellular immunity.

Q

A 28-year-old African-American woman is seen by her physician for a new-onset, painful rash. She noticed the erythematous nodules on both lower legs 3 days ago. She has a history of uveitis. What is the next best step to identify the underlying cause of this rash?

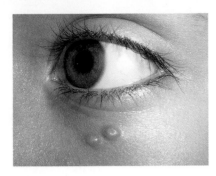

FIGURE 2.2-17. **Molluscum contagiosum.** (Reproduced with permission from Dr. Richard Usatine.)

DIAGNOSIS

- Characteristic exam findings and history are sufficient.
- **Most accurate test:** If the diagnosis is uncertain, the most accurate test is the presence of large inclusion or molluscum bodies seen under the microscope.

TREATMENT

- **Local destruction:** Curetting, freezing, or applying cantharidin (a blistering agent) to the lesions.
- In children, lesions resolve spontaneously over months to years and are occasionally left untreated.

Verrucae (Warts)

Warts are caused by human papillomavirus (HPV) and can occur on skin, mucous membranes, and other epithelia. Although usually benign, some subtypes of HPV (especially 16 and 18) lead to squamous malignancies. Spread is by direct contact.

HISTORY/PE

- Common warts are most often seen on the hands, though they can occur anywhere.
- Classic genital warts (condyloma acuminatum, caused by HPV subtypes 6 and 11) are cauliflower-like papules or plaques appearing on the penis, vulva, or perianal region (see Figure 2.2-18).
- Mothers with genital HPV can transmit laryngeal warts to the infant by aspiration during delivery.

DIAGNOSIS

- Characteristic exam findings and history are sufficient. Acetic acid turns lesions white and can be used to visualize mucosal lesions.
- **Most accurate test:** PCR of the lesion for HPV.

TREATMENT

Genital warts are treated locally with cryotherapy, podophyllin, trichloroacetic acid, imiquimod, or 5-FU. Cervical lesions are monitored for evidence of malignancy (see Gynecology chapter).

CXR to look for bilateral hilar adenopathy, which is suggestive of sarcoidosis. Erythema nodosum is the most common nonspecific cutaneous manifestation of sarcoidosis, after cutaneous sarcoidosis.

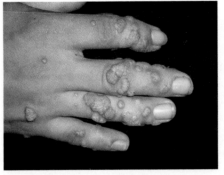

A

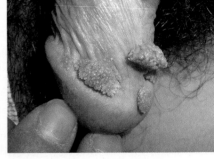

B

FIGURE 2.2-18. **Verrucae (warts) caused by HPV.** **(A)** Soft, tan-colored, cauliflower-like papules on hands. **(B)** Condyloma acuminatum on genitals. (Reproduced with permission from Dr. Richard Usatine.)

BACTERIAL INFECTIONS

Skin and soft-tissue bacterial infections are a diverse group of diseases that manifest in different ways: red, inflamed papules, and pustules centered around hair follicles are characteristic of folliculitis, while rapidly expanding crepitant dusky plaques suggest necrotizing fasciitis. Often, the clinical manifestation and treatment approach are dictated by the causative organism and the location of the infectious process within the layers of the skin and soft tissues. See Figure 2.2-19 for an illustration of the layers of the skin.

Impetigo

Local infection of the epidermis that primarily occurs in children and is caused by both group A streptococcal and staphylococcal organisms. It is transmitted by direct contact. Streptococcal impetigo can be complicated by poststreptococcal glomerulonephritis.

HISTORY/PE

- **Common type:** Pustules and honey-colored crusts on an erythematous base, often on the face around the mouth, nose, or ears (see Figure 2.2-20).
- **Bullous type:** Characterized by bulla in addition to crusts that can involve the acral surfaces. Bullous impetigo is almost always caused by S *aureus* and can evolve into SSSS.

DIAGNOSIS

Clinical. Obtaining a culture is rarely useful.

TREATMENT

- Use antibiotics with antistaphylococcal activity based on severity and suspicion of methicillin-resistant *Staphylococcus aureus* (MRSA):
    - **Mild localized disease:** Topical antibiotics (mupirocin) are sufficient.
    - **Severe disease (non-MRSA):** Oral cephalexin, dicloxacillin, or erythromycin.

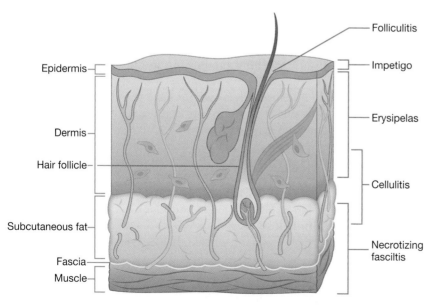

FIGURE 2.2-19. Skin layers (blue) and depths of infection (red).

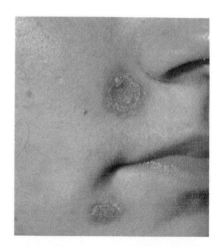

FIGURE 2.2-20. **Impetigo.** Dried pustules with a superficial golden-brown crust are most commonly found around the nose and mouth. (Reproduced with permission from Bondi EE. *Dermatology: Diagnosis and Therapy.* Stamford, CT: Appleton & Lange; 1991.)

KEY FACT

Scarlet fever: "Sandpaper" rash or "sunburn with goose bumps" appearance; strawberry tongue. Caused by *Streptococcus pyogenes*. Treat with penicillin.

KEY FACT

Salmonella typhi: Small pink papules on the trunk ("rose spots") in groups of 10–20 plus fever and GI involvement. Treat with fluoroquinolones and third-generation cephalosporins. Consider cholecystectomy for chronic carrier state.

KEY FACT

Ludwig angina is a bilateral cellulitis of the submental, submaxillary, and sublingual spaces that usually results from an infected tooth. It presents with dysphagia, drooling, fever, and a red, warm mouth, and can lead to death from asphyxiation.

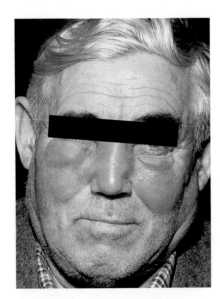

FIGURE 2.2-21. Erysipelas of the face. (Reproduced from Goldsmith LA et al. *Fitzpatrick's Dermatology in General Medicine,* 8th ed. New York, NY: McGraw-Hill; 2012.)

■ **Severe disease (MRSA likely):** Oral trimethoprim-sulfamethoxazole, clindamycin, or doxycycline.

Cellulitis

A deeper skin infection involving dermis and subcutaneous tissue. Commonly caused by staphylococci or group A streptococci originating from damaged skin or a systemic source. Community-acquired MRSA is an increasingly common cause of purulent cellulitis. Risk factors include diabetes mellitus (DM), IV drug use, venous stasis, and immune compromise.

HISTORY/PE

■ Presents with red, hot, swollen, tender skin. Fever and chills are common.
■ Erysipelas is a type of cellulitis usually caused by streptococcus that is confined to the dermis and lymphatic tissue, creating a characteristically raised, indurated, well-demarcated, erythematous area of skin (see Figure 2.2-21).

DIAGNOSIS

■ Characteristic exam findings and history are sufficient. Wound and/or blood cultures may aid in diagnosis and help determine antibiotic sensitivities.
■ Rule out abscess, osteomyelitis, and necrotizing fasciitis.

TREATMENT

■ Topical antibiotics are ineffective due to depth of infection.
■ Use 5–10 days of oral antibiotics. IV antibiotics are used if there is evidence of systemic toxicity, comorbid conditions, DM, extremes of age, or hand or orbital involvement. Antibiotic choices like those used to treat impetigo.

Necrotizing Fasciitis

Deep infection along a fascial plane causing severe pain followed by anesthesia and necrosis. It is usually caused by a mixed infection of anaerobic and aerobic bacteria that includes *S aureus, Escherichia coli,* and *Clostridium perfringens.* Ten percent of cases are caused by *S pyogenes.* A history of trauma or recent surgery to the affected area is sometimes elicited.

HISTORY/PE

■ Acute onset of pain and swelling progressing to anesthesia at the site of trauma or surgery.
■ An area of erythema quickly spreads over the course of hours to days. Margins move out into normal skin, and skin becomes dusky or purplish near the site of insult, ultimately leading to necrosis (see Figure 2.2-22).
■ If a necrotic area is open, gloved fingers can easily pass between two layers to reveal yellow-green necrotic fascia (infection spreads quickly in deep fascia).
■ Important signs of tissue necrosis are gas production (crepitus on physical exam), a putrid discharge, bullae, severe pain, lack of inflammatory signs, and intravascular volume loss.

DIAGNOSIS

Strong suspicion of necrotizing fasciitis based on clinical exam and imaging (showing gas in soft tissue) requires immediate surgical exploration and debridement; tissue culture helps determine the organisms involved.

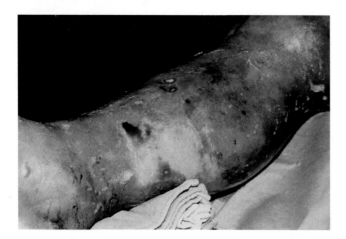

FIGURE 2.2-22. **Necrotizing fasciitis of the lower extremity.** Patient presented with hypotension due to late necrotizing fasciitis and myositis due to β-hemolytic streptococcal infection. (Reproduced with permission from Brunicardi FC et al. *Schwartz's Principles of Surgery*, 9th ed. New York, NY: McGraw-Hill; 2010.)

TREATMENT

- **Surgical emergency:** Early and aggressive surgical debridement is critical.
- In most cases, broad-spectrum coverage is necessary. If *Streptococcus* is the principal organism involved, penicillin G is the drug of choice. Clindamycin is added to ↓ exotoxin production. For anaerobic coverage, give metronidazole or a third-generation cephalosporin.

Folliculitis

Inflammation and/or infection of a hair follicle. Typically caused by infection with *Staphylococcus*, *Streptococcus*, and gram ⊖ bacteria. Occasionally can be caused by yeast such as *Candida albicans* or *Malassezia furfur*. Can occur on any body area with follicles.

HISTORY/PE

- Presents as a tiny pustule at the opening of a hair follicle with a hair penetrating it. When the infection is deeper, a furuncle, or hair follicle abscess, develops. Furuncles may disseminate to adjacent follicles to form a carbuncle (see Figure 2.2-23).
- Patients with DM or immunosuppression are at ↑ risk. Eosinophilic folliculitis can occur in AIDS patients, in whom the disease is intensely pruritic and resistant to therapy.

DIAGNOSIS

Characteristic exam findings and history are sufficient. KOH prep or biopsy may be needed if fungus or eosinophilic folliculitis is suspected.

TREATMENT

Topical antibiotics (mupirocin) treat mild superficial disease. More severe disease is treated similarly to impetigo, with cephalexin or dicloxacillin orally, escalating to clindamycin or doxycycline if MRSA is suspected.

Acne Vulgaris

A skin disease common among adolescents. The pathogenesis involves hormonal activation of sebaceous glands, the development of the comedo

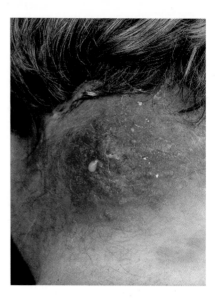

FIGURE 2.2-23. **Carbuncle due to methicillin-sensitive *S aureus*.** A very large, inflammatory plaque studded with pustules, draining pus, on the nape of the neck. Infection extends down to the fascia and has formed from a confluence of many furuncles. (Reproduced with permission from Wolff K et al. *Fitzpatrick's Color Atlas & Synopsis of Clinical Dermatology*, 7th ed. New York, NY, McGraw-Hill; 2013.)

 KEY FACT

Fournier gangrene is a form of necrotizing fasciitis that is localized to the genital and perineal area.

 KEY FACT

Pseudomonas aeruginosa infection leads to "hot tub folliculitis."

Q

A 7-year-old girl presents with fever, sore throat, and a facial rash. Physical exam reveals an erythematous pharynx without exudates and a red, painful patch on the child's cheek that the mother notes has been expanding. What is the appropriate therapy?

(plugged pilosebaceous unit), and involvement of *Propionibacterium acnes* in the follicle, causing inflammation. Acne lesions can be caused by medications (lithium, corticosteroids) or by topical occlusion (cosmetics).

History/PE

- There are three stages of acne lesions as follows:
    - **Comedonal:** Open ("blackheads") or closed ("whiteheads") comedones.
    - **Inflammatory:** The comedones rupture, creating inflammatory papules, pustules, nodules, and cysts.
    - **Scar:** May develop as inflammation heals. Picking at lesions exacerbates scarring.
- Acne develops at puberty and typically persists for several years. Male adolescents are more likely to have severe cystic acne than are their female contemporaries.
- Women in their 20s can have a variant that flares cyclically with menstruation, with fewer comedones but more painful lesions on the chin.
- Drug-induced acne is a common side effect of glucocorticoid use. These lesions are monomorphic papules without comedones, nodules, or cysts, and do not respond to standard acne therapy. However, they usually resolve with discontinuation of the steroids.

Diagnosis

Characteristic exam findings and history are sufficient.

Treatment

- **Mild–moderate acne:** Topical retinoids are the most effective topical agent for comedonal acne. Topical benzoyl peroxide kills *Propionibacterium acnes.* Consider adding a topical antibiotic (clindamycin, erythromycin) if response to other topicals is inadequate.
- **Moderate–severe acne:** In addition to topical treatment as above, add oral antibiotics such as doxycycline or minocycline. When acne is severe and all treatments are failing, oral retinoids (isotretinoin) are the most effective treatment. All other medications are stopped.
    - Isotretinoin is a teratogen and elevates LFTs. Patients require periodic blood tests to check liver function, cholesterol, and triglycerides. Given the teratogenicity of isotretinoin, female patients must be monitored with baseline and serial pregnancy tests.

Pilonidal Cysts

Abscesses in the sacrococcygeal region. Thought to be a foreign body reaction to entrapped hairs. Most common in 20- to 40-year-old men.

History/PE

Presents as an abscess at the superior gluteal cleft that can be tender, fluctuant, and warm—sometimes associated with purulent drainage or cellulitis. Systemic symptoms are uncommon, but cysts can develop into perianal fistulas.

Diagnosis

Characteristic exam findings and history are sufficient.

Treatment

- Treat with incision and drainage of the abscess followed by sterile packing of the wound.
- Good local hygiene and shaving of the sacrococcygeal skin can help prevent recurrence.

KEY FACT

Ironically, erythromycin does not cause erythema with sun exposure. It is tetracycline and doxycycline that can cause photosensitivity!

KEY FACT

General progression of acne treatment based on severity: topical benzoyl peroxide, retinoid, or antibiotic → oral antibiotic → oral isotretinoin.

KEY FACT

Antibiotics are not needed for pilonidal cysts unless cellulitis is present; if antibiotics are prescribed, both aerobic and anaerobic coverage is required.

This child has erysipelas, a rash commonly caused by group A streptococci. It can present as a small red patch on the cheek or extremities that turns into a painful, shiny red plaque. Patients often have a history of chronic cutaneous ulcers, lymphedema, or pharyngitis. Treat with penicillin.

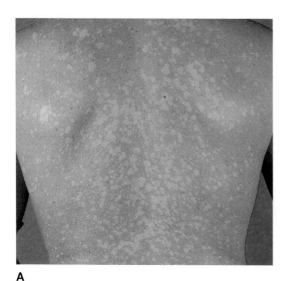

A

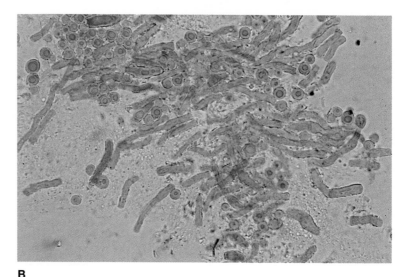

B

FIGURE 2.2-24. **Tinea versicolor.** (**A**) Note the discrete, hypopigmented patches extensively involving the patient's back. Tinea versicolor may also present as hyperpigmented macules or patches in some individuals. (**B**) KOH preparation shows the characteristic "spaghetti and meatballs" pattern. (Image A reproduced with permission from Tintinalli JE et al. *Tintinalli's Emergency Medicine: A Comprehensive Study Guide*, 7th ed. New York, NY: McGraw-Hill; 2011. Image B reproduced with permission from Wolff K et al. *Fitzpatrick's Dermatology in General Medicine*, 7th ed. New York, NY: McGraw-Hill; 2008.)

Leprosy

Disease of skin and peripheral nerves, found in southwest United States and developing countries. Caused by acid-fast bacterium *Mycobacterium leprae* and causes chronic granuloma formation. Patients present with loss of peripheral sensation and muscle atrophy. Treat with dapsone and rifampin.

FUNGAL INFECTIONS

Tinea Versicolor

Caused by *Malassezia* species, a yeast that is part of normal skin flora. Humid and sweaty conditions as well as oily skin can make the organism pathogenic. Cushing syndrome and immunosuppression are also risk factors.

HISTORY/PE

- Presents with small scaly patches of varying color on the chest or back (see Figure 2.2-24A).
- Patches can be hypopigmented as a result of interference with melanin production, or hyperpigmented/pink due to inflammation.

DIAGNOSIS

- Characteristic exam findings and history are sufficient.
- **Best initial test:** KOH preparation of the scale revealing "spaghetti and meatballs" pattern of hyphae and spores (see Figure 2.2-24B).

TREATMENT

Treat lesions with topical ketoconazole or selenium sulfide.

Candidiasis

Yeast infection or thrush, candidiasis can be caused by any *Candida* species but is most commonly caused by *C albicans*. In immunocompetent patients, it typically presents as eroded erythematous papules and plaques in moist areas such as the groin, skin folds, axillae, vagina, and below the breasts. Oral thrush is common in infancy, but in adults it is often a sign of a weakened immune system.

Q

A 42-year-old man is admitted for cellulitis after injuring his leg while swimming. He is febrile and has a well-demarcated area of erythema on the anterior aspect of his right knee. Antibiotics are started. Six hours later, the patient is in excruciating pain. The erythema has spread circumferentially around the knee, and the anterior aspect of the knee now has a purplish hue. What is the next best step?

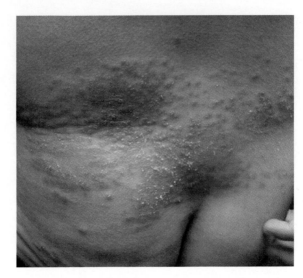

FIGURE 2.2-25. **Cutaneous candidiasis with satellite lesions.** (Reproduced with permission from Goldsmith LA et al. *Fitzpatrick's Dermatology in General Medicine,* 8th ed. New York, NY: McGraw-Hill; 2012.)

History/PE

- Patients often have history of antibiotic or steroid use, DM, or immunocompromise.
- **Oral candidiasis:** Presents with painless white plaques that can be easily scraped off to reveal erosions.
- **Candidiasis of the skin:** Presents as markedly erythematous papules and plaques with occasional erosions and smaller satellite lesions (see Figure 2.2-25) seen nearby, often in skin folds. In infants, infection is often seen in the diaper area and along the inguinal folds.

Diagnosis

- Characteristic exam findings and history are sufficient.
- **Best initial test:** KOH preparation of a scraping of the affected area. KOH dissolves the skin cells but leaves the *Candida* untouched such that candidal spores and pseudohyphae become visible.
- **Most accurate test:** Fungal culture.

Treatment

- **Oral candidiasis:** Oral fluconazole tablets; nystatin swish and swallow, clotrimazole troches.
- **Superficial (skin) candidiasis:** Topical antifungals; keep skin clean and dry.
- **Diaper rash:** Topical nystatin.

Dermatophyte Infections

Dermatophytes only live in tissues with keratin (skin, nails, and hair) and are commonly seen. Causative organisms include *Trichophyton* (most common), *Microsporum*, and *Epidermophyton* species. Risk factors include DM, ↓ peripheral circulation, immune compromise, and chronic maceration of skin (from athletic activities).

History/PE

Varies according to subtype:

- **Tinea corporis:** Scaly, pruritic eruption with a sharp, irregular border, often with central clearing (see Figure 2.2-26). Can be seen in

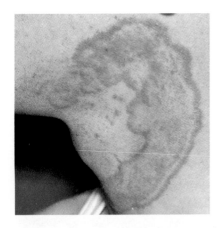

FIGURE 2.2-26. **Tinea corporis.** Note the ringworm-like rash with a scaly, erythematous, distinct border and central clearing. (Reproduced with permission from Wolff K et al. *Fitzpatrick's Dermatology in General Medicine,* 7th ed. New York, NY: McGraw-Hill; 2008.)

Emergent surgical consult for debridement given the clinical suspicion for necrotizing fasciitis, a surgical emergency.

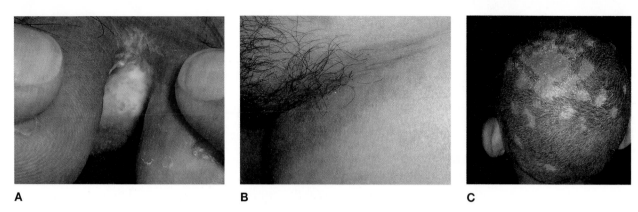

A   **B**   **C**

FIGURE 2.2-27. **Cutaneous mycoses.** (A) Tinea pedis; (B) tinea cruris; (C) tinea capitis. (Reproduced with permission from Dr. Richard Usatine.)

immunocompromised patients or in children following contact with infected pets.

- **Tinea pedis/manuum** (see Figure 2.2-27A): Presents as chronic interdigital scaling with erosions between the toes (athlete's foot) or as a thickened, scaly skin on the soles (moccasin distribution). In addition, involvement of one hand is typical in the "one hand two feet syndrome."
- **Tinea cruris (jock itch)** (see Figure 2.2-27B): A fungal infection of the groin (typically sparing the scrotum) that is usually associated with tinea pedis.
- **Tinea capitis** (see Figure 2.2-27C): A fungal scalp infection causing scaling and hair loss with scarring. A large inflammatory boggy mass caused by tinea capitis is called a kerion.

DIAGNOSIS

- Clinical.
- **Best initial test:** KOH skin scraping showing hyphae.
- **Most accurate test:** Fungal culture.

TREATMENT

Start with topical antifungals; escalate to oral griseofulvin or terbinafine if infection is widespread or unresponsive to topicals. Treat tinea capitis with oral medications to penetrate into hair follicles; consider oral treatment for immunocompromised patients.

Sporotrichosis

Infection caused by *Sporothrix schenckii*, a fungus found in plant matter. Often called "rose-gardener disease." Acquired by direct contact, which causes a papule that drains odorless fluid. Additional lesions form over time along lines of lymphatic drainage, although lymphadenopathy is absent. Treat with itraconazole.

PARASITIC INFECTIONS

Lice

Lice live off blood and on specific parts of the body, depending on their species (head lice, body lice, pubic lice). Lice are spread through body contact or by the sharing of bedclothes and other garments or hair accessories. They secrete local toxins that lead to pruritus.

HISTORY/PE

- Patients with lice often experience severe pruritus, and 2° bacterial infection of the excoriations is a risk. Classroom breakouts of head lice are common.
- Body lice are seen in persons with inadequate hygiene or in those with crowded living conditions. Pubic lice (called "crabs" because of their squat, crablike body shape) contain anticoagulant in their saliva, so their bites often become ecchymotic.

DIAGNOSIS

Lice and their eggs (nits) can be seen on hairs or in clothes with the naked eye. Microscopy can reveal the arthropods, their eggs, and their droppings.

TREATMENT

- **Head lice:** Treat with topical permethrin, pyrethrin, benzyl alcohol, and mechanical removal.
- **Body lice:** Wash body, clothes, and bedding thoroughly. Rarely, topical permethrin is needed.
- **Pubic lice:** Treat with the same medications as for head lice.

Scabies

Caused by *Sarcoptes scabiei*. The burrowing of this arthropod into the epidermis leads to pruritus that ↑ in intensity once an allergy to the mite or its products develops. 2° Bacterial infections due to scratching are common. Scabies mites are spread through close contact.

HISTORY/PE

- Patients present with intense pruritus, especially at night and after hot showers, and erythematous papules with linear tracks, representing the burrows of the mite.
- The most commonly affected sites are the skin folds of the hands (often includes the interdigital finger webs), wrists, axillae, and genitals.

DIAGNOSIS

A history of pruritus in several family members is suggestive. The mite may be identifiable by scraping an intact tunnel and looking under the microscope for the arthropods, their eggs, and their droppings.

TREATMENT

- Patients should be treated with 5% permethrin from the neck down (head to toe for infants) for at least two treatments separated by 1 week, and their close contacts should be treated as well. Oral ivermectin is also effective.
- Pruritus can persist up to 2 weeks after treatment.
- Clothes and bedding should be thoroughly washed as for lice.

Cutaneous Marva Migrans

Erythematous, serpentine, migratory rash due to infection with hookworm larvae, commonly acquired by walking barefoot on grass or sand. Treat with ivermectin.

KEY FACT

Lice can be seen with the naked eye. Scabies are too small and can only be identified with a microscope/dermatoscope.

Ischemic Skin Disorders

DECUBITUS ULCERS

Result from ischemic necrosis following continuous pressure on an area of skin that restricts microcirculation.

HISTORY/PE

Ulcers are commonly seen in bedridden patients who lie in the same spot for too long. An underlying bony prominence or lack of fat ↑ the likelihood of ulcer formation (sacrum, heels). Patients lacking mobility or cutaneous sensation are also at ↑ risk. Incontinence of urine or stool may macerate the skin, facilitating ulceration.

DIAGNOSIS

Characteristic exam findings and history are sufficient. Occasionally, a biopsy can be performed on a nonhealing ulcer to rule out infection and/or pyoderma gangrenosum.

TREATMENT

- **Prevention is key:** Routinely reposition bedridden patients (at least once every 2 hours); special beds can distribute pressure.
- If an ulcer develops, low-grade lesions can be treated with routine wound care, including hydrocolloid dressings. High-grade lesions require surgical debridement.

GANGRENE

Necrosis of body tissue. There are three subtypes as follows:
- **Dry gangrene:** Due to insufficient blood flow to tissue, typically from atherosclerosis.
- **Wet gangrene:** Involves bacterial infection, usually with skin flora.
- **Gas gangrene:** Due to *C perfringens* infection.

HISTORY/PE

- **Dry gangrene:** Early signs are a dull ache, cold, and pallor of the flesh. As necrosis sets in, the tissue (toes, fingers) becomes bluish-black, dry, and shriveled. Diabetes, vasculopathy, and smoking are risk factors.
- **Wet gangrene:** The tissue appears bruised, swollen, or blistered with pus.
- **Gas gangrene:** Occurs at sites of large trauma/surgery compromising blood flow to a region, bringing about an anaerobic environment. Bacteria rapidly destroy tissue, producing gas that separates healthy tissue and exposes it to infection. Associated with dirty wounds contaminated with dirt or bowel/fecal matter. Subcutaneous injection of black tar heroin is a risk factor. Presents with swelling and pale or dark-red skin around the injury. A medical emergency.

DIAGNOSIS

Characteristic exam findings and history are sufficient. Air in soft tissue on x-ray is very suggestive of necrosis (see Figure 2.2-28).

Q

A 17-year-old girl is seen by a dermatologist for severe cystic acne that has been refractory to both topical and systemic antibiotics. She inquires about isotretinoin. Given this drug's potentially hazardous side effects, what laboratory tests would be performed monthly if this patient were to be placed on isotretinoin?

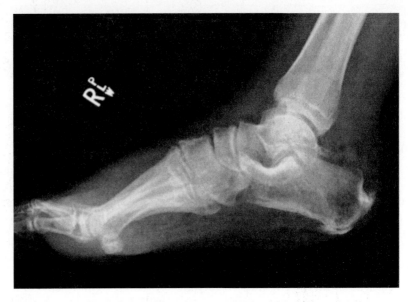

FIGURE 2.2-28. **Gas gangrene.** X-ray of the foot showing gas tracking through soft tissues, most clearly seen overlying the calcaneus. (Reproduced with permission from Tintinalli JE et al. *Tintinalli's Emergency Medicine: A Comprehensive Study Guide,* 7th ed. New York, NY: McGraw-Hill; 2011.)

TREATMENT

- Emergency surgical debridement, with amputation if necessary, is the mainstay of treatment. Antibiotics alone do not suffice by virtue of inadequate blood flow, but they should be given as an adjuvant to surgery.
- Hyperbaric oxygen (toxic to the anaerobic *C perfringens*) can be used after debridement to help with treatment.

Miscellaneous Skin Disorders

ACANTHOSIS NIGRICANS

- A condition in which the skin in the intertriginous zones (neck folds, genitals, axillae) becomes hyperkeratotic and hyperpigmented with a velvety appearance (see Figure 2.2-29).
- Associated with DM, Cushing disease, polycystic ovarian syndrome, and obesity. May also be a paraneoplastic sign of underlying adenocarcinoma (usually GI).
- **Tx:** Typically not treated. Encourage weight loss, and treat the underlying endocrinopathy.

LICHEN PLANUS

- A self-limited, recurrent, or chronic inflammatory disease affecting the skin, oral mucosa, and genitalia. Lesions classically described using the 6 **P**'s (planar, purple, polygonal, pruritic, papules, and plaques). It may be induced by drugs (thiazides, quinines, β-blockers) and is associated with HCV infection.
- **Hx/PE:** Presents with violaceous, flat-topped, polygonal papules (see Figure 2.2-30). Wickham striae (lacy white lines) may be present on the lesion. Lesions may demonstrate prominent Koebner phenomenon (lesions that appear at the site of trauma).

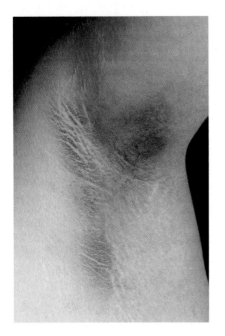

FIGURE 2.2-29. Acanthosis nigricans. Velvety, dark-brown epidermal thickening of the armpit is seen with prominent skin fold and feathered edges. (Reproduced with permission from Wolff K et al. *Fitzpatrick's Color Atlas & Synopsis of Clinical Dermatology,* 7th ed. New York, NY: McGraw-Hill; 2013.)

A

Serum or urine β-human chorionic gonadotrophin (to rule out pregnancy), liver function tests (LFTs), cholesterol, and triglycerides.

- **Tx:** Mild cases are treated with topical corticosteroids. For severe disease, systemic corticosteroids and phototherapy may be used.

ROSACEA

A chronic disorder of pilosebaceous units of which the etiology is unclear.

DIAGNOSIS

Presentation can vary depending on the subtype as follows:

- **Erythematotelangiectatic rosacea:** Presents with central facial erythema with telangiectasias.
- **Papulopustular rosacea:** Develops papules and pustules.
- **Phymatous rosacea:** May lead to severe overgrowth of nasal connective tissue known as rhinophyma (see Figure 2.2-31).
- **Ocular rosacea:** Can predispose to blepharitis, stye, and chalazion formation.

HISTORY/PE

- Patients are middle-aged with fair skin and often have an abnormal flushing response to hot drinks, spicy foods, alcohol, and sun. There is a female predominance.
- Often referred to as "adult acne" because it can present similarly to acne but involves an older age group.

TREATMENT

Topical metronidazole. For severe or ocular disease, use oral doxycycline.

PITYRIASIS ROSEA

An acute dermatitis of unknown etiology that has been hypothesized to represent a reaction to a viral infection with human herpesvirus (HHV) 7 because it tends to occur in mini-epidemics among young adults.

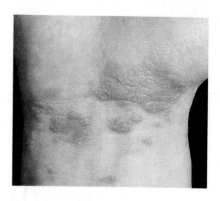

FIGURE 2.2-30. Lichen planus. Flat-topped, polygonal, sharply defined papules of violaceous color are grouped and confluent. The surface is shiny and reveals fine white lines (Wickham striae). (Reproduced with permission from Wolff K et al. *Fitzpatrick's Dermatology in General Medicine,* 7th ed. New York, NY: McGraw-Hill; 2008.)

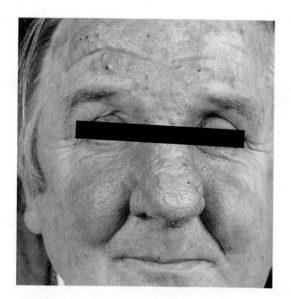

FIGURE 2.2-31. Rhinophyma. (Reproduced with permission from Wolff K et al. *Fitzpatrick's Color Atlas & Synopsis of Clinical Dermatology,* 7th ed. New York, NY: McGraw-Hill; 2008.)

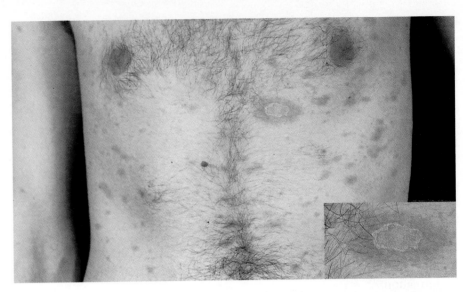

FIGURE 2.2-32. **Pityriasis rosea.** The round to oval erythematous plaques are often covered with a fine white scale ("cigarette paper") and are often found on the trunk and proximal extremities. Plaques are often preceded by a larger herald patch (inset). (Reproduced with permission from Tintinalli JE et al. *Tintinalli's Emergency Medicine: A Comprehensive Study Guide,* 7th ed. New York, NY: McGraw-Hill; 2011.)

HISTORY/PE

- Initial lesion is classically a herald patch that is erythematous with a peripheral scale.
- Days to weeks later, a 2° eruption appears: multiple scaling papules and plaques with a fine "cigarette paper" scale (see Figure 2.2-32). Papules are arranged along skin lines, giving a classic "Christmas tree" pattern on the patient's back.

DIAGNOSIS

Diagnosis is clinical. Confirm with KOH exam to rule out fungus (the herald patch may be mistaken for tinea corporis). Consider testing for secondary syphilis, which can present similarly.

TREATMENT

Rash heals in 6–8 weeks without any treatment. Supportive therapy to manage symptoms includes emolliation and antihistamines.

VITILIGO

Autoimmune destruction of melanocytes leading to well-demarcated areas of depigmentation. Frequently associated with other autoimmune diseases, such as hypothyroidism and type I DM.

- **Hx/PE:** Sharply demarcated, depigmented macules or patches on otherwise normal skin, often on the hands, face, or genitalia (see Figure 2.2-33). Vitiligo can present at any age and vary from small areas of involvement with or without progression to large areas of depigmentation.
- **Dx:** Many patients have serologic markers of autoimmune disease (eg, antithyroid antibodies, DM, pernicious anemia) and occasionally present with these diseases.
- **Tx:** Topical steroids, tacrolimus ointment, UV and laser therapy are used. Sunscreen prevents burns. Cover-up makeup can help with cosmetic concerns.

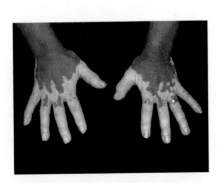

FIGURE 2.2-33. **Vitiligo of the hands.** (Reproduced with permission from Dr. Richard Usatine.)

EYELID LESIONS

- **Xanthelasma:** Soft yellow plaques seen on the medial aspects of the eyelids bilaterally, occasionally associated with hyperlipidemia and 1° biliary cirrhosis. Serum total cholesterol is often normal.
- **Hordeolum:** Painful acute eyelid gland infection (stye), usually due to *S aureus* and located on the edge of the lid.
- **Chalazion:** Chronic inflammatory painless cyst due to a blocked eyelid gland.

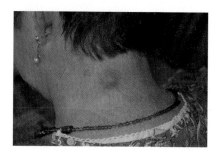

FIGURE 2.2-34.   Inflamed epidermal inclusion cyst. (Reproduced with permission from Steven Fruitsmaak.)

EPIDERMAL INCLUSION CYSTS

- Dome-shaped, firm or freely movable cyst often surrounding a hair follicle (see Figure 2.2-34). Erythema, mild tenderness, and cheeselike discharge may be seen.
- Does not dimple when pinched (in contrast with dermatofibroma).
- Usually resolves spontaneously but can recur, thus excision of large cysts is preferred.

DERMATOFIBROMA

- Dome-shaped, firm, brown-pink, nontender nodule, < 1 cm in diameter resulting from fibroblast proliferation (see Figure 2.2-35).
- Dimples when pinched (dimple or buttonhole sign).
- Benign. Treatment with shave biopsy or excision for cosmetic reasons.

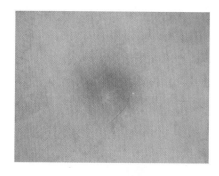

FIGURE 2.2-35.   Dermatofibroma. (Reproduced with permission from Diluvio L, Torti C, Terrinoni A, et al. Dermoscopy as an adjuvant tool for detecting skin leiomyomas in patient with uterine fibroids and cerebral cavernomas. *BMC Dermatol.* 2014;14:7.doi:10.1186/1471-5945-14-7.)

HIDRADENITIS SUPPURATIVA

- Chronic inflammation of folliculopilosebaceous units causing inflamed, painful nodules that may progress to form sinus tracts and scars that secrete a malodorous discharge (see Figure 2.2-36). It is more common in African-Americans, smokers, diabetics, and the obese.
- Common in intertriginous areas (axilla, groin), and often has a chronic relapsing course.
- **Dx:** Clinical. No biopsy needed.
- **Tx:** Oral antibiotics, drainage, and marsupialization of sinus tracts and wound care.

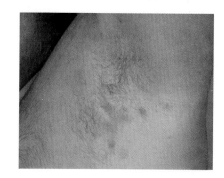

FIGURE 2.2-36.   Hidradenitis suppurativa. (Reproduced with permission from Alharbi Z, Kauczok J, Pallua N. A review of wide surgical excision of hidradenitis suppurativa. *BMC Dermatol.* 2012;12:9.)

ICHTHYOSIS VULGARIS

- Disorder of diffuse, dry dermal scaling that resembles fish scales (ichthyosis means "fishlike" in Greek). See Figure 2.2-37.
- Inherited mutation in filaggrin gene; worse in homozygous individuals.
- Diagnosis is clinical.
- Treat with emollients, keratolytics, and topical retinoids.

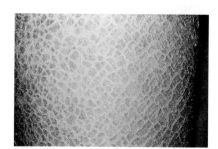

FIGURE 2.2-37.   Ichthyosis vulgaris. (Reproduced with permission from Dr. Richard S. Hibbets, Centers for Disease Control and Prevention, Atlanta, GA.)

AGE-RELATED SKIN CHANGES

The elastic fibers in perivascular connective tissue deteriorate with age, causing wrinkles. Chronically photoaged skin will develop solar elastosis (thickened yellow skin with deep wrinkles). Botulinum toxin may be used for cosmetic purposes to reduce development of wrinkles. Senile purpura (ecchymoses in elderly patients in areas exposed to repetitive trauma such as extensor surfaces) is a benign finding and does not warrant further workup.

Ultraviolet radiation from the sun causes hyperpigmentation and destruction of dermal structural proteins, such as collagen and elastin. Sun avoidance is the best way to prevent sun-associated skin damage. When going outside, apply sunblock of at least sun protection factor (SPF) 30, 30 minutes prior to exposure in order for a protective film to develop that prevents sunburn. SPF of greater than 50 has diminishing returns on effective sun protection.

SUNBURN

Erythematous, occasionally blistering lesions caused by prolonged exposure to ultraviolet radiation. Fever, headache, vomiting, and symptoms of heat exhaustion may also be seen. Treat with cool, moist compresses and NSAIDs for mild cases. Consider hospitalization, intravenous fluids, and wound care for severe cases.

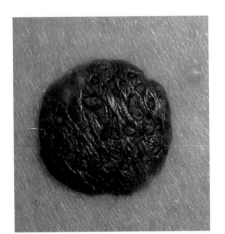

FIGURE 2.2-38. Seborrheic keratosis. (Reproduced with permission from Dr. Richard Usatine.)

Neoplasms of the Skin

SEBORRHEIC KERATOSIS

A very common skin tumor that appears in almost all persons after 40 years of age. The etiology is unknown. Lesions have no malignant potential (see Figure 2.2-38).

History/PE

- Present as exophytic, waxy brown papules and plaques with superficial keratin cysts (see Figure 2.2-38). Lesions may appear in great numbers and have a "stuck on" appearance.
- Lesions can become irritated either spontaneously or by external trauma.

Diagnosis

Characteristic exam findings and history are sufficient. As some may appear similar to melanoma, a biopsy may be prudent in these cases.

Treatment

Cryotherapy, shave excision, or curettage.

ACTINIC KERATOSIS

Flat areas of erythema and scale caused by exposure to the sun. These lesions should be treated to prevent the possible transformation into squamous cell carcinoma.

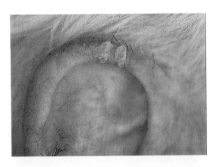

FIGURE 2.2-39. Actinic keratosis. The discrete patch above has an erythematous base and a rough white scale. (Reproduced with permission from Hurwitz RM. *Pathology of the Skin: Atlas of Clinical-Pathological Correlation*, 2nd ed. Stamford, CT: Appleton & Lange; 1998.)

- **Hx/PE:** Lesions appear on sun-exposed areas (face, arms) and primarily affect older patients, who often have multiple such lesions. They are erythematous with a gritty texture that can become thick and crusted (see Figure 2.2-39).
- **Dx:** Clinical.
- **Tx:** Cryosurgery, topical 5-FU, or topical imiquimod can be used to destroy the lesion. If carcinoma is suspected, perform a biopsy. Patients should be advised to use sun protection.

CUTANEOUS SQUAMOUS CELL CARCINOMA

The second most common skin cancer, with locally destructive effects as well as the potential for metastasis and death. Sun exposure is the most common causative factor, but exposure to chemical carcinogens, prior radiation therapy, sites of burns or chronic trauma (as in draining infectious sinuses in osteomyelitis), and chronic immunosuppression (as in transplant recipients) also predispose patients to developing SCC.

History/PE

- SCCs have many forms, and a single patient will often have multiple variants.
- Most SCCs occur in older adults with sun-damaged skin, arising from actinic keratoses, presenting as an erythematous, ulcerated papule or nodule (see Figure 2.2-40).
- Marjolin ulcer is a type of rare SCC that arises in sites of scars, burns, or ulcers.
- Arsenic exposure is a rare cause of multiple SCCs in a palmoplantar distribution.
- SCCs from actinic keratoses rarely metastasize, but those that arise on lips and ulcers are more likely to do so. SCC occurs on the lower lip more commonly than basal cell carcinoma.

Diagnosis

Characteristic exam findings and history are sufficient. Confirm with shave biopsy, which may show keratin pearls and full-thickness atypical keratinocytes with invasion into the dermis.

Treatment

Surgical excision or Mohs surgery (very thin slices are excised and examined with a microscope via frozen section, ideally used for cosmetically sensitive areas such as face and distal extremities). Lesions with high metastatic potential may need radiation or chemotherapy.

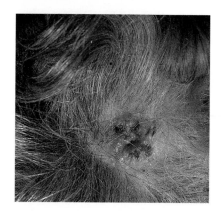

FIGURE 2.2-40. Squamous cell carcinoma. Note the crusting and ulceration of this erythematous plaque. Most lesions are exophytic nodules with erosion or ulceration. (Reproduced with permission from Hurwitz RM. *Pathology of the Skin: Atlas of Clinical-Pathological Correlation*, 2nd ed. Stamford, CT: Appleton & Lange; 1998.)

BASAL CELL CARCINOMA

The most common malignant skin cancer, basal cell carcinoma (BCC) is slow growing and locally destructive but has virtually no metastatic potential. Cumulative sun exposure is the main risk factor. Most lesions appear on the face or other sun-exposed areas. Multiple BCCs appearing early in life and on non–sun-exposed areas are suggestive of inherited basal cell nevus syndrome.

History/PE

There are many types of BCC with varying degrees of pigmentation, ulceration, and depth of growth (see Figure 2.2-41). Nodular, superficial, and sclerosing are the three main types.

Diagnosis

Confirm with shave biopsy, which will show nests of basophilic cells invading into the dermis.

Treatment

Excision via curettage, cautery, cryotherapy, superficial radiation, and Mohs surgery.

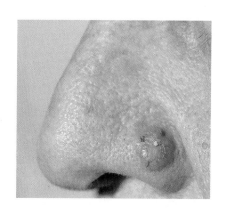

FIGURE 2.2-41. Nodular basal cell carcinoma. A smooth, pearly nodule with telangiectasias. (Reproduced with permission from Wolff K et al. *Fitzpatrick's Color Atlas & Synopsis of Clinical Dermatology*, 5th ed. New York, NY: McGraw-Hill; 2005.)

MNEMONIC

The ABCDEs of melanoma—

Asymmetric
Irregular **B**order
Variations in **C**olor
Diameter > 6 mm
Evolution: changing or new lesions

KEY FACT

Bacillary angiomatosis, caused by *Bartonella henselae* and *Bartonella quintana*, can mimic Kaposi sarcoma (KS) and should be excluded in suspected KS patients; erythromycin is the treatment of choice.

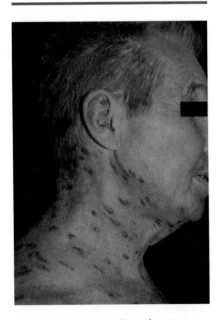

FIGURE 2.2-42. Kaposi sarcoma. Note the multiple violaceous papules on the neck, back, and face. (Reproduced with permission from Wolff K et al. *Fitzpatrick's Color Atlas & Synopsis of Clinical Dermatology*, 5th ed. New York, NY: McGraw-Hill; 2005.)

MELANOMA

The most common life-threatening dermatologic disease. Risk factors include fair skin and a tendency to burn; intense bursts of sun exposure (especially in childhood and with intermittent exposure); and the presence of large congenital melanocytic nevi, an ↑ number of nevi, or dysplastic nevi. Immunosuppression also ↑ risk. Some patients inherit a predisposition to melanoma with the familial atypical mole and melanoma (FAM-M) syndrome. There are several subtypes (see Table 2.2-4).

HISTORY/PE

- Malignant melanomas begin in the epidermal basal layer, where melanocytes are found.
- Malignant melanomas may metastasize anywhere in the body (eg, lung, liver, brain, fat). Three percent to 5% of patients with metastatic melanoma have no known 1° lesion.

DIAGNOSIS

- Early recognition and treatment are essential. Screening exams using the ABCDE criteria, and dermoscopy may detect melanoma early when it is curable (see Table 2.2-4). An excisional biopsy should be performed on any suspicious lesion. Malignancy is determined histologically.
- A biopsy should be performed on a mole that is substantially different from nearby moles to assess for melanoma. This is the "ugly duckling sign" and has greater than 90% sensitivity for melanoma.
- Malignant melanomas are staged by Breslow thickness (depth of invasion in millimeters) and by tumor-node-metastasis (TNM) staging. Ulceration is a poor prognostic sign.

TREATMENT

- Lesions confined to the skin are treated by excision with margins. Sentinel lymph node biopsy is useful for staging but does not ↑ survival. Chemotherapy, biologic therapy, and radiation therapy may be used for recurrent or metastatic melanoma.
- Patients with early melanoma are at low risk for recurrence but are at high risk for the development of subsequent melanomas. More advanced melanomas may recur or metastasize at a higher rate. Patient surveillance is thus essential.

KAPOSI SARCOMA

A vascular proliferative disease that has been attributed to a herpesvirus (HHV-8), also called Kaposi sarcoma–associated herpesvirus (KSHV).

HISTORY/PE

- Presents with multiple red to violaceous macules, papules, or nodules that can progress to plaques on the lower limbs, back, face, mouth, and genitalia (see Figure 2.2-42).
- Plaques can also be found in the GI tract and lung.
- HIV-associated (epidemic) KS is an aggressive form of the disease, and although less common since the advent of HAART, it remains the most common HIV-associated malignancy.

DIAGNOSIS

Diagnosed by history, clinical impression, and histology.

TABLE 2.2-4. Types of Melanoma

Type	Presentation
Superficial spreading	60% of all melanomas; can occur at any age but is seen in young adults
	Often presents on the trunk in men and on the legs in women
	A prolonged horizontal growth (see Image A) allows for early diagnosis when it is still confined to the epidermis
Nodular	Lesions have a rapid vertical growth phase and appear as a fast-growing reddish-brown nodule with ulceration (see Image B)
Acral lentiginous	Begins on the palms, soles (see Image C), and nailbed as a slowly spreading, pigmented patch
	Most commonly seen in Asians and African-Americans
Lentigo maligna	Arises in a solar lentigo
	Usually found on sun-damaged skin of the face (see Image D)
Amelanotic	Presents as a lesion without clinical pigmentation
	Difficult to identify; this variant of melanoma can be further classified into any of the above types

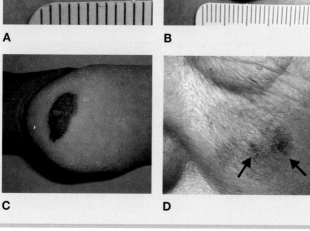

Images reproduced with permission from Dr. Richard Usatine.

TREATMENT

Start HAART therapy if patient is HIV⊕. Small local lesions can be treated with radiation or cryotherapy. Widespread or internal disease is treated with systemic chemotherapy (doxorubicin, paclitaxel, or interferon-α [IFN-α]).

Q

A 72-year-old man presents to a new internist after moving to Florida. The internist notes a chronic wound on the patient's right lower leg. The patient states that the wound followed an episode of cellulitis and has been present for 3 years. What is the next best step?

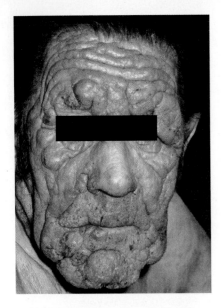

FIGURE 2.2-43. Mycosis fungoides. Massive nodular infiltration of the face leads to a leonine facies. (Reproduced with permission from Wolff K et al. *Fitzpatrick's Dermatology in General Medicine*, 7th ed. New York, NY: McGraw-Hill; 2008.)

MYCOSIS FUNGOIDES (CUTANEOUS T-CELL LYMPHOMA)

Not a fungus but a slow, progressive neoplastic proliferation of epidermotropic T cells. The disease is chronic and more common in men.

HISTORY/PE

- Early lesions are nonspecific, psoriatic-appearing plaques or patches that are often pruritic with a predilection for the trunk and buttocks. Later lesions are characterized by skin tumors with palpable lymph nodes (see Figure 2.2-43).
- Patients may have dermatopathic lymphadenopathy without tumor involvement of the node. However, the internal organs can be involved, including the lymph nodes, liver, and spleen.
- Sézary syndrome is the leukemic phase of cutaneous T-cell lymphoma, characterized by circulating Sézary cells in the peripheral blood, erythroderma, and lymphadenopathy.

DIAGNOSIS

- Diagnosed by clinical features and histology, with immunophenotypic characterization showing clonal T cells and electron microscopy showing the typical Sézary or Lutzner cells (cerebriform lymphocytes).
- Early lesions are clinically indistinguishable from dermatitis, so histologic diagnosis is indicated for any dermatitis that is chronic and resistant to treatment.

TREATMENT

Phototherapy and skin-directed topical treatments are the mainstay of treatment for many patients. Early localized disease is amenable to total skin electron beam irradiation. For more extensive or advanced disease, radiation therapy is an effective option. Treatment modalities, including steroids, chemotherapy, retinoids, monoclonal antibodies, and IFN-α, are often combined.

CHERRY ANGIOMAS (HEMANGIOMAS)

Small, vascular, red papules that can appear anywhere on the body (see Figure 2.2-44). It is the most common benign vascular tumor, and it often appears with age. No treatment necessary, but can be excised for cosmetic reasons.

Similar lesions known as infantile hemangiomas are seen in infants during the first few weeks of life. They are also benign and usually regress spontaneously after an initially rapid growth phase. Involution typically begins at 9 months to 1 year of age. Persistent lesions may be treated with topical or oral β-blockers.

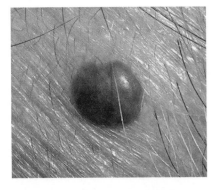

FIGURE 2.2-44. Cherry hemangioma. (Reproduced with permission from Dr. Richard Usatine.)

A

Perform a biopsy to rule out squamous cell carcinoma.

ENDOCRINOLOGY

Disorders of Glucose Metabolism

TYPE 1 DIABETES MELLITUS

Type 1 diabetes mellitus (DM) is caused by autoimmune pancreatic β-cell destruction, leading to insulin deficiency and abnormal glucose metabolism.

TABLE 2.3-1.   **Treatment of Type 2 Diabetes Mellitus**

LIFESTYLE MODIFICATIONS

Diet	Personalized diet to encourage weight loss; avoid saturated fats and added sugars
Exercise	Moderate-intensity exercise for 30-60 minutes 5 days per week

PHARMACOTHERAPY (MONOTHERAPY OR COMBINATION THERAPY IF POOR GLYCEMIC CONTROL)

DRUG	MECHANISM	SIDE EFFECTS	CONTRAINDICATIONS
Metformin (first-line)	Inhibits hepatic gluconeogenesis and ↑ peripheral sensitivity to insulin	Weight loss, GI upset, and rarely, lactic acidosis	Contraindicated in the elderly (age > 80 years) and in renal insufficiency, hepatic failure, or heart failure
Sulfonylureas (glipizide, glyburide, glimepiride)	↑ Endogenous insulin secretion	Hypoglycemia and weight gain	
Thiazolidinediones (rosiglitazone, pioglitazone)[a]	↑ Insulin sensitivity	Weight gain, edema, hepatotoxicity, and bone loss	Contraindicated in patients with heart failure
DPP-4 inhibitors (sitagliptin, linagliptin, and other -liptins)	Inhibit degradation of GLP-1; ↑ insulin secretion and ↓ glucagon secretion	Weight neutral	
Incretins (exenatide, liraglutide, and other -tides)	GLP-1 agonists. Delay absorption of food; ↑ insulin secretion and ↓ glucagon secretion	Injected subcutaneously. Slow GI motility, nausea, and, rarely, pancreatitis. Can cause weight loss	
SGLT2 inhibitors (dapagliflozin and other -flozins)	Inhibit SGLT2 in proximal tubule to ↓ glucose reabsorption	UTIs, vulvovaginal candidiasis. Can cause weight loss and ↓ blood pressure	
α-glucosidase inhibitors (acarbose, miglitol)	↓ Intestinal absorption of carbohydrates	Flatulence, diarrhea, and hypoglycemia	
Insulin	Given alone or in conjunction with oral agents. Types of insulin include regular, short-acting (lispro, aspart, glulisine), NPH, long-acting (detemir, glargine), and combination preparations (longer + shorter-acting agents like 70 NPH/30 regular)	Weight gain and hypoglycemia	

[a]In September 2010, the US Food and Drug Administration restricted access to rosiglitazone because of concern for increased cardiovascular risks. The drug is still available but is restricted to patients currently on the medication who acknowledge that they understand the risks and to patients who cannot achieve adequate glycemic control with other medication.

HISTORY/PE

- Classically presents with polyuria, polydipsia, polyphagia, and rapid, unexplained weight loss. Patients may also present with ketoacidosis.
- Usually affects nonobese children or young adults.
- Associated with HLA-DR3 and -DR4.
- Type 1 DM diagnosed as an adult is known as latent autoimmune diabetes of adults (LADA).

DIAGNOSIS

- At disease onset, anti–islet cell, anti–glutamic acid decarboxylase (anti-GAD) antibodies, anti–insulin or anti–Zn transporter antibodies may be present in serum.
- At least one of the following is required to make the diagnosis:
  - A random plasma glucose level ≥ 200 mg/dL plus symptoms.
  - A fasting (> 8-hour) plasma glucose level ≥ 126 mg/dL on two separate occasions.
  - A 2-hour postprandial glucose level ≥ 200 mg/dL following an oral glucose tolerance test. Hemoglobin A_{1c} (HbA_{1c}) > 6.5%.

TREATMENT

- Insulin injections (see Table 2.3-1 and Figure 2.3-1) to maintain blood glucose in the normal range (80–130 mg/dL preprandial levels, < 180 mg/dL postprandial levels).
- Consider the use of an insulin pump, which provides a continuous, short-acting insulin infusion.
- Encourage routine HbA_{1c} testing every 3 months. Goal HbA_{1c} < 7% (< 7.5% in children). Higher blood glucose and HbA_{1c} levels can be tolerated, particularly in the very young and the very old, or those with multiple medical problems considering the ↑ risk for hypoglycemia.
- Table 2.3-2 outlines general health maintenance guidelines.

KEY FACT

Microalbuminuria cannot be detected on routine UA protein dipstick. Instead, do a spot urine albumin:creatinine ratio (microalbuminuria = 30–300 mg/g).

KEY FACT

Diabetic ketoacidosis (DKA) and hyperosmolar hyperglycemic state (HHS) often present with paradoxic hyperkalemia. Serum potassium may be elevated, but total body potassium stores are depleted (acidosis causes extracellular shift of potassium).

KEY FACT

Use normal saline for initial fluid resuscitation in DKA and HHS. Add 5% dextrose to fluids once glucose is < 250 mg/dL.

TABLE 2.3-2. Diabetes Mellitus General Health Maintenance

Cardiovascular risk modification	The presence of diabetes is equivalent to the highest risk for cardiovascular disease regardless of all other risk factors All diabetic patients 40–75 years of age should be placed on a statin regardless of lipid levels. Use the AHA risk calculator to determine whether moderate or high-intensity statin is recommended.[a]
BP management	Strict BP control to < 140/80 mm Hg; ACEIs/ARBs are first-line agents
Screening exams	Annual physical exam to screen for cardiovascular disease (BP and lipid monitoring), nephropathy (test for microalbuminuria), retinopathy (dilated-eye exams), and neuropathy (foot care evaluations)
Other	All diabetic patients > 19 years of age should receive the pneumonia vaccine Tight glucose control decreases the risk for microvascular complications (nephropathy, retinopathy), but the effect on macrovascular complications (stroke, myocardial infarction) and all-cause mortality is unknown

[a]https://professional.heart.org/professional/GuidelinesStatements/PreventionGuidelines/UCM_457698_Prevention-Guidelines.jsp

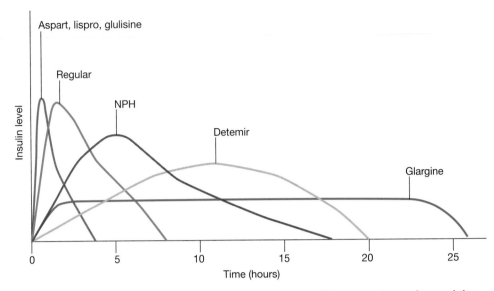

FIGURE 2.3-1. **Pharmacokinetics of insulin preparations.** Short acting (aspart, lispro, glulisine): onset in 5–20 minutes, peak in 0.5–3 hours, duration 3–8 hours. Regular: onset in 30 minutes, peak in 2–4 hours, duration 5–8 hours. NPH: onset in 2–4 hours, peak in 6–10 hours, duration 18–28 hours. Long acting (detemir, glargine): onset in 2 hours, peak none, duration 20–24 hours.

COMPLICATIONS

Tables 2.3-3 and 2.3-4 outline the acute and chronic complications of DM.

TYPE 2 DIABETES MELLITUS

A dysfunction in glucose metabolism caused by varying degrees of insulin resistance in peripheral tissues combined with insufficient insulin secretion.

TABLE 2.3-3. **Acute Complications of Diabetes Mellitus: Comparing DKA with HHS**

	DKA	HHS
Patient characteristics	Type 1 > type 2 diabetics	Type 2 diabetics
Precipitants	Infections, trauma, alcohol, or noncompliance with insulin therapy	Same but includes dietary indiscretion
Symptoms	Abdominal pain, nausea, vomiting, Kussmaul respirations, mental status changes, fruity, acetone breath odor	Profound dehydration, mental status changes (more prominent in HHS than in DKA)
Lab values	Glucose > 250 mg/dL Metabolic acidosis (bicarbonate < 18 mEq/L) ↑ Urine and serum ketones ↑ Anion gap Serum osmolality normal	Glucose > 600 mg/dL No acidosis (bicarbonate > 18 mEq/L) No ketones Normal anion gap Serum osmolality > 320 mOsm/kg
Treatment	Fluids and continuous insulin (caution: will ↓ potassium, monitor and replace). Bicarbonate rarely used (only if pH is < 6.9). Treat initiating event. Monitor response to treatment by closure of the anion gap	Aggressive fluids, electrolyte replacement, and insulin. Treat the initiating event

TABLE 2.3-4. **Chronic Complications of Diabetes Mellitus**

Complication	Description
Retinopathy (nonproliferative, proliferative)	Appears when diabetes has been present for at least 3–5 years (see Figure 2.3-2). Preventive measures include control of hyperglycemia and hypertension, annual eye exams, anti-VEGF (nonproliferative), and laser photocoagulation therapy (focal for nonproliferative vs panretinal for proliferative)
Diabetic nephropathy	Characterized by glomerular hyperfiltration followed by microalbuminuria, macroproteinuria, and progression to CKD. Seen in patients with diabetes for > 10 years. Preventive measures include ACEIs or ARBs. BP control more effective than glucose control. Kimmelstiel-Wilson nodules seen on kidney biopsy
Neuropathy	Peripheral nerves: Most common neuropathy. Symmetric sensorimotor polyneuropathy leading to burning pain, foot trauma, infections, and ulcers Small fiber neuropathy: Pain and paresthesia Large fiber neuropathy: Absence of sensation Ischemic CN III damage: down-and-out eye, ptosis, diplopia, with preserved pupil response Treat with preventive foot care and analgesics (amitriptyline, gabapentin, NSAIDs). Monofilament testing predicts ulcer risk GI: Gastroparesis with delayed gastric emptying. Treat with metoclopramide or erythromycin. Can also get esophageal dysmotility, diarrhea/constipation GU: Neurogenic bladder with decreased sensation to void, overflow incontinence, high postvoid residuals. Can also have erectile dysfunction Cardiovascular: Orthostatic hypotension
Macrovascular complications	Cardiovascular, cerebrovascular, and peripheral vascular disease. Cardiovascular disease is the most common cause of death in diabetic patients. See Table 2.3-2 for risk modification guidelines

VEGF, Vascular endothelial growth factor.

History/PE

- Patients may present with symptoms of hyperglycemia (polyuria, polydipsia, polyphagia, blurred vision, fatigue).
- Onset is more insidious than that of type 1 DM, and patients often present with complications.

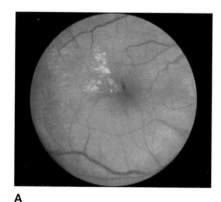
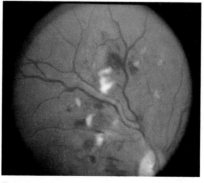

A   B

FIGURE 2.3-2. **Diabetic retinopathy.** (**A**) Nonproliferative retinopathy presents with exudates, dot-blot hemorrhages, and microaneurysms. (**B**) Proliferative retinopathy presents with macular edema, vitreous traction, and neovascularization of the retinal vasculature. (Reproduced with permission from USMLE-Rx.com.)

- Nonketotic hyperosmolar hyperglycemic state (HHS) may be seen in the setting of poor glycemic control (see Table 2.3-3).
- Usually occurs in older adults with obesity (often abdominal) and has a strong genetic predisposition; diagnosed increasingly in obese children.
- Risk factors include obesity, rapid weight gain, ⊕ family history, sedentary lifestyle, increasing age, ethnicity (Asian, Hispanic, and African-American), and other components of metabolic syndrome (see later).

DIAGNOSIS

- Diagnostic criteria are the same as those for type 1 DM.
- Anti–islet cell and anti-GAD antibodies will be ⊖.
- **Screening recommendations:**
  - **Screening tests:** Fasting glucose (first-line due to cost-effectiveness), HbA_{1c} level (> 6.5% is diagnostic), and 2-hour oral glucose tolerance test.
  - Consider screening all patients with risk factors for diabetes (eg, hypertension, obesity, family history, racial/ethnic minorities).
  - **Patients with no risk factors:** Test HbA_{1c} at 45 years of age; retest every 3 years if HbA_{1c} is < 5.7% and no other risk factors develop.
  - **Patients with impaired fasting glucose** (> 100 mg/dL but < 126 mg/dL) or impaired glucose tolerance: Follow up with frequent retesting.

TREATMENT

See Table 2.3-1 and 2.3-2 for treatment options and general health maintenance guidelines. Treat to goal HbA_{1c} level < 7% (corresponds to an average glucose of 154 mg/dL) with more liberal goals in patients > 65 years of age who are at risk for hypoglycemia.

COMPLICATIONS

See Tables 2.3-3 and 2.3-4 for an outline of the complications associated with DM.

MNEMONIC

Diabetes complications—

KNIVE

Kidney (nephropathy)
Neuromuscular (peripheral neuropathy)
Infectious (UTIs, pneumonia, soft-tissue infections, TB)
Vascular (coronary/cerebrovascular/ peripheral artery disease)
Eye (cataracts, retinopathy)

MNEMONIC

Criteria for metabolic syndrome—

WEIGHHT

Waist **E**xpanded
Impaired **G**lucose
Hypertension
HDL ↓
Triglycerides ↑

METABOLIC SYNDROME

Also known as insulin resistance syndrome or syndrome X, metabolic syndrome is associated with an ↑ risk for CAD and mortality from a cardiovascular event.

HISTORY/PE

Presents with abdominal obesity, high BP, impaired glycemic control, and dyslipidemia.

DIAGNOSIS

Three out of five of the following criteria must be met:

- Abdominal obesity (↑ waist girth): ≥ 40 inches (102 cm) in men and ≥ 35 inches (88 cm) in women.
- Triglycerides ≥ 150 mg/dL.
- HDL < 40 mg/dL in men and < 50 mg/dL in women.
- BP ≥ 130/85 mm Hg or a requirement for antihypertensive drugs.
- Fasting glucose ≥ 100 mg/dL.

TREATMENT

- **Best initial treatment:** Lifestyle modifications (diet, exercise, intensive weight loss).

- Also consider additional prevention of diabetes with metformin and mitigation of cardiovascular risk with aggressive cholesterol management and BP control.

Thyroid Disorders

See Figure 2.3-3 for an overview of thyroid hormone synthesis and Figure 2.3-4 for a review of the hypothalamic-pituitary-thyroid axis.

TESTING OF THYROID FUNCTION

Thyroid function tests (TFTs) include the following (see also Table 2.3-5):

- **TSH measurement:** Single best test for the screening of thyroid disease and for the assessment of thyroid function, unless there is a history of brain injury (eg, tumor, radiation, trauma), in which case free T_4 should also be checked.
- **Free T_4 measurement:** Preferred screening test for thyroid hormone levels.
- **Total T_4 measurement:** Not an adequate screening test. Ninety-nine percent of circulating T_4 is bound to thyroxine-binding globulin (TBG). Total T_4 levels can be altered by changes in levels of binding proteins.
- **Radioactive iodine uptake (RAIU) test and scan:** Measures the thyroid's level and distribution of iodine uptake. Determines if a nodule is functioning, in the case of hyperthyroidism, or nonfunctioning, and requires a biopsy for malignancy workup. See Table 2.3-6.

KEY FACT

↑TBG can be found in pregnancy, estrogen administration, and infection. You do not need to treat.

KEY FACT

Exophthalmos, pretibial myxedema, and thyroid bruits are specific for Graves disease.

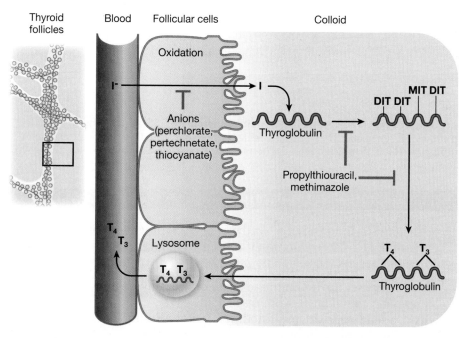

FIGURE 2.3-3. **Overview of thyroid synthesis and mechanism of antithyroid medications.** Iodide (I^-) is taken up from the bloodstream by follicular thyroid cells, transported to the colloid of the follicle, and oxidized to iodine (I). I combines with thyroglobulin to form monoiodotyrosine (MIT) and diiodotyrosine (DIT). Two DIT molecules combine to form T_4; MIT and DIT combine to form T_3. Iodinated thyroglobulin is transported back to the follicular cells and is cleaved in lysosomes; T_4 and T_3 are then released into the circulation.

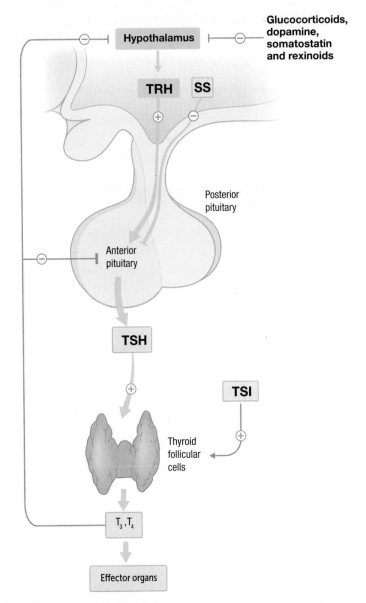

FIGURE 2.3-4. **The hypothalamic-pituitary-thyroid axis.** SS, somatostatin; T_3, triiodo-thyronine; T_4, thyroxine; TSH, thyroid-stimulating hormone; TSI, thyroid-stimulating immu-noglobulin; TRH, thyrotropin-releasing hormone. (Reproduced with permission from USMLE-Rx.com.)

KEY FACT

TSH receptor–stimulating antibodies are found in patients with Graves disease.

KEY FACT

When screening for thyroid dysfunction, measure serum TSH:
- If normal—no further tests
- If high—measure free T_4
- If low—measure free T_4 and T_3

HYPERTHYROIDISM/THYROTOXICOSIS

Hyperthyroidism is a state of ↑ synthesis of T_3/T_4; thyrotoxicosis is a state of ↑ levels of T_3/T_4. Most commonly caused by Graves disease, but can also result from other causes (see Table 2.3-5).

- **Graves disease:** An autoimmune cause of hyperthyroidism. TSH receptor-stimulating antibodies ↑ synthesis of T_3/T_4.
- **Toxic adenoma/toxic multinodular goiter:** Result in hyperthyroidism caused by autonomous hyperactive thyroid nodules.
- **Thyroiditis:** Caused by transient inflammation of the thyroid gland with release of previously synthesized thyroid hormone; causes a temporary ↑ in circulating T_3/T_4. A hypothyroid phase may follow the hyperthyroid phase with eventual return to normal in many patients.
- **Fetal thyrotoxicosis:** Classically in an infant born to a mother with Graves disease. TSH-stimulating antibodies are IgG and can cross the placenta.

TABLE 2.3-5.   Thyroid Function Tests in Thyroid Disease

DIAGNOSIS	TSH	T$_4$	T$_3$	CAUSES
1° Hyperthyroidism	↓	↑	↑	Graves disease, toxic multinodular goiter, toxic adenoma, amiodarone, postpartum thyrotoxicosis, postviral thyroiditis
2° Hyperthyroidism	Nl/↑	↑	↑	Rare. Caused by TSH-producing pituitary adenoma. TSH often inappropriately normal (not suppressed)
1° Hypothyroidism	↑	↓	↓	Hashimoto thyroiditis, iatrogenic (radioactive ablation, excision), drugs (lithium, amiodarone)
2° Hypothyroidism	↓	↓	↓	Often caused by pituitary nonfunctioning macroadenomas, infiltrative diseases, or post–pituitary surgery
Subclinical hypothyroidism	↑	Nl	Nl	Often with mild elevations in TSH, asymptomatic
Euthyroid sick syndrome	Nl	Nl/↓	↓	Caused by any serious illness. Will have ↑ reverse T$_3$ (nonfunctional), as T$_4$ is converted to rT$_3$ instead of T$_3$. Thought to be caused by caloric deprivation and increased cytokines. May have transient ↑ in TSH during recovery period

KEY FACT

Thyroid storm is an acute, life-threatening form of thyrotoxicosis that may present with AF, fever, and delirium. Administer β-blockers and antithyroid drugs initially, followed by iodine. Consider steroids if necessary.

HISTORY/PE

- Presents with weight loss, heat intolerance, anxiety, palpitations, ↑ bowel frequency, myopathy/proximal muscle weakness, insomnia, and menstrual abnormalities.
- Exam reveals warm, moist skin, goiter, hypertension, sinus tachycardia, or atrial fibrillation (AF), fine tremor, lid lag, and hyperactive reflexes. Exophthalmos (direct stimulation of orbital fibroblasts by antibodies), pretibial myxedema, acropachy, and thyroid bruits are seen only in Graves disease (see Figure 2.3-5).
- Cardiac findings are a result of increased heart rate and contractility.

DIAGNOSIS

Best initial test: Serum TSH level, followed by T$_4$ levels and, rarely, T$_3$ (unless TSH is low and free T$_4$ is not elevated). May need additional information provided by RAI scans (see Figure 2.3-6) and thyroglobulin levels. See Tables 2.3-5 and 2.3-6.

TREATMENT

- **Symptomatic treatment:** Propranolol (or metoprolol, atenolol) to manage adrenergic symptoms.
- **Pharmacologic treatment:** Antithyroid medications (methimazole or propylthiouracil). Generally used for mild disease, and for stabilizing treatment before definitive treatment.

Q   **1**

A 24-year-old woman with hypothyroidism presents at 10 weeks' gestation for a prenatal visit. Her only medication is levothyroxine. What adjustment is probably needed to her levothyroxine dose?

Q   **2**

A 10-year-old boy presents to the ED with 2 weeks of polyuria and polydipsia and new-onset lethargy. Physical exam reveals signs of severe dehydration, and labs reveal a blood glucose level of 500 mg/dL. A diagnosis of DKA is made, and the patient is started on insulin and non–dextrose-containing IV fluids. His glucose on recheck is 250 mg/dL. What is the next best step in management?

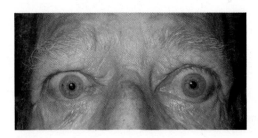

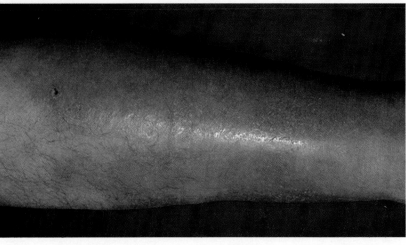

FIGURE 2.3-5. Physical signs of Graves disease. (A) Graves ophthalmopathy. (B) Pretibial myxedema. (Reproduced with permission from USMLE-Rx.com.)

- **Definitive treatment:** Radioactive ^{131}I thyroid ablation or total thyroidectomy (less common in the United States). Radioactive iodine may worsen ophthalmopathy from Graves disease.
- Administer levothyroxine (oral T_4 replacement) to prevent hypothyroidism in patients who have undergone ablation or surgery.
- Administer steroids to treat severe ophthalmopathy (if causing diplopia or threatening vision).

See Table 2.3-7 for adverse drug reactions associated with antithyroid medications.

COMPLICATIONS

Thyroid storm is an acute, life-threatening form of thyrotoxicosis. Admit to ICU and treat immediately with β-blockers and high-dose antithyroid medications (propylthiouracil or methimazole). Give high-dose potassium iodide (SSKI) 1 hour after use of an antithyroid medication. The addition of corticosteroids may also be effective. Untreated hyperthyroidism can also lead to long-term bone loss.

> **KEY FACT**
>
> Myxedema coma can be triggered in a hypothyroid patient by acute events such as infections, MI, stroke, trauma, sedative drugs, surgery, and levothyroxine noncompliance.

1 A

Her dose will probably have to be ↑ (sometimes by up to 50%!). ↑ TBG levels in pregnancy lead to ↓ free T_3/T_4 levels and ↑ TSH.

2 A

Add 5% dextrose to the IV fluids. In the management of DKA, it is important to start IV fluids and insulin immediately. Initially, the goal is to rehydrate the patient and ↓ blood glucose, but as blood glucose reaches 250–300 mg/dL, it is important to add 5% dextrose to ↓ the risk for hypoglycemia.

TABLE 2.3-6. Radioactive Iodine Findings in Hyperthyroidism

DIAGNOSIS	RAI % UPTAKE	RAI SCAN FINDINGS	THYROGLOBULIN
Graves disease	↑	Diffuse uptake	N/A
Multinodular goiter	NI/↑	Multiple nodules of ↑ uptake	N/A
Toxic adenoma	NI/↑	One area of ↑ uptake	N/A
Thyroiditis, iodine exposure, extraglandular production	↓	Low uptake	↑
Exogenous thyroid hormone	↓	Low uptake	↓

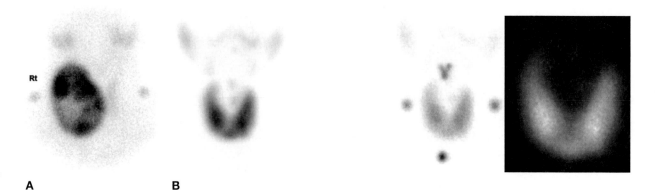

A **B**

FIGURE 2.3-6. **Radioactive iodine uptake scans.** 99m-Technetium pertechnetate thyroid scans showing **(A)** multinodular areas of increased uptake and **(B)** diffuse uptake as seen in Graves disease. (Image A reproduced with permission from Cho EA, et al. A case of masked toxic adenoma in a patient with non-thyroidal illness. *BMC Endocr Disord.* 2014;14:1. Image B reproduced with permission from Coutinho E, et al. Graves' disease presenting as pseudotumor cerebri: a case report. *J Med Case Reports.* 2011;5:68.)

HYPOTHYROIDISM

A state involving ↓ levels of T_3/T_4. Most commonly caused by Hashimoto thyroiditis, but can result from other causes (see Table 2.3-5).

- **Hashimoto thyroiditis (autoimmune hypothyroidism):** Associated with ⊕ antithyroglobulin and antithyroid peroxidase (anti-TPO) antibodies that precipitate thyroid destruction.
- **Thyroiditis (postpartum, postviral, subacute/de Quervain):** Can have a hypothyroid phase that follows the hyperthyroid phase. Hypothyroidism can be permanent. Subacute thyroiditis is usually painful.
- **Secondary hypothyroidism:** Caused by pituitary tumors or pituitary surgery.
- **Congenital hypothyroidism:** Most common etiology is thyroid dysgenesis. Presents as failure to thrive, hypotonia, umbilical hernias, prolonged jaundice.
- **Generalized resistance to thyroid hormone:** Rare. Elevated T_3/T_4, normal to elevated TSH.

HISTORY/PE

- Presents with weakness, fatigue, cold intolerance, constipation, weight gain, depression, hair loss, menstrual irregularities, myopathy, and hoarseness.
- Exam reveals dry, cold, puffy skin accompanied by edema, bradycardia, and delayed relaxation of deep tendon reflexes.

TABLE 2.3-7. **Adverse Drug Reactions for Thyrotoxicosis Treatments**

DRUG/TREATMENT	ADVERSE REACTIONS
Propylthiouracil	Allergic reaction, rash, arthralgias, agranulocytosis, vasculitis, liver failure (black box warning). Safe to use in pregnancy
Methimazole	Allergic reaction. Contraindicated in pregnancy. Agranulocytosis. Cholestasis
Radioactive ¹³¹I thyroid ablation	Most common side effect is hypothyroidism (most common when treating patients with Graves disease). Contraindicated in pregnancy. Will initially worsen ophthalmopathy
Total thyroidectomy	Hypothyroidism, hypoparathyroidism, damage to nearby structures (recurrent laryngeal nerve)

DIAGNOSIS

Best initial test: Serum TSH level, followed by free T_4 levels. See Table 2.3-5. Other lab abnormalities include high LDL, ↑ triglycerides, ↑ CK, hyponatremia.

TREATMENT

For uncomplicated hypothyroidism (eg, Hashimoto disease), administer levothyroxine. In subclinical hypothyroidism (↑ TSH, normal T_4), treat with levothyroxine if TSH > 10 mU/L.

COMPLICATIONS

- Increased risk for thyroid lymphoma in patients with Hashimoto disease.
- **Myxedema coma:** Severe hypothyroidism with ↓ mental status, hypothermia, hypotension, bradycardia, hypoglycemia, and hypoventilation. Mortality is 30–60%. Admit to the ICU and treat urgently with IV levothyroxine and IV hydrocortisone (if adrenal insufficiency not excluded).

THYROIDITIS

Inflammation of the thyroid gland. Common subtypes include subacute granulomatous, radiation-induced, autoimmune, postpartum, infectious, and drug-induced (eg, amiodarone) thyroiditis.

HISTORY/PE

- The subacute form presents with a tender thyroid, malaise, and URI symptoms.
- All other forms are associated with painless goiter.

DIAGNOSIS

Thyroid dysfunction (typically thyrotoxicosis followed by hypothyroidism), with ↓ uptake on RAI scan during the hyperthyroid phase.

TREATMENT

- β-blockers for hyperthyroidism; levothyroxine for hypothyroidism if TSH > 10 mU/L.
- Subacute thyroiditis is usually self-limited; for severe cases, treat with NSAIDs or with oral corticosteroids.

THYROID NEOPLASMS

Thyroid nodules are very common and show an ↑ incidence with age. Most (~ 95%) are benign.

HISTORY/PE

- Usually asymptomatic on initial presentation; discovered incidentally.
- Hyperfunctioning nodules present with hyperthyroidism.
- Large nodules adjacent to the trachea/esophagus may cause dysphagia, dyspnea, cough, and choking sensation.
- An ↑ risk for malignancy is associated with a history of childhood neck irradiation, "cold" nodules (minimal uptake on RAI scan), female sex, age < 20 or > 70, firm and fixed solitary nodules, ⊕ family history, and rapidly growing nodules with hoarseness.
- Check for anterior cervical lymphadenopathy. Carcinoma (see Table 2.3-8) may be firm and fixed.

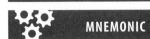

KEY FACT

Subacute thyroiditis is not a "cute" thyroiditis—it is painful!

MNEMONIC

Thyroid neoplasms—

The most Popular is Papillary

Papillae (branching)
Palpable lymph nodes
"**P**upil" nuclei ("Orphan Annie" nuclei)
Psammoma bodies within lesion (often)
Also has a **P**ositive **P**rognosis

TABLE 2.3-8.   **Types of Thyroid Carcinoma**

TYPE[A]	CHARACTERISTICS	PROGNOSIS
Papillary	Represents 75–80% of thyroid cancers. The female-to-male ratio is 3 : 1. Slow growing; found in thyroid hormone–producing follicular cells. Associated with psammoma bodies. Lymphatic spread	90% of patients survive ≥ 10 years after diagnosis; the prognosis is poorer in patients > 45 years of age or those with large tumors
Follicular	Accounts for 17% of thyroid cancers; found in thyroid hormone–producing follicular cells. Hematologic spread	Same as above
Medullary	Responsible for 6–8% of thyroid cancers. Found in calcitonin-producing C cells; the prognosis is related to degree of vascular invasion	80% of patients survive at least 10 years after surgery. Consider MEN 2A or 2B based on family history
Anaplastic	Accounts for < 2% of thyroid cancers; rapidly enlarges and metastasizes	10% of patients survive for > 3 years

[A]Tumors may contain mixed papillary and follicular pathologies.

- Medullary thyroid carcinoma is associated with multiple endocrine neoplasia (MEN) type 2.

DIAGNOSIS

See Figure 2.3-7 for a diagnostic workup of thyroid nodules.

TREATMENT

- **Benign fine-needle aspiration (FNA):** Follow with physical exam/ ultrasonography to assess for continued nodule growth or for development of suspicious characteristics (eg, microcalcifications, ↑ vascular flow).

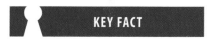

KEY FACT

Check calcitonin levels if medullary cancer is suspected!

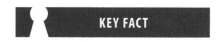

KEY FACT

Hyperfunctioning (hot) thyroid nodules are not malignant.

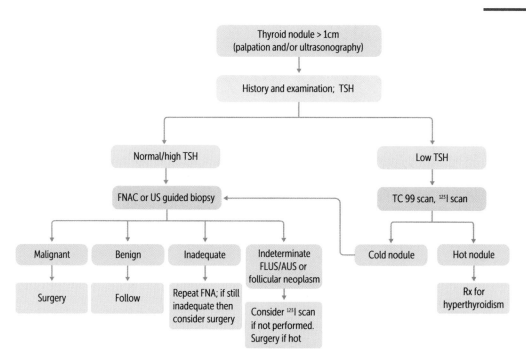

FIGURE 2.3-7.   **Diagnostic steps in the workup of a thyroid nodule.** (Reproduced with permission from USMLE-Rx.com.)

- **Malignant FNA:** Surgical resection with hemi- or total thyroidectomy is **best initial treatment;** adjunctive radioiodine ablation following excision is appropriate for some follicular lesions.
- **Indeterminate FNA:** Watchful waiting vs hemithyroidectomy (10–30% chance of malignancy). If resected, await final pathology to guide further treatment.

KEY FACT

Do not confuse osteoporosis with osteomalacia. Osteomalacia is a mineralization defect often caused by severe vitamin D deficiency that presents with bone pain, ↓ calcium/phosphate, and 2° hyperparathyroidism.

Bone and Mineral Disorders

Figure 2.3-8 reviews calcium and phosphate regulation.

OSTEOPOROSIS

A common metabolic bone disease characterized by low bone mass. It most often affects thin postmenopausal women, especially white and Asian individuals, with risk doubling after 65 years of age. Men are also at risk for osteoporosis, but the diagnosis is often overlooked.

HISTORY/PE

- Commonly asymptomatic even in the presence of a vertebral fracture.
- **Risk factors:** Smoking, advancing age, excessive alcohol intake, a history of estrogen-depleting conditions in women (eg, amenorrhea, eating disorders, early menopause) or hypogonadism in men, physical inactivity, uncontrolled hyperthyroidism, hyperparathyroidism, chronic inflammatory disease, corticosteroid use, Cushing syndrome.

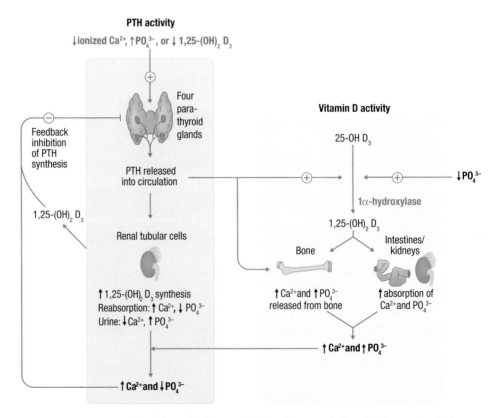

FIGURE 2.3-8. **Overview of calcium and phosphate regulation.** PTH, parathyroid hormone. (Reproduced with permission from USMLE-Rx.com)

- Exam may reveal hip fractures, vertebral compression fractures (loss of height and progressive thoracic kyphosis), and/or distal radius fractures (Colles fracture) following minimal trauma (see Figure 2.3-9).

DIAGNOSIS

- **Diagnostic test:** Dual-energy x-ray absorptiometry (DEXA). Recommended as screening test for all women > 65 years of age and men > 70 years of age, and those with other risk factors for osteoporosis.
  - **Osteoporosis:** Bone mineral density (T-score) is 2.5 standard deviations (SDs) less than normal.
  - **Osteopenia:** T-score between 1 and 2.5 SDs below normal.
- **Lab tests:** Look for secondary causes by measuring calcium, phosphate, parathyroid hormone (PTH), TSH, free T_4, liver enzymes, creatinine, and electrolytes. If estrogen deficiency or hypogonadism is suspected, measure FSH, LH, estradiol, and testosterone.

TREATMENT

- **Lifestyle modifications:** Adequate calcium and vitamin D intake (supplementation can be used for prevention), smoking cessation, avoiding heavy alcohol use, and weight-bearing exercises.
- **Best initial treatment:** Bisphosphonates (eg, alendronate, risedronate, ibandronate, zoledronic acid) are used in the treatment of osteoporosis, not osteopenia.
- **Other drugs:** Teriparatide (PTH analogue), denosumab (a monoclonal antibody to RANK-L), selective estrogen receptor modulators (eg, raloxifene).

COMPLICATIONS

Fracture is the most devastating consequence of low bone mineral density/osteoporosis, carrying a 50% ↑ in mortality in the year following hip fracture.

KEY FACT

Osteoporosis is the most common cause of pathologic fractures in thin women and men > 60 years of age.

KEY FACT

Upper gastrointestinal side effects such as reflux, esophagitis, and esophageal ulcers are common reasons for oral bisphosphonate (alendronate and risedronate) intolerance.

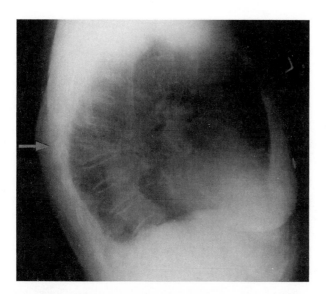

FIGURE 2.3-9. **Radiographic findings in osteoporosis.** Lateral thoracic spine radiograph shows osteoporosis and an anterior wedge deformity of a lower thoracic vertebral body with associated kyphosis. This is a typical insufficiency fracture in osteoporotic patients. (Reproduced with permission from Fauci AS, et al. *Harrison's Principles of Internal Medicine,* 17th ed. New York, NY: McGraw-Hill; 2008.)

Increased serum alkaline phosphatase with normal gamma-glutamyl transpeptidase (GGT) points to bone etiology, not a liver etiology.

MNEMONIC

Symptoms and signs of Paget disease of bone—

PANICS

Pain
Arthralgia
Nerve compression/**N**eural deafness
Increased bone density
Cardiac failure
Skull involvement/**S**clerotic vertebra

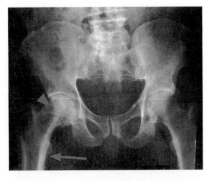

FIGURE 2.3-10. Radiographic findings in Paget disease. Pelvic radiograph demonstrates a thickened cortex (*arrow*), thickened trabeculae (*arrowhead*), and expansion of the right femoral head, classic signs of Paget disease. (Reproduced with permission from Fauci AS, et al. *Harrison's Principles of Internal Medicine,* 17th ed. New York, NY: McGraw-Hill; 2008.)

PAGET DISEASE OF BONE

Characterized by an ↑ rate of bone turnover with both excessive resorption and formation of bone, leading to a "mosaic" lamellar bone pattern appearance on x-ray. Suspected to be caused by the effects of a latent viral infection in genetically susceptible individuals. Associated with 1° hyperparathyroidism and ↑ risk for osteosarcoma. The disease can affect one (monostotic) or more (polystotic) bones, with the skull, vertebral bodies, pelvis, and long bones most commonly affected.

HISTORY/PE

- Usually asymptomatic.
- May present with aching bone or joint pain, bony deformities, fracture at a pagetoid site, nerve entrapment, headaches, and hearing loss (latter two occur if involving the skull).

DIAGNOSIS

- **Best initial test:** Plain film x-rays (lytic and sclerotic lesions; see Figure 2.3-10) usually diagnostic.
- Radionuclide bone scan necessary to characterize extent and sites of disease (see Figure 2.3-11).

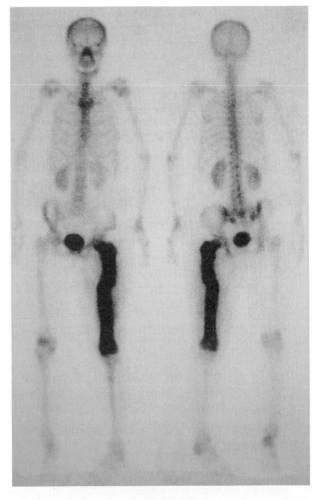

FIGURE 2.3-11. Radionuclide bone scan in Paget disease. Dark areas represent increased bone-seeking isotope uptake and depicts severe disease in the left femur. (Reproduced with permission from Takigami I, et al. Functional bracing for delayed union of a femur fracture associated with Paget's disease of the bone in an Asian patient: a case report. *J Orthop Surg Res.* 2010;5:33.)

- **Lab values:** ↑ Serum alkaline phosphatase with normal calcium and phosphate levels. Must be distinguished from metastatic bone disease.

TREATMENT

- Most patients are asymptomatic and require no treatment.
- There is no cure, but goal is to reduce pain and disease progression.
- **Pharmacologic:** Bisphosphonates (first-line), calcitonin (if intolerant to bisphosphonates), calcium and vitamin D supplementation, analgesics (NSAIDs and acetaminophen).
- **Adjunctive therapy:** Physiotherapy, occupational therapy.
- **Surgery:** If necessary in the case of fractures, severe deformities, and osteoarthritis.

COMPLICATIONS

Osteoarthritis, pathologic fractures, high-output cardiac failure (from AV connections), osteosarcoma (up to 1%).

HYPERPARATHYROIDISM

See Figure 2.3-8 for the effects of PTH on serum calcium and phosphate regulation. For a more thorough review of hypo- and hypercalcemia, see the Renal/Genitourinary chapter.

- **1° Hyperparathyroidism:** Most cases (80%) are caused by a single hyperfunctioning adenoma, with the rest (15%) resulting from parathyroid hyperplasia and, rarely (5%), parathyroid carcinoma.
- **2° Hyperparathyroidism:** A physiologic ↑ of PTH in response to renal insufficiency (caused by ↓ production of 1-25 dihydroxyvitamin D), calcium deficiency, or vitamin D deficiency.
- **3° Hyperparathyroidism:** Seen in dialysis patients with long-standing 2° hyperparathyroidism that leads to hyperplasia of the parathyroid glands. When one or more of the glands become autonomous, 3° hyperparathyroidism results.
- **Pseudohypoparathyroidism:** PTH resistance. ↑ PTH levels but ineffective at target organs. Hypocalcemia and hyperphosphatemia. Associated with Albright hereditary osteodystrophy (may have shortened fourth and fifth metatarsal or metacarpal bones).

HISTORY/PE

Most cases of 1° hyperparathyroidism are asymptomatic but may show signs and symptoms of hypercalcemia (see Renal/Genitourinary chapter).

DIAGNOSIS

- Lab results in 1° hyperparathyroidism reveal hypercalcemia, hypophosphatemia, and hypercalciuria. Intact PTH is inappropriately ↑ relative to total and ionized calcium (see Table 2.3-9).
- A ^{99m}Tc sestamibi scan, in conjunction with thyroid ultrasonography, can help localize a solitary adenoma.
- DEXA may reveal low bone mineral density or frank osteoporosis in the distal radius or other sites.
- Consider renal imaging to look for nephrocalcinosis and nephrolithiasis.

TREATMENT

- **Best initial treatment:** For acute hypercalcemia, IV fluids and calcitonin. Consider IV bisphosphonates for long term.
- Parathyroidectomy if the patient is symptomatic or if certain criteria are met (↑↑ calcium, ↑ creatinine, ↓ Bone mineral density, < 50 years of age). In the case of a solitary adenoma, 1 gland can be removed. In the setting of hyperplasia, 3.5 glands must be removed.

KEY FACT

Bone pain and hearing loss → think Paget disease.

KEY FACT

Hypercalcemia is associated with "stones, bones, moans, groans, and psychiatric overtones." Administer IV fluids (first-line) and calcitonin. Add bisphosphonates if malignancy.

KEY FACT

Etiologies of hypoparathyroidism include iatrogenic (postsurgical), autoimmune, congenital (DiGeorge), infiltrative (hemochromatosis, Wilson) diseases.

TABLE 2.3-9.   Lab Values in Hyperparathyroidism

	PTH	CALCIUM	PO₄
1°	↑	↑	↓
2°	↑	Nl/↓	↑ (when etiology is renal failure)
3°	↑	↑	↑
Ectopic PTHrP[a]	↓	↑	Nl/↓

[a]PTH-related peptide (PTHrP) is a member of the PTH family and acts on the same PTH receptors. Some tumors (eg, breast, lung) produce PTHrP, causing hypercalcemia of malignancy.

- In patients with chronic kidney disease, administer oral phosphate binders (calcium salts, sevelamer hydrochloride, and lanthanum carbonate) and restrict dietary phosphate intake to prevent 2° hyperparathyroidism.
- Cinacalcet is a calcimimetic that acts to lower serum PTH levels and is approved for use in hyperparathyroidism caused by renal failure or in patients who cannot undergo surgery.

COMPLICATIONS

Hypercalcemia is the most severe complication of 1° hyperparathyroidism. Postparathyroidectomy, watch for hungry bone syndrome (severe and prolonged hypocalcemia caused by acute reversal of PTH and ↑ in bone uptake of calcium, phosphate, and magnesium).

Pituitary and Hypothalamic Disorders

Figure 2.3-12 illustrates the hypothalamic-pituitary axis. The following sections outline the manner in which the components of this axis interact with target organs in various pathologic states.

HYPOPITUITARISM

Caused by mass lesions (tumors, cysts), surgery, radiation, Sheehan syndrome (pituitary infarction seen in severe postpartum hemorrhage), apoplexy

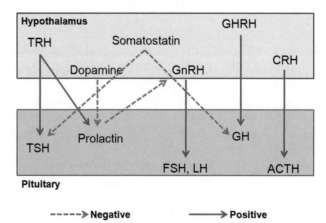

FIGURE 2.3-12.   The hypothalamic-pituitary axis. ACTH, adrenocorticotropic hormone; CRH, corticotropin-releasing hormone; FSH, follicle-stimulating hormone; GH, growth hormone; GHRH, growth hormone-releasing hormone; GnRH, gonadotropin-releasing hormone; LH, luteinizing hormone ; TRH, thyrotropin-releasing hormone; TSH, thyroid-stimulating hormone. (Reproduced with permission from USMLE-Rx.com.)

(hemorrhage), infiltrative disorders (hemochromatosis), infections. Gonadotropins and growth hormone are often affected first.

HISTORY/PE

See corresponding sections for presentation of pituitary hormone deficiencies. May present suddenly (apoplexy, Sheehan syndrome) or gradually (radiation, infiltrative diseases).

DIAGNOSIS

Measure 8 AM cortisol (on at least two separate occasions), free T_4 (TSH not diagnostic), testosterone/estradiol levels, insulin-like growth factor 1 (IGF-1).

TREATMENT

Treat underlying disorder. See corresponding sections for treatments of specific hormone deficiencies.

CUSHING SYNDROME

Elevated serum cortisol levels and most frequently from prolonged treatment with exogenous corticosteroids. The most common endogenous cause is hypersecretion of ACTH from a pituitary adenoma (known as Cushing disease; see Figure 2.3-13). Other endogenous causes include excess adrenal secretion of cortisol (eg, bilateral adrenal hyperplasia, adrenal adenoma, adrenal cancer) and ectopic ACTH production from an occult neoplasm (eg, carcinoid tumor, medullary thyroid cancer, small cell lung cancer).

HISTORY/PE

See Figure 2.3-14 for classic signs and symptoms of Cushing syndrome.

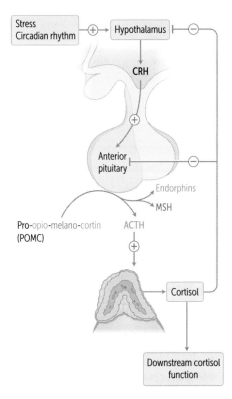

FIGURE 2.3-13. **The hypothalamic-anterior pituitary axis (hypophyseal portal system): Cushing disease.** ACTH, adrenocorticotropic hormone; CRH, corticotropin-releasing hormone. (Reproduced with permission from USMLE-Rx.com.)

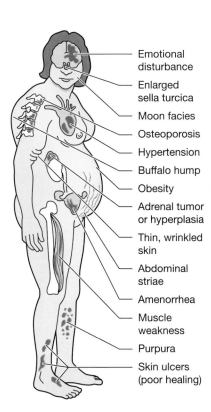

- Emotional disturbance
- Enlarged sella turcica
- Moon facies
- Osteoporosis
- Hypertension
- Buffalo hump
- Obesity
- Adrenal tumor or hyperplasia
- Thin, wrinkled skin
- Abdominal striae
- Amenorrhea
- Muscle weakness
- Purpura
- Skin ulcers (poor healing)

FIGURE 2.3-14. **Physical findings in Cushing syndrome.** (Reproduced with permission from USMLE-Rx.com.)

KEY FACT

Cushing syndrome: Too much cortisol.
Cushing disease: Too much cortisol from an ACTH-producing pituitary adenoma.

Q

An asymptomatic 36-year-old man presents for his annual physical. Routine labs reveal a serum calcium level of 11.3 mg/dL. He returns in 2 weeks, and his serum calcium level remains elevated. Additional studies show a normal serum PTH level and a low 24-hour urinary calcium level. What is the most likely diagnosis?

In Cushing disease, cortisol secretion remains elevated with the low-dose (1 mg) dexamethasone test but is suppressed with the high-dose (8 mg) dexamethasone test.

MNEMONIC

Cushing syndrome symptoms—

CUSHINGOID

Cataracts
Ulcers
Skin (striae, bruising, thinning, ulcer)
Hirsutism, hypertension
Infections
Necrosis (femur head)
Glycosuria
Obesity, osteoporosis
Immunosuppression
Diabetes

A

Familial hypocalciuric hypercalcemia (FHH), an inherited disorder caused by mutations in a calcium-sensing receptor present in the parathyroid and kidney, presents with elevated serum calcium levels. Unlike patients with 1° hyperparathyroidism, these patients are asymptomatic and have low urinary calcium levels. No treatment is required.

DIAGNOSIS

Diagnosis follows a stepwise progression of tests. See Figure 2.3-15 for the diagnostic algorithm. Table 2.3-10 outlines important lab findings that aid in diagnosis.

TREATMENT

- **Exogenous:** Gradually withdraw and stop glucocorticoids.
- **Endogenous:** Surgical resection of the source (pituitary, adrenal, ectopic neoplasm). Permanent hormone replacement therapy to correct deficiencies after treatment or resection of the 1° lesion.

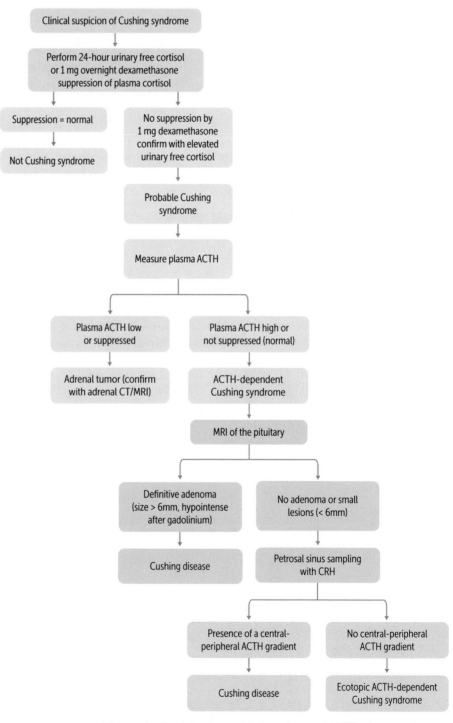

FIGURE 2.3-15. **Diagnostic algorithm for Cushing syndrome.** ACTH, adrenocorticotropic hormone. (Reproduced with permission from USMLE-Rx.com.)

TABLE 2.3-10. Laboratory Findings in Cushing Syndrome

	CUSHING DISEASE (PITUITARY HYPERSECRETION)	EXOGENOUS STEROID USE	ECTOPIC ACTH SECRETION	ADRENAL CORTISOL HYPERSECRETION
24-hour urinary free cortisol	↑	↑	↑	↑
Salivary cortisol	↑	↑	↑	↑
ACTH	↑	↓	↑	↓
Dexamethasone suppression test morning cortisol level:		N/Aª		N/Aª
Low dose	↑		↑	
High dose	↓		↑	

ªA dexamethasone suppression test is not required once the diagnosis of ACTH-independent Cushing syndrome is made.

ACROMEGALY

Elevated growth hormone (GH) levels in adults, most commonly caused by a benign pituitary GH-secreting adenoma (see Figure 2.3-16). Children with excess GH production present with gigantism.

HISTORY/PE

- Presents with enlargement of the skull (frontal bossing, wide-spaced teeth), hands, and feet, coarsening of facial features, large tongue, and skin tags. Associated with an ↑ risk for carpal tunnel syndrome, obstructive sleep apnea, type 2 DM, heart disease (diastolic dysfunction), hypertension, colon cancer, and arthritis.
- Bitemporal hemianopsia may result from compression of the optic chiasm by a pituitary adenoma.
- Excess GH may also lead to glucose intolerance, diabetes, and cardio-myopathy.

DIAGNOSIS

- **Lab tests:** Measure IGF-1 levels (↑ with acromegaly); confirm diagnosis with an oral glucose suppression test (GH levels will remain elevated despite glucose administration). Baseline GH is not a reliable test.
- **Imaging:** MRI shows a sellar lesion.

TREATMENT

- **Surgery:** Transsphenoidal surgical resection.
- **Medical therapy:** Octreotide or lanreotide (somatostatin analogues) can be used to suppress GH secretion; pegvisomant (a GH receptor antagonist) can be used to block the peripheral actions of GH.
- **Radiation:** Effective when surgical and medical therapies fail.

COMPLICATIONS

The leading cause of death is from cardiovascular complications (congestive heart failure).

KEY FACT

Measure IGF-1 levels to confirm acromegaly, not GH levels!

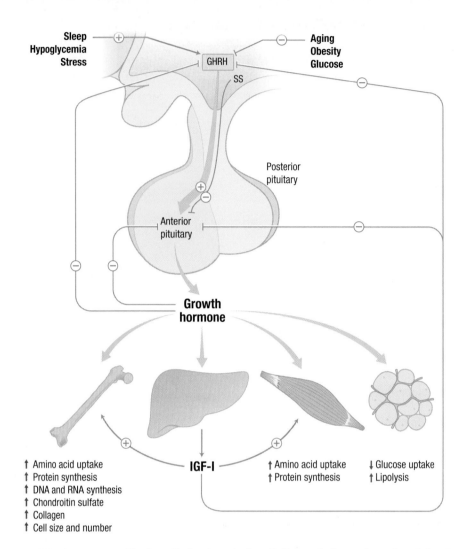

FIGURE 2.3-16. **The hypothalamic–anterior pituitary axis (hypophyseal portal system): acromegaly.** GHRH, growth hormone-releasing hormone; IGF-1, insulin-like growth factor 1. (Reproduced with permission from USMLE-Rx.com.)

HYPERPROLACTINEMIA

Elevated prolactin levels, most commonly caused by a pituitary adenoma (see Figure 2.3-17). Prolactinoma is the most common functioning pituitary tumor. Other causes include pituitary stalk compression from other masses (eg, craniopharyngioma, meningioma, nonsecreting pituitary tumor), drugs (eg, dopamine antagonists), renal failure, and cirrhosis.

HISTORY/PE

Elevated prolactin inhibits GnRH secretion and consequently lowers LH and FSH secretion, manifesting as infertility, galactorrhea, gynecomastia, impotence, and amenorrhea. Bitemporal hemianopsia may also be present.

DIAGNOSIS

- Serum prolactin level is typically > 200 ng/mL.
- Pregnancy test (exclude pregnancy).
- MRI shows a sellar lesion.

KEY FACT

Rule out pregnancy in all cases of hyperprolactinemia!

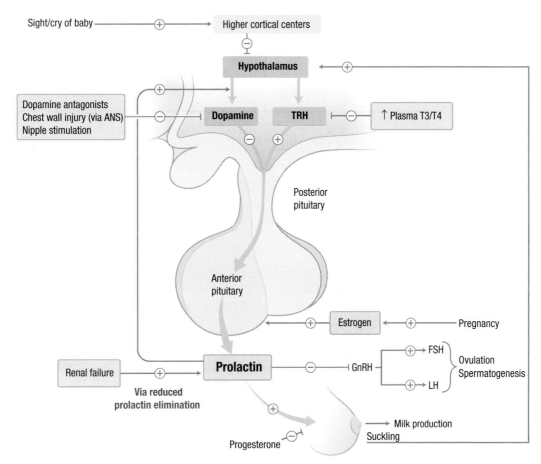

FIGURE 2.3-17. **The hypothalamic–anterior pituitary axis (hypophyseal portal system): prolactin regulation.** ANS, autonomic nervous system; FSH, follicle-stimulating hormone; GnRH, gonadotropin-releasing hormone; LH, luteinizing hormone; TRH, thyrotropin-releasing hormone. (Reproduced with permission from USMLE-Rx.com.)

TREATMENT

■ **Best initial treatment:** Dopamine agonists (eg, cabergoline, bromocriptine).
■ **Surgery:** Indicated in adenomas refractory to medical management or with compressive effects (eg, visual loss).
■ **Radiation:** Rarely indicated.

DIABETES INSIPIDUS

Inability to produce concentrated urine as a result of antidiuretic hormone (ADH) dysfunction. The two subtypes of diabetes insipidus (DI) are as follows:

■ **Central DI (ADH deficiency):** The posterior pituitary gland fails to secrete ADH. Causes include tumor, ischemia (Sheehan syndrome), pituitary hemorrhage, traumatic brain injury, infection, metastatic disease, and autoimmune disorders (see Figure 2.3-18).
■ **Nephrogenic DI (ADH resistance):** The kidneys fail to respond to circulating ADH. Causes include renal disease and drugs (eg, lithium, demeclocycline).

HISTORY/PE

■ Presents with polydipsia, polyuria, and persistent thirst with dilute urine. Most cases are normonatremic.
■ If access to water is limited (eg, in the institutionalized or elderly), patients may present with dehydration and severe hypernatremia leading to altered mental status, lethargy, seizures, and coma.

KEY FACT

In patient suspected of diabetes insipidus, ensure to check serum or urinary glucose to rule out diabetes mellitus.

DIAGNOSIS

- **Lab tests:** Serum osmolality > urine osmolality, ↓ urinary sodium, and possible hypernatremia.
- **Water deprivation test:** In psychogenic polydipsia and normal renal physiology, water restriction will lead to more concentrated urine. In central and nephrogenic DI, patients excrete a high volume of inappropriately dilute urine.
- **Desmopressin acetate replacement test:**
  - Also known as DDAVP, a synthetic analogue of ADH.
  - **Central DI:** ↓ Urine output and ↑ urine osmolarity (by 50–100%).
  - **Nephrogenic DI:** No effect is seen on urine output or urine osmolarity.
- MRI may show a pituitary or hypothalamic mass in central DI.

TREATMENT

- Treat the underlying cause.
- **Central DI:** Administer DDAVP intravenously, intranasally, or orally.
- **Nephrogenic DI:** Salt restriction, reduced water intake, hydrochlorothiazide, amiloride.

SYNDROME OF INAPPROPRIATE ANTIDIURETIC HORMONE SECRETION

Syndrome of inappropriate antidiuretic hormone secretion (SIADH) is a common cause of euvolemic hyponatremia that results from persistent ADH release independent of serum osmolality (see Figure 2.3-19).

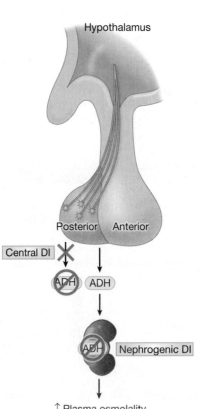

FIGURE 2.3-18. **The hypothalamic-pituitary axis: diabetes insipidus.** ADH, antidiuretic hormone; DI, diabetes insipidus.

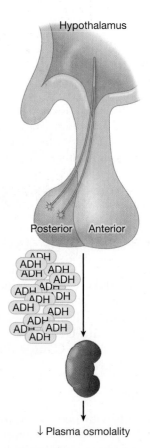

FIGURE 2.3-19. **The hypothalamic-pituitary axis: SIADH.** ADH, antidiuretic hormone.

HISTORY/PE

May be associated with: CNS disease (eg, head injury, tumor), pulmonary disease (eg, sarcoid, COPD, pneumonia), ectopic tumor production/paraneoplastic syndrome (eg, small cell lung carcinoma), and drugs (eg, antipsychotics, antidepressants, NSAIDs). Euvolemic on physical exam.

DIAGNOSIS

- Serum osmolality < 280 mOsm/kg (hypotonic).
- Urine osmolality > 100 mOsm/kg in the setting of serum hypoosmolarity without a physiologic reason for ↑ ADH (eg, congestive heart failure, cirrhosis, hypovolemia).
- Urinary sodium level often ≥ 20 mEq/L.

TREATMENT

- Explore and address the underlying cause.
- **Best initial treatment:** Restrict fluid.
- **Persistent or symptomatic hyponatremia (< 120 mEq/L):** IV hypertonic saline therapy.
- **Severe SIADH:** ADH antagonists (eg, tolvaptan, conivaptan).
- **Chronic SIADH:** Demeclocycline.

Adrenal Gland Disorders

See Figure 2.3-20 for an overview of adrenal anatomy, regulatory control, and secretory products.

ADRENAL INSUFFICIENCY

Inadequate production of adrenal hormones, including glucocorticoids and/or mineralocorticoids. Adrenal insufficiency (AI) may be 1° or 2°/3°. Etiologies are as follows:

- **1°:** In the United States, most commonly caused by autoimmune adrenal cortical destruction (Addison disease). Other causes include congenital enzyme deficiencies, adrenal hemorrhage (Waterhouse-Friderichsen syndrome from *Neisseria meningitidis*), and infections (HIV, histoplasmosis, TB).

> **KEY FACT**
>
> Fluid restriction is the cornerstone of SIADH treatment.

> **KEY FACT**
>
> Correct hyponatremia slowly to prevent osmotic demyelination syndrome.

> **KEY FACT**
>
> Dehydroepiandrosterone (DHEAS) is produced only by the adrenal gland.

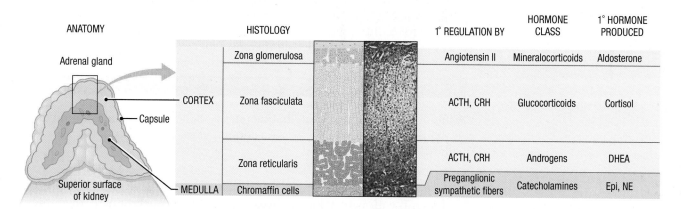

FIGURE 2.3-20. **Overview of adrenal anatomy, regulatory control, and secretory products.** ACTH, adrenocorticotropic hormone; CRH, corticotropin-releasing hormone; DHEA, dehydroepiandrosterone; Epi, epinephrine; NE, norepinephrine. (Reproduced with permission from USMLE-Rx.com.)

TABLE 2.3-11. Laboratory Findings in Adrenal Insufficiency

	CORTISOL	ALDOSTERONE	ACTH	SODIUM	POTASSIUM
1° Adrenal insufficiency	↓	↓	↑	↓	↑↑
2°/3° Adrenal insufficiency	↓	Normal	↓	Nl/↓	Nl

- **2°/3°:** Caused by ↓ ACTH production by the pituitary gland or ↓ CRH production by the hypothalamus; most often caused by cessation of long-term glucocorticoid treatment (often during higher doses and longer duration of therapy).

HISTORY/PE

- Most symptoms are nonspecific.
- Weakness, fatigue, and anorexia with weight loss are common.
- Hyperpigmentation (caused by ↑ ACTH secretion) and non–anion gap metabolic acidosis (caused by ↓ aldosterone deficiency) is seen in Addison disease.
- Hypotension, confusion, and coma is seen in acute adrenal crisis (eg, stopping long-term steroids).

DIAGNOSIS

- **Lab tests:** Hypoglycemia, electrolyte imbalances (see Table 2.3-11).
- 8 AM plasma cortisol levels and ACTH levels (see Table 2.3-11). An 8 AM plasma cortisol level < 3 μg/dL in the absence of exogenous glucocorticoid administration is diagnostic of AI.
- A synthetic ACTH stimulation (cosyntropin) test is the test of choice if morning cortisol levels are nondiagnostic. Failure of cortisol to rise > 20 μg/dL following ACTH administration confirms the diagnosis.

TREATMENT

- **1°:** Glucocorticoid and mineralocorticoid replacement.
- **2°/3°:** Only glucocorticoid replacement is necessary (mineralocorticoid production is not ACTH dependent).
- **Acute adrenal crisis:** Provide IV steroids, correct electrolyte abnormalities as needed, provide 50% dextrose to correct hypoglycemia, and initiate aggressive volume resuscitation.
- ↑ Steroids during periods of stress (eg, major surgery, trauma, infection).
- In patients on chronic steroid therapy, taper slowly to prevent 2°/3° AI.

PHEOCHROMOCYTOMA

A tumor of chromaffin tissue that secretes catecholamines and is found either in the adrenal medulla or in extra-adrenal sites. Most commonly associated with MEN 2A and 2B.

HISTORY/PE

- Presents with paroxysmal tachycardia, palpitations, chest pain, diaphoresis, hypertension, headache, tremor, and anxiety.
- Obtain a family history to rule out genetic causes of pheochromocytoma (eg, MEN 2A/2B, von Hippel–Lindau disease, neurofibromatosis).

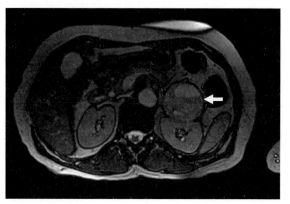

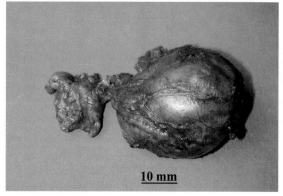

A   **B**

FIGURE 2.3-21. **Pheochromocytoma.** (A) MRI showing left suprarenal mass (*arrow*). (B) Pheochromocytoma post-surgical resection. (Reproduced with permission from Roghi A, et al. Adrenergic myocarditis in pheochromocytoma. *J Cardiovasc Magn Reson.* 2011;13:4.)

DIAGNOSIS

- **Best initial test:** Look for ↑ 24-hour urine metanephrines and catecholamines or plasma-fractionated metanephrines.
- **Imaging (only after labs):** CT or MRI of adrenal glands (see Figure 2.3-21). A nuclear metaiodobenzylguanidine (MIBG) scan can localize extra-adrenal lesions and metastatic disease.

TREATMENT

- Surgical resection.
- Preoperatively, use α-adrenergic blockade first (phenoxybenzamine) to control hypertension, followed by β-blockade to control tachycardia. Never give β-blockade first, as unopposed α-adrenergic stimulation can lead to severe hypertension.

HYPERALDOSTERONISM

Results from excessive secretion of aldosterone from the zona glomerulosa of the adrenal cortex. It is usually caused by bilateral adrenocortical hyperplasia (60–70%) but can also result from unilateral adrenal adenoma (Conn syndrome).

HISTORY/PE

- Presents with hypertension, headache, polyuria, and muscle weakness (caused by hypokalemia).
- Consider hyperaldosteronism in younger adults who are diagnosed with hypertension without risk factors or a family history of hypertension.

DIAGNOSIS

- **Lab tests:** Hypokalemia, metabolic alkalosis, hypomagnesemia, hyperaldosteronism, ↑ aldosterone-to-plasma renin activity ratio (usually > 30).
- **Imaging:** Only after labs. CT or MRI may reveal an adrenal mass.
- Adrenal venous sampling (will show ↑ aldosterone) may be needed to localize the adenoma or to confirm bilateral adrenal hyperplasia.

TREATMENT

- **Adenoma:** Surgical resection (after correction of BP and potassium).
- **Bilateral hyperplasia:** Aldosterone receptor antagonist (eplerenone preferred over spironolactone as has fewer side effects).

MNEMONIC

The 5 P's of pheochromocytoma—

Pressure (BP)
Pain (headache)
Perspiration
Palpitations
Pallor

KEY FACT

In pheochromocytoma, administer α-blockers before β-blockers to prevent hypertensive crisis.

Q   **1**

A 23-year-old man with a history of schizophrenia presents with complaints of fatigue, weakness, cramps, and headache for the past several days. He denies any other symptoms, although he had to urinate several times while in the office. Routine labs reveal hyponatremia. With water deprivation, his urine osmolality ↑. What is the most likely diagnosis?

Q   **2**

An asymptomatic 36-year-old woman presents with a 2-cm thyroid mass. TFTs are unremarkable, but FNA reveals medullary carcinoma. Total thyroidectomy with thyroid hormone replacement is recommended. What is the most important screening test to perform prior to surgery?

TABLE 2.3-12.   Overview of Congenital Adrenal Hyperplasia

Enzyme Deficiency	Mineralocorticoids	Cortisol	Sex Hormones	BP	[K⁺]	Laboratory tests	Presentation
17α-hydroxylase[a]	↑	↓	↓	↑	↓	↓ Androstenedione	XY: pseudohermaphroditism (ambiguous genitalia, undescended testes) XX: lack secondary sexual development
21-hydroxylase[a]	↓	↓	↑	↓	↑	↑ Renin activity ↑ 17-hydroxyprogesterone ↓ Sodium ↓ Chloride	Most common Presents in infancy (salt wasting) or childhood (precocious puberty) XX: virilization
11β-hydroxylase[a]	↓ Aldosterone ↑ 11-deoxycorticosterone (results in ↑ BP)	↓	↑	↑	↓	↓ Renin activity	XX: virilization

[a]All congenital adrenal enzyme deficiencies are characterized by an enlargement of both adrenal glands caused by ↑ ACTH stimulation (caused by ↓ cortisol).

Reproduced with permission from Le T, Bhushan V. *First Aid for the USMLE Step 1 2018*. New York, NY: McGraw-Hill; 2018.

1   **A**

1° (psychogenic) polydipsia, a condition in which patients consume large volumes of fluid, resulting in polyuria. It most often occurs in patients with psychiatric disorders. Patients present with symptoms similar to DI, but following a water deprivation test, urine osmolality ↑ (vs DI, in which urine remains dilute).

2   **A**

VMA and metanephrines. Medullary carcinoma of the thyroid is associated with MEN type 2A/2B, an autosomal dominant condition that predisposes patients not only to medullary carcinoma but also to parathyroid adenomas and pheochromocytomas. Screening for pheochromocytoma with urine VMA and metanephrines prior to surgery can prevent potentially life-threatening hypertensive crises during thyroidectomy.

CONGENITAL ADRENAL HYPERPLASIA

Inherited enzyme defects that impair cortisol synthesis and result in the accumulation of cortisol precursors. Most cases are caused by 21-hydroxylase deficiency (95%, autosomal recessive), but other causes include 11- and 17-hydroxylase deficiencies.

History/PE
See Table 2.3-12.

Diagnosis
- **Lab tests:** Electrolyte abnormalities (see Table 2.3-12). In severe cases, mineralocorticoid deficiency may lead to life-threatening salt wasting.
- Elevated serum 17-hydroxyprogesterone level is diagnostic of 21-hydroxylase deficiency.

Treatment
- Immediate fluid resuscitation and salt repletion. Administer cortisol to ↓ ACTH and adrenal androgens. Fludrocortisone is appropriate for severe 21-hydroxylase deficiency.
- Possible surgical correction of ambiguous genitalia.
- Refer to the Gynecology chapter for information on the diagnosis and treatment of late-onset CAH.

Multiple Endocrine Neoplasias

A family of tumor syndromes with autosomal dominant inheritance (see Figure 2.3-22).

- **MEN type 1 (Wermer syndrome):**
  - Pancreatic islet cell tumors.
  - Gastrinomas: Zollinger-Ellison syndrome.
  - Insulinomas: Recurrent hypoglycemia with elevated insulin and C-peptide levels.
  - VIPomas: Watery diarrhea, hypokalemia, hypochlorhydria.
  - Glucagonoma: New-onset diabetes, necrolytic migratory erythema.
  - Parathyroid hyperplasia.
  - Pituitary adenomas.
- **MEN type 2A (Sipple syndrome):** Medullary carcinoma of the thyroid, pheochromocytoma or adrenal hyperplasia, parathyroid gland hyperplasia. Caused by mutations in the RET proto-oncogene.
- **MEN type 2B:** Medullary carcinoma of the thyroid, pheochromocytoma, oral and intestinal ganglioneuromatosis (mucosal neuromas), marfanoid habitus. Caused by mutations in the RET proto-oncogene.

KEY FACT

Congenital aromatase deficiency will present similarly to CAH in female newborns with external virilization and ambiguous external genitalia. However, the patient will have no electrolyte or blood pressure abnormalities.

MNEMONIC

MEN 1 affects "P" organs—

Pancreas
Pituitary
Parathyroid

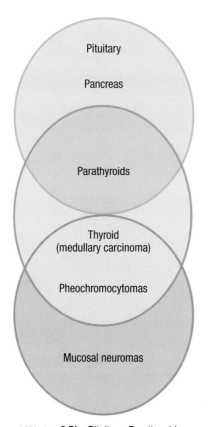

MEN 1 = **3 P's: P**ituitary, **P**arathyroids, and **P**ancreas
MEN 2A = **2 P's: P**arathyroids and **P**heochromocytomas
MEN 2 B = **1 P: P**heochromocytomas

FIGURE 2.3-22. **Multiple endocrine neoplasias (MEN).** (Reproduced with permission from UMSLE-Rx.com.)

EPIDEMIOLOGY

KEY FACT

Incidence can be measured in a cohort study; prevalence can be measured in a cross-sectional study.

KEY FACT

As the mortality of a disease ↓, the prevalence of that disease ↑ (eg, HIV infection), because the duration of disease has lengthened. Remember: P = I × D.

KEY FACT

Accuracy (and validity) measures bias. Accuracy requires correct measurements. Precision (and reliability) measures random error. Precision ↑ with ↑ sample size.

MNEMONIC

SNOUT—**SeN**sitive tests rule **OUT** disease.
SPIN—**SP**ecific tests rule **IN** disease.

Assessment of Disease Frequency

The prevalence of a disease is the number of existing cases in the population at a specific moment in time.

$$\text{Prevalence} = \frac{\text{total number of cases in the population at one point in time}}{\text{total population}}$$

The incidence of a disease is the number of new cases in the disease-free population ("population at risk") that develop over a period of time.

$$\text{Incidence} = \frac{\text{number of new cases in the population over a given time period}}{\text{total population at risk during the specified time period}}$$

Prevalence depends on incidence and duration.

$$\text{Prevalence (P)} = \text{incidence (I)} \times \text{average duration of disease (D)}$$

For incidence, remember to subtract any preexisting cases of the disease from the total population at risk, as these individuals are no longer at risk.

Assessment of Diagnostic Studies

SENSITIVITY AND SPECIFICITY

Physicians often use tests to narrow and confirm possible diagnoses. The sensitivity and specificity of these tests allow physicians to determine how often false⊕ and false⊖ results occur (see Figure 2.4-1). Both sensitivity and specificity are independent of disease prevalence.

- **Sensitivity:** The probability that a patient with a disease will have a ⊕ test result.
    - A sensitive test will rarely miss people with the disease and is therefore good at ruling out those who do not have the disease. A high sensitivity means there is a low false⊖ rate.
    - Desirable early in a diagnostic workup or screening test, when it is necessary to reduce a broad differential diagnosis.
    - Example: An initial ELISA test for HIV infection.

$$\text{False}\ominus \text{ ratio} = 1 - \text{sensitivity}$$

- **Specificity:** The probability that a patient without a disease will have a ⊖ test result.
    - A specific test will rarely determine that someone has the disease when in fact they do not and is therefore good at ruling in those who have the disease. A high specificity means there is a low false⊕ rate.

	Disease present	No disease	
Positive test	a	b	PPV = a / (a + b) LR+ = Sensitivity / (a − Specificity)
Negative test	c	d	NPV = d / (c + d) LR− = (1 Sensitivity) / Specificity

Sensitivity = a / (a + c)   Specificity = d / (b + d)
Prevalence = (a + b) / (a + b + c + d)

FIGURE 2.4-1.   Sensitivity, specificity, positive predictive value (PPV), and negative predictive value (NPV). Presence or absence of disease is typically assessed using a "gold standard" test, or the most accurate test available for a given disease.

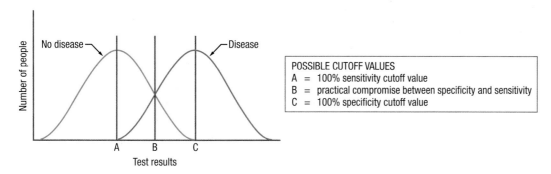

FIGURE 2.4-2. **Effect of cutoff values on sensitivity and specificity.** (Modified with permission from USMLE-RX.com.)

- Desirable when confirming a likely diagnosis. ↑ Specificity ↓ the number of false⊕ results.
- Example: A Western blot confirmatory HIV test.

$$\text{False} \oplus \text{ratio} = 1 - \text{specificity}$$

The ideal test is both sensitive and specific, but a trade-off must often be made between sensitivity and specificity (see Figure 2.4-2). For a given test, when sensitivity ↑, specificity ↓ (and vice versa).

Occasionally, you will be asked to compare different diagnostic tests using their receiver operating characteristic (ROC) curves, where sensitivity is plotted on the *y*-axis and 1 – specificity is plotted on the *x*-axis (see Figure 2.4-3). The best diagnostic test will have a curve that "hugs" the *x*- and *y*-axes (curve X).

POSITIVE AND NEGATIVE PREDICTIVE VALUES

Once a test has been administered and a patient's result has been made available, that result must be interpreted through use of predictive values. Remember, unlike sensitivity and specificity, positive predictive value (PPV) and negative predictive value (NPV) depend both on the test characteristics and the underlying disease prevalence.

- **PPV:** The probability that a patient with a ⊕ test result truly has the disease. The higher the disease prevalence, the higher the PPV of the test for that disease. A change in test cutoff point which ↑ both TP and FP will ↓ the PPV.

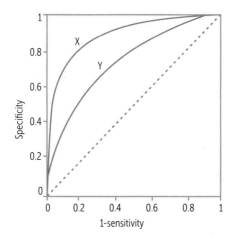

FIGURE 2.4-3. **Receiver operating characteristic (ROC) curves.** Curve X represents a better diagnostic test than curve Y. (Reproduced with permission of USMLE-Rx.com.)

Q

Your hospital is considering adopting a new diagnostic test for pheochromocytoma. In Figure 2.4-2, the current diagnostic test (urinary metanephrines) falls close to point B. The new test falls closer to point A. How will the false positive and false negative rates of this new test compare to urinary metanephrines?

- **NPV:** The probability that a patient with a $\ominus$ test result truly does not have the disease. The lower the disease prevalence, the higher the NPV of the test for that disease.

LIKELIHOOD RATIO

The likelihood ratio (LR) expresses the extent to which a given test result is likely in diseased people as opposed to people without disease:

- $\oplus$ LR shows how much the odds (or probability) of disease are $\uparrow$ if the test result is $\oplus$.
- $\ominus$ LR shows how much the odds (or probability) of disease are $\downarrow$ if the test result is $\ominus$.

$$LR+ = \text{sensitivity}/(1 - \text{specificity})$$

$$LR- = (1 - \text{sensitivity})/\text{specificity}$$

$$\text{Posttest odds} = \text{pretest odds} \times LR$$

Measures of Effect

A central aim of epidemiology is to assess the relationship between an exposure event and an outcome measure. The likelihood or risk of observing an outcome following an exposure is quantified using measures of effect. There are several ways to express and compare risk. These include the following:

- **Absolute risk:** The incidence of disease.
- **Attributable risk (or risk difference):** The difference in risk between the exposed and unexposed groups.

$$\text{Attributable risk} = \text{incidence of disease in exposed} - \text{incidence in unexposed}$$
$$= (RR - 1)/RR$$

- **Number needed to treat (NNT):** Number of individuals that need to be treated for one patient to benefit.

$$NNT = 1/\text{absolute risk reduction}$$

- **Relative risk (or risk ratio; RR):** Expresses how much more likely an exposed person is to get the disease in comparison to an unexposed person. This indicates the relative strength of the association between exposure and disease, making it useful when one is considering disease etiology.

$$RR = \frac{\text{incidence in exposed}}{\text{incidence in unexposed}}$$

$$RR > 1 \text{ suggests } \uparrow \text{ risk}$$

$$RR < 1 \text{ suggests } \downarrow \text{ risk}$$

- **Odds ratio (OR):** An estimate of relative risk that is used in case-control studies. The OR tells how much more likely it is that a person with a disease has been exposed to a risk factor than someone without the disease. The lower the disease prevalence, the more closely it approximates RR. In case-control studies, the OR also describes how many times more likely an exposed individual is to have disease compared to an unexposed individual (see Figure 2.4-4).
- **Hazard ratio (HR):** An estimate of the chances that an event occurs in the treatment arm of a trial vs the nontreatment arm. Calculated similarly to

---

A

The false positive rate will $\uparrow$ (capturing more of the "no disease" cohort), but the false negative rate will $\downarrow$ (capturing the little tail of the "disease" cohort).

	Disease develops	No disease
Exposure	a	b
No exposure	c	d

$RR = \dfrac{a/(a+b)}{c/(c+d)}$ Absolute risk = $(a+c)/(a+b+c+d)$
$OR = ad/bc$ Attributable risk = $a/(a+b) - c/(c+d)$
Number needed to treat = $1/AR$

FIGURE 2.4-4. **Relative risk (RR) vs odds ratio (OR).**

OR. Values < 1 indicate that the treatment arm had a ↓ event rate and values > 1 indicate the event rate ↑.

$$OR = \frac{\text{odds that a diseased person is exposed}}{\text{odds that a nondiseased person is exposed}}$$

Survival Curves

Once a diagnosis has been established, it is important to be able to describe the associated prognosis. Survival analysis is used to summarize the average time from one event (eg, presentation, diagnosis, or start of treatment) to any outcome that can occur only once during follow-up (eg, death or recurrence of cancer). The usual method is with a Kaplan-Meier curve (see Figure 2.4-5) describing the survival in a cohort of patients, with the probability of survival ↓ over time as patients die or drop out from the study.

Types of Clinical Studies

Studies are typically used to evaluate diagnosis, treatment, and screening for a disease. Although the gold standard for such evaluation is a randomized, double-blind controlled trial, other types of studies may be used as well (eg, an observational study, in which the exposure in question is a therapeutic intervention). In descending order of strength of evidence, published studies regarding treatment options include randomized controlled trials (RCTs),

KEY FACT

Randomization minimizes bias and confounding; double-blind studies prevent observation bias.

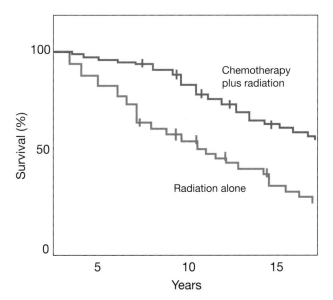

FIGURE 2.4-5. **Example of a Kaplan-Meier curve.** Tick marks indicate right-censoring, or patients who did not fulfill the outcome measure during follow-up. In this example, the blue curve represents a more favorable prognosis compared to the red curve.

observational studies, and case series/case reports. Meta-analyses are often used to systematically synthesize information across studies to help summarize the totality of the evidence. Randomization is successful when the baseline characteristics of patients in each group are statistically similar.

CROSS-SECTIONAL STUDY

A cross-sectional study is an observational study that assesses risk factors and outcomes at a snapshot in time. This study does not prove temporal relationships because it measures correlation, not causation.

Advantages of cross-sectional studies are as follows:

- Provide an efficient means of examining a population, allowing simultaneous assessment of people with the disorder and those without it.
- Can be used as a basis for diagnostic testing.

Disadvantages include the following:

- Causal relationships cannot be determined because information is obtained only at a single point in time.
- Risk or incidence of disease cannot be directly measured.

COHORT STUDY

In a cohort study, a group of people sharing certain characteristics (eg, age, gender, occupation, or date of birth) is assembled to study the relationships between exposures and outcomes of interest. For each possible risk factor, the members of the cohort are classified as either exposed or unexposed. All the cohort members are then followed over time, and the incidence of outcome events is compared in the two exposure groups. Example: The Framingham Heart Study followed a group of men and women over time to see how different exposures (eg, diet, exercise, aspirin) affected the incidence of heart disease.

Advantages of cohort studies are as follows:

- Only way to directly determine incidence (because they follow a cohort over time to assess disease development).
- Can be used to assess the relationship of a given exposure to many diseases.
- In prospective studies, exposure is elicited without bias from a known outcome.

Disadvantages include the following:

- Can be time-consuming and expensive.
- Studies assess only the relationship of the disease to the few exposure factors recorded at the start of the study.
- Requirements for many subjects makes it difficult to study rare diseases.

Cohort studies can be either prospective, in which a cohort is assembled in the present and followed into the future, or retrospective, in which a cohort is identified from past records and is followed to the present.

CASE-CONTROL STUDY

In a case-control study, a series of cases are identified and a set of controls are sampled from the underlying population to estimate the frequency of exposure in the population at risk for the outcome. In such a study, a researcher compares the frequency of exposure to a possible risk factor between the case

KEY FACT

A cross-sectional study that is undertaken to estimate prevalence is called a prevalence study.

KEY FACT

Cohort studies are also known as longitudinal studies or incidence studies, from which both OR and RR can be calculated.

KEY FACT

In cohort studies, the researcher determines whether the participants are exposed or unexposed and follows them over time for disease development.

and control groups. Example: A study examines patients with heart disease (cases) and without heart disease (controls) and compares exposures to red meat between both groups.

- Validity depends on appropriate selection of cases and controls, the way exposure is measured, and the way with which confounding variables are dealt.
- External validity (also known as generalizability) is the applicability of the results to a new population.
- Cases and controls should be comparable in terms of opportunity for exposure (ie, they should be members of the same base population with an equal opportunity of risk factor exposure).
- "Matching" occurs when the researcher chooses controls that match cases on a particular characteristic.
  - Example: If matching on gender, female cases would be matched to female controls and male cases would be matched to male controls.
  - The purpose of matching is to ↓ confounding.

Advantages of case-control studies are as follows:

- Use smaller groups than cohorts, thereby reducing cost.
- Can be used to study rare diseases and can easily examine multiple risk factors. This is because in case-control studies the odds ratio is a close approximation of relative risk, known as "rare disease assumption."

Disadvantages include the following:

- Studies cannot calculate disease prevalence, or incidence, or directly estimate the relative risk because the numbers of subjects with and without a disease are determined artificially by the investigator, not by nature. However, an OR can be used to estimate a measure of RR, if the prevalence is low.
- Retrospective data can be inaccurate because of recall or survivorship biases.

RANDOMIZED CONTROLLED TRIAL

An experimental, prospective study in which subjects are randomly assigned to a treatment or control group. Random assignment helps remove confounding and ensure that the two groups are truly comparable. The control group may be treated with a placebo or with the accepted standard of care.

The study can be masked in one of two ways: single blind, in which patients do not know which treatment group they are in, or double blind, in which neither the patients nor their physicians know who is in which group.

- Double-blind studies are the gold standard for studying treatment effects.
- Factorial design involves several rounds of randomization with two or more variables.
- Example: A trial studies the role of aspirin in preventing MI by giving one randomized group a baby aspirin daily and the control group a placebo. The rates of MI are then measured.

Advantages of RCTs are as follows (see also Table 2.4-1):

- Minimize bias.
- Have the potential to demonstrate causal relationships, because exposure is assigned randomly, which minimizes confounding.

Disadvantages include the following:

- Costly and time-intensive.
- Some interventions (eg, surgery) are not amenable to masking.

KEY FACT

In case-control studies, the researcher controls the number of cases and controls. Only ORs can be calculated from case-control studies.

Q 1

A local child care center that was built before the 1950s was found to have elevated lead levels in its paint. A student organization at your medical school is hosting a lead-screening event to test all children at the center. Which initial screening test would be more appropriate: a test that has high sensitivity or one that has high specificity?

Q 2

What happens to the PPV and NPV when prevalence ↓?

TABLE 2.4-1.   Comparison of Study Designs

VARIABLE	RCT	COHORT	CROSS-SECTIONAL	CASE CONTROL
Purpose	Tests causality through random assignment of exposure	Follows groups of patients over a specified period to capture the association of risk factors to the development of disease	Determines prevalence in a snapshot of time	Tests association (usually retrospectively, but outcome first, then looks for risk factors)
Measures	Varied, including response to treatment, adverse effects, survival during follow-up	RR, OR, incidence, prevalence	Prevalence (not incidence)	OR
Design	Subjects are randomly assigned to be in treatment or placebo arms	Subjects are not assigned to groups. Determines if subjects are in exposed or unexposed groups and follows them until they develop the disease (or do not)	Determines disease prevalence at one point in time; cannot determine the directionality of association between exposure and outcome	Identifies cases (disease) and controls (no disease) groups first and then goes backward to determine if they are exposed or not (the opposite of RCT and cohort studies)
Advantages	Can determine causality; minimizes bias and confounding	Temporality can be determined; incidence can be determined	Less time-consuming and costly	Predetermined number of cases; less time-consuming and costly
Disadvantages	RCT is not possible when: ▪ Treatment has a known adverse outcome ▪ Disease is very rare ▪ Treatment is in widespread use or represents the best option (because it is unethical to withhold treatment)	Follows large groups over long periods. Selection bias in retrospective cohort studies	Directionality of association cannot be determined. Incidence cannot be determined	Recall bias, selection bias

1 **A**

A test with high sensitivity, such as a fingerstick lead test (capillary blood), is preferred for initial screening because it can ensure that no children who might have the disease—and who might benefit from further testing and treatment—will be missed. The children with a ⊕ fingerstick test should subsequently have a serum blood level drawn (higher specificity).

2 **A**

PPV ↓ and NPV ↑. Remember that if prevalence is low, even a test with high sensitivity or specificity will have a low PPV.

Evaluating Clinical Studies

BIAS

Any process that causes results to systematically differ from the truth. Common types of bias include the following:

▪ **Selection bias:** Occurs when samples or participants are selected that differ from other groups in additional determinants of outcome.
  ▪ Example: Individuals concerned about a family history of breast cancer may be more likely to self-select in entering a mammography program, giving the impression of a prevalence that is higher than it is in reality.
  ▪ Example: If a substantial portion of subjects in one group are lost to follow-up (attrition bias), the study may overestimate the association. This is a special type of selection bias.

- **Measurement bias:** Occurs when measurement or data-gathering methods differ between groups.
  - Example: One group is assessed by CT, while another group is assessed by MRI.
- **Confounding bias:** Occurs when a third variable is either positively or negatively associated with both the exposure and outcome variables, inducing an incorrect association.
  - Example: Fishermen in an area may experience a higher incidence of lung cancer than that found in the general population. However, if smokers are more likely to become fishermen and are also more likely to develop lung cancer than nonsmokers, becoming a fisherman will not in itself lead to lung cancer. Rather, it is the smoking to which those fishermen are exposed that causes the association.
  - Effect modification, on the other hand, occurs when a third variable disproportionately affects two groups. Effect modification shows a meaningful difference, whereas confounding does not.
  - Example: A new chemotherapeutic agent is shown to improve survival in non-Hodgkin lymphoma, but only in patients who are undergoing radiation therapy, whereas those not receiving radiation show no benefit.
- **Recall bias:** Results from a difference between two groups in the retrospective recall of past factors or outcomes.
  - Example: A patient with cancer may be more motivated to recall past episodes of chemical exposure than would a healthy individual.
- **Observer bias:** Results from investigator's awareness of the population being studied and its exposure status.
  - Example: A trial for new blood pressure management in the ICU is biased when the attending physician knows which patients are enrolled in the treatment arm.
- **Hawthorne effect:** Results from study subjects' awareness that they are being studied, causing them to change aspects of their behavior.
  - Example: Employees at an automotive factory may work more productively when they realize that their superiors are conducting random audits.
- **Lead-time bias:** Results from earlier detection of disease, giving an appearance of prolonged survival when in fact the natural course is not altered.
  - Example: A new and widely used screening test that detects cancer 5 years earlier may yield the impression that patients are living longer with the disease.
- **Length bias:** Occurs when screening tests detect a disproportionate number of slowly progressive diseases but miss rapidly progressive ones, leading to overestimation of the benefit of the screen.
  - Example: A better prognosis for patients with cancer is celebrated following the implementation of a new screening program. However, this test disproportionately detects slow-growing tumors, which generally tend to be less aggressive.

STATISTICAL TESTING

Even with bias reduction, unsystematic random error is unavoidable because of chance variation in studied data. Types of errors are as follows:

- **Type I (α) error:**
  - The probability of concluding that there is a difference in treatment effects between groups when in fact there is not (ie, a false⊕ conclusion)—in other words, rejecting the null hypothesis (of no effect) when it should not be rejected.

KEY FACT

Studies that are masked and randomized are better protected from the effects of bias, whereas observational studies are particularly susceptible to bias.

KEY FACT

Confounding variables reduce the internal validity of a study.

Q

Assume that the data below are from a hypothetical case-control study. Calculate and interpret the OR.

	Exposed	Not exposed
Cases	283	263
Controls	182	210

- The **P** value is an estimate of the probability that differences in treatment effects in a study could have happened by chance alone if no true association exists. Often, differences associated with a **P**<0.05 are statistically significant. A **P** value alone does not give any information about the direction or size of the effect.
- **Type II (β) error:**
  - The probability of concluding that there is no difference in treatment effects when in fact a difference exists (ie, a false⊖ conclusion)—in other words, not rejecting the null hypothesis (of no effect) when it should be rejected.
  - Power is the probability that a study will find a statistically significant difference when one is truly there. Increasing the number of subjects in a study ↑ the power.

$$\text{Power} = 1 - \text{type II error } (\beta)$$

The confidence interval (CI) is a way of expressing statistical significance (P value) that shows the size of the effect and the statistical power (the narrower the CI, the greater the statistical power). CIs are interpreted as follows:

- If one is using a 95% CI, there is a 95% chance that the interval contains the true value.
- Larger sample sizes produce more power and narrower CIs. If the CI includes the null value (RR of 1.0% or 0%), the results are not statistically significant.
- Example: An RCT studying aspirin to prevent myocardial infarction shows a relative risk of 0.9 with a 95% CI of 0.85 to 0.95 in a sample of 3000 patients, whereas in a sample of 30 patients the 95% CI is 0.1 to 1.7. The first example shows a significant difference, whereas the second does not.

PREVENTION

There are three levels of prevention:

- **1° Prevention:** Includes preventive measures to ↓ the incidence of disease in unaffected individuals.
- **2° Prevention:** Focuses on identifying the disease early, when it is asymptomatic or mild, and implementing measures that can halt or slow disease progression. Includes screening tests that are designed to identify subclinical disease.
- **3° Prevention:** Includes measures that ↓ morbidity or mortality resulting from the presence of disease.

Prevention may be accomplished by a combination of immunization, chemoprevention, behavioral counseling, and screening. A good screening test has the following characteristics:

- High sensitivity and specificity (usually more important to have high sensitivity to rule out those who do not have the disease).
- High PPV.
- Inexpensive, easy to administer, and safe.
- Treatment after screening is more effective than subsequent treatment without screening.

VACCINATION

Vaccines work by mimicking infections and triggering an immune response in which memory cells are formed to recognize and fight any future infection. There are several different vaccine formulations, as indicated in Table 2.4-2.

A

OR = ad/bc
  = (283 × 210)/(263 × 182) = 1.24

Interpretation: The exposed group had 1.24 times the odds of having disease compared to the unexposed group.

TABLE 2.4-2.   Types of Vaccinations

VACCINE TYPE	TARGETED DISEASES
Live attenuated	Measles, mumps, rubella, polio (Sabin), yellow fever, influenza (nasal spray), varicella
Inactivated (killed)	Cholera, HAV, polio (Salk), rabies, influenza (injection)
Toxoid	Diphtheria, tetanus
Subunit	HBV, pertussis, *Streptococcus pneumoniae*, HPV, meningococcus
Conjugate	Hib, *S pneumoniae*

Recommended vaccination schedules for children and adults are outlined in Figures 2.4-6 and 2.4-7.

Live vaccines should not be administered to immunosuppressed patients (see Figure 2.4-8). They are also contraindicated in pregnant women owing to a theoretical risk for maternal-fetal transmission. A possible exception to this rule can be some asymptomatic HIV/AIDS patients who may be candidates for the MMR vaccine.

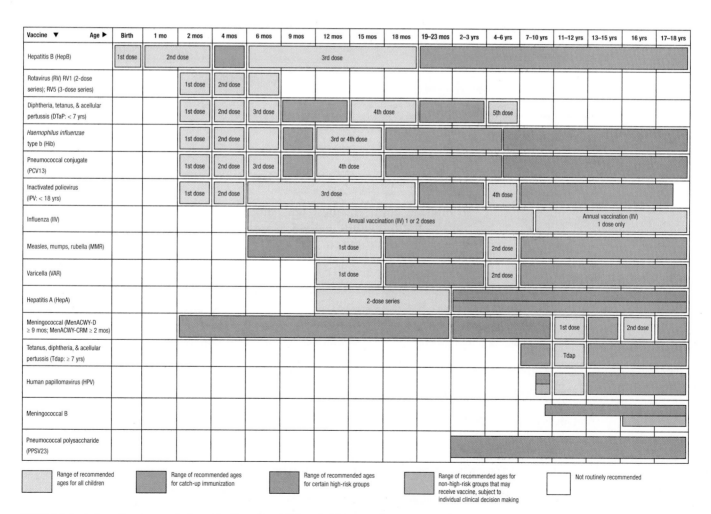

FIGURE 2.4-6.   Recommended vaccinations for children 0–18 years of age. (Reproduced courtesy of the Centers for Disease Control and Prevention, Atlanta, GA, https://www.cdc.gov/vaccines/schedules/downloads/child/0-18yrs-child-combined-schedule.pdf. Data from 2017.)

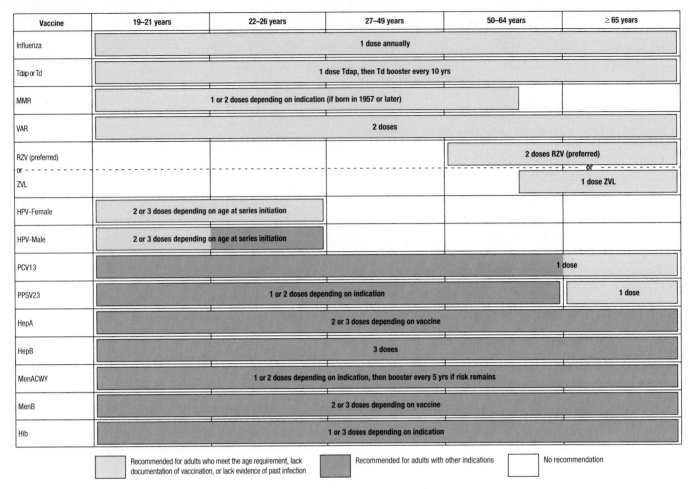

FIGURE 2.4-7.   Recommended vaccinations for adults. (Reproduced courtesy of the Centers for Disease Control and Prevention, Atlanta, GA, https://www.cdc.gov/vaccines/schedules/downloads/adult/adult-combined-schedule.pdf. Data from 2017.)

Behavioral Counseling

In offering counsel, physicians should tailor their education and suggestions to the individual patient as well as to his or her stage of change (see Table 2.4-3 and Figure 2.4-9).

TABLE 2.4-3.   Stages of Change in Behavioral Counseling

STAGE OF CHANGE	CHARACTERIZATION	EXAMPLE
Precontemplation	Denial or ignorance of the problem	A heroin addict has not even thought about cessation
Contemplation	Ambivalence or conflicted emotions; assessing benefits and barriers to change	The heroin addict considers treatment for his addiction
Preparation	Experimenting with small changes; collecting information about change	The heroin addict visits his doctor to ask questions about quitting
Action	Taking direct action toward achieving a goal	The heroin addict enters a rehabilitation facility for treatment of addiction
Maintenance	Maintaining a new behavior; avoiding temptation	The heroin addict continues to visit recovery meetings to gain support and reinforcement against relapse

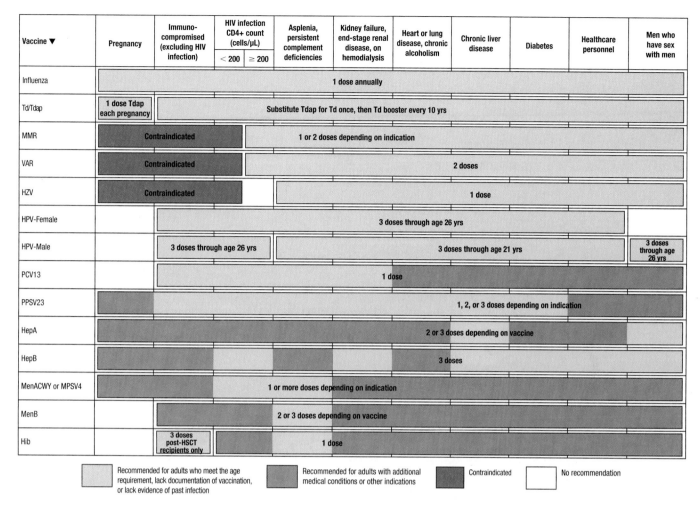

Vaccine ▼	Pregnancy	Immuno-compromised (excluding HIV infection)	HIV infection CD4+ count (cells/μL)		Asplenia, persistent complement deficiencies	Kidney failure, end-stage renal disease, on hemodialysis	Heart or lung disease, chronic alcoholism	Chronic liver disease	Diabetes	Healthcare personnel	Men who have sex with men
			< 200	≥ 200							
Influenza	1 dose annually										
Td/Tdap	1 dose Tdap each pregnancy	Substitute Tdap for Td once, then Td booster every 10 yrs									
MMR	Contraindicated			1 or 2 doses depending on indication							
VAR	Contraindicated			2 doses							
HZV	Contraindicated			1 dose							
HPV-Female		3 doses through age 26 yrs									
HPV-Male		3 doses through age 26 yrs			3 doses through age 21 yrs						3 doses through age 26 yrs
PCV13		1 dose									
PPSV23		1, 2, or 3 doses depending on indication									
HepA		2 or 3 doses depending on vaccine									
HepB		3 doses									
MenACWY or MPSV4		1 or more doses depending on indication									
MenB		2 or 3 doses depending on vaccine									
Hib		3 doses post-HSCT recipients only	1 dose								

☐ Recommended for adults who meet the age requirement, lack documentation of vaccination, or lack evidence of past infection   ☐ Recommended for adults with additional medical conditions or other indications   ☐ Contraindicated   ☐ No recommendation

FIGURE 2.4-8. **Recommended vaccines for special populations.** (Reproduced courtesy of the Centers for Disease Control and Prevention, Atlanta, GA, https://www.cdc.gov/vaccines/schedules/downloads/adult/adult-combined-schedule.pdf. Data from 2017.)

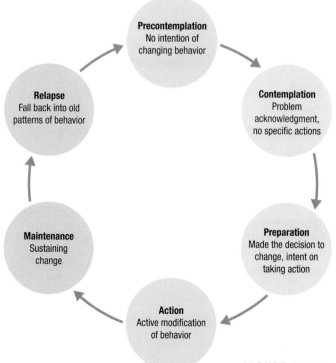

FIGURE 2.4-9. **Stages of change model.** (Reproduced with permission from USMLE-Rx.com.)

Screening Recommendations

Tables 2.4-4 and 2.4-5 outline recommended health care screening measures by gender and age.

TABLE 2.4-4. Health Screening Recommendations for Women by Age

AGE IN	RECOMMENDATION		
YEARS	CARDIOVASCULAR	BREAST/REPRODUCTIVE	OTHER
19–39	BP screening at least once every 2 years Cholesterol screening starting at 20 years of age for patients at ↑ risk of heart disease	Pap test every 3 years starting at 21 years of age; co-testing (Pap + HPV) may be done every 5 years starting at 30 years of age Chlamydia test yearly until 24 years of age if sexually active. Women ≥ 25 years of age should be tested only if there is an ↑ risk HIV test at least once to ascertain status Test for gonorrhea and syphilis if at ↑ risk	Diabetes: Blood glucose or HbA$_{1c}$ screening starting if BP > 135/80 mm Hg or taking medication for hypertension
40–49	BP screening at least once every 2 years Cholesterol screening for patients at ↑ risk for heart disease	Pap test every 3 years or co-testing every 5 years Pelvic exam yearly; chlamydia test if patient has new or multiple partners HIV test at least once to ascertain status Test for gonorrhea and syphilis if at ↑ risk	Diabetes: Blood glucose or HbA$_{1c}$ screening starting if BP > 135/80 mm Hg or taking medication for hypertension
50–64	BP screening at least once every 2 years Cholesterol screening for patients at ↑ risk for heart disease	Mammogram once every 1–2 years (can start at 40 years of age, if patient chooses) Pap test every 3 years Chlamydia test if patient has new or multiple partners HIV test at least once to ascertain status Test for gonorrhea and syphilis if at ↑ risk	Diabetes: Blood glucose or HbA$_{1c}$ screening starting if BP > 135/80 mm Hg or taking medication for hypertension Bone: Discuss BMD test with physician or nurse Colorectal: FOBT yearly; flexible sigmoidoscopy every 5 years or colonoscopy every 10 years
≥ 65	BP screening at least once every 2 years Cholesterol screening for patients at ↑ risk for heart disease	Mammogram once every 1–2 years until 75 years of age Discuss Pap test with physician or nurse Chlamydia test if patient has new or multiple partners Discuss HIV test with physician or nurse Test for gonorrhea and syphilis if at ↑ risk	Diabetes: Blood glucose or HbA$_{1c}$ screening starting if blood pressure higher than 135/80 or taking medication for hypertension Bone: BMD test at least once Colorectal: Screening with fecal occult blood testing, sigmoidoscopy, or colonoscopy every 10 years until 75 years of age

Modified with permission from the US Department of Health and Human Services, Washington, DC.

TABLE 2.4-5. **Health Screening Recommendations for Men by Age**

AGE IN YEARS	RECOMMENDATION		
	CARDIOVASCULAR	REPRODUCTIVE	OTHER
19–39	BP screening at least once every 2 years Cholesterol screening starting at 20 years of age for patients at ↑ risk for heart disease. Screen all men > 35 years of age	Both partners should be tested for STDs, including HIV, before initiating sexual intercourse Test for syphilis if at ↑ risk	N/A
40–49	BP screening at least once every 2 years Cholesterol screening for all men > 35 years of age	Discuss DRE and PSA with physician or nurse HIV test at least once to ascertain status Test for syphilis if at ↑ risk	Diabetes: Blood glucose or HbA$_{1c}$ screening starting if BP > 135/80 mm Hg or taking medication for hypertension
50–64	BP screening at least once every 2 years Cholesterol screening for all men > 35 years of age	Discuss DRE and PSA with physician or nurse HIV test at least once to ascertain status Test for syphilis if at ↑ risk	Diabetes: Blood glucose or HbA$_{1c}$ screening starting if BP > 135/80 mm Hg or taking medication for hypertension Colorectal: Screening with fecal occult blood testing yearly; flexible sigmoidoscopy every 5 years or colonoscopy every 10 years
≥ 65	BP screening at least once every 2 years Cholesterol screening for all men > 35 years of age	Discuss DRE and PSA with physician or nurse Discuss HIV test with physician Test for syphilis if at ↑ risk	Diabetes: Blood glucose or HbA$_{1c}$ screening starting if BP > 135/80 mm Hg or taking medication for hypertension Colorectal: Screening with fecal occult blood testing; flexible sigmoidoscopy every 5 years or colonoscopy every 10 years (patients > 75 years of age should discuss with physician) Abdominal aortic aneurysm: One-time screening for men who have ever smoked

Modified with permission from the US Department of Health and Human Services, Washington, DC.

Causes of Death

The leading cause of cancer mortality in the United States is lung cancer. Prostate and breast cancers are the most prevalent cancers in men and women, respectively, with lung and colorectal cancers ranking second and third most common in both sexes. Table 2.4-6 lists the principal causes of death in the United States by age group.

Q

A hypothetical study finds a ⊕ association between poor sleep habits and the risk for Parkinson disease. The RR is 10, and the *P* value is 0.4. How do you interpret these results?

TABLE 2.4-6. **Leading Causes of Death by Gender**

RANK	MEN	WOMEN
1	Heart disease (24%)	Heart disease (22%)
2	Cancer (23%)	Cancer (21%)
3	Unintentional injuries (7%)	Chronic lower respiratory diseases (6%)
4	Chronic lower respiratory diseases (7%)	Cerebrovascular diseases (6%)
5	Cerebrovascular diseases (4%)	Alzheimer disease (6%)
6	Diabetes (3%)	Unintentional injuries (4%)
7	Suicide (2%)	Diabetes (3%)
8	Alzheimer disease (2%)	Influenza and pneumonia (2%)
9	Influenza and pneumonia (2%)	Kidney disease (2%)
10	Chronic liver disease and cirrhosis (2%)	Septicemia (2%)

Modified with permission from the Centers for Disease Control and Prevention, Atlanta, GA, https://www.cdc.gov/nchs/data/hus/hus16.pdf. Data from 2015.

Reportable Diseases

By law, disease reporting is mandated at the state level, and the list of diseases that must be reported to public health authorities varies slightly by state. The CDC has a list of nationally notifiable diseases that states voluntarily report to the CDC. These diseases include but are not limited to those listed in Table 2.4-7.

TABLE 2.4-7. **Common Reportable Diseases**

DISEASE CATEGORY	EXAMPLES
STDs	HIV, AIDS, syphilis, gonorrhea, chlamydia, chancroid, HCV
Tick-borne disease	Lyme disease, ehrlichiosis, Rocky Mountain spotted fever
Potential bioweapons	Anthrax, smallpox, plague
Vaccine-preventable disease	Diphtheria, tetanus, pertussis, measles, mumps, rubella, polio, varicella, HAV, HBV, *H influenzae* (invasive), meningococcal disease
Water-/food-borne disease	Cholera, giardiasis, *Legionella*, listeriosis, botulism, shigellosis, shiga toxin–producing *E coli*, salmonellosis, trichinellosis, typhoid
Zoonoses	Tularemia, psittacosis, brucellosis, rabies
Miscellaneous	TB, leprosy, toxic shock syndrome, SARS, West Nile virus, VRSA, coccidioidomycosis, cryptosporidiosis. MRSA is reportable in several states

There is no sufficient evidence to reject the null hypothesis, and therefore there is insufficient evidence to support an association between poor sleep habits and the risk for Parkinson disease. Remember that the null hypothesis always assumes that there is no association between the exposure and outcome variables. If the **P** value is > 0.05, then you cannot reject the null hypothesis.

ETHICS AND LEGAL ISSUES

General Principles

- **Respect for autonomy:** Clinicians are obligated to respect patients as individuals and to honor their preferences.
  - Example: A pregnant women has the right to refuse cesarean section despite potential risk to the fetus. This is called the principle of maternal autonomy—so long as the mother has capacity, she has ultimate rights over her unborn child (in the United States).
- **Beneficence:** Physicians have a responsibility to act in the patient's best interest. Respect for patient autonomy may conflict with beneficence. In general, if a patient is mentally competent, respect for patient autonomy supersedes beneficence even if the physician believes the patient is not acting in his or her best interest.
  - Example: The physician has a responsibility to recommend a lifesaving transfusion to a Jehovah's Witness (beneficence) and respect the patient's autonomy if he or she should refuse.
- **Nonmaleficence:** "Do no harm." All medical interventions involve benefits and risks, and physicians should generally only recommend treatments where the likely benefits outweigh the known risks.
  - Example: A surgeon declines to perform a procedure, because she thinks the patient will die intraoperatively.
- **Justice:** Health care is a scarce resource. Fairness and equality in distribution and delivery of health care are ongoing challenges for health policy and in the clinical arena.

Informed Consent

- Willing and voluntary acceptance of a medical intervention by a patient after adequate discussion with a physician about the nature of the intervention along with its indications, risks, benefits, and potential alternatives (including no treatment).
- Patients may change their minds at any time.
- Informed consent is required for significant procedures except for the following:
  - Emergency treatment is required.
    - Example: An unconscious patient presents with cerebral edema after a motor vehicle collision, or a patient without previously indicated DNR/DNI (do not resuscitate/do not intubate) status undergoes cardiac arrest.
  - Patient lacks decision-making capacity. Consent is still required but must be obtained from a surrogate decision maker.
    - Example: Minors generally require surrogate decision makers until they demonstrate adequate decision-making capacity or are of legal age.

Minors

In general, minors (persons < 18 years of age) cannot consent for their own medical treatment and require parents or guardians to consent on their behalf (one parent is sufficient as long as that parent has custody), except in the following situations:

- **Life-threatening emergencies** when parents cannot be contacted.
- **Legal emancipation:** Emancipated minors do not require parental consent for medical care. Although emancipation laws vary from state to state,

in general minors are emancipated if they are married, are in the armed services, or are financially independent of their parents and have obtained legal emancipation.

- **Sexually transmitted infections and substance abuse treatment:** Rules concerning contraception, pregnancy, and abortion services and treatment for drug and alcohol dependency vary across the United States. In some states, the physician is left with the decision of informing parents about adolescent use of confidential services in the interest of best serving the patient; other states limit disclosure.

- **Refusal of treatment:** A parent has the right to refuse treatment for his or her child as long as those decisions do not pose a serious threat to the child's well-being (eg, refusing immunizations is not considered a serious threat). If a parental decision is not in the best interest of the child, a physician may provide treatment against parental wishes. In emergent situations, if withholding treatment jeopardizes the child's safety, treatment can be initiated on the basis of legal precedent. In nonemergent situations, the provider should seek a court order.
  - Example: A physician provides blood transfusion to save the life of a 6-year-old child seriously injured in a motor vehicle collision despite parental requests to withhold such a measure.

- **Prenatal care:** Some states allow, but do not require, parental disclosure when a minor seeks prenatal care.

Competence and Decision-Making Capacity

- **Competence:** A person's global and legal capacity to make decisions and to be held accountable in a court of law. Competence is assessed by the courts and is distinct from the term decision-making capacity.
  - Incompetent patients, as assessed by the courts, or temporarily incapacitated patients may still be able to provide assent for treatment or refuse treatment. However, the need to treat supersedes the refusal of an incapacitated patient in emergency situations.
    - Example: An extremely hypertensive patient with altered mental status who refuses treatment may receive antihypertensive therapy, as this constitutes a medical emergency.

- **Decision-making capacity:** The ability of a patient to understand relevant information, appreciate the severity of the medical situation and its consequences, communicate a choice, and deliberate rationally about his or her values in relation to the decision being made. This can be assessed by the physician.
  - Decision-making capacity is best understood as varying with the complexity of the decision involved.
    - Example: The level of capacity needed for a decision about liver transplantation is different from that needed to choose between two types of pain medication for fracture-related pain.
  - In general, patients who have decision-making capacity have the right to refuse or discontinue treatment.
    - Example: Jehovah's Witnesses can refuse blood products. When a Jehovah's Witness lacks decision-making capacity (eg, altered mental status or unconscious), the physician is allowed to provide a blood transfusion in an emergency situation.
  - A patient's decision to refuse treatment can be overruled if the choice endangers the health and welfare of others.
    - Example: A patient with active TB must undergo antibiotic treatment, because not treating would pose a public health threat.

KEY FACT

Brain death is the irreversible loss of all brain activity and is equivalent to cardiopulmonary death. If a patient is brain dead, no consent is needed to stop therapy. Two physicians are required to perform a brain death exam to legally declare a patient brain dead.

Q   1

A 47-year-old man is diagnosed with pancreatic cancer. His diagnosis and treatment options are discussed, but the patient refuses any intervention. He states that he would like to go home to his wife and children to die peacefully. What is the most appropriate next step in management?

Q   2

A 5-year-old girl with hydrocephalus needs another revision of her ventriculoperitoneal shunt. There are no satisfactory alternatives available to relieve her symptoms. Her father consents, but her mother refuses, arguing that she has been through enough procedures in her young life. What is the most appropriate next step in management?

Q   3

A 51-year-old man is brought to the emergency department after he was struck by a motor vehicle. He is unresponsive and in need of emergent surgery. His wife and children cannot be reached. What is the most appropriate next step in treatment?

End-of-Life Issues

WRITTEN ADVANCE DIRECTIVES

- **Living will:** Addresses a patient's wishes to maintain, withhold, or withdraw life-sustaining treatment in the event of terminal disease or a persistent vegetative state when the patient has lost the capacity to make decisions. DNR and DNI orders are based on patient preferences regarding CPR and intubation only. Patients can refuse all nonpalliative treatments or specific therapies (eg, CPR, intubation, antibiotics, feeding tubes). A living will overrides the wishes of the family.
- **Durable power of attorney for health care:** Legally designates a surrogate health care decision maker if a patient lacks decision-making capacity. More flexible than a living will. Surrogates should make decisions consistent with the person's stated wishes.
- **No living will:** If no living will or durable power of attorney for health care exists, decisions should be made by close family members (spouse, adult children, parents, and adult siblings) or friends, in that order.
- Ethics committees or court orders can be helpful when the patient lacks capacity, has no proxy or advance directives, and there is disagreement among family members, or when there is disagreement between the family and health care providers (eg, in cases of medical futility or parental refusal of necessary treatment for minors).

WITHDRAWAL OF CARE

1   **A**

Respectfully ask the patient about his reasons for not wanting to pursue treatment. Patients often need clarification and reassurance. If he continues to decline treatment, abide by his decision (respect for autonomy).

2   **A**

Proceed with the shunt revision. The consent of one parent is sufficient to proceed with the treatment of a minor, particularly when it is unequivocally clear that the decision is in the child's best interest.

3   **A**

Proceed with the surgery. A physician may give emergent treatment in the absence of informed consent when immediate intervention is necessary to prevent serious harm or death.

- Patients and their decision makers have the right to forego or withdraw life-sustaining treatment. Nevertheless, physicians should seek to understand patients and their reasons for refusing beneficial treatments.
- No ethical distinction is made between withholding a treatment and withdrawing a treatment, because a patient may choose to refuse an intervention either before or after it is initiated. This can include ventilation, fluids, nutrition, and medications such as antibiotics.
- Hospice care is focused on palliation of symptoms for patients with a prognosis of < 6 months of life. The focus is on pain management, quality of life, and bereavement.
- If the intent is to relieve suffering and medications administered are titrated for that purpose, it is considered ethical to provide palliative treatment to relieve pain and suffering even if it may hasten a patient's death (principle of double effect).
    - Example: A physician may prescribe a high-dose opioid analgesic to a patient who is expected to die within 1 day, even though it may suppress respiration and hasten death.

EUTHANASIA AND PHYSICIAN-ASSISTED SUICIDE

- Euthanasia is the administration of a lethal agent with the intent to end life.
    - It is opposed by the AMA Code of Medical Ethics and is illegal in all states.
    - Patients who request euthanasia should be evaluated for inadequate pain control and comorbid depression.
- Physician-assisted suicide consists of prescribing a lethal agent to a patient who will self-administer it to end his or her own life. This is currently

illegal except in the states of Oregon, Washington, Vermont, Colorado, and California. This is also legal via court order in Montana. Though legal in the aforementioned states, according to the AMA Code of Medical Ethics, physician-assisted suicide is "fundamentally incompatible with the physician's role as healer."

FUTILE TREATMENT

Physicians are not ethically obligated to provide treatment and may refuse a patient's or family member's request for further intervention on the grounds of futility under any of the following circumstances:

- There is no evidence or pathophysiologic rationale for the treatment.
- The intervention has already failed.
- Maximal intervention is currently failing.
- Treatment will not achieve the goals of care.

ALTERNATIVE TREATMENT

If a patient is interested in alternative/nontraditional treatment, the physician should obtain more information as to why the patient is interested. While the physician should provide as much information as possible, he or she should not dismiss the patient.

Disclosure

FULL DISCLOSURE

- Patients have a right to know about their medical status, prognosis, and treatment options (full disclosure). They have the legal right to obtain copies of their medical records within a specified timeframe.
- A patient's family cannot require that a physician withhold information from the patient without the knowledge and consent of the patient. A physician should explore why the family member does not want the diagnosis revealed, but ultimately the patient should be told.
- A physician may withhold information only if the patient requests not to be told, or in the rare and controversial case in which a physician determines that disclosure would cause severe and immediate harm to the patient (therapeutic privilege).

MEDICAL ERRORS

- Physicians are obligated to inform patients of mistakes made in their medical treatment.
- It is not appropriate for a physician to blame another physician for a medical error without obtaining additional information from the original physician.
- If the cause of a specific error or series of errors is not known, the physician should communicate this with the family promptly and maintain contact with the patient as investigations reveal more facts.
  - One of the largest contributors to medical error is failure to communicate during sign-out and hand-off processes. The best way to avoid communication breakdown is to implement a checklist for hand-off.

KEY FACT

Potential signs of elder abuse and neglect:
- Cuts, bruises, pressure ulcers, burns.
- Uncommon fractures.
- Malnutrition or dehydration.
- Anogenital injury or infection.
- Evidence of poor caretaking or financial exploitation.

KEY FACT

Signs of suspected child abuse:
- History given not consistent with injury.
- Unusual child or parental behavior.
- Delay in seeking medical care.
- Subdural hematomas.
- Retinal hemorrhages.
- Spiral, bucket-handle, or rib fractures.
- Injuries in different stages of healing.

Q

A 35-year-old woman visits a primary care physician after hurting her wrist. Physical exam reveals circumferential bruises of her wrist, neck, and arms. The patient admits that the injuries were inflicted by her husband. What is the most appropriate next step in management?

MNEMONIC

Overriding confidentiality—

WAIT a SEC before letting a dangerous patient go!

Wounds
Automobile-driving impairment
Infectious disease
Tarasoff (violent crimes) and Human
   Trafficking
Suicide
Elder abuse and neglect
Child abuse

KEY FACT

Guiding principles for overriding confidentiality:

- There is an identifiable third party at risk for harm.
- The harm is significant and probable.
- Disclosure will help prevent or mitigate the harm.
- Other measures, such as convincing the patient to self-disclose, have failed.

KEY FACT

Mandatory reporting of intimate-partner violence is controversial and varies by state. Nonetheless, physicians should document the encounter, offer support, and have resources available for assistance.

Offer support, and acknowledge the courage it takes to discuss abuse. Assess the safety of the woman and of any children involved, introduce the concept of an emergency plan, and encourage the use of community resources. If the patient consents, report the abuse to relevant authorities.

CLINICAL RESEARCH

- Physicians are obligated to inform patients considering involvement in a clinical research protocol about the purpose of the research study and the entire study design as it will affect the patient's treatment. This includes the possible risks, benefits, and alternatives to the research protocol.
- An informed consent form approved by the overseeing research institutional review board must be completed for participation in any clinical research protocol.
  - Newly deceased patients may be used for training health care providers. The physician must obtain permission from the family (or patient prior to death), and training must occur as part of a structured training program.

Confidentiality

- Information disclosed by a patient to his or her physician and information about a patient's medical condition are strictly confidential and should be discussed and accessed only by those directly involved in the patient's care, with few exceptions (described later).
- A patient may waive the obligation of the physician to protect confidentiality (eg, with insurance companies, authorized family members), preferably by way of written or verbal consent. The physician should disclose only the minimally necessary information.
- It is ethically and legally necessary to override confidentiality in the following situations:
  - **Patient intent to commit a violent crime (*Tarasoff* decision):** Physicians have a duty to protect the intended victim through reasonable means (eg, warn the victim, notify police).
  - **Suicidal patients.**
  - **Child abuse/neglect and elder abuse/neglect.**
  - **Reportable infectious diseases** (eg, HIV, sexually transmitted infections, tuberculosis). Duty to warn public officials and identifiable people at risk. It is normally best to encourage patients themselves to inform sexual contacts who are at risk for contracting the illness.
  - **Gunshot and knife wounds** (duty to notify the police).
  - **The patient is a danger to others** (eg, impaired automobile drivers). Currently, only six states have mandatory physician reporting laws.
    - Example: A patient begins to drive 1 week after hospitalization for seizures, although the department of motor vehicles in his state requires that licensed drivers be without seizures for at least 3 months.

Conflict of Interest

- Occurs when physicians find themselves having a personal interest in a given situation that influences their professional obligations.
  - Example: A physician may own stock in a pharmaceutical company (financial interest) that produces a drug he is prescribing to his patient (patient care interest).
- Physicians should disclose existing conflicts of interest to affected parties (eg, patients, institutions, audiences of journal articles or scientific meetings).
  - Accepting gifts from pharmaceutical companies can influence a physician's practice and should generally be avoided. Nonmonetary gifts should be accepted only if they will directly benefit patient care and are of small monetary value. A physician should never accept cash.

Malpractice

The essential elements of a civil suit under negligence include the **4 D's:**

- The physician has a **Duty** to the patient.
- **Dereliction** of duty occurs.
- There is **Damage** to the patient.
- Dereliction is the **Direct** cause of damage.

Unlike a criminal suit, in which the burden of proof is "beyond a reasonable doubt," the burden of proof in a malpractice suit is "a preponderance of the evidence."

Physicians may refuse inappropriate requests, such as demanding to be seen after hours. The physician should set clear limits and professional boundaries while remaining calm. If the patient has a nonurgent condition, the physician should not recommend that the patient visit the emergency department.

 KEY FACT

Physicians are not obligated to accept everyone coming to them as a patient. Furthermore, physicians have the right to end a doctor-patient relationship but must give the patient the resources and time to find another physician.

 MNEMONIC

The 4 D's of malpractice—

Duty
Dereliction
Damage
Direct cause

NOTES

GASTROINTESTINAL

KEY FACT

In an immunocompromised person with odynophagia, consider candidiasis.

KEY FACT

Esophageal webs are associated with iron deficiency anemia and glossitis (Plummer-Vinson syndrome).

Esophageal Disease

DYSPHAGIA/ODYNOPHAGIA

Difficulty swallowing (dysphagia) or pain with swallowing (odynophagia) caused by abnormalities of the oropharynx or esophagus.

Oropharyngeal Dysphagia

- Problem with initiation of swallowing; may lead to aspiration of food into the lungs.
- **Etiology:** Neurologic or muscular, including stroke, Parkinson disease, myasthenia gravis, prolonged intubation, and Zenker diverticula.
- Usually more of a problem with liquids than with solids.
- **Best initial test:** Modified barium swallow (video fluoroscopic swallowing exam). Esophagogastroduodenoscopy (EGD) may also be appropriate.

Esophageal Dysphagia

- Can be caused by an obstruction (eg, strictures, Schatzki rings, webs, carcinoma) or motility disorder (eg, achalasia, scleroderma, esophageal spasm).
- Obstructions usually more of a problem with solids than with liquids; while motility disorders cause both solid and liquid food dysphagia.
- **Best initial test:** EGD; consider pre-EGD barium swallow (aka esophagram) if history of esophageal radiation or strictures as these patients may be at higher risk for esophageal perforation (Boerhaave syndrome). May be followed by manometry in some cases.

INFECTIOUS ESOPHAGITIS

Seen in immunocompromised patients. Table 2.6-1 outlines the etiology, diagnosis, and treatment of infectious esophagitis.

TABLE 2.6-1. Causes of Infectious Esophagitis

ETIOLOGIC AGENT	EXAM FINDINGS	UPPER ENDOSCOPY	TREATMENT
Candida albicans **A**	± oral thrush (see Image A)	Yellow-white plaques adherent to the mucosa	Fluconazole PO (treat with more than a topical agent alone)
Herpes simplex virus	Oral ulcers	Small, deep ulcerations; multinucleated giant cells with intranuclear inclusions on biopsy + Tzanck smear	Acyclovir IV
Cytomegalovirus	Retinitis, colitis	Large, linear, superficial ulcerations; intranuclear and intracytoplasmic inclusions on biopsy	Ganciclovir IV

Image reproduced with permission from Kantarjian HM, et al. *MD Anderson Manual of Medical Oncology.* New York: McGraw-Hill; 2006.

Remember that esophagitis may also be caused by medications, especially tetracyclines, bisphosphonates, NSAIDs, and potassium chloride.

DIFFUSE (DISTAL) ESOPHAGEAL SPASM

Motility disorder in which normal peristalsis is periodically interrupted by high-amplitude nonperistaltic contractions (see Figure 2.6-1A).

HISTORY/PE

Presents with heartburn, chest pain, dysphagia, and odynophagia. Often precipitated by ingestion of hot or cold liquids; relieved by nitroglycerin.

DIAGNOSIS

- **Barium swallow:** Shows a corkscrew-shaped esophagus.
- **Esophageal manometry (most accurate test):** High-amplitude, simultaneous contractions in greater than 20% of swallows.

TREATMENT

- **Symptomatic relief:** Calcium channel blockers, tricyclic antidepressants (TCAs), or nitrates.
- **Severe, incapacitating symptoms:** Surgery (esophageal myotomy) but has limited utility.

ACHALASIA

- Motility disorder of the esophagus characterized by impaired relaxation of the lower esophageal sphincter (LES) and loss of peristalsis in the distal two-thirds of the esophagus.
- **Etiology:** Degeneration of the inhibitory neurons in the myenteric (Auerbach) plexus.

HISTORY/PE

Progressive dysphagia (solids and liquids), chest pain, regurgitation of undigested food, weight loss, and nocturnal cough.

KEY FACT

Candida esophagitis is an AIDS-defining illness.

KEY FACT

The musculature of the upper one-third of the esophagus is skeletal, whereas that of the lower two-thirds is smooth muscle.

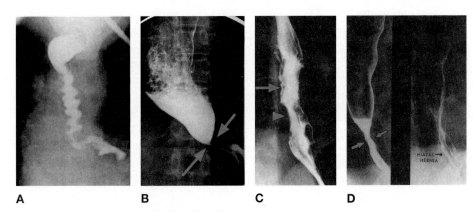

A   **B**   **C**   **D**

FIGURE 2.6-1. **Esophageal disease on barium esophagram.** (**A**) Esophageal spasm. (**B**) Achalasia. Note the dilated esophagus tapering to a "bird's beak" narrowing (*arrows*) at the LES. (**C**) Barrett esophagus with adenocarcinoma. Note the nodular mucosa of Barrett esophagus (*arrow*) and the raised filling defect (*arrowhead*) representing adenocarcinoma in this patient. (**D**) Peptic stricture (*arrows*) 2° to GERD above a hiatal hernia (*right*). (Image A reproduced with permission from USMLE-Rx.com. Image B reproduced with permission from Doherty GM. *Current Diagnosis & Treatment: Surgery,* 13th ed. New York, NY: McGraw-Hill; 2010. Images C and D reproduced with permission from Chen MY et al. *Basic Radiology,* 1st ed. New York, NY: McGraw-Hill; 2004.)

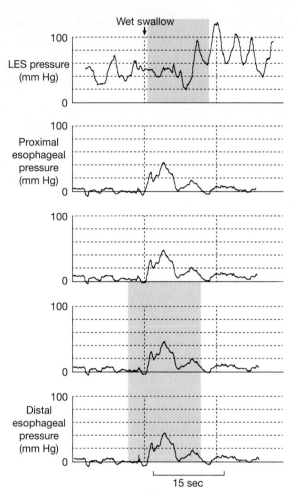

FIGURE 2.6-2. **Achalasia.** Manometry with incomplete LES relaxation. (Reproduced with permission from Farrokhi F, Vaezi MF. Idiopathic (primary) achalasia. *Orphanet J Rare Dis.* 2007;2:38.)

DIAGNOSIS

- **Best initial test:** Barium swallow; shows esophageal dilation with a "bird's beak" tapering of the distal esophagus (see Figure 2.6-1B).
- **Most accurate test:** Manometry; shows ↑ resting LES pressure, incomplete LES relaxation upon swallowing, and ↓ peristalsis in the body of the esophagus (see Figure 2.6-2).
- EGD to rule out structural disorders beyond achalasia (ie, mechanical obstruction) that may present similarly to achalasia (pseudoachalasia), especially cancer.

TREATMENT

- **Short term:** Nitrates, calcium channel blockers, or endoscopic injection of botulinum toxin into the LES.
- **Long term:** Pneumatic balloon dilation or surgical (Heller) myotomy.

ESOPHAGEAL DIVERTICULA

- Diverticula can be present in any location. Zenker diverticulum is defined as cervical outpouching through the cricopharyngeus muscle and is a posterior, false diverticulum (outpouching only through submucosa and mucosa).

- **Hx/PE:** Chest pain, dysphagia, halitosis, and regurgitation of undigested food.
- **Dx:** Barium swallow will demonstrate outpouchings.
- **Tx:** If symptomatic, treat with surgical excision of the diverticulum. For Zenker diverticulum, myotomy of the cricopharyngeus is required to relieve the high-pressure zone.

ESOPHAGEAL CANCER

- Squamous cell carcinoma (SCC) is the most common type of esophageal cancer worldwide. Adenocarcinoma is the most common type of esophageal cancer in United States, Europe, and Australia.
- **Risk factors:**
  - **SCC:** Alcohol, tobacco use, and nitrosamines.
  - **Adenocarcinoma:** Barrett esophagus (columnar metaplasia of the distal esophagus 2° to chronic GERD).

HISTORY/PE

Progressive dysphagia, initially to solids and later to liquids, is common. Weight loss, odynophagia, GERD, GI bleeding, and vomiting are also seen.

DIAGNOSIS

- **Best initial test:** Barium study. Narrowing of esophagus with an irregular border protruding into the lumen (see Figure 2.6-1C).
- **Most accurate test:** EGD with biopsy; required to establish the diagnosis.
- CT and endoscopic ultrasound for tumor staging.

TREATMENT

- **Best initial treatment:** Chemoradiation and surgical resection.
- Resection is also indicated in cases of high-grade Barrett dysplasia. Has a poor prognosis.

GASTROESOPHAGEAL REFLUX DISEASE

Symptomatic reflux of gastric contents into the esophagus, most commonly from transient LES relaxation. Can also result from an incompetent LES, gastroparesis, or hiatal hernia.

HISTORY/PE

- **Hx:** Heartburn that commonly occurs 30–90 minutes after a meal, worsens with reclining, and often improves with antacids, sitting, or standing; sour taste; a globus sensation; unexplained cough; morning hoarseness; and chest pain mimicking coronary artery disease.
- **PE:** Normal unless a systemic disease (eg, scleroderma) is present.

DIAGNOSIS

- Primarily a clinical diagnosis, with empirical treatment first (see below for lifestyle modification and medical treatment).
- **Most accurate test:** 24-hour pH monitoring with impedance; indicated if the diagnosis is uncertain.
- **EGD with biopsy:** Performed in patients whose symptoms are the following:
  - Refractory to initial empiric therapy.
  - Long-standing (to rule out Barrett esophagus and adenocarcinoma; see Figure 2.6-3).

KEY FACT

Esophageal cancer metastasizes early, because the esophagus lacks a serosa.

KEY FACT

SCC of the esophagus tends to occur in the upper and middle thirds of the esophagus, whereas adenocarcinoma occurs in the lower third.

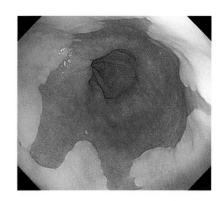

FIGURE 2.6-3. Barrett esophagus on upper endoscopy. Shown is an irregular Z line (squamocolumnar junction between the esophagus and stomach) caused by columnar metaplasia of the lower esophagus. (Reproduced with permission from Fauci AS et al. *Harrison's Principles of Internal Medicine,* 17th ed. New York, NY: McGraw-Hill; 2008.)

KEY FACT

GERD can also mimic angina or myocardial infarction.

KEY FACT

GERD is not a result of the presence of *Helicobacter pylori*. GERD arises from a transient relaxation of the LES.

- Associated with alarm symptoms like blood in the stool, weight loss, dysphagia/odynophagia (signs of obstruction), or chest pain.
- **Other studies:** Indicated for refractory symptoms or if concern for other causes. May include barium swallow (may demonstrate reflux see Figure 2.6-1D) or esophageal manometry.

TREATMENT

- **Lifestyle modifications:** Indicated for all patients. Includes weight loss, head-of-bed elevation, small but frequent meals, avoidance of nocturnal meals, avoidance of substances like alcohol, chocolate, or coffee that ↓ LES tone.
- **Pharmacologic:**
    - **Mild/intermittent:** Antacids.
    - **Chronic/frequent:** H_2-receptor antagonists (cimetidine, ranitidine) or proton pump inhibitors (PPIs) (omeprazole, lansoprazole).
    - **Severe/erosive:** PPIs first; if refractory, Nissen fundoplication surgery may be of benefit.
    - **Complications:** Erosive esophagitis, esophageal peptic stricture, aspiration pneumonia, upper GI bleeding, Barrett esophagus.

HIATAL HERNIA

- Herniation of stomach upward into the chest through the diaphragm.
- **Common types:**
    - **Sliding hiatal hernia (95%):** Gastroesophageal junction and a portion of the stomach are displaced above the diaphragm (see Figure 2.6-4).
    - **Paraesophageal hiatal hernia (5%):** Gastroesophageal junction remains below the diaphragm, while the fundus herniates into the thorax (see Figure 2.6-4).
- **Hx/PE:** May be asymptomatic. Patients with sliding hernias may present with GERD; paraesophageal hernias can cause strangulation.
- **Dx:** Incidental finding on chest x-ray (CXR); also frequently diagnosed by barium swallow or EGD.
- **Tx:**
    - **Sliding hernias:** Medical therapy and lifestyle modifications to ↓ GERD symptoms.
    - **Paraesophageal hernias:** Surgical gastropexy to prevent gastric volvulus.

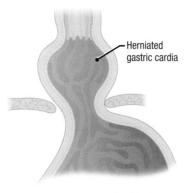

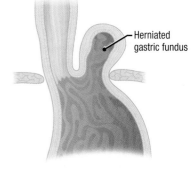

A

B

FIGURE 2.6-4. (A) Sliding hiatal and (B) paraesophageal hiatal hernia. (Reproduced with permission from USMEL-Rx.com.)

Disorders of the Stomach and Duodenum

GASTRITIS

Inflammation of the gastric mucosa. Subtypes:

- **Acute gastritis:** Rapidly developing, superficial or deep erosive lesions, often caused by NSAID use, alcohol, *H pylori* infection, and stress from severe illness (eg, burns, CNS injury). Toxic ingestion can also cause acute gastritis along with possible gastric outlet stricture.
- **Chronic gastritis:**
  - **Type A (10%):** Occurs in the fundus and is caused by autoantibodies to parietal cells. Causes pernicious anemia and is associated with other autoimmune disorders and ↑ risk for gastric adenocarcinoma and carcinoid tumors.
  - **Type B (90%):** Occurs in the antrum and may be caused by NSAIDs or *H pylori* infection. Often asymptomatic, but associated with ↑ risk for peptic ulcer disease (PUD) and gastric cancer. Note: *H pylori* infection can but does not always cause gastritis.

HISTORY/PE

Asymptomatic or symptoms of epigastric pain, nausea, vomiting, hematemesis, or melena.

DIAGNOSIS

Upper endoscopy is required to diagnose acute gastritis. Different tests for *H pylori* are shown in the Table 2.6-2.

TREATMENT

- Stop intake of exacerbating agents such as NSAIDs or alcohol.
- Antacids, sucralfate, H_2 receptor blockers, and/or PPIs may help.

TABLE 2.6-2. Tests for *H pylori*

TEST	DESCRIPTION	TEST CHARACTERISTICS
Serology	Detects IgG antibodies to *H pylori*	High sensitivity, high specificity. Cannot distinguish between treated and active disease
Urea breath test	*H pylori* urease converts radio-labeled urea (C14 or C13) to CO_2 and ammonia; this test detects CO_2 formed from urea metabolism	High specificity, lower sensitivity. PPIs may cause false ⊖ results
Stool antigen test	Detects *H pylori* antigens in stool	High specificity, high sensitivity. Cost-effective initial test for *H pylori*
Endoscopic biopsy	Detects *H pylori* on histology or culture. Can also detect intestinal metaplasia, mucosa-associated lymphoid tissue (MALT), or widespread gastritis	Gold standard for diagnosis of gastritis and *H pylori*. Most invasive test

KEY FACT

Type A gastritis is associated with pernicious anemia caused by lack of intrinsic factor necessary for the absorption of vitamin B_{12}.

KEY FACT

Stress ulcers include Curling ulcers, which are associated with burn injuries, and Cushing ulcers, which are associated with traumatic brain injury.

KEY FACT

H pylori antibodies stay ⊕ even when the infection is cleared. Use the urea breath test or a repeat stool antigen as a test of cure.

KEY FACT

Consider peptic ulcer disease or gastritis in elderly patients who are taking medications for arthritis or heart disease (eg, NSAIDs) who present with abdominal pain or GI bleeding.

KEY FACT

A gastric adenocarcinoma that metastasizes to the ovary is called a Krukenberg tumor.

KEY FACT

MALT lymphoma is a rare gastric tumor that presents in patients with chronic *H pylori* infection. It is the only malignancy that can be cured with antibiotics. Treat with triple therapy.

KEY FACT

Gastric cancer may present with Virchow node (an enlarged left supraclavicular lymph node) or a Sister Mary Joseph node (a palpable lymph node near the umbilicus).

KEY FACT

After a meal, pain from a **G**astric ulcer is **G**reater, whereas **D**uodenal pain **D**ecreases.

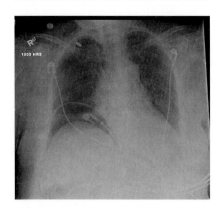

FIGURE 2.6-5. **Pneumoperitoneum.** Upright chest x-ray (CXR) reveals free air under the diaphragm. (Reproduced with permission from USMLE-Rx.com.)

- Administer triple therapy (amoxicillin, clarithromycin, omeprazole) to treat *H pylori* infection unless the patient is allergic to penicillin, in which case metronidazole should be substituted for amoxicillin.
- Give prophylactic PPIs to patients at risk for stress ulcers (eg, ICU patients).

GASTRIC CANCER

- Malignant tumor (mostly adenocarcinoma) with a poor prognosis that is particularly common in Korea and Japan.
- **Risk factors:** Diet high in nitrites and salt and low in fresh vegetables (antioxidants), *H pylori* colonization, and chronic gastritis.
- **Hx/PE:** Early-stage disease is usually asymptomatic but may be associated with indigestion and loss of appetite.
  - Late-stage disease presents with alarm symptoms: abdominal pain, weight loss, and upper GI bleeding.
- **Dx:** Upper endoscopy with biopsy (most accurate test) to rule out other etiologies and confirm the diagnosis.
- **Tx:** If detected early, treatment is surgical resection. Most patients present with late-stage, incurable disease. Five-year survival rate is < 10% for advanced disease.

PEPTIC ULCER DISEASE

- Results from damage to the gastric or duodenal mucosa caused by impaired mucosal defense and/or ↑ acidic gastric contents.
- **Risk factors:** *H pylori* (> 90% of duodenal ulcers and 70% of gastric ulcers), NSAIDs, alcohol, and tobacco use; concomitant use of corticosteroids and NSAIDs; male gender.

HISTORY/PE

- **Presentation:** Chronic or periodic dull, burning epigastric pain that is often related to meals and can radiate to the back; nausea; hematemesis ("coffee-ground" emesis); or melena (blood in the stool).
- **PE:** Usually normal but may reveal epigastric tenderness and stool guaiac.
- **Risks:** Acute perforation (rigid abdomen, rebound tenderness, and/or guarding).

DIAGNOSIS

- **Most accurate test:** Upper endoscopy with biopsy is the most accurate test. It can also be used to test for *H pylori* infection and to rule out active bleeding or gastric adenocarcinoma (10% of gastric ulcers without perforation).
- *H pylori* testing. See Table 2.6-2.
- If perforation is suspected, perform upright CXR (see Figure 2.6-5) to evaluate air under the diaphragm or CT scan of the abdomen.
- In recurrent or refractory cases, check serum gastrin levels to screen for Zollinger-Ellison syndrome.

TREATMENT

- **Acute management:**
  - **If perforation is suspected:** Perform x-ray of the abdomen (initial test) to rule out free air under the diaphragm. Consider CT (definitive test) if x-ray of the abdomen shows no perforation but there is high clinical suspicion. Then, surgery if perforation is confirmed on CT. Carefully monitor BP.

- Rule out active bleeding: Serial hematocrits (initially), rectal vault exam, NG suction. Monitor BP and treat with IV hydration, blood transfusion, and IV PPIs. Then, perform an urgent EGD (definitive) to control suspected bleeding.
- **Long-term management:**
  - **Medical therapy goals:** Protect the mucosa, ↓ acid production, and eradicate *H pylori* infection.
    - Mild disease: Treat with antacids, PPIs, or H₂-blockers.
    - *H pylori* infection: Triple therapy (omeprazole, clarithromycin, and amoxicillin).
    - Discontinue exacerbating agents (alcohol, tobacco).
  - **Endoscopy with targeted biopsy:** Indicated in patients with symptoms refractory to medical therapy to rule out gastric cancer.
  - **Surgical therapy (eg, parietal cell vagotomy):** Severe cases refractory to medical therapy.

COMPLICATIONS

Hemorrhage (most likely from posterior ulcers that erode into the gastroduodenal artery), gastric outlet obstruction (presenting with succussion splash), perforation, intractable pain.

ZOLLINGER-ELLISON SYNDROME

- Rare condition characterized by gastrin-producing tumors in the duodenum and/or pancreas that lead to excessive secretion of gastrin and recurrent or intractable ulcers.
- **Hx/PE:** Unresponsive, recurrent gnawing, burning abdominal pain; diarrhea; nausea; vomiting; fatigue; weakness; weight loss; and GI bleeding.
- **Dx:** ↑ Fasting serum gastrin levels and ↑ gastrin with the administration of secretin are diagnostic; CT is indicated to characterize and stage disease. Nuclear octreotide scan can also be used to facilitate localization of gastrinomas.
- **Tx:** Moderate- to high-dose PPIs to control symptoms. Surgical resection of the gastrinoma if not metastatic.

Disorders of the Small Bowel

DIARRHEA

- The most common mechanisms are malabsorption/osmotic, secretory, inflammatory/infectious, and ↑ motility. (See also Tables 2.6-3 and 2.6-4).

KEY FACT

A biopsy must be performed on all gastric ulcers to rule out malignancy.

KEY FACT

Misoprostol can help patients with PUD who require NSAID therapy (eg, for arthritis).

KEY FACT

Zollinger-Ellison syndrome:
- Hypercalcemia from hyperparathyroidism (In 20%, gastrinomas are associated with MEN type 1).
- Epigastric pain (peptic ulcer).
- Diarrhea (caused by mucosal damage and pancreatic enzyme inactivation leading to malabsorption).

TABLE 2.6-3. **Types of Stool Osmotic Gap**

STOOL OSMOTIC GAP	DESCRIPTION	EXAMPLES
Low osmotic gap (< 50 mOsm/kg)	Secretory diarrhea: ↑ Secretion or inhibition of absorption of water	Bacterial toxins (eg, cholera, *Escherichia coli*), VIPoma, gastrinoma, medullary cancer of thyroid
High osmotic gap (> 100 mOsm/kg)	Osmotic diarrhea: Osmotically active compounds in bowel draw in water	Celiac disease, Whipple disease, pancreatic insufficiency, laxative abuse

KEY FACT

Cryptosporidium and *Isospora* are associated with chronic diarrhea in patients with HIV/AIDS.

- **Stool electrolytes:** Primarily sodium and potassium (normal stool osmotic gap is 50–100 mOsm/kg).

$$\text{Stool osmotic gap} = 290 - 2 \times (\text{stool Na} + \text{stool K})$$

History/PE

- **Acute diarrhea:** Acute onset with a duration of < 2 weeks; usually infectious and self-limited.
  - Multiple pathogens may be responsible (see Table 2.6-4).

TABLE 2.6-4. Causes of Infectious Diarrhea

INFECTIOUS AGENT	HISTORY	EXAM AND TEST RESULTS (NOTE: ALL HAVE FECAL RBCs AND WBCs)	COMMENTS	TREATMENT
Campylobacter	The most common etiology of bacterial diarrhea Caused by ingestion of contaminated food or water Affects young children and young adults; generally lasts 7–10 days	Frequently presents with bloody diarrhea	Rule out appendicitis and inflammatory bowel disease (IBD)	Supportive treatment first, then fluoroquinolones (eg, ciprofloxacin) or azithromycin
Clostridium difficile	Associated with recent treatment with antibiotics (penicillins, quinolones, clindamycin) Affects hospitalized adult patients Watch for toxic megacolon (seen on x-ray of the abdomen)	Presents with fever, abdominal pain, and possible systemic toxicity	Most commonly causes colitis, but can involve the small bowel Identify *C difficile* toxin in the stool Sigmoidoscopy shows pseudomembranes	Cessation of the inciting antibiotic Treat with PO metronidazole (mild disease), PO vancomycin (moderate-severe disease), or IV metronidazole ± rectal vancomycin (if ileus) PO fidaxomicin useful when there are multiple relapses on previous antibiotics
Echinococcus granulosus	Contracted from close contact with dogs, definitive host for tapeworm. Causes simple liver cysts	"Eggshell calcification" on CT scan Usually found incidentally, but may cause mild right upper quadrant (RUQ) pain caused by compression of other structures	Cyst aspiration may cause cyst rupture and anaphylactic shock	Surgical resection and albendazole
Entamoeba histolytica	Caused by ingestion of contaminated food or water; look for a history of travel in developing countries The incubation period can last up to 3 months	Presents with severe abdominal pain and fever Endoscopy shows "flask-shaped" ulcers	Chronic amebic colitis mimics IBD	Steroids can lead to fatal perforation Treat with metronidazole

(continues)

TABLE 2.6-4. **Causes of Infectious Diarrhea** *(continued)*

INFECTIOUS AGENT	HISTORY	EXAM AND TEST RESULTS (NOTE: ALL HAVE FECAL RBCs AND WBCs)	COMMENTS	TREATMENT
E coli O157:H7	Caused by ingestion of contaminated food (raw meat) Affects children and the elderly; generally lasts 5–10 days	Presents with severe abdominal pain, low-grade fever, and vomiting	It is important to rule out GI bleeding and ischemic colitis Hemolytic uremic syndrome (HUS) is a potential complication, primarily in children	Avoid antibiotic or antidiarrheal therapy, which ↑ HUS risk
Salmonella	Caused by ingestion of contaminated poultry or eggs Affects young children and the elderly; generally lasts 2–5 days	Presents with a prodromal headache, fever, myalgia, and abdominal pain	Sepsis is a concern, as 5–10% of patients become bacteremic Sickle cell patients are susceptible to invasive disease leading to osteomyelitis	First fluids. Treat bacteremia or at-risk patients (eg, sickle cell patients) with oral quinolone or TMP-SMX
Shigella	Extremely contagious; transmitted between people by the fecal-oral route Affects young children and institutionalized patients		May lead to severe dehydration Can also cause febrile seizures in the very young	Treat with TMP-SMX to ↓ person-to-person spread
Taenia solium	Pork tapeworm. Acquired by ingestion of undercooked pork	Presents with signs of elevated intracranial pressure (headaches, vomiting, seizures, visual changes)	Diagnosed via CT or magnetic resonance imaging (MRI) showing several cysts with edema	Treat with albendazole and with symptomatic management of CNS symptoms
Trichinella	Acquired by ingestion of undercooked meat in developing countries (especially Mexico and Thailand)	Classic triad of myositis, periorbital edema, and eosinophilia	Multiorgan involvement is possible	

- Common causes of pediatric diarrhea are rotavirus, Norwalk virus, and enterovirus infection.
- **Chronic diarrhea:** Insidious onset with a duration of > 4 weeks.
    - **Secretory:** Carcinoid tumors, VIPomas.
    - **Malabsorption/maldigestive/osmotic:** Bacterial overgrowth, pancreatic insufficiency, mucosal damage, lactose intolerance, celiac disease, laxative abuse (presents with dark brown colonic discoloration), postsurgical short bowel syndrome.
    - **Inflammatory/infectious:** Inflammatory bowel disease (IBD), giardiasis, amoebic dysentery.
    - **Increased motility:** Irritable bowel syndrome (IBS).

DIAGNOSIS

- **Acute diarrhea:** No further studies are indicated unless the patient has a high fever, bloody diarrhea, or diarrhea lasting > 4–5 days.

KEY FACT

Organisms that cause bloody diarrhea include *Salmonella*, *Shigella*, *E coli* (EHEC), and *Campylobacter*.

KEY FACT

Organisms that cause watery diarrhea include *Vibrio cholerae*, rotavirus, *E coli* (ETEC), *Cryptosporidium*, *Giardia*, and norovirus.

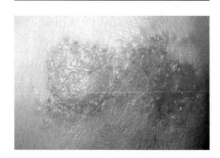

FIGURE 2.6-6. Dermatitis herpetiformis. Grouped, papulovesicular, pruritic skin lesions are shown. Lesions tend to be symmetrically located on the extensor surfaces of the elbows, knees, buttocks, and posterior scalp, and are associated with celiac disease. (Reproduced with permission from Caproni M et al. Celiac disease and dermatologic manifestations: many skin clues to unfold gluten-sensitive enteropathy. *Gastroenterol Res Pract.* 2012;2012:952753.)

- **Chronic diarrhea:** History/physical exam to narrow the differential diagnosis. Additional studies include the following:
    - **Stool analysis:** Leukocytes, culture, *C difficile* toxin, and ova and parasite exam (O&P).

TREATMENT

- **Acute diarrhea:** Oral rehydration is key. Antibiotics are not indicated (except in *C difficile* infection, or in the epidemic setting), because they do not shorten the course of illness.
- **Chronic diarrhea:** Treatment is etiology specific.

MALABSORPTION/MALDIGESTION

- Inability to absorb macro- and/or micronutrients. Common etiologies include the following:
    - **Mucosal abnormalities:** Celiac disease (associated with dermatitis herpetiformis; see Figure 2.6-6), Whipple disease (also presents with arthritis, lymphadenopathy, cardiac issues, PAS positive granules in lamina propria on biopsy), tropical sprue.
    - **Bile salt deficiency:** Ileal disease in Crohn disease or small bowel resections (> 100 cm of terminal ileum), bacterial overgrowth.
    - **Other:** Pancreatic insufficiency, short bowel syndrome.
- **Hx/PE:** Presents with pale, foul-smelling, bulky stools (steatorrhea or fat maldigestion) associated with abdominal pain, flatus, bloating, weight loss, nutritional deficiencies, and fatigue.
- **Dx:** Multiple laboratory tests based on the clinical suspicion. Biopsy is definitive.
- **Tx:** Etiology dependent. In severe cases, patients may require TPN, immunosuppressants, and anti-inflammatory medications.

LACTOSE INTOLERANCE

- Common among populations of African, Asian, and Native American descent, also transiently after an acute episode of gastroenteritis.
- **Hx/PE:** Presents with abdominal bloating, flatulence, cramping, and watery diarrhea following milk ingestion.
- **Dx:** Often treated empirically with lactose-free diet. Hydrogen breath test reveals ↑ hydrogen following the ingestion of lactose.
- **Tx:** Avoidance of dairy products; oral lactase enzyme replacement.

CARCINOID SYNDROME

- Carcinoid syndrome is caused by metastasis of carcinoid tumors, which most commonly arise from the ileum and appendix and produce serotonin. Prior to metastasis, most secreted hormones undergo first-pass metabolism by the liver and do not cause systemic symptoms.
- **Hx/PE:** Cutaneous flushing, diarrhea, abdominal cramps, wheezing, and right-sided cardiac valvular lesions are the most common manifestations.
- **Dx:** High urine levels of the serotonin metabolite 5-HIAA (best initial test) are diagnostic. CT and In-111 octreotide scans are used to localize the tumor.
- **Tx:** Treatment includes octreotide and surgical resection.

IRRITABLE BOWEL SYNDROME

An idiopathic functional disorder that commonly affects women in their 20s to 30s; often patients have comorbid psychiatric disorders like depression, anxiety, and fibromyalgia.

HISTORY/PE

- Patients present with abdominal pain that is relieved by bowel movements, diarrhea and/or constipation, abdominal distention, and mucous stools. Symptoms often worsen with stress.
- **No alarm symptoms:** Rarely awakens patients from sleep; vomiting, significant weight loss, and constitutional symptoms are uncommon.
- **PE:** Usually unremarkable.

DIAGNOSIS

- **Definition (per Rome III diagnostic criteria):** At least 3 days in 3 months of episodic abdominal discomfort that is (two or more criteria): (1) relieved by defecation; (2) associated with a change in stool frequency or consistency; (3) associated with a change in stool appearance.
- Exclude organic disorders such as IBD; increased prevalence of celiac disease in IBS, so celiac should be ruled out when IBS is suspected.

TREATMENT

- **Psychosocial:** Patients benefit from a strong patient-physician relationship. Physicians should offer reassurance and should not dismiss the symptoms.
- **Diet:** Fiber supplements (psyllium); exclude gas-producing foods.
- Chronic constipation may lead to anal fissures. Treat with topical anesthetics and vasodilators.
- **Pharmacologic:** Symptomatic treatment with antispasmodics. TCAs and SSRIs may help. Long-term medical therapy is usually not indicated.

> **KEY FACT**
>
> In the United States, the leading cause of SBO in children is hernia. The leading cause of SBO in adults is adhesions.

SMALL BOWEL OBSTRUCTION

Partial or complete blockage of passage of bowel contents through the small bowel.

- **Etiologies:** Adhesions (60% of cases), hernias (10–20%), neoplasms (10–20%), intussusception, gallstone ileus, stricture caused by IBD, and volvulus.
- **Partial small bowel obstruction (SBO):** Continued passage of flatus, but no stool.
- **Complete SBO:** No passage of flatus or stool (obstipation).

HISTORY/PE

- **Hx:** Crampy abdominal pain at 4- to 5-minute intervals; vomiting typically follows the pain.
- **Abdominal exam:** Distention, tenderness, prior surgical scars, or hernias, hyperactive bowel sounds (high-pitched tinkles and peristaltic rushes).
- **Complications:** Ischemic necrosis and bowel rupture with prolonged or complete obstruction. Patients present with peritonitis manifested by fever, hypotension, rebound tenderness, and tachycardia.

> **Q**
>
> A 53-year-old woman with a history of carcinoid tumor of the appendix (status post-resection) presents to a local clinic with symmetric, dry, hyperpigmented skin lesions and persistent diarrhea. Her husband expresses concern that the patient does not seem to be herself anymore; he reports that she has been irritable, confused, and forgetful. What is the most likely diagnosis?

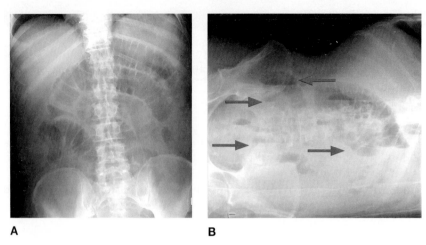

A   **B**

FIGURE 2.6-7. **Small bowel obstruction.** **(A)** Supine x-ray of the abdomen shows dilated air-filled small bowel loops with relatively little gas in the colon. **(B)** Left lateral decubitus x-ray on the same patient demonstrates multiple air-fluid levels *(arrows)* at different levels. These are typical plain film findings of complete SBO. (Reproduced with permission from Doherty GM. *Current Diagnosis & Treatment: Surgery*, 13th ed. New York, NY: McGraw-Hill; 2010.)

DIAGNOSIS

- **Best initial test:** Abdominal x-ray demonstrates a stepladder pattern of dilated small bowel loops, air-fluid levels (see Figure 2.6-7), and a paucity of gas in the colon.
- **Most accurate test:** CT scan of the abdomen to further characterize obstruction and evaluate for etiology.
- CBC may demonstrate leukocytosis if there is ischemia or necrosis of bowel.
- Lab tests often reveal dehydration. Lactic acidosis is a prognostic sign, as it suggests necrotic bowel.

TREATMENT

- **Best initial treatment:** Fluid resuscitation.
- **Partial obstruction:** Supportive care may be sufficient and should include NPO status, NG suction, IV hydration, correction of electrolyte abnormalities, Foley catheterization to monitor fluid status, and pain management; avoid opioids and anticholinergics (slow GI motility).
- **Complete obstruction:** Exploratory laparotomy indicated in complete SBO, ischemic necrosis, or refractory SBO symptoms.

KEY FACT

Gallstone ileus is a form of SBO that occurs when a gallstone lodges at the ileocecal valve.

Pellagra, a deficiency of vitamin B$_3$ (niacin), 2° to a recurrent carcinoid tumor. Carcinoid tumors produce serotonin, which is a derivative of tryptophan. However, tryptophan is also the precursor of niacin. In patients with carcinoid tumors, the tumor can be so active that most tryptophan is used for serotonin production, resulting in niacin deficiency.

ILEUS

- Loss of peristalsis without structural obstruction.
- **Risk factors:** Recent surgery/GI procedures, severe medical illness, immobility, hypokalemia or other electrolyte imbalances, hypothyroidism, diabetes mellitus (DM), and medications that slow GI motility (eg, anticholinergics, opioids).

HISTORY/PE

- **Hx:** Diffuse, constant abdominal discomfort, nausea and vomiting, and an absence of flatus or bowel movements.
- **PE:** Diffuse tenderness, abdominal distention, and ↓ or absent bowel sounds; rectal exam required to rule out fecal impaction in elderly patients.

DIAGNOSIS

- Must consider clinical history in diagnosis.
- **Best initial test:** Abdominal film shows distended loops of small and large bowel, with air seen throughout the colon and rectum (SBO has no air distal to the obstruction).
- **Most accurate test:** CT scan of the abdomen.

TREATMENT

- ↓ or discontinue the use of narcotics and any other drugs that reduce bowel motility.
- **Bowel rest:** Temporarily ↓ or discontinue oral feeds.
- **Bowel decompression:** Initiate NG suction/parenteral feeds as necessary.
- **Supportive care:** Replete electrolytes as needed; hydrate with IV fluids.

KEY FACT

In ileus, there is air present throughout the small and large bowel on x-ray of the abdomen.

MESENTERIC ISCHEMIA

Insufficient blood supply to the small intestine, resulting in ischemia and, potentially, necrosis. The most common causes are as follows:

- **Embolism:** Emboli most commonly originate in the heart. Risk factors include atrial fibrillation and stasis from ↓ ejection fraction.
- **Acute arterial occlusion from thrombosis:** Most commonly occurs in the proximal SMA. The 1° risk factor is atherosclerosis.
- **Other causes:** Nonocclusive arterial disease (atherosclerosis of mesenteric vessels, arteriolar vasospasm), venous thrombosis (caused by hypercoagulable states), or shock state.

HISTORY/PE

- Presents with severe abdominal pain out of proportion to the exam, nausea, vomiting, diarrhea, bloody stools, prior episodes of abdominal pain after eating ("intestinal angina").

DIAGNOSIS

- **Best initial test:** x-ray or CT scan of the abdomen may reveal bowel wall edema ("thumbprinting") and air within the bowel wall (pneumatosis intestinalis).
- **Most accurate test:** Mesenteric/CT angiography; gold standard for diagnosis of arterial occlusive disease, but conventional angiography allows for intervention of thrombosis/embolism.

TREATMENT

- **Best initial treatment:** Volume resuscitation, broad-spectrum antibiotics.
- **For acute arterial thrombosis or embolism:** Anticoagulation and either laparotomy or angioplasty.
- **For venous thrombosis:** Anticoagulation.
- **Surgery:** Resect infarcted bowel.

COMPLICATIONS

Sepsis/septic shock, multisystem organ failure, death

KEY FACT

Cholesterol embolism may occur following cardiac catheterization, and ischemia of multiple organs may be seen (bowel, kidney, pancreas, lower extremity skin causing livedo reticularis).

APPENDICITIS

See the Surgery and Emergency Medicine chapter.

Disorders of the Large Bowel

KEY FACT

Diverticulosis is the most common cause of acute lower GI bleeding in patients > 40 years of age.

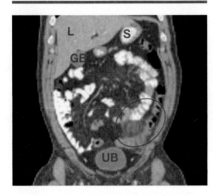

FIGURE 2.6-8. Acute diverticulitis. Coronal reconstruction from a contrast-enhanced CT demonstrates sigmoid diverticula with presigmoid inflammatory "fat stranding." The area of abnormality is circled in red. L, liver; S, stomach; GB, gallbladder; UB, urinary bladder. (Reproduced with permission from USMLE-Rx.com.)

 KEY FACT

Sigmoidoscopy should be avoided in the initial stages of diverticulitis because of the risk for perforation.

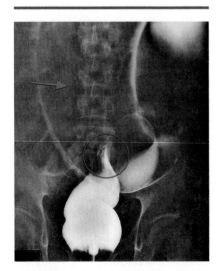

FIGURE 2.6-9. Large bowel obstruction. Anteroposterior x-ray from a barium enema in a patient with an LBO reveals a massively dilated sigmoid colon (*arrow*) and a "bird's beak" appearance of the barium column at the site of volvulus (*circle*). (Reproduced with permission from Doherty GM. *Current Diagnosis & Treatment: Surgery*, 13th ed. New York, NY: McGraw-Hill; 2010.)

DIVERTICULAR DISEASE

- **Diverticula:** Outpouching of mucosa and submucosa (false diverticula) that herniate through the colonic muscle layers in areas of high intraluminal pressure; most commonly found in the sigmoid colon.
- **Diverticulosis:** Many diverticula, most common cause of acute lower GI bleeding in patients > 40 years of age.
- **Diverticulitis:** Inflammation and, generally, microperforation of a diverticulum 2° to fecalith impaction.
- **Risk factors:** Low-fiber and high-fat diet, advanced age (65% occur in those > 80 years of age), and connective tissue disorders.

HISTORY/PE

- **Diverticulosis:** Often asymptomatic until patients present with sudden, intermittent, painless bleeding, which can cause symptoms of anemia when bleeding is severe. Associated with chronic constipation.
- **Diverticulitis:** LLQ abdominal pain, fever, nausea, and vomiting. Perforation is a serious complication that presents with peritonitis and shock.

DIAGNOSIS

- Clinical history is important to diagnosis.
- CBC may show leukocytosis or anemia.
- **Most accurate test:** Colonoscopy provides definitive diagnosis in diverticular disease, however, avoid sigmoidoscopy/colonoscopy in patients with acute diverticulitis because of the risk for perforation.
- In acute diverticulitis, CT scan is best test for diagnosis; it may reveal inflammation or abscess (see Figure 2.6-8).

TREATMENT

- **Uncomplicated diverticulosis:** Routine follow-up. Encourage a high-fiber diet or fiber supplements.
- **Diverticular bleeding:** Bleeding usually stops spontaneously; transfuse and hydrate as needed. If bleeding does not stop, hemostasis by colonoscopy, angiography with embolization, or surgery is indicated.
- **Diverticulitis:** Treat with bowel rest (NPO), NG tube placement (if severe), and broad-spectrum antibiotics (metronidazole and a fluoroquinolone or a second- or third-generation cephalosporin), colonoscopy after initial stage.
- **Hospitalization** is required if there is evidence of peritonitis or systemic signs of infection.
- **For perforation:** Immediate surgical resection of diseased bowel via a Hartmann procedure with a temporary colostomy.

COMPLICATIONS

Diverticulitis may cause fistulas in other organs, leading to pneumaturia, fecaluria, or fecal discharge from the vagina. Diagnose with CT and treat with surgical resection.

LARGE BOWEL OBSTRUCTION

Table 2.6-5 describes features that distinguish SBO from large bowel obstruction (LBO). Figure 2.6-9 demonstrates the classic radiographic findings of LBO.

TABLE 2.6-5. Characteristics of Small and Large Bowel Obstruction

VARIABLE	SMALL BOWEL OBSTRUCTION	LARGE BOWEL OBSTRUCTION
History	Moderate to severe acute abdominal pain; copious emesis Cramping pain with distal SBO Fever, signs of dehydration, and hypotension may be seen	Constipation/obstipation, deep and cramping abdominal pain (less intense than SBO), nausea/vomiting (less than that of SBO, but more commonly feculent)
Exam	Abdominal distention (distal SBO), abdominal tenderness, visible peristaltic waves, fever, hypovolemia Look for surgical scars/hernias; perform a rectal exam High-pitched "tinkly" bowel sounds; later, absence of bowel sounds	Significant distention, tympany, and tenderness; examine for peritoneal irritation or mass Fever or signs of shock suggest perforation/peritonitis or ischemia/necrosis High-pitched "tinkly" bowel sounds; later, absence of bowel sounds
Etiologies	Adhesions (postsurgery), hernias, neoplasm, volvulus, intussusception, gallstone ileus, foreign body, Crohn disease, cystic fibrosis (CF), stricture, hematoma	Colon cancer, diverticulitis, volvulus, fecal impaction, benign tumors Assume colon cancer until proven otherwise
Differential	LBO, paralytic ileus, gastroenteritis	SBO, paralytic ileus, appendicitis, IBD, Ogilvie syndrome (pseudo-obstruction)
Diagnosis	CBC, electrolytes, lactic acid, x-ray of the abdomen (see Figure 2.6-7), contrast studies (determine if it is partial or complete), CT scan	CBC, electrolytes, lactic acid, x-ray of the abdomen (see Figure 2.6-9), CT scan, water contrast enema (if perforation is suspected), sigmoidoscopy/colonoscopy if stable
Treatment	Hospitalize. Partial SBO can be treated conservatively with NG decompression and NPO status Patients with complete SBO should be managed aggressively with NPO status, NG decompression, IV fluids, electrolyte replacement, and surgical correction	Hospitalize. Obstruction can be relieved with a Gastrografin enema, colonoscopy, or a rectal tube; however, surgery is usually required. Ischemic colon usually requires partial colectomy with a diverting colostomy Treat the underlying cause (eg, neoplasm)

COLORECTAL CANCER

The second leading cause of cancer mortality in the United States. There is an ↑ incidence with age, with a peak incidence at 70–80 years of age. Risk factors and screening recommendations are summarized in Tables 2.6-6 and 2.6-7.

HISTORY/PE

Most patients are asymptomatic. When they are symptomatic, symptoms depend on the location of the lesion:

- **Right-sided lesions:** Often bulky, ulcerating masses that lead to anemia from chronic occult blood loss. Patients may complain of weight loss, anorexia, diarrhea, weakness, or vague abdominal pain. Obstruction is rare. (Right colon has a larger diameter than left colon.)
- **Left-sided lesions:** Typically, "apple-core" obstructing masses (see Figure 2.6-10). Patients complain of obstruction, change in bowel habits (eg, ↓ stool caliber, constipation, obstipation), and/or blood-streaked stools. (Left side has smaller diameter and thus is easier to obstruct.)
- **Rectal lesions:** Usually present with bright-red blood per rectum, often with tenesmus and/or rectal pain. Rectal cancer must be ruled out in all patients with rectal bleeding. However, ⊖ FOBT has insufficient sensitivity to exclude the possibility of cancer.

MNEMONIC

Bovis in blood = Cancer in butt

Q

A 60-year-old man with no past medical history presents with fever, dyspnea, and orthopnea of 2 weeks' duration. Physical exam reveals splinter hemorrhages and a new IV/VI diastolic decrescendo murmur. Echocardiogram confirms aortic valve endocarditis, and IV antibiotics are started. Blood cultures are ⊕ for *Streptococcus bovis*. What is the next diagnostic step?

TABLE 2.6-6. Risk Factors for Colorectal Cancer

Risk Factor	Comments
Age	Risk ↑ with age; peak incidence is at 70–80 years of age
Hereditary polyposis syndromes	Familial adenomatous polyposis (FAP; 100% risk by 40 years of age); hereditary nonpolyposis colorectal cancer (HNPCC, also known as Lynch syndrome. Also risk for endometrial and ovarian cancers.)
⊕ Family history	Especially first-degree relatives < 60 years of age
IBD	Ulcerative colitis > Crohn disease
Adenomatous polyps	Villous > tubular; sessile > pedunculated
High-fat, low-fiber diet	—

DIAGNOSIS

- **Most accurate test:** Colonoscopy with biopsy.
- **Evaluate for metastases:** CXR, liver function tests (LFTs), and an abdominal/pelvic CT.
- Staging is based on the depth of tumor penetration into the bowel wall and the presence of lymph node involvement and distant metastases.

TREATMENT

- **Best initial treatment:** Surgical resection of the tumor.
- Adjuvant chemotherapy is appropriate in cases with ⊕ lymph nodes.
- Follow with serial CEA levels to detect recurrence, colonoscopy, LFTs, CXR, and abdominal CT to screen for metastases.

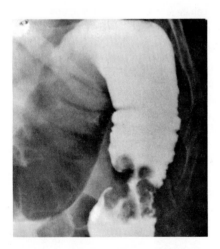

FIGURE 2.6-10. Colon carcinoma. The encircling carcinoma appears as an "apple-core" filling defect in the descending colon on barium enema x-ray. (Reproduced with permission from Way LW. *Current Surgical Diagnosis & Treatment,* 10th ed. Stamford, CT: Appleton & Lange; 1994.)

Colonoscopy. Although the mechanism of association has yet to be determined, there is a well-established association between *S bovis* and colon cancer. *Clostridium septicum* is also associated with colon cancer.

TABLE 2.6-7. Screening Recommendations for Colorectal Cancer

Risk Category	Recommendations
No past medical or family history	Starting at 50 years of age: - Annual digital rectal exam (DRE) and home fecal occult blood test (FOBT) - Colonoscopy every 10 years or - Sigmoidoscopy every 5 years
First-degree relative with colon cancer	Colonoscopy every 5 years starting at 40 years of age or Colonoscopy every 5 years starting 10 years before the age of affected family member at time of diagnosis (whichever comes first)
Ulcerative colitis	Colonoscopy every 1–2 years starting 8–10 years after diagnosis
Hereditary nonpolyposis colon cancer syndrome	Colonoscopy every 1–2 years starting at 25 years of age
Familial adenomatous polyposis	Sigmoidoscopy every year starting at 12 years of age
Previous large adenomas	Colonoscopy every 3–5 years

ISCHEMIC COLITIS

- Insufficient blood supply to the colon that results in ischemia and, potentially, necrosis. Most commonly affects the left colon, particularly the "watershed area" at the splenic flexure. Usually occurs in the setting of atherosclerosis.

HISTORY/PE

- Presents with crampy lower abdominal pain followed by bloody diarrhea after meals or exertion or in the heat. Fever and peritoneal signs suggest bowel necrosis.

DIAGNOSIS

- **Best initial test:** CT scan with contrast may show thickened bowel wall, atherosclerosis.
- **Most accurate test:** Angiography.
- Colonoscopy may show a pale mucosa with petechial bleeding.

TREATMENT

- Supportive therapy with bowel rest, IV fluids, and broad-spectrum antibiotics.
- Surgical bowel resection is indicated for infarction, fulminant colitis, or obstruction.

PILONIDAL DISEASE

Painful, fluctuant masses that develop in anal area of obese individuals with sedentary lifestyles. May present with purulent, bloody, or mucoid discharge. Treat with surgical drainage.

Gastrointestinal Bleeding

- GI bleeding presents as hematemesis, hematochezia, and/or melena.
- **Upper GI tract bleeding:** Bleeding from lesions proximal to the ligament of Treitz (the anatomic boundary between the duodenum and jejunum). Table 2.6-8 presents the features of upper and lower GI bleeding.

Inflammatory Bowel Disease

Includes Crohn disease (see Figure 2.6-11) and ulcerative colitis (see Figure 2.6-12). Most common in whites and Ashkenazi Jews, with onset most

KEY FACT

One unit of packed RBCs should ↑ hemoglobin by 1 g/dL and hematocrit by 3–4 units.

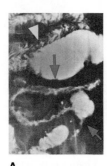 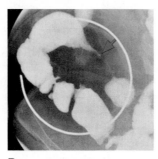 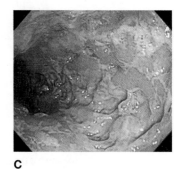

A   B   C

FIGURE 2.6-11. Crohn disease. (A) Small bowel follow-through (SBFT) barium study shows skip areas of narrowed small bowel with nodular mucosa (*arrows*) and ulceration. Compare with normal small bowel (*arrowhead*). **(B)** Spot compression image from SBFT shows "string sign" narrowing (*arrow*) caused by stricture. **(C)** Deep ulcers in the colon of a patient with Crohn disease, seen at colonoscopy. (Image A reproduced with permission from Chen MY et al. *Basic Radiology,* 1st ed. New York, NY: McGraw-Hill; 2004. Image B reproduced with permission from USMLE-Rx.com. Image C reproduced with permission from Fauci AS et al. *Harrison's Principles of Internal Medicine,* 17th ed. New York, NY: McGraw-Hill; 2008.)

TABLE 2.6-8. **Features of Upper and Lower GI Bleeding**

VARIABLE	UPPER GI BLEEDING	LOWER GI BLEEDING
History/exam	Hematemesis ("coffee-ground" emesis), melena > hematochezia, hypovolemia (eg, elevated BUN, tachycardia, lightheadedness, hypotension)	Hematochezia > melena, but can be either
Diagnosis	NG tube and lavage (may be ⊖ in 15% of upper GI bleeds); endoscopy is definitive	Rule out upper GI hemorrhage with NG lavage if brisk Anoscopy/sigmoidoscopy for patients < 45 years of age with small-volume bleeding Colonoscopy if stable; arteriography or exploratory laparotomy if unstable
Etiologies	PUD, esophagitis/gastritis, Mallory-Weiss tear, esophageal/gastric varices, gastric antral vascular ectasia, Dieulafoy lesions	Diverticulosis (60%), angiodysplasia, IBD, hemorrhoids/fissures, neoplasm, arteriovenous malformation
Initial management	Protect the airway (intubation may be needed) Stabilize the patient with IV fluids and packed RBCs (hematocrit may be normal early in acute blood loss)	Stabilize the patient with IV fluids and packed RBCs (hematocrit may be normal early in acute blood loss)
Long-term management	Endoscopy followed by therapy directed at the underlying cause	Depends on the underlying etiology. Endoscopic therapy (eg, epinephrine injection, cauterization, or clip placement), intra-arterial vasopressin infusion or embolization, or surgery for diverticular disease or angiodysplasia

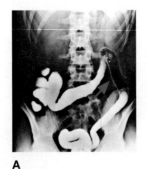

A

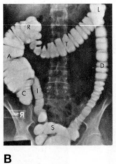

B

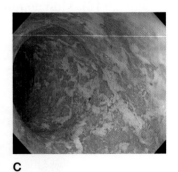

C

FIGURE 2.6-12. **Ulcerative colitis.** (A) X-ray from a barium enema showing a featureless ("lead pipe") colon with small mucosal ulcerations *(arrow)*. Compare with normal haustral markings in (**B**). (**C**) Diffuse mucosal ulcerations and exudates at colonoscopy in chronic ulcerative colitis. (Image A reproduced with permission from Doherty GM. *Current Diagnosis & Treatment: Surgery,* 13th ed. New York, NY: McGraw-Hill; 2010. Image B reproduced with permission from Chen MY et al. *Basic Radiology.* New York, NY: McGraw-Hill; 2004. Image C reproduced with permission from Fauci AS et al. *Harrison's Principles of Internal Medicine,* 17th ed. New York, NY: McGraw-Hill; 2008.)

TABLE 2.6-9. Features of Ulcerative Colitis and Crohn Disease

VARIABLE	ULCERATIVE COLITIS	CROHN DISEASE
Site of involvement	Rectum is always involved. May extend proximally in a continuous fashion Inflammation and ulceration are limited to the mucosa and submucosa	May involve any portion of the GI tract, particularly the ileocecal region, in a discontinuous pattern ("skip lesions"); rectum is often spared Transmural inflammation is seen, sometimes leading to fistulas to other organs
History/exam	Bloody diarrhea, lower abdominal cramps, tenesmus, urgency Exam may reveal orthostatic hypotension, tachycardia, abdominal tenderness, frank blood on rectal exam, and extraintestinal manifestations Toxic megacolon may be presenting finding (avoid tubes or scopes in view of the risk for perforation)	Abdominal pain, abdominal mass, low-grade fever, weight loss, watery diarrhea Exam may reveal fever, abdominal tenderness or mass, perianal fissures or tags, fistulas, and extraintestinal manifestations
Extraintestinal manifestations	Aphthous stomatitis, episcleritis/uveitis, arthritis, primary sclerosing cholangitis, erythema nodosum, and pyoderma gangrenosum	Same as ulcerative colitis in addition to fistulas to the skin, to the bladder, or between bowel loops
Diagnosis	CBC, x-ray of the abdomen, stool cultures, O&P, stool assay for *C difficile* Colonoscopy can show diffuse and continuous rectal involvement, friability, edema, and pseudopolyps Definitive diagnosis can be made with biopsy	Same lab workup as that of ulcerative colitis; upper GI series with small bowel follow-through Colonoscopy may show aphthoid, linear, or stellate ulcers, strictures, noncaseating granulomas, "cobblestoning," and "skip lesions" "Creeping fat" may also be present during laparotomy Definitive diagnosis can be made with biopsy
Treatment	5-ASA agents (eg, sulfasalazine, mesalamine), topical or oral; corticosteroids for flare-ups and immunomodulators (eg, azathioprine) or biologics (eg, infliximab) for refractory or moderate to severe disease Total proctocolectomy can be curative for long-standing or fulminant colitis or toxic megacolon; also ↓ cancer risk	Similar to UC: 5-ASA agents; corticosteroids for flare-ups. May require immunomodulators (eg, azathioprine) or biologics (eg, infliximab) for refractory or moderate to severe disease and for maintenance therapy Surgical resection may be necessary for suspected perforation, stricture, fistula, or abscess
Incidence of cancer	Markedly ↑ risk for colorectal cancer in long-standing cases (monitor with frequent FOBT and yearly colonoscopy with multiple biopsies after 8 years of disease)	Incidence of 2° malignancy is lower than that of ulcerative colitis but is greater than that of the general population

frequently occurring in the teens to early 30s or in the 50s. Table 2.6-9 summarizes the features of IBD. In patients with a history of Crohn disease and acute abdominal pain, suspect SBO, which is caused by the fistula formation. Ulcerative colitis does not cause fistulas.

Hernias

Inguinal hernias are protrusions of abdominal contents (usually the small intestine) into the inguinal region through a weakness or defect in the

KEY FACT

The Hesselbach triangle is an area bounded by the inguinal ligament, the inferior epigastric artery, and the rectus abdominis.

TABLE 2.6-10.   Types of Hernias

Hernia Type	Location	Etiology	Prevalence
Indirect	Herniation of abdominal contents through both external and internal rings, lateral to inferior epigastric vessels (see Figure 2.6-13)	Results from congenital patent processus vaginalis	Most common
Direct	Herniation through floor of Hesselbach triangle, medial to epigastric vessels (see Figure 2.6-13)	Mechanical breakdown in transversalis fascia resulting from age	
Femoral	Herniation below inguinal ligament through femoral canal, below and lateral to the pubic tubercle	Increased intra-abdominal pressure, weakened pelvic floor	More common in women than in men

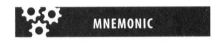

MNEMONIC

MDs Don't LIE

Direct hernias lie **Me**D**ial** and indirect lie **L**ateral to the **I**nferior **E**pigastric vessels.

abdominal wall. Classified as either direct or indirect. There are also femoral hernias. See Table 2.6-10 and Figure 2.6-13.

TREATMENT

Because of the risk for incarceration and strangulation, surgical correction is indicated.

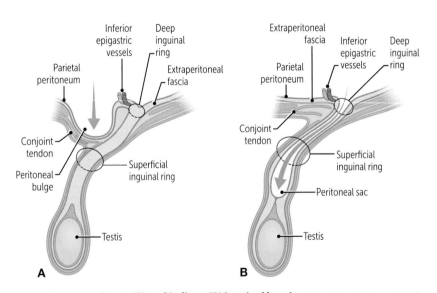

FIGURE 2.6-13.   Direct (A) and indirect (B) inguinal hernias. (Reproduced with permission from USMLE-Rx.com.)

Biliary Disease

CHOLELITHIASIS AND BILIARY COLIC

Colic results from transient cystic duct blockage from impacted stones. Although risk factors include the **four F's** (Female, Fat, Fertile, and Forty), the disorder is common and can occur in any patient. Additional risk factors include OCP use, rapid weight loss, chronic hemolysis (pigment stones in sickle cell disease), small bowel resection (loss of enterohepatically circulated bile), and TPN. Table 2.6-11 details the forms of biliary disease and contrasts the lab findings associated with each.

KEY FACT

Pigmented gallstones result from hemolysis (black) or infection (brown).

TABLE 2.6-11. **Disorders Caused by Gallstones**

DISORDER	DEFINITION	PRESENTATION	LABS	DIAGNOSIS	MANAGEMENT
Cholelithiasis	Stones in the gallbladder	May be asymptomatic, or may cause biliary colic; transient RUQ pain commonly seen after eating fatty meals; caused by temporary occlusion of the cystic duct by a stone	Normal total bilirubin/alkaline phosphatase, serum amylase	Ultrasonography	If asymptomatic, observation; if symptomatic, laparoscopic chole-cystectomy
Cholecystitis	Inflammation of the gallbladder, typically caused by stone occluding the cystic duct	RUQ pain, fever (maybe), Murphy sign (cessation of inspiration with palpation of RUQ)	↑WBC, normal total bilirubin/alkaline phos-phatase, amylase	Ultrasonography, HIDA scan	Laparoscopic cholecystectomy; if patient is too ill to undergo surgery, transcuta-neous drainage of gallbladder
Choledocholithiasis	Stone in the common bile duct (CBD)	Jaundice, ± RUQ pain, afebrile	Normal/↑WBC, ↑total bili-rubin/alkaline phosphatase, ↑amylase/lipase (if pancreatitis is present)	Ultrasonography often does not show the stone but may show dilated CBD. Magnetic resonance cholangiopan-creatography (MRCP) and endoscopic retrograde cholangiopancreatography (ERCP) are definitive	ERCP to remove stone, followed by cholecystectomy
Cholangitis	Infection of the CBD, usually caused by stone in the CBD	Charcot triad: RUQ pain, fever, jaundice, Reyn-olds pentad: Charcot triad + shock and altered mental status	↑WBC, ↑total bilirubin/alkaline phosphatase	Clinical diagnosis con-firmed by biliary dilation on imaging; or ERCP (both diagnostic and therapeutic)	ERCP; surgery if patient toxic

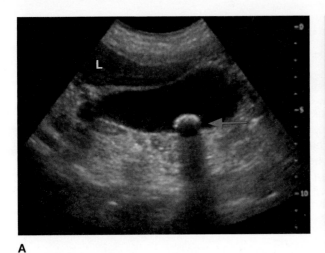
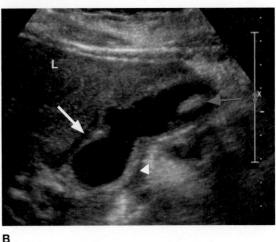

FIGURE 2.6-14. **Gallstone disease.** (A) **Cholelithiasis.** Ultrasound image of the gallbladder shows a gallstone (*arrow*) with posterior shadowing. (B) **Acute cholecystitis.** Ultrasound image shows a gallstone (*red arrow*), a thickened gallbladder wall (*arrowhead*), and pericholecystic fluid (*white arrow*). L, liver. (Reproduced with permission from USMLE-Rx.com.)

KEY FACT

Sphincter of Oddi dysfunction: Look for RUQ pain following opiate administration.

KEY FACT

Immunosuppressed patients (especially diabetics) are at risk for emphysematous cholecystitis (infection of the gallbladder with gas-forming bacteria). This requires emergent cholecystectomy.

KEY FACT

Most gallstones are precipitations of cholesterol and are not radiopaque.

HISTORY/PE

- Postprandial abdominal pain (usually in the RUQ) that radiates to the right subscapular area or the epigastrium, often associated with nausea and vomiting, dyspepsia, and flatulence.
- **Gallstones:** May have RUQ tenderness and a palpable gallbladder or be asymptomatic.

DIAGNOSIS

RUQ ultrasound is the best initial and most accurate test (see Figure 2.6-14).

TREATMENT

- Cholecystectomy is curative and recommended for patients with symptomatic gallstones. Asymptomatic gallstones do not require treatment.
- Porcelain gallbladder is an incidental finding of peripheral gallbladder calcifications that places the patient at higher risk for gallbladder adenocarcinoma. Emergent cholecystectomy is needed.

COMPLICATIONS

Postcholecystectomy syndrome can be caused by retained stones, strictures, or extrabiliary causes. Symptoms include early satiety, bloating, and dyspepsia after cholecystectomy. Diagnosis is made with additional abdominal imaging (ultrasound, ERCP, MRCP).

ACUTE CHOLECYSTITIS

Prolonged blockage of the cystic duct by a gallstone that leads to progressive distention, inflammation, and infection. Acalculous cholecystitis occurs in the absence of cholelithiasis in patients who are chronically debilitated or critically ill.

HISTORY/PE

- **Hx:** RUQ pain, nausea, vomiting, and fever.
- **Physical Exam:** RUQ tenderness, inspiratory arrest with deep palpation of the RUQ (Murphy sign), and low-grade fever.

DIAGNOSIS

- **Best initial test:** Ultrasound; may demonstrate stones, bile sludge, pericholecystic fluid, a thickened gallbladder wall, gas in the wall of the gallbladder, and/or an ultrasonic Murphy sign (see Figure 2.6-14).
- When ultrasound is equivocal, obtain a HIDA scan. In this nuclear medicine scan, which uses a radiotracer excreted through the biliary system, nonvisualization of the gallbladder suggests acute cholecystitis.

TREATMENT

- Broad-spectrum IV antibiotics and IV fluids.
- Cholecystectomy is indicated.

CHOLEDOCHOLITHIASIS

- Gallstones in the common bile duct (CBD). Symptoms vary according to the degree of obstruction, the duration of the obstruction, and the presence/severity of infection.
- **Hx/PE:** Biliary colic, jaundice, afebrile unless current infection, and/or pancreatitis.
- **Dx:** ↑ Alkaline phosphatase and total and direct bilirubin (see Table 2.6-11).
- **Tx:** Management consists of ERCP with sphincterotomy followed by cholecystectomy.

ACUTE CHOLANGITIS

- An acute bacterial infection of the biliary tree that commonly occurs 2° to obstruction, usually from gallstones (choledocholithiasis).
- **Other etiologies:** Bile duct stricture, primary sclerosing cholangitis, and malignancy. Gram ⊖ enterics are commonly identified pathogens.

HISTORY/PE

- Charcot triad—RUQ pain, jaundice, and fever/chills—is classic.
- Reynolds pentad—Charcot triad plus septic shock and altered mental status—may be present in acute suppurative cholangitis.

DIAGNOSIS

- **Labs:** Leukocytosis, ↑ bilirubin, and ↑ alkaline phosphatase (see Table 2.6-11); blood cultures.
- **Best initial test:** Ultrasound; diagnostic for CBD dilation.
- **Most accurate test:** ERCP; diagnostic and therapeutic.

TREATMENT

- Patients often require ICU admission for monitoring, hydration, BP support, and broad-spectrum IV antibiotic treatment.
- Patients with acute suppurative cholangitis require emergent bile duct decompression via ERCP/sphincterotomy, percutaneous transhepatic drainage, or open decompression.

GALLSTONE ILEUS

- Mechanical obstruction resulting from the passage of a large (> 2.5 cm) stone into the bowel through a cholecystoduodenal fistula. Obstruction is often at the ileocecal valve.
- **Hx/PE:** The classic presentation is a subacute SBO in an elderly woman. Patients may have no history of biliary colic.

KEY FACT

Charcot triad consists of RUQ pain, jaundice, and fever/chills. Reynolds pentad consists of RUQ pain, jaundice, fever/chills, shock, and altered mental status.

Q

A 35-year-old man with a 12-year history of ulcerative colitis presents to a clinic for annual follow-up. He has no current complaints. What is the most important screening test he should undergo?

- **Dx:** X-ray of the abdomen with characteristics of SBO and pneumobilia (gas in the biliary tree) confirms the diagnosis. Upper GI barium contrast images will demonstrate no contrast in the colon.
- **Tx:** Laparotomy with stone extraction; closure of the fistula and cholecystectomy.

Liver Disease

ABNORMAL LIVER FUNCTION TESTS

Liver diseases can be divided into several patterns based on LFT results as follows:

- **Hepatocellular injury:** ↑ AST and ALT.
- **Cholestasis:** ↑ Alkaline phosphatase and bilirubin.
- **Mixed:** Combination of hepatocellular and cholestatic picture.
- **Isolated hyperbilirubinemia:** ↑ Bilirubin.

Jaundice is a clinical sign that occurs when bilirubin levels exceed 2.5 mg/dL. Figures 2.6-15 and 2.6-16 summarize the clinical approaches toward cholestasis and isolated hyperbilirubinemia.

HEPATITIS

Inflammation of the liver leading to cell injury and necrosis. Hepatitis can be either acute or chronic.

- **Acute:** The most common causes are viruses (HAV, HBV, HCV, HDV, HEV) and drugs (alcohol, acetaminophen, INH, methyldopa).
    - Fulminant: Also known as acute liver failure. Severe liver injury with INR > 1.5 and hepatic encephalopathy in a patient without underlying chronic liver disease.
- **Chronic:** The most common causes are chronic viral infection (HCV most common in United States, HBV worldwide), alcohol, autoimmune hepatitis, and metabolic syndromes (Wilson disease, hemochromatosis, α_1-antitrypsin deficiency).

KEY FACT

HCV is **C**hronic; 70–80% of patients with HCV infection will develop chronic hepatitis.

Colonoscopy. Patients with ulcerative colitis are at a significantly ↑ risk for colon cancer. Thus, colonoscopies are recommended for such patients every 1–2 years beginning 8–10 years after diagnosis. If dysplasia is present on random biopsy, total colectomy is recommended.

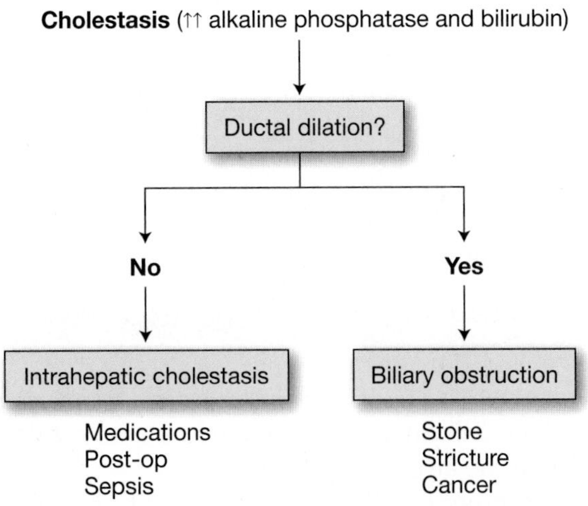

Cholestasis (↑↑ alkaline phosphatase and bilirubin)

↓

Ductal dilation?

No / Yes

No → Intrahepatic cholestasis
Medications
Post-op
Sepsis

Yes → Biliary obstruction
Stone
Stricture
Cancer

FIGURE 2.6-15.   Approach to cholestasis.

TABLE 2.6-12. Types of Hepatitis

Virus Type	Mode of Transmission	Presentation	Notes
HAV	Fecal-oral	Typically self-limited acute hepatitis May lead to fulminant hepatic failure	Most common cause of acute viral hepatitis worldwide
HBV	Bodily fluids	May be asymptomatic, but may present as viral pro-drome (this is listed above) and/or jaundice May lead to fulminant hepatic failure and require treatment with antivirals or liver transplant in severe cases	< 10% of infections in adults become chronic, while most vertically transmitted become chronic Extremely high transmission rate
HCV	Bodily fluids	Asymptomatic or viral prodrome and/or jaundice	80% become chronic. Less likely to be sexually transmitted than HBV; may present with very mild acute phase Very rarely leads to acute liver failure If palpable purpura, arthralgia, and low complement levels are seen, consider cryoglobulinemia
HDV	Bodily fluids	Co-infection with HBV or superinfection in patient with prior HBV (more severe)	Requires HBV surface antigen. H**D**V is **D**ependent on HBV
HEV	Fecal-oral	Typically self-limited acute hepatitis similar to HAV	High mortality rate in pregnant women May become chronic in immunosuppressed patients

History/PE

- **Acute hepatitis:**
  - Often begins with a nonspecific viral prodrome (malaise, fever, joint pain, nausea, vomiting, changes in bowel habits) followed by jaundice and RUQ tenderness. Exam often reveals jaundice, scleral icterus, and tender hepatomegaly.
  - HAV and HEV have only a self-limited acute phase; HBV and HCV may feature a mild acute phase or none at all. Acetaminophen toxicity can cause a life-threatening hepatitis. Table 2.6-12 outlines further distinctions among these.
- **Chronic hepatitis:** May be asymptomatic, but may cause fatigue and joint and muscle pains. Jaundice and complications of portal hypertension typically occur only when the disease progresses to cirrhosis. At least 80% of those infected with HCV and 10% of those with HBV in adulthood will develop persistent infection with chronic active hepatitis.

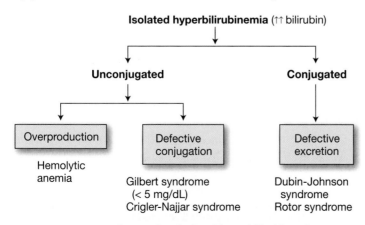

FIGURE 2.6-16. Approach to isolated hyperbilirubinemia.

TABLE 2.6-13.   **Key Hepatitis Serologic Markers**

SEROLOGIC MARKER	DESCRIPTION
IgM HAVAb	IgM antibody to HAV; the best test to detect acute HAV
HBsAg	Antigen found on the surface of HBV; continued presence indicates carrier state
HBsAb	Antibody to HBsAg; indicates immunity to HBV
HBcAg	Antigen associated with core of HBV. Not measured in clinical practice
HBcAb	Antibody to HBcAg; IgM ⊕ during the window period IgG HBcAb is an indicator of prior or current infection
H**Be**Ag	A different antigenic determinant in the HBV core An important indicator of transmissibility (**Be**ware!)
HBeAb	Antibody to e antigen; indicates low transmissibility

1 **A**

Gallstone pancreatitis results from a gallstone that travels through the CBD and lodges at the ampulla of Vater, thus obstructing the flow of both pancreatic exocrine enzymes and bile. It most commonly occurs in women, who often report a history of biliary colic. Treatment involves management of the pancreatitis with supportive care and elective cholecystectomy.

2 **A**

Gilbert syndrome is an autosomal recessive disorder of bilirubin glucuronidation caused by ↓ activity of the enzyme glucuronyl transferase. Patients present with unconjugated hyperbilirubinemia but have a normal CBC, blood smear, and LFTs. The condition is benign, and no treatment is indicated.

DIAGNOSIS

- **Acute hepatitis:** Labs reveal markedly ↑ ALT and AST, ↑ GGT, ↑ ferritin, and ↑ bilirubin/alkaline phosphatase.
- **Chronic hepatitis:** ALT and AST are either mildly elevated or even normal/low for > 3–6 months. Contrast this with the marked elevation of acute hepatitis as above.
- Diagnosis of viral hepatitis is made by hepatitis serology (see Table 2.6-13 and Figure 2.6-17 for a description and timing of serologic markers). May require liver biopsy if diagnosis is uncertain or to rule out other causes of liver disease in chronic or severe cases.

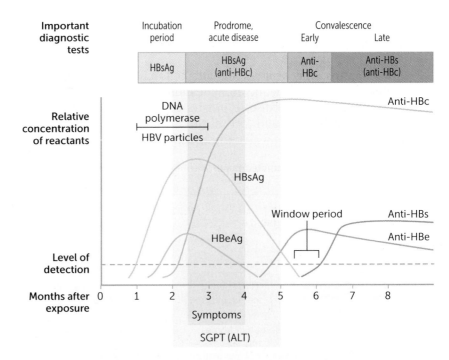

FIGURE 2.6-17.   **Time course of hepatitis B with serologic markers.** (Reproduced with permission from USMLE-Rx.com.)

- Other diagnostic studies include the following:
    - **Autoimmune hepatitis:** ⊕ Anti–nuclear and anti–smooth muscle antibodies (type 1) and anti–liver-kidney microsomal-1 antibodies and anti–liver cytosol antibodies (type 2). May also present with elevated serum gamma globulins (IgG) and p-ANCA.
    - **Hemochromatosis:** ↑ Ferritin and transferrin saturation > 50%. Liver biopsy showing high hepatic iron index.
    - **Wilson disease:** ↓ Ceruloplasmin, ↑ urine copper, Kayser-Fleischer rings. Liver biopsy if diagnosis is uncertain.

TREATMENT

- **Acute hepatitis:** Generally supportive care. Acute HBV may require treatment with antivirals.
- **Hepatitis B postexposure prophylaxis:** Nonimmunized individuals requires both vaccination and immunoglobulins. Hepatitis B–immunized individuals and those exposed to hepatitis C do not require any postexposure prophylaxis.
- **Chronic hepatitis:** Treatment is etiology specific.
    - **Chronic HBV infection:** Tenofovir and entecavir are most commonly used and have the least viral resistance. Other agents include telbivudine, adefovir, and lamivudine, but they are not recommended because of a high rate of resistance.
    - **Chronic HCV infection:** Medications and treatment duration vary based on genotype, cirrhosis status, and history of prior treatment. Typically, either two direct-acting antivirals (DAAs) or one DAA plus ribavirin. Interferon is still used occasionally today. This field is rapidly evolving. Previously, interferon and ribavirin, plus a protease inhibitor for some genotypes.
    - **Most definitive treatment:** Liver transplantation for patients with end-stage liver failure. Emergent transplantation is indicated in cases of fulminant hepatic failure.

KEY FACT

The sequelae of chronic hepatitis include cirrhosis, portal hypertension, liver failure, and hepatocellular carcinoma.

COMPLICATIONS

Cirrhosis, liver failure, hepatocellular carcinoma (3–5%).

CIRRHOSIS

- Bridging fibrosis and nodular regeneration resulting from chronic hepatic injury.
- Most common etiologies in the United States are alcohol, chronic HCV, and nonalcoholic steatohepatitis. Etiologies can be as follows:
    - **Intrahepatic:** All causes of chronic hepatitis.
    - **Extrahepatic:**
        - Biliary tract disease (primary biliary cirrhosis, primary sclerosing cholangitis).
        - Posthepatic causes include right-sided heart failure, constrictive pericarditis, and Budd-Chiari syndrome (hepatic vein thrombosis 2° to hypercoagulability).

KEY FACT

Spontaneous bacterial peritonitis is a common complication in patients with cirrhosis and ascites, and if they present with signs and symptoms suggestive of infection, paracentesis should be performed. Spontaneous bacterial peritonitis is diagnosed by > 250 PMNs/mL in the ascitic fluid.

HISTORY/PE

- **Hx:** May be asymptomatic, though may present with jaundice, easy bruising (coagulopathy), and complications of portal hypertension such as ascites, hepatic encephalopathy (asterixis, altered mental status), gastroesophageal varices, hepatic hydrothorax (transudative pleural effusion) and thrombocytopenia. Ascites can be complicated by spontaneous bacterial peritonitis.
- **PE:** May reveal an enlarged, palpable, or firm liver and other signs of portal hypertension and liver failure (see Figures 2.6-18 and 2.6-19).

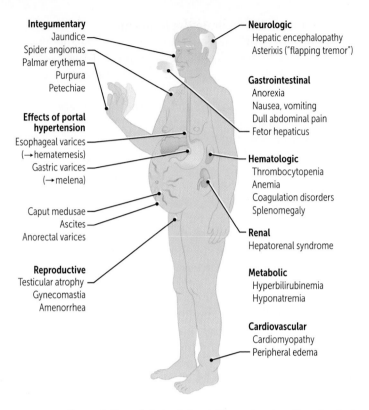

FIGURE 2.6-18.   Presentation of cirrhosis/portal hypertension. (Reproduced with permission from USMLE-Rx.com.)

DIAGNOSIS

- **Synthetic dysfunction (best initial tests):** ↓ Albumin, ↑ PT/INR, and ↑ bilirubin.
- **Portal hypertension:** Thrombocytopenia (2° to hypersplenism, sequestration of platelets in the liver, and ↓ thrombopoietin production), varices, ascites (paracentesis).

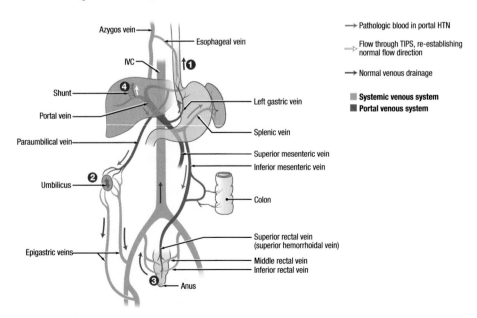

FIGURE 2.6-19.   Portosystemic anastomoses. 1. Esophageal varices: left gastric ↔ azygos. 2. Caput medusae: paraumbilical ↔ small epigastric veins of the anterior abdominal wall. 3. Anorectal varices: superior rectal ↔ middle and inferior rectal. 4. Treatment with transjugular intrahepatic portosystemic shunt (TIPS): portal vein ↔ hepatic vein.

TABLE 2.6-14. **Etiologies of Ascites by SAAG**

SAAG > 1.1	SAAG < 1.1
Related to portal hypertension:	Not related to portal hypertension:
▪ Presinusoidal: Splenic or portal vein thrombosis, schistosomiasis	▪ Nephrotic syndrome
▪ Sinusoidal: Cirrhosis	▪ TB
▪ Postsinusoidal: Right heart failure, constrictive pericarditis, Budd-Chiari syndrome	▪ Malignancy with peritoneal carcinomatosis (eg, ovarian cancer)

- **Most accurate test:** Liver biopsy shows bridging fibrosis and nodular regeneration.
- **Etiology:** Hepatitis serologies, autoimmune markers, serum ferritin, ceruloplasmin, and α_1-antitrypsin.
- If ascites is present, the etiology of ascites can be determined by the serum-ascites albumin gradient (SAAG = serum albumin – ascites albumin); see Table 2.6-14.

TREATMENT

The goal is to treat and prevent the progression of cirrhosis and minimize factors that can lead to decompensation (see Table 2.6-15). All cirrhotic patients should receive vaccinations for hepatitis A, hepatitis B, and PPSV-23 (pneumonia).

PRIMARY SCLEROSING CHOLANGITIS

- An idiopathic disorder characterized by progressive inflammation and fibrosis accompanied by strictures of extrahepatic and intrahepatic bile ducts. The disease usually presents in young men with ulcerative colitis. Patients are at ↑ risk for cholangiocarcinoma.
- **Hx/PE:** Presents with progressive jaundice, pruritus, and fatigue.
- **Dx:**
    - Laboratory findings include ↑ alkaline phosphatase and ↑ bilirubin; primary sclerosing cholangitis is also associated with P-ANCA antibodies.
    - **Most accurate test:** MRCP/ERCP show multiple bile duct strictures and dilatations ("beading").
    - Liver biopsy reveals periductal sclerosis ("onion skinning").
    - All newly diagnosed patients should undergo colonoscopy to evaluate for IBD.
- **Tx:** ERCP with dilation and stenting of strictures. Liver transplantation is the definitive treatment. Ursodeoxycholic acid has been shown to improve the liver function profile in some patients.

KEY FACT

Primary sclerosing cholangitis is strongly associated with ulcerative colitis.

PRIMARY BILIARY CHOLANGITIS

- Autoimmune disorder characterized by destruction of intrahepatic bile ducts. Most commonly presents in middle-aged women with other autoimmune conditions.
- **Hx/PE:** Presents with progressive jaundice, pruritus, and fat-soluble vitamin deficiencies (A, D, E, K).
- **Dx:** Laboratory findings include ↑ alkaline phosphatase, ↑ bilirubin, ⊕ antimitochondrial antibody, and ↑ cholesterol.
    - **Most accurate test:** Liver biopsy.

TABLE 2.6-15. **Complications of Cirrhosis**

COMPLICATION	MECHANISM/HISTORY	MANAGEMENT
Ascites	↑ Portal hypertension results in transudative effusion Physical exam reveals abdominal distention, fluid wave, and shifting dullness to percussion	Sodium restriction and diuretics (furosemide, spironolactone); large-volume paracentesis. **TIPS** (**T**ransjugular **I**ntrahepatic **P**ortosystemic **S**hunt) Treat underlying liver disease if possible
Spontaneous bacterial peritonitis	Presents with fever, abdominal pain, chills, nausea, and vomiting Treatment indicated if diagnostic paracentesis reveals > 250 PMNs/mL	IV antibiotics acutely (third-generation cephalosporin), IV albumin; prophylaxis with a fluoroquinolone to prevent recurrence Development of SBP is associated with poor 1-year prognosis
Hepatorenal syndrome	Prerenal failure in the setting of severe liver disease A diagnosis of exclusion Caused by splanchnic vasodilation and decreased blood flow to the kidneys Urinary sodium < 10 mEq/L "Healthy kidneys in an unhealthy environment"	Initially trial of volume repletion and rule out other causes of renal failure May use octreotide (decrease splanchnic vasodilation) and midodrine (increase blood pressure) May require dialysis Poor prognosis Liver transplantation can be curative
Hepatic encephalopathy	↓ Clearance of ammonia; often precipitated by dehydration, infection, electrolyte abnormalities, and GI bleeding	Lactulose, and/or rifaximin Correct underlying triggers
Esophageal varices	Portal hypertension leads to ↑ flow through portosystemic anastomoses	Endoscopic surveillance in all patients with cirrhosis; medical prophylaxis with nonselective β-blockers or endoscopic band ligation to prevent bleeding in patients with known varices For acute bleeding, endoscopy with band ligation or sclerotherapy is indicated. Urgent TIPS in refractory cases (associated with high mortality)
Coagulopathy	Impaired synthesis of all clotting factors (except VIII)	For acute bleeding, administer fresh frozen plasma Vitamin K will not correct coagulopathy

KEY FACT

Primary biliary cholangitis is an autoimmune disease that presents with jaundice and pruritus in middle-aged women.

- **Tx:** Ursodeoxycholic acid (slows progression of disease); cholestyramine for pruritus; liver transplantation.

NONALCOHOLIC FATTY LIVER DISEASE

- Steatosis of hepatocytes leads to liver injury. Some patients progress to nonalcoholic steatohepatitis (NASH) and are at risk for liver fibrosis and cirrhosis.
- Associated with insulin resistance and metabolic syndrome.
- **Dx:** Largely a diagnosis of exclusion. Liver biopsy may show steatosis or steatohepatitis.
- **Tx:** Weight loss, diet, and exercise. If nonalcoholic steatohepatitis is present, consider vitamin E and pioglitazone.

HEPATOCELLULAR CARCINOMA

- One of the most common cancers worldwide despite its relatively low incidence in the United States.

- Remember that metastatic disease (especially from colon cancer) is much more common than primary hepatic cancer.
- **Risk factors:** In the United States, risk factors are cirrhosis (from alcohol, HCV, and nonalcoholic steatohepatitis) and chronic hepatitis B (even without cirrhosis). In developing countries, HBV infection and aflatoxins (in various food sources) are major risk factors.

HISTORY/PE

- Patients commonly present with RUQ tenderness, abdominal distention, and signs of chronic liver disease such as jaundice, easy bruisability, and coagulopathy. May present as decompensation of previously compensated cirrhosis.
- Exam may reveal tender enlargement of the liver.

DIAGNOSIS

Often suggested by the presence of a mass on ultrasound or CT as well as by abnormal LFTs and significantly elevated α-fetoprotein (AFP) levels. Biopsy is required if diagnosis is uncertain.

TREATMENT

- **Surgical:** Partial hepatectomy if technically feasible and synthetic function preserved; orthotopic liver transplantation in patients with cirrhosis is preferred treatment if there are only a few small tumors (Milan criteria: single lesion < 5 cm or 3 lesions < 3 cm).
- **Nonsurgical:** Transarterial chemoembolization (TACE) and/or radiofrequency ablation. Sorafenib for advanced metastatic disease.
- May monitor AFP levels (if previously elevated) and serial surveillance imaging (ultrasound, CT) to screen for recurrence.

KEY FACT

Hepatic adenomas (caused by oral contraceptives) are benign tumors and do not transform into malignancy.

HEMOCHROMATOSIS

A state of iron overload in which hemosiderin accumulates in the liver, pancreas (islet cells), heart, adrenal glands, testes, and pituitary gland.

- **1° Hemochromatosis:** An autosomal recessive disease characterized by mutations in the *HFE* gene that result in excessive absorption of dietary iron.
- **2° Hemochromatosis:** Occurs in patients receiving chronic transfusion therapy (eg, sickle cell disease or α-thalassemia).

HISTORY/PE

- **Hx:** Patients may present with abdominal pain, DM, hypogonadism, arthropathy of the metacarpophalangeal joints, heart failure, impotence, or cirrhosis.
- **PE:** Bronze skin pigmentation, cardiac dysfunction (CHF), hepatomegaly, and testicular atrophy. Labs may reveal evidence of DM.
- Hemochromatosis does not affect the lung, kidney, or eye.

DIAGNOSIS

- **Best initial tests:** Iron studies showing ↑ serum iron, percent saturation of iron, and ferritin with ↓ serum transferrin. A transferrin saturation (serum iron divided by TIBC) > 45% is highly suggestive of iron overload.
- **Most accurate tests:** *HFE* gene mutation screen (C282Y/H63D) and MRI; liver biopsy (most accurate test) to determine hepatic iron index.

Q

A 36-year-old woman with a past medical history of hypercholesterolemia and type 2 DM presents with intermittent dull RUQ discomfort. The patient does not drink alcohol. Her physical exam is unremarkable. Lab studies show elevated AST and ALT but are otherwise normal. Hepatitis serologies are ⊖. What is the most likely diagnosis?

TREATMENT

- Weekly phlebotomy to normalize serum iron levels, and then maintenance phlebotomy every 2–4 months.
- Iron chelating agents such as deferoxamine, deferiprone, or deferasirox can be used for maintenance therapy.

COMPLICATIONS

Cirrhosis, hepatocellular carcinoma, restrictive cardiomyopathy, arrhythmias, DM, impotence, arthropathy, hypopituitarism. Patients with hemochromatosis have increased susceptibility to *Vibrio vulnificus*, *Listeria monocytogenes*, and *Yersinia enterocolitica* infections.

WILSON DISEASE (HEPATOLENTICULAR DEGENERATION)

- An autosomal recessive disorder that results in defective copper transport and subsequent accumulation and deposition of copper in the liver and brain. Usually occurs in patients < 30 years of age.
- **Hx:** Patients present with hepatitis/cirrhosis, neurologic dysfunction (ataxia, tremor), and psychiatric abnormalities (psychosis, anxiety, mania, depression).
- **PE:** May reveal Kayser-Fleischer rings (green-to-brown copper deposits in the Descemet membrane; see Figure 2.6-20) as well as jaundice, hepatomegaly, asterixis, choreiform movements, and rigidity.
- **Dx:**
  - **Best initial test:** Slit-lamp exam. Other tests that may aid in diagnosis includes ↓ serum ceruloplasmin level, liver biopsy.
  - **Most accurate test:** ↑ 24-hour urinary copper excretion after giving penicillamine.
- **Tx:** Penicillamine or trientine (copper chelators that ↑ urinary copper excretion), dietary copper restriction (avoid shellfish, liver, legumes), and zinc (↑ fecal excretion).

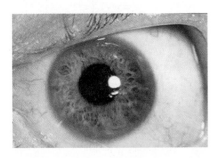

FIGURE 2.6-20. Kayser-Fleischer ring. Note the brown ring encircling the iris. This is a result of copper deposits in the Descemet membrane and is a classic finding in Wilson disease. (Reproduced with permission from USMLE-Rx.com.)

Pancreatic Disease

INSULINOMA

- Results from insulin-producing tumor, associated with MEN type 1, usually benign.
- **Hx:** Hypoglycemia satisfying Whipple triad: (1) documented hypoglycemia on a venipuncture; (2) with associated symptoms including sweating, palpitations, anxiety, tremors, headache, confusion; and (3) resolution of symptoms with correction of hypoglycemia.
- **Dx:**
  - **Best initial test:** Lab tests: fasting serum insulin (elevated), C-peptide (elevated).
  - **Most accurate test:** 72-hour fasting. Patient develops profound or symptomatic hypoglycemia after prolonged fast. Once hypoglycemia is reached, labs drawn to determine etiology: glucose, serum insulin level (elevated), C-peptide level (elevated), sulfonylurea screen (⊖), serum beta hydroxybutyrate level (low), serum cortisol level (normal/elevated).
- **Tx:** Surgery to resect tumor.

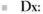

Nonalcoholic fatty liver disease (NAFLD), a condition that is associated with insulin resistance and metabolic syndrome.

VIPOMA

- Results from VIP-producing tumor; highly malignant.
- **Hx:** Watery diarrhea, dehydration, muscle weakness, flushing.
- **Dx:**
    - **Stool sample:** Low stool osmotic gap (ie, secretory diarrhea).
    - **Lab tests:** High VIP levels, achlorhydria (since VIP inhibits gastrin secretion), hyperglycemia, hypercalcemia, hypokalemia.
    - **CT scan:** Localize the tumor.
- **Tx:** Initially, replace fluid and electrolyte losses. Surgery to resect tumor. May also consider octreotide.

PANCREATITIS

Table 2.6-16 outlines the features of acute and chronic pancreatitis.

PANCREATIC CANCER

Most (75%) are adenocarcinomas in the head of the pancreas. Risk factors include smoking, chronic pancreatitis, and a first-degree relative with pancreatic cancer. Incidence ↑ after 45 years of age; slightly more common in men.

HISTORY/PE

- **Presentation:** Abdominal pain radiating toward the back, obstructive jaundice, loss of appetite, nausea, vomiting, weight loss, weakness, fatigue, and indigestion. Often asymptomatic, and thus presents late in the disease course. In some patients, depression may be the most prominent symptom.
- **PE:** May reveal a palpable, nontender gallbladder (Courvoisier sign) or migratory thrombophlebitis (Trousseau syndrome).

DIAGNOSIS

- **Best initial test:** CT scan with contrast. Localize the tumor, and assess the extent of local invasion and distant metastases. Ultrasound of the abdomen is the initial test of choice if the patient suspected of having pancreatic cancer also has jaundice.
- If a mass is not visualized on CT/ultrasound, use ERCP.
- CA-19-9 is often elevated but is neither sensitive nor specific.

TREATMENT

- **Locally advanced or metastatic disease:** Most frequent presentation. Palliative chemotherapy or best supportive care.
- **Small tumors in the pancreatic head with no metastasis or major vessel involvement:** Whipple procedure (pancreaticoduodenectomy).
- **Tumors in the body or tail of the pancreas with no metastasis or celiac artery involvement:** Distal pancreatotomy and splenectomy.
- Chemotherapy with 5-FU and gemcitabine may improve short-term survival, but long-term prognosis is poor (5–10% 5-year survival).
- ERCP with stenting to relieve patients presenting with obstructive symptoms.

KEY FACT

The hallmark finding in pancreatic cancer is a nontender, palpable gallbladder and jaundice.

TABLE 2.6-16. Features of Acute and Chronic Pancreatitis

VARIABLE	ACUTE PANCREATITIS	CHRONIC PANCREATITIS
Pathophysiology	Leakage of activated pancreatic enzymes into pancreatic and peripancreatic tissue	Irreversible parenchymal destruction leading to pancreatic dysfunction and insufficiency
Time course	Abrupt onset of severe pain	Persistent, recurrent episodes of severe pain
Etiology/risk factors	Gallstones, alcohol abuse, hypercalcemia, hypertriglyceridemia, trauma (most common cause of acute pancreatitis in children), drug side effects (thiazide diuretics), viral infections, post-ERCP, scorpion bites	Alcohol abuse (90%), gallstones, CF, smoking, pancreatic divisum, family history
History/PE	Severe epigastric pain (radiating to the back); nausea, vomiting, weakness, fever, shock, pleural effusions, ARDS Flank bruising (Grey Turner sign) and periumbilical discoloration (Cullen sign) may be evident on exam	Recurrent episodes of persistent epigastric pain; anorexia, nausea, constipation, flatulence, steatorrhea, weight loss, DM
Diagnosis	↑ Lipase (more sensitive and specific than amylase), ↑ amylase, ↓ calcium if severe; "sentinel loop" or "colon cutoff sign" on x-ray of the abdomen Ultrasound of the abdomen or CT may show an enlarged pancreas with peripancreatic fluid and fat stranding (arrows in Image A), abscess, hemorrhage, necrosis, or pseudocyst	↑ To normal amylase and lipase, ↓ stool elastase, pancreatic calcifications (arrows in Image B), and alternating stenosis and dilation (arrowheads in Image B) of the main pancreatic duct on CT or ultrasound ("chain of lakes")
Treatment	Removal of the offending agent if possible Supportive care, including IV fluids/electrolyte replacement, analgesia, bowel rest, NG suction, nutritional support, and O_2 Infected pancreatic necrosis should be treated with antibiotics, though prophylactic antibiotics are not recommended Endoscopic, percutaneous, or surgical debridement may be considered	Analgesia, pancreatic enzyme replacement, avoidance of causative agents (EtOH), celiac nerve block; endoscopic dilation of pancreatic duct; surgery for intractable pain or structural causes
Prognosis	Roughly 85–90% are mild and self-limited; 10–15% are severe, requiring ICU admission Mortality may approach 50% in severe cases	Patients can have chronic pain and pancreatic dysfunction
Complications	Pancreatic pseudocyst, fistula formation, hypocalcemia, renal failure, pleural effusion, chronic pancreatitis, sepsis, and ARDS Mortality 2° to acute pancreatitis can be predicted with Ranson criteria	Chronic pain, opiate addiction, diabetes mellitus, malnutrition/weight loss, splenic vein thrombosis, pancreatic cancer

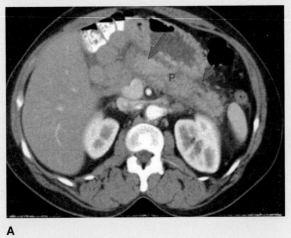

A

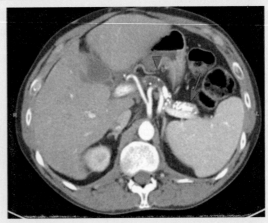

B

P, pancreas. (Images reproduced with permission from USMLE-Rx.com.)

HEMATOLOGY/ONCOLOGY

Coagulation Disorders

NORMAL HEMOSTASIS

Divided into three phases: vascular phase (spasm), platelet phase (plug), and coagulation phase.

The coagulation phase can be further subdivided into extrinsic (outside the blood vessel, fewer factor[s], shorter prothrombin time [PT]) and intrinsic (inside the blood vessel, more factors, longer partial thromboplastin time [PTT]) pathways, both leading to the common pathway.

Vascular injury leads to the release of von Willebrand factor (vWF) and tissue factor from subendothelial vessel walls.

- vWF facilitates attachment and aggregation of platelets, forming a platelet plug.
- Tissue factor triggers the coagulation cascade via the extrinsic pathway with factor VII.

Ultimately the platelet plug and coagulation cascade create a fibrin mesh, as shown in Figure 2.7-1. Drugs affecting the cascade are shown in Table 2.7-1.

Heparin-to-warfarin bridge is necessary because proteins C and S have shorter half-lives than the other vitamin K–dependent factors (II, VII, IX, and X), leading to a transient period of paradoxic hypercoagulability before proper anticoagulation.

> **KEY FACT**
>
> Enteric bacteria synthesize vitamin K. Neonates lack these bacteria and are prone to bleeding unless given a vitamin K shot at birth.

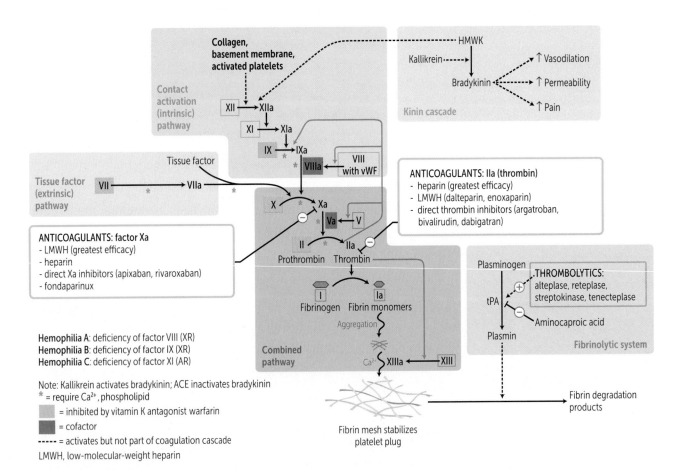

Hemophilia A: deficiency of factor VIII (XR)
Hemophilia B: deficiency of factor IX (XR)
Hemophilia C: deficiency of factor XI (AR)

Note: Kallikrein activates bradykinin; ACE inactivates bradykinin
* = require Ca²⁺, phospholipid
▨ = inhibited by vitamin K antagonist warfarin
▨ = cofactor
----- = activates but not part of coagulation cascade
LMWH, low-molecular-weight heparin

FIGURE 2.7-1. Coagulation cascade. HMWK, high-molecular-weight kininogen; low-molecular-weight-heparin; vWF, von Willebrand factor. (Reproduced with permission from USMLE-Rx.com.)

TABLE 2.7-1. **Coagulation Pharmacology**

Medication	Mechanism	Lab Values	Miscellaneous
Unfractionated heparin	Activates antithrombin Activated antithrombin then inactivates factor Xa, thrombin (IIa), and other proteases	↑ Partial thrombo-plastin time (PTT)	Antidote is protamine sulfate Low-molecular-weight heparin (LMWH) has more effect on factor Xa, can be given subcutaneously, and does not ↑ PTT
Warfarin	Inhibits synthesis of vitamin K–dependent coagulation factors (II, VII, IX, X, and to a lesser extent proteins C and S) by blocking vitamin K epoxide reductase	↑ Prothrombin time (PT)	For rapid reversal, give FFP; otherwise give vitamin K Teratogenic
Tissue plasminogen activators (tPAs)	Aid conversion of plasminogen to plasmin, which breaks down fibrin Include alteplase, reteplase, and tenecteplase	↑ PT, ↑ PTT No change in platelet count	Treat toxicity with aminocaproic acid
Factor **Xa** inhibitors (Api**XA**ban, Rivaro**XA**ban)	Directly inhibit factor Xa New/novel oral anticoagulant (NOAC)	PT/PTT not monitored	Antidote/reversal agent to factor Xa inhibitor is andexanet alfa
LMWH (enoxaparin, dalteparin)	Mainly inhibits factor Xa	Antifactor Xa, although typically unmonitored	Protamine less effective at reversal than for heparin LMWH has better bioavailability and 2–4 times longer half-life than unfractionated heparin (UFH) Can be administered subcutaneously
Direct thrombin inhibitors (dabigatran, argatroban)	Directly inhibit factor II (thrombin) NOAC		Antidote/reversal agent to dabigatran is idarucizumab
Glycoprotein IIb/IIIa inhibitors (abciximab, eptifibatide, tirofiban)	Reversibly binds to the glycoprotein receptor IIb/IIIa on activated platelet, preventing aggregation		Abciximab is made from monoclonal antibody Fab fragments

HEMOPHILIA

Clotting factor deficiencies of factors VIII (hemophilia A, 80% of cases), IX (hemophilia B), and XI (hemophilia C) that result in an ↑ tendency to bleed. X-linked recessive pattern of inheritance (1:10000 male births). Rarely, hemophilias can be acquired if antibodies against these factors are produced as a result of autoimmune, lymphoproliferative, or postpartum states.

History/PE

- Presents as a young boy with spontaneous bleeding into the tissues, muscles, and joints (hemarthrosis) that, if untreated, can lead to crippling arthropathy and joint destruction caused by hemosiderin deposition and fibrosis.

KEY FACT

Hemophilia C is most common in Ashkenazi Jews and is often autosomal recessive.

- Spontaneous intracerebral, renal, retroperitoneal, and GI hemorrhages are also seen.
- Mild cases may have major hemorrhage after surgery, trauma, or dental procedures, but are otherwise asymptomatic.

DIAGNOSIS

- PTT is prolonged (VIII, IX, XI are all intrinsic pathway) on basic bleeding workup. PT and bleeding time are normal.
- **Best initial test:** Mixing study. Mixing the patient's plasma with normal plasma will correct the PTT in hemophilia patients as it contains all clotting factors.
- **Most accurate test:** Obtain specific factor assays for factors VII, VIII, IX, XI, and XII.

TREATMENT

- If bleeding is severe or factor level is ≤ 1% of normal (severe), immediately transfuse missing factor, or if unavailable, use cryoprecipitate.
- If bleeding is not severe and factor level is > 5% of normal (mild) or 1–5% of normal (moderate), hemophilia may be treated with desmopressin, which releases factor VIII from endothelial cells.
- Genetic counseling may be required.
- Prophylactic application of clotting factor concentrates is the basis of modern treatment of severe hemophilia A.

VON WILLEBRAND DISEASE

An autosomal dominant defect or deficiency in vWF with ↓ levels of factor VIII, which is carried by vWF (see Figure 2.7-2). The three main roles of vWF are to (1) bring platelets to exposed subendothelium; (2) aggregate platelets; and (3) bind to factor VIII. Symptoms are caused by platelet dysfunction and deficient factor VIII, but are milder than in hemophilia. vWD is the most common inherited bleeding disorder (1% of the population), and the most common form of vWD is type 1 vWD (mild to moderate deficiency in vWF). Type 2 includes qualitative defects in vWF, and type 3 is absence of functional vWF.

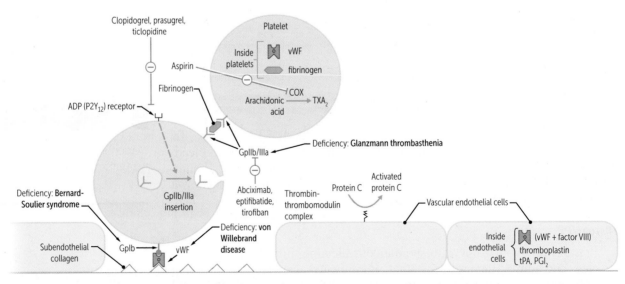

FIGURE 2.7-2. Thrombogenesis deficiencies. ADP, adenosine diphosphate; COX, cyclooxygenase; PGI_2, prostacyclin; tPA, tissue plasminogen activator; TXA_2, thromboxane A_2; vWF, von Willebrand factor. (Adapted with permission from Le T, et al. *First Aid for the USMLE Step 1 2018.* New York, NY: McGraw-Hill; 2018.)

HISTORY/PE

- Often presents in childhood with recurrent and prolonged mucosal bleeding (epistaxis, gums, gingival, menorrhagia) and bleeding after dental or surgical procedures.
- Often a family history is present.
- Symptoms worsen with acetylsalicylic acid (ASA) use.

DIAGNOSIS

- Ristocetin cofactor assay of patient plasma is diagnostic. It measures the capacity of vWF to agglutinate platelets and detects vWF dysfunction.
- **vWF antigen level:** ↓ Levels of antigen may be present.
- Initial bleeding workup will show an ↑ bleeding time in all vWD types. ↑ PTT as in hemophilia may be seen caused by low factor VIII levels. PT and platelet count will be normal.

TREATMENT

- **Best initial treatment:** Desmopressin for mild to moderate disease.
- Use factor VII replacement or vWF concentrate for severe disease, disease that does not respond to desmopressin, or for major bleeds and surgery.
- Control menorrhagia with oral contraceptive pills (OCPs). Avoid ASA, NSAIDs, and platelet function inhibitors.

HYPERCOAGULABLE STATES

Hypercoagulable states (thrombophilias or prothrombotic states) is an all-inclusive term describing conditions that ↑ a patient's risk for developing thrombosis, usually venous thromboembolism (VTE) disease.

ETIOLOGY

Causes can be genetic, acquired, or physiologic (see Table 2.7-2). Three commonly tested causes are highlighted here, but all present similarly:

- **Activated protein C (APC) resistance/factor V Leiden:** The most common cause of inherited thrombophilia. A single point mutation in factor V, rendering it resistant to inactivation/breaking down by activated protein C.

TABLE 2.7-2. Causes of Hypercoagulable States

GENETIC	ACQUIRED	PHYSIOLOGIC
Antithrombin III deficiency	Surgery	Pregnancy
Protein C deficiency	Trauma	Age
Protein S deficiency	OCPs/HRT	
Factor V Leiden	Malignancy	
Hyperhomocysteinemia (*MTHFR* gene mutation)	Immobilization	
Dysfibrinogenemia	Antiphospholipid syndrome	
Plasminogen deficiency	Nephrotic syndrome	
Prothrombin G20210A mutation	Inflammatory bowel disease	
	Smoking	
	Obesity	
	Varicose veins	
	Paroxysmal nocturnal hemoglobinuria	

KEY FACT

↓ Agglutination seen on the ristocetin cofactor assay (detects vWF dysfunction) is diagnostic of vWD.

KEY FACT

ASA ↑ the risk for bleeding in patients with vWD.

KEY FACT

VWD types 1 and 2 are generally inherited in an autosomal-dominant pattern. VWD type 3 is inherited in an autosomal-recessive pattern.

Q

An 8-year-old boy from Eastern Europe presents with severe swelling and warmth of his knee several hours after a minor "bump" against a lamppost. What is the most accurate diagnostic test for his presentation?

KEY FACT

Protein C or S deficiency: hypercoagulable state with skin or tissue necrosis following warfarin administration.

KEY FACT

Suspect PE in a patient with rapid onset of dyspnea, pleuritic chest pain, hypoxia, tachycardia, and an ↑ alveolar-arterial oxygen gradient without another obvious explanation.

MNEMONIC

Antiphospholipid syndrome effects—

CLOTS

Coagulation defect
Livedo reticularis
Obstetric (recurrent miscarriage)
Thrombocytopenia (↓ platelets)
SLE (association)

Risk for DVT or pulmonary embolism (PE) is ↑ 5-fold if heterozygous and 50-fold if homozygous.

- **Heparin-induced thrombocytopenia (HIT):** More common with use of unfractionated heparin. It can happen with heparin or enoxaparin. An immunologic reaction to the administration of heparin creates platelet-activating antibodies, which leads to the formation of blood clots and a rapid (> 30%) drop in platelet count. Usually occurs 5–10 days after starting heparin. Often presents as skin necrosis at the injection site of subcutaneous heparin. HIT rarely causes bleeding. Venous and arterial thromboses can occur, however, VTE is more common.

- **Antiphospholipid syndrome (APS):** Often associated with SLE (20–30%) and rheumatoid arthritis. The two main APS antibodies are the lupus anticoagulant and anticardiolipin. APS predisposes to both arterial and venous thrombi formation and spontaneous abortion (particularly associated with anticardiolipin antibodies). Laboratory testing shows a paradoxically prolonged PTT (only thrombophilia with an abnormality in the PTT).

HISTORY/PE

- Can present with recurrent thrombotic complications: DVT, PE, arterial thrombosis, MI, and stroke. Women may have recurrent miscarriages.
- **Factor V Leiden:** Young, white patients (< 45 years of age) with a personal and family history of thrombosis (eg, multiple VTEs, unusual location, atypically young age).
- **Heparin-induced thrombocytopenia:** Hospitalized patients on anticoagulation (heparin) with a marked drop in platelets 5–10 days after commencing anticoagulation.
- **Antiphospholipid syndrome:** Young and middle-aged women with recurrent miscarriages or thrombosis.

DIAGNOSIS

- Rule out acquired causes of thrombosis before thrombophilia screening.
- **Thrombophilia screening:** Consider in patients with a history of VTE that occurred in the absence of risk factors that were not estrogen- or pregnancy-related, and in patients with a first-degree relative with a VTE that occurred < 50 years of age or with a diagnosis of thrombophilia.
- Hereditary abnormality is confirmed with two abnormal values obtained while the patient is asymptomatic and untreated, with similar values obtained in two other family members.
- **Lab tests:** Complete blood count (CBC), PT, thrombin time, PTT, fibrinogen, and assays for antithrombin and protein C and S deficiency.
- **Disease-specific tests:** Factor V Leiden (APC resistance test), HIT (platelet factor 4 antibody or serotonin release assay), APS (lupus anticoagulant and anticardiolipin antibodies).

TREATMENT

- Patients with a hypercoagulable state with DVT or pulmonary embolism should be treated with heparin immediately followed by 3–6 months of warfarin anticoagulation for the first event and lifelong anticoagulation for subsequent events.
- If anticoagulation is contraindicated (ie, recent trauma, hemorrhage, severe hypertension), an inferior vena cava filter is the **next best step** and is also considered for patients who have recurrent DVTs on anticoagulation.

A

This boy (X-linked) probably has hemophilia A (most common), which is most accurately diagnosed with a specific factor VIII level.

- For factor V Leiden mutation, warfarin is used for 6 months with a target INR of 2 to 3. Avoid OCPs in patients with factor V Leiden.
- **HIT:** Discontinue heparin immediately. Start a direct thrombin inhibitor (eg, fondaparinux, argatroban, and bivalirudin). Warfarin should be commenced after a direct thrombin inhibitor is started. Starting nonheparin anticoagulation is crucial to prevent arterial and venous clots.
- **APS:** Treat with heparin and warfarin. May require lifelong anticoagulation.

DISSEMINATED INTRAVASCULAR COAGULATION

An acquired coagulopathy caused by deposition of fibrin in small blood vessels, leading to thrombosis and end-organ damage. Depletion of clotting factors and platelets leads to a bleeding diathesis. It is associated with many severe illnesses and is often seen in hospitalized patients.

HISTORY/PE

- **Common associations with DIC:** Obstetric complications (eg, amniotic fluid embolism, abruptio placentae), sepsis, malignancy (AML, pancreatic cancer), burns, acute promyelocytic leukemia, pancreatitis, hemolysis, vascular disorders (aortic aneurysm), massive trauma, snake bites, drug reactions, acidosis, transfusion reactions, transplant rejections, and acute respiratory distress syndrome (ARDS).
- **Clinical presentation:**
  - **Acute:** Bleeding from venipuncture sites, into organs, with ecchymoses and petechiae.
  - **Chronic:** Bruising and mucosal bleeding, thrombophlebitis, renal dysfunction, respiratory dysfunction, hepatic dysfunction, shock, and transient neurologic syndromes.

DIAGNOSIS

- **Lab tests:** ↑ PT and PTT, ↓ platelets (thrombocytopenia), ↑ D-dimer and fibrin, ↓ fibrinogen.
- DIC may be confused with liver disease, but unlike liver disease, factor VIII is depressed.

TREATMENT

Reverse the underlying cause; transfuse red blood cells (RBCs), platelets, and FFP; and manage shock as necessary.

THROMBOTIC THROMBOCYTOPENIC PURPURA

Thrombotic thrombocytopenic purpura (TTP) is a deficiency of the vWF-cleaving enzyme (ADAMTS-13) resulting in abnormally large vWF multimers that aggregate platelets and create platelet microthrombi. These block off small blood vessels, leading to end-organ damage. RBCs are fragmented by contact with the microthrombi, leading to hemolysis (microangiopathic hemolytic anemia).

Hemolytic uremic syndrome (HUS) and thrombotic thrombocytopenic purpura have overlap and are considered a spectrum of the same disease that is caused by ADAMTS-13 deficiency, which is either inherited or often acquired secondary to infection. TTP is more common in adults, and HUS is frequently seen in children (associated with *Escherichia coli* 0157:H7).

KEY FACT

DIC is characterized by both thrombosis and hemorrhage.

Q

A 33-year-old woman was admitted to the hospital for anticoagulation after a PE. On day 4 of her stay, her platelet level ↓ from 150,000 to 60,000/mm³ and her INR remains < 2. What is the next best step, and what complications can result from this condition?

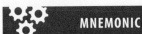

MNEMONIC

Pentad of features for TTP—

LMNOP

Low platelet count (thrombocytopenia)
Microangiopathic hemolytic anemia
Neurologic changes
'Obsolete' renal function
Pyrexia

MNEMONIC

DICk's **HoUS**e got **TTP**ed because he caused microangiopathic hemolytic anemia.

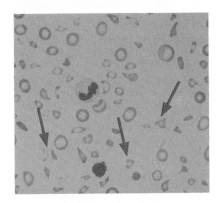

FIGURE 2.7-3. Schistocytes. These fragmented RBCs (*arrows*) can be seen in microangiopathic hemolytic anemia and in mechanical hemolysis. (Reproduced with permission from Dr. Peter McPhedran, Yale Department of Hematology.)

A

This patient is experiencing HIT, which occurs 2° to the formation of antibodies that activate platelets. Because HIT can lead to a hypercoagulable state and subsequent thrombotic complications, heparin must be stopped immediately and the patient must be switched to argatroban, bivalirudin, or fondaparinux.

HISTORY/PE

- **TTP:** Associated with SLE, malignancy, pregnancy, cyclosporine, quinidine, clopidogrel, ticlopidine, and AIDS. Classic description involves a pentad of features. Suspect TTP if three of five of the following symptoms are present:
  - Low platelet count (thrombocytopenia).
  - Microangiopathic hemolytic anemia with schistocytes (severe, often with jaundice).
  - Neurologic changes (delirium, seizure, stroke, ↓ consciousness, ↓ vision).
  - Impaired renal function (acute kidney injury [AKI]).
  - Fever.
- **HUS:** Can present similarly to TTP with the absence of neurologic features.
  - > 90% of cases in children caused by O157:H7 *E coli* hemorrhagic diarrhea preceding the syndrome (eating undercooked contaminated meat).
  - Atypical HUS (aHUS) if caused by Shiga toxin–producing *E coli* (STEC) infection or as secondary HUS with a coexisting disease including infections, especially those caused by *Streptococcus pneumoniae*, and the influenza virus.
  - Characterized by renal failure, microangiopathic hemolytic anemia, and low platelets without neurologic symptoms.
  - Abdominal pain, bloody diarrhea, and AKI are seen. Severe ↑ in creatinine levels are more typical of HUS than of TTP.
  - Schistocytes (fragmented RBCs) are seen in both HUS and TTP.

DIAGNOSIS

- **Lab tests:** ↓ Platelets, ↓ Hb, ↑ creatinine, normal clotting/coagulation screen.
- **Blood film:** Presence of schistocytes (fragmented RBCs) (see Figure 2.7-3).

TREATMENT

- **TTP:** Plasma exchange is the best initial treatment. Steroids can be added to ↓ microthrombus formation.
- **HUS:** Dialysis for AKI may be needed. Plasma exchange is used for severe persistent disease.
- Platelet transfusion is contraindicated, as additional platelets are consumed by the disease process, potentially worsening the patient's condition.

IDIOPATHIC THROMBOCYTOPENIC PURPURA (IMMUNE THROMBOCYTOPENIA)

IgG antibodies (antiplatelet antibodies) are formed against the patient's platelets. The platelet-antibody complex is destroyed by the spleen. Bone marrow production of platelets is ↑, with ↑ megakaryocytes in the marrow. It is the most common immunologic disorder in women of childbearing age.

HISTORY/PE

- Patients often feel well with no systemic symptoms. They may have minor mucocutaneous bleeding, easy bruising, petechiae, hematuria, or melena. Generally there is no splenomegaly.
- Idiopathic thrombocytopenic purpura (ITP) is associated with a range of conditions, including lymphoma, leukemia, SLE, HIV infection, and HCV infection. Can present acutely or as a chronic illness.
  - **Acute:** Abrupt onset of hemorrhagic complications following a viral illness with sudden, self-limiting purpura. Commonly affects children 2–6 years of age, with boys and girls affected equally.
  - **Chronic:** Insidious onset of symptoms or incidental thrombocytopenia on CBC. There is a fluctuating course of bleeding, purpura, epistaxis, and menorrhagia. Affects adults 20–40 years of age and women more than men.

DIAGNOSIS

- Diagnosis of exclusion. Once other causes of thrombocytopenia have been ruled out, diagnose by history and PE, a CBC, and a peripheral blood smear showing normal RBC morphology.
- Antiplatelet antibody often present.
- Bone marrow biopsy would show ↑ megakaryocytes but is done only in atypical cases or patients > 60 years of age.
- **Additional tests for all patients with ITP:** *Helicobacter pylori* testing, hepatitis C testing, direct antiglobulin test, blood type.

TREATMENT

- **Platelet count > 30,000 and no bleeding:** No treatment required.
- **Platelet count < 30,000 or clinically significant bleeding symptoms:** Corticosteroids or IVIG.
- If platelet count fails to improve or bleeding recurs, consider splenectomy ± rituximab ± thrombopoietin (TPO) receptor agonist to ↑ platelet production (romiplostim or eltrombopag).
- Platelet transfusions are not used (except during splenectomy or life-threatening hemorrhage) as the platelets are quickly destroyed by autoantibodies.
- If caused by HCV or HIV, treatment of underlying infection can improve platelet count.
- In pregnant patients, severe thrombocytopenia may occur in the fetus.

Red Blood Cell Disorders

ANEMIAS

A disorder of low hematocrit and hemoglobin. Subtypes are classified according to RBC mean corpuscular volume (MCV) and reticulocyte count (see Figure 2.7-4).

Iron Deficiency Anemia

Anemia in which iron loss exceeds intake. May occur as a result of ↑ demand (growth phase, pregnancy, erythropoietin [EPO] therapy) or ↓ iron (chronic menorrhagia, GI bleeding, malnutrition/absorption disorders like celiac). Toddlers, adolescent girls, and women of childbearing age are most commonly affected.

HISTORY/PE

- **Symptoms:** Fatigue, dyspnea, tachycardia, angina, syncope, and pica.
- If the anemia develops slowly, patients are generally asymptomatic.
- **Physical findings:** Glossitis, conjunctival pallor, cheilosis, and koilonychia ("spoon nails," see Figure 2.7-5).

DIAGNOSIS

- **Best initial test:** CBC (↓ MCV, ↓ MCH, ↓ MCHC) with iron studies (see Table 2.7-3). No single value is diagnostic, but the constellation of the following points to the correct diagnosis:
    - ↓ Ferritin (↓ iron stores).
    - ↑ RBC distribution width (RDW), reflecting high RBC size variation caused by poor erythropoiesis.

Q

An 8-year-old girl presents to the ED with 2 days of fever, vomiting, bloody diarrhea, and irritability. She began feeling unwell after attending a classmate's birthday party. Her labs reveal thrombocytopenia, an ↑ creatinine level, and schistocytes. What is the next best step?

Iron deficiency anemia in an elderly patient may be caused by colorectal cancer until proven otherwise and must therefore be evaluated to rule out malignancy.

MNEMONIC

Causes of microcytic anemia—

IRON LAST

IRON deficiency
Lead poisoning
Anemia of chronic disease
Sideroblastic anemia
Thalassemia

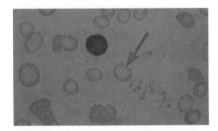

FIGURE 2.7-5. **Koilonychia (spoon nails).** The fingernail plate is concave. (Reproduced with permission from Wolff K, et al. *Fitzpatrick's Color Atlas and Synopsis of Clinical Dermatology.* New York, NY: McGraw-Hill; 2013.)

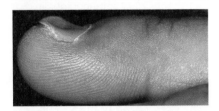

FIGURE 2.7-6. **Iron deficiency anemia.** Note the microcytic, hypochromic RBCs ("doughnut cells") with enlarged areas of central pallor (*arrow*). (Reproduced with permission from Dr. Peter McPhedran, Yale Department of Hematology.)

HUS is the most common cause of acute renal failure in children. Supportive therapy includes IV fluids, BP control, blood transfusion, and, if necessary, dialysis. Antibiotics are not indicated, as they are thought to ↓ expulsion of the toxin and may ↑ toxin from the destruction of bacteria.

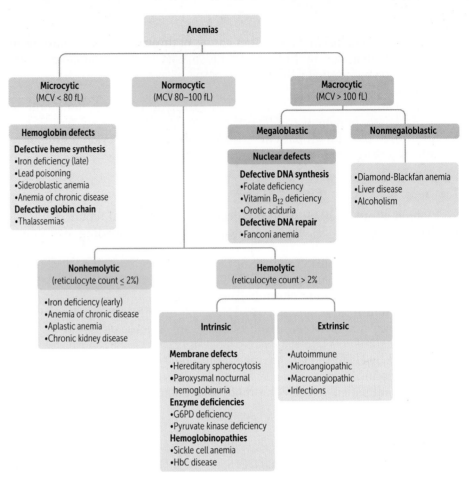

FIGURE 2.7-4. **Anemia algorithm.** (Reproduced with permission from Le T, et al. *First Aid for the USMLE Step 1 2018.* New York, NY: McGraw-Hill; 2018.)

- ↑ Total iron-binding capacity (TIBC); ↓ iron means many empty receptors, so binding capacity is ↑.
- ↓ Serum iron.
- **Most accurate test:** Bone marrow biopsy is seldom performed.
- Peripheral blood smear shows microcytic, hypochromic RBCs (see Figure 2.7-6) with anisocytosis, poikilocytosis, and a low reticulocyte count.

TABLE 2.7-3. **Iron Deficiency Anemia vs Anemia of Chronic Disease**

	IRON DEFICIENCY	**CHRONIC DISEASE**	**BOTH/MIXED DISEASE**
Serum iron	↓	↓	↓
TIBC or transferrin	↑	↓	Normal/↑
Ferritin	↓	↑	Normal/↓
Serum transferrin receptor	↑	Normal	Normal/↑
RDW	↑	Normal	Normal/↑

TREATMENT

- Replace iron orally until normal and for at least 4–6 months to replenish stores. Oral iron sulfate may lead to nausea, constipation, diarrhea, abdominal pain, and black stools. Antacids may interfere with iron absorption.
- If the oral route is insufficient, use intramuscular iron.
- IV iron circumvents gastrointestinal absorption and is therefore only considered as a preferred agent if the oral route is ineffective, such as with gluten sensitivity, inflammatory bowel disease, gastrointestinal malabsorption, post–gastric bypass surgery, hyperemesis gravidarum, and a history of oral iron intolerance.
- IV iron is superior to oral iron in achieving a sustained Hb response, reducing the need for packed RBC transfusions, and improving the quality of life for patients with chronic heart failure, inflammatory bowel disease, chronic kidney disease and hemodialysis, and cancer-related anemia.
- IV iron dextran is associated with a small risk for serious side effects, including anaphylaxis. Iron sucrose may be associated with a lower risk for allergy.

Anemia of Chronic Inflammation/Disease

To limit bacterial proliferation, the body "hides" or "locks" its iron in situations of chronic inflammation such as infection, malignancy, RA, or SLE. Iron is trapped in macrophages or in ferritin ($\uparrow$ in inflammation). This results in a micro- or normocytic anemia with normal or $\uparrow$ levels of iron storage in the form of ferritin, but $\downarrow$ serum iron and $\downarrow$ TIBC (see Table 2.7-3). Treatment consists of treating the underlying disease. Anemia associated with end-stage renal disease (ESRD) responds to erythropoietin replacement.

Sideroblastic Anemia

A microcytic anemia caused by defects in heme metabolism that can be hereditary or acquired. The most common cause is alcohol (suppresses bone marrow). Less common causes include lead poisoning, chloramphenicol, isoniazid (INH), vitamin B_6 deficiency, and malignancy.

- **Hx/PE:** Presents with $\downarrow$ hemoglobin, $\uparrow$ serum iron, and basophilic stippling (in lead poisoning).
- **Dx:** Prussian blue staining for ringed sideroblasts on a smear is diagnostic (see Figure 2.7-7).
- **Tx:** Treat the underlying cause. Treat acquired causes with vitamin B_6 or pyridoxine replacement.

Megaloblastic Anemia

Impaired DNA synthesis secondary to vitamin B_{12} (cobalamin) or folate deficiency leads to megaloblastic anemia. Vitamin B_{12} deficiency is caused by intestinal malabsorption, traditionally from pernicious anemia (autoimmune destruction of parietal cells, which produce the intrinsic factor needed for cobalamin absorption), gastrectomy, pancreatic insufficiency, Crohn disease, celiac disease, topical sprue, tapeworms, or low dietary intake (eg, vegetarian or vegan diet). Folate deficiency results from alcoholism, low dietary folate, malabsorption, psoriasis, sulfa drugs, and phenytoin. Drugs that interfere with DNA synthesis, including chemotherapeutic agents (methotrexate, 6-mercaptopurine), may lead to megaloblastic anemia.

HISTORY/PE

- Presents with fatigue, pallor, glossitis, cheilosis, diarrhea, loss of appetite, and headache.

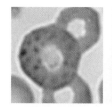
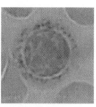

A   **B**

FIGURE 2.7-7. Pathogenic RBC forms. (A) Basophilic stippling. **(B)** Ringed sideroblasts. (Image A reproduced courtesy of van Dijk HA, Fred HL. Images of memorable cases: case 81. OpenStax website. June 18, 2018. Available at https://cnx.org/contents/57cfLKUe@7.2:MZa_Ph4e@4/Images-of-Memorable-Cases-Case. Image B reproduced with permission of Paulo Henrique Orlandi Mourao.)

 KEY FACT

Anemia secondary to end-stage renal disease is caused by deficiency of erythropoietin. Treatment with recombinant EPO is effective, but often leads to worsening of hypertension.

 KEY FACT

Sideroblastic anemia is the only form of microcytic anemia in which the serum iron level is elevated.

 KEY FACT

Subacute combined degeneration of the cord seen in B_{12} deficiency presents as peripheral neuropathy, vibration and proprioception dysfunction, dementia, and spasticity.

 Q

A 49-year-old man comes into the clinic complaining of "tiredness" over the last several months. His past medical history is significant for hypertension, diabetes mellitus, and alcohol abuse. A CBC reveals a low hemoglobin and an MCV of 115. What is the most likely cause of his anemia?

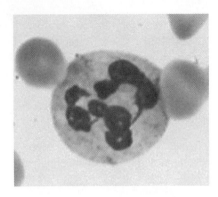

FIGURE 2.7-8. Hypersegmentation. The nucleus of this hypersegmented neutrophil has six lobes (six or more nuclear lobes are required). This is a characteristic finding of megaloblastic anemia. (Reproduced with permission from Dr. Ed Uthman.)

KEY FACT

B_{12} deficiency can be caused by infection by a tapeworm, *Diphyllobothrium latum*. Folate deficiency can occur secondary to chronic phenytoin use, causing malabsorption.

KEY FACT

Although many factors $\uparrow$ MCV (macrocytic anemia), only megaloblastic anemia is associated with hypersegmented neutrophils (ie, alcohol can cause macrocytic anemia but is not associated with hypersegmented neutrophils).

KEY FACT

Pernicious anemia increases the risk for gastric cancer and is the most common cause of B_{12} deficiency in Europeans.

The patient has a megaloblastic anemia caused by either a B_{12} or folate deficiency. His history of alcohol dependence strongly suggests folate deficiency, as that is the most common cause of megaloblastic anemia in alcoholics.

- B_{12} deficiency affects the nervous system. Neurologic and neuropsychiatric signs and symptoms can be present (eg, irritability, depression, psychosis, dementia, paraesthesia, and peripheral neuropathy).
- Patients may develop a demyelinating disorder and present with subacute combined degeneration of the cord. There is a combination of symmetrical posterior (dorsal) column loss, causing sensory and lower motor neuron (LMN) signs, and symmetrical corticospinal tract loss, causing motor and upper motor neuron (UMN) signs.

DIAGNOSIS

- **Best initial test:** CBC with smear showing RBCs with an elevated MCV and hypersegmented (six or more lobes) neutrophils (see Figure 2.7-8). B_{12} and folate deficiency are identical hematologically and on blood smear.
- $\downarrow$ Hb, $\uparrow$ MCV, $\downarrow$ B_{12} and folate levels, $\downarrow$ reticulocyte count, pancytopenia if severe, $\uparrow$ LDH, $\uparrow$ indirect bilirubin levels.
- Serum vitamin levels should be measured and adjunctive tests, including methylmalonic acid (MMA) and homocysteine levels can be assessed if vitamin levels are nondiagnostic and clinical suspicion persists:
  - **B_{12} deficiency:** $\uparrow$ MMA and $\uparrow$ homocysteine.
  - **Folate deficiency:** Normal MMA and $\uparrow$ homocysteine.
- Bone marrow sample reveals giant neutrophils and hypersegmented mature neutrophils.
- Anti-intrinsic factor and antiparietal cell antibodies in pernicious anemia.
- Schilling test measures the absorption of cobalamin via ingestion of radiolabeled cobalamin with and without intrinsic factor. This test is rarely performed, but its interpretation is tested. The patient is given an unlabeled B_{12} IM shot to saturate B_{12} receptors in the liver and an oral challenge of radiolabeled B_{12}. The radiolabeled B_{12} will pass into the urine if properly absorbed, as the liver's B_{12} receptors will be saturated from the IM dose.
  - **Radiolabeled B_{12} in urine:** Dietary B_{12} deficiency.
  - **No radiolabeled B_{12} in urine:** Consider pernicious anemia, bacterial overgrowth, or pancreatic enzyme deficiency; test the hypothesis with the addition of intrinsic factor, antibiotics, or pancreatic enzymes to radiolabeled B_{12}.

TREATMENT

Correct the underlying cause of the anemia. If B_{12} deficiency is caused by malabsorption, replenish stores with IM hydroxycobalamin. If the cause is dietary, give oral B_{12}. Folate replacement corrects the hematologic problems of B_{12}, but not the neurologic problems.

Hemolytic Anemia

Occurs when bone marrow production is unable to compensate for $\uparrow$ destruction of circulating blood cells. Etiologies include the following:

- Glucose 6-phosphate dehydrogenase (G6PD) deficiency, paroxysmal nocturnal hemoglobinuria (PNH), spherocytosis (see Figure 2.7-9), sickle cell disease, and autoimmune anemia (discussed separately later).
- **Microangiopathic hemolytic anemia:** TTP, HUS, DIC.
- **Mechanical hemolysis:** Associated with mechanical heart valves.
- **Other:** Malaria, hypersplenism.

HISTORY/PE

- Present with pallor, fatigue, tachycardia, and tachypnea.
- Patients are often jaundiced. Hepatosplenomegaly, pigmented gallstones (pigmented caused by $\uparrow$ indirect bilirubin), and leg ulcers (poor blood flow) may be noted.

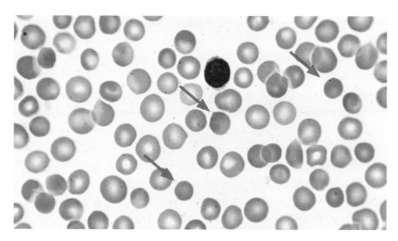

FIGURE 2.7-9. **Spherocytes.** These RBCs *(arrows)* lack areas of central pallor. Spherocytes are seen in autoimmune hemolysis and in hereditary spherocytosis. (Reproduced with permission from Bun HF, Aster JC. *Pathophysiology of Blood Disorders.* New York, NY: McGraw Hill; 2011.)

DIAGNOSIS

- **Lab tests:** FBC, reticulocytes, electrolytes, liver function test (LFT), haptoglobin, urinary urobilinogen.
- ↓ Hematocrit, ↑ LDH, ↑ indirect bilirubin, ↑ reticulocyte count, ↓ haptoglobin, are commonly seen. Folate deficiency (folate is used from increased cell production) and hyperkalemia (↑ cell breakdown) may be seen. Urine is dark with hemoglobinuria, and there is ↑ excretion of urinary and fecal urobilinogen. A slight ↑ MCV (macrocytosis) caused by large reticulocytes.
- **Blood films:** Hypochromic microcytic anemia (thalassemia), sickle cells (sickle-cell anemia), schistocytes (microangiopathic hemolytic anemia), abnormal cells (hematologic malignancy), spherocytes (hereditary spherocytosis or autoimmune hemolytic anemia), Heinz bodies/bite cells (G6PD deficiency).
- Direct antiglobulin (Coombs) test can be used to identify autoimmune hemolytic anemia.

TREATMENT

Varies with the cause of hemolytic anemia (see later), but often includes corticosteroids to address immunologic causes and iron supplementation to replace losses. Splenectomy or transfusions are helpful in severe cases.

G6PD Deficiency

An X-linked recessive defect in G6PD causing the inability to generate glutathione reductase, leaving RBCs susceptible to hemolytic anemia following oxidant stress.

- **Hx/PE:** Patients are often Mediterranean or African men presenting with sudden anemia, episodic dark urine, and jaundice who have a normal-sized spleen with an infection or use drugs that induce oxidative damage to RBCs. Common triggers include: infections (most common), fava beans, isoniazid, nitrofurantoin, dapsone, sulfa-drugs (TMP-SMX), and antimalarials (quinines).
- **Dx:**
  - **Best initial test:** CBC with smear showing hemolytic anemia with bite cells and Heinz bodies.
  - **Most accurate test:** G6PD level 1 to 2 months after an episode (often normal during acute episode since G6PD-deficient RBCs are hemolyzed first).

MNEMONIC

Causes of hemolytic anemia—

MOM PASS me the GLUCOSE

Microangiopathic hemolytic anemia (TTP, HUS, DIC)
Other: malaria, hypersplenism
Mechanical hemolysis
Paroxysmal nocturnal hemoglobinuria
Autoimmune anemia
Sickle cell disease
Spherocytosis
me the
GLUCOSE 6-phosphate dehydrogenase deficiency

KEY FACT

A classic presentation of G6PD deficiency is a black male patient presenting with fatigue, dark urine, and SOB after taking TMP-SMX for a cold.

Causes of oxidative stress in G6PD deficiency—

Sell FAVA BEANS in INDIA

Sulfa-drugs
FAVA Beans
Infections (most common cause)
Nitrofuratoin
Dapsone
Isoniazid
Antimalarials (quinines)

KEY FACT

Patients who had a splenectomy for any reason are at an increased lifelong risk for sepsis (for up to 30 years) from encapsulated bacteria and thus require pneumococcal, meningococcal, and *Haemophilus* vaccinations before the operation.

KEY FACT

Sickling occurs with dehydration, deoxygenation, and at high altitude. If it happens in the vasa rectae (vessels supplying the inner medulla of the kidneys), sickle cell patients can have ↓ ability to concentrate urine, presenting as polyuria or nocturia.

- **Tx:** There is no reversal to the hemolysis. Avoiding triggers is the main stay of treatment.

Paroxysmal Nocturnal Hemoglobinuria

CD55/CD59 proteins (also known as decay accelerating factor) found on the surface of RBCs protect them from complement-mediated hemolysis. Paroxysmal nocturnal hemoglobinuria (PNH) is a deficiency in glycosylphosphatidylinositol-anchor molecules that inhibit CD55/CD59 attachment or binding to RBCs, resulting in complement-mediated hemolysis and thrombosis.

- **Hx/PE:** PNH can manifest as iron deficiency anemia, episodic dark urine, venous thrombosis (most commonly mesenteric and hepatic vein thrombosis), pancytopenia, and abdominal pain.
- **Dx:** Most accurate diagnostic test is CD55/CD59 absence via flow cytometry.
- **Tx:** Prednisone is the best initial therapy. Allogeneic bone marrow transplant is curative. Eculizumab, a complement inhibitor, can be used for hemolysis and thrombosis.

Hereditary Spherocytosis

Autosomal dominant defect or deficiency in spectrin or ankyrin, an RBC membrane protein resulting in a loss of RBC membrane surface area and characteristic biconcave disc. RBCs are forced to take spherical shapes and are trapped and destroyed by the spleen.

- **Hx/PE:** Clinically presents as an extravascular hemolytic anemia with splenomegaly and jaundice. Acute cholecystitis from pigmented gallstones is a common complication.
- **Dx:**
  - **Best initial test:** CBC with a ↓ MCV, ↑ MCHC, and ⊖ Coombs test. A blood smear shows spherocytes (see Figure 2.7-9).
  - **Most accurate test:** Eosin-5 maleimide flow cytometry (replaced osmotic fragility test) and acidified glycerol lysis test.
- **Tx:** Manage with a splenectomy (stops hemolysis) and chronic folic acid replacement (assists in RBC production). Patients with HS have a characteristically increased mean cell hemoglobin concentration and RBC distribution widths.

Sickle Cell Disease

An autosomal recessive disorder caused by a mutation of adult hemoglobin (the β-chain has Glu replaced by Val causing production of abnormal β globin chain) resulting in the production of HbS rather than HbA. HbA₂ and HbF are still produced. It is common in patients of African descent. The homozygote (SS) has sickle-cell anemia (HbSS), and the heterozygote (HbAS) has sickle-cell trait, which causes no disability (uniquely protects from *Plasmodium falciparum* malaria). Signs and symptoms are caused by ↓ RBC survival and a tendency of sickled cells to aggregate and cause vaso-occlusion.

HISTORY/PE

- **Classic presentation:** African-American patient with sudden onset of severe chest pain, back pain, or thigh pain. May be accompanied by fever.
- **Acute chest syndrome:** Pulmonary infiltrates involving complete lung segments causing pain, fever, wheeze, cough, and tachypnea. Chief causes of infiltrates are fat embolism from bone marrow or infection with *Mycoplasma*, *Chlamydia*, or viruses.

- **Presentation:** May first present with dactylitis in childhood (bilateral hand/foot swelling). Lifelong hemolysis results in anemia, jaundice, pigmented cholelithiasis, ↑ CO (murmur, eventual CHF), and delayed growth.
- Chronic hemolysis is usually well-tolerated, except in acute painful vaso-occlusive crisis (VOC; commonly caused by microvascular occlusion), which is caused by infection/fever, hypoxia, dehydration, and cold temperatures.
- **Painful VOC:** Dactylitis (occurs < 3 years of age), mesenteric ischemia (mimics acute abdomen), CNS infarction (leads to stroke, cognitive defects, or seizures), priapism, and avascular necrosis of the femoral head. Leads to ischemic organ damage, especially splenic infarction (typically occurs < 2 years of age), which predisposes to infection from encapsulated organisms, particularly pneumococcal sepsis and acute chest syndrome (pneumonia and/or pulmonary infarction; see Figure 2.7-10). Also, susceptible to osteomyelitis.
- **Other complications:** Splenic sequestration (sudden pooling of blood into the spleen resulting in hypovolemia) and aplastic crisis (2° to infection with viruses such as parvovirus B19). Both complications present with ↓ hematocrit but are distinguished clinically by ↓ reticulocytes in aplastic crisis (2° to bone marrow involvement) and normal to ↑ reticulocytes in splenic sequestration.
- Sickle cell trait (HbAS) is relatively benign. Patients have normal Hb and RBC morphology. However, renal complications include hematuria (renal papillary necrosis), defect in the ability to concentrate urine (hyposthenuria), and ↑ risk for urinary tract infections.

DIAGNOSIS

- **Best initial test:** CBC (↑ reticulocytes, ↑ indirect bilirubin) with peripheral smear showing sickle cells and Howell-Jolly bodies (see Figure 2.7-11A, B).
- **Most accurate test:** Hemoglobin electrophoresis.

KEY FACT

The most common cause of osteomyelitis in patients with sickle cell disease is *Staphylococcus aureus; Salmonella* is the second most common cause. Patients are also at ↑ risk for avascular necrosis of the femoral head.

MNEMONIC

Causes/triggers of acute VOC in sickle cell disease—

HIDe in the COLD

Hypoxia
Infections/fever
Dehydration
COLD temperatures

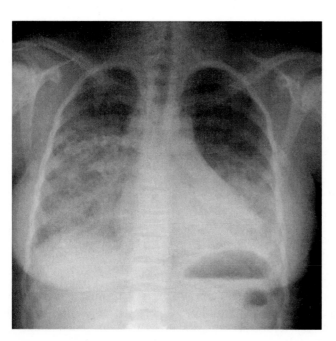

FIGURE 2.7-10. **Acute chest syndrome.** Frontal chest x-ray (CXR) of a 19-year-old woman with sickle cell disease and acute chest pain. Note the bilateral lower and midlung opacities and mild cardiomegaly. (Reproduced with permission from USMLE-Rx.com.)

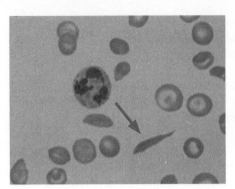
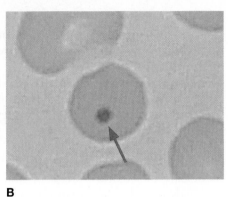

A　　　　　　　　　　　　　**B**

FIGURE 2.7-11. **Sickle cell disease.** (**A**) Sickle-shaped RBCs (*arrow*) are almost always seen on blood smear, regardless of whether the patient is having a sickle cell crisis. (**B**) Howell-Jolly bodies, which suggest functional hyposplenia or asplenia. (Image A reproduced with permission from Dr. Peter McPhedran, Yale Department of Hematology. Image B reproduced with permission from Paulo Henrique Orlandi Mourao and Mikael Häggström.)

TREATMENT

- **Management of chronic disease:**
  - Treat with hydroxyurea, which stimulates the production of fetal hemoglobin and helps prevent the recurrence of sickle cell crises. Hydroxyurea is teratogenic and may cause mild myelosuppression (important to monitor WBCs).
  - If hydroxyurea does not prove effective, chronic transfusion therapy, which carries the risk for iron overload, can be attempted.
  - Folic acid supplementation is often required to prevent macrocytic anemia caused by frequent RBC turnover.
  - Risk for septicemia in febrile patients or in leukocytosis. Give antibiotics (use ceftriaxone, levofloxacin, or moxifloxacin).
  - Prophylactic pneumococcal vaccination and antibiotics (penicillin in patients < 5 years of age) caused by autosplenectomy (↑ risk for infection from encapsulated bacteria). Treat recurrent cholelithiasis with cholecystectomy.
- **Management of sickle cell crises:**
  - VOC must be treated with adequate analgesia (pain management), O_2 therapy, IV fluid rehydration, and antibiotics (if infection is suspected to be the trigger).
  - If there is concern of a VOC progressing to acute chest syndrome, initiate aggressive hydration, antibiotics, and incentive spirometry. Keep the sickle variant < 40%. This can be done with simple transfusions or, if necessary, exchange transfusion in an ICU setting. Bronchodilators may be helpful.
- No treatment is required for sickle cell trait (HbAS).

Autoimmune Hemolytic Anemia

Autoantibodies against RBC membrane destroy blood cells, causing extravascular hemolysis.

- **Two types:**
  - **Warm:** IgG, associated with SLE, chronic lymphocytic leukemia (CLL), lymphoma, penicillin, rifampin, phenytoin, and α-methyldopa.
  - **Cold:** IgM, associated with *Mycoplasma pneumonia*, Epstein-Barr virus, and Waldenström macroglobulinemia.
- **Hx/PE:** Presents as a hemolytic anemia.

KEY FACT

The indirect Coombs test detects antibodies to RBCs in the patient's serum. The direct Coombs test detects sensitized erythrocytes.

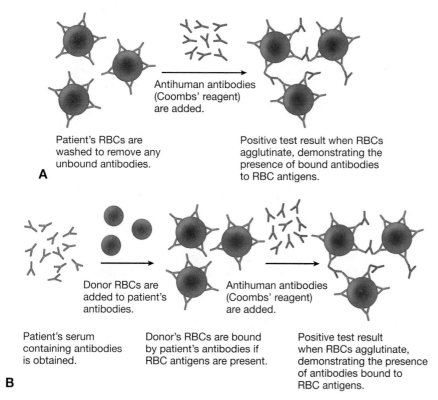

FIGURE 2.7-12. **(A) Direct and (B) indirect Coombs tests.**

- **Dx:** Direct Coombs test (see Figure 2.7-12). Autoimmune hemolytic anemia (AIHA) is also associated with spherocytes. Cold agglutinin is the most effective test in cold AIHA.
- **Tx:** If AIHA is mild, no treatment is necessary. Warm AIHA is treated with steroids; recurrent episodes respond to splenectomy. Severe, nonresponsive hemolysis is controlled with IVIG. Severe cold AIHA is managed by avoiding exposure to cold (keep patient warm) ± rituximab (anti-CD20 antibody).

Aplastic Anemia

Failure of blood cell production (pancytopenia) caused by destruction of bone marrow cells. It may be hereditary, as in Fanconi anemia (genetic analysis will show chromosomal breaks); may have an autoimmune or viral etiology (HIV, parvovirus B19, EBV, CMV, hepatitis); or may result from exposure to toxins (cleaning solvents, insecticides, benzene), radiation, or drugs (sulfa, chloramphenicol, propylthiouracil, carbamazepine, alcohol, methimazole, chemotherapy).

History/PE

Patients are pancytopenic, with symptoms resulting from a lack of RBCs, WBCs, and platelets: pallor, fatigue, weakness, a tendency to infection, petechiae, bruising, and bleeding.

Diagnosis

- Diagnosed by clinical presentation and CBC.
- **Most accurate test:** Bone marrow biopsy revealing hypocellularity and space occupied by fat.

KEY FACT

Both AIHA and hereditary spherocytosis can present with spherocytes and positive osmotic fragility tests, but only AIHA will have a ⊕ direct Coombs test.

KEY FACT

Patients with Fanconi anemia can be identified on physical exam by café-au-lait spots, short stature, and radial/thumb hypoplasia/aplasia.

KEY FACT

Diamond-Blackfan syndrome presents with pure red cell aplasia and congenital anomalies, such as triphalangeal thumbs and cleft lip.

TREATMENT

- **Supportive therapy:** Blood transfusion for anemia, antibiotics for infection, platelets for bleeding.
- Consider allogenic bone marrow transplantation (BMT) in young patients with a matched donor. In severe cases, in patients without a stem cell donor, or patients too old for BMT (> 50 years of age), immunosuppress with cyclosporine, antithymocyte globulin (ATG), and eltrombopag to prevent autoimmune marrow destruction. Tacrolimus is an alternative to cyclosporine. Treat infections aggressively.

THALASSEMIAS

Hereditary disorders involving ↓ or absent production of normal globin chains of hemoglobin. α-thalassemia is caused by a gene deletion of one or more of the four genes that encode α-hemoglobin. β-thalassemia results from a point mutation of one or both of the two genes encoding β-hemoglobin.

HISTORY/PE

Thalassemia is most common among people of African, Middle Eastern, and Asian descent. Disease presentation varies with the number of genes missing (see Table 2.7-4). A typical case can be an asymptomatic or fatigued individual with a microcytic anemia and normal iron studies.

DIAGNOSIS

Most accurate test is hemoglobin electrophoresis (normal in α trait, α silent carrier). For α-thalassemia, genetic studies are the most accurate tests. All

TABLE 2.7-4. **Differential Diagnosis of Thalassemias**

SUBTYPE	NUMBER OF GENES PRESENT	CLINICAL FEATURES
β-thalassemia major (Cooley anemia)	0/2 β	Patients develop severe microcytic anemia and failure to thrive in the first year of life and need chronic transfusions lifelong or marrow transplant to survive. Extramedullary hemopoiesis occurs in response to anemia (ie, skull bossing, hepatosplenomegaly)
β-thalassemia minor	1/2 β	Patients are asymptomatic with mild-moderate, well-tolerated anemia, but their cells are microcytic and hypochromic on peripheral smear Often confused with iron deficiency anemia Common in the Mediterranean region
Hydrops fetalis (Bart's hydrops)	0/4 α	Patients die in utero
Hemoglobin H disease	1/4 α	Patients have severe hypochromic, microcytic anemia with chronic hemolysis, splenomegaly, jaundice, and cholelithiasis The reticulocyte count ↑ to compensate, and one-third of patients have skeletal changes caused by expanded erythropoiesis
α-thalassemia trait	2/4 α	Patients have low MCV but are usually asymptomatic
Silent carrier	3/4 α	Patients have no signs or symptoms of disease. Normal clinical state

forms of thalassemia have a normal RDW. Only 3-gene deletion α-thalassemia is associated with hemoglobin H and ↑ reticulocyte count.

TREATMENT

- Most patients do not require treatment (trait is not treated).
- Those with β-thalassemia major and hemoglobin H disease are often transfusion dependent (chronic, lifelong transfusion) and require oral iron chelators (deferasirox or deferiprone) or a parenteral iron chelator (deferoxamine) to prevent overload.

POLYCYTHEMIAS

Erythrocytosis (an abnormal elevation of hematocrit) may be either absolute (↑ RBC production) or relative (↓ plasma volume and hemoconcentration). Absolute polycythemia causes are primary (polycythemia rubra vera) or secondary (caused by hypoxia) or inappropriately ↑ erythropoietin secretion (EPO-producing tumors).

HISTORY/PE

- Characterized by ↑ hematocrit, ↓ tissue blood flow and oxygenation, and ↑ cardiac work.
- Absolute erythrocytosis is associated with hypoxia (lung disease, heavy smoking, high altitudes, obstructive sleep apnea, cyanotic congenital heart disease, or poor intrauterine environment); neoplasia (renal carcinoma, hepatocellular carcinoma); or polycythemia vera (PCV).
- **PCV:** Results from clonal proliferation of a pluripotent marrow stem cell caused by a mutation in the *JAK2* protein, which regulates marrow production. There is excess proliferation of RBCs, WBCs, and platelets → hyperviscosity and thrombosis, but RBCs are most significantly affected and proliferate at an exceedingly high rate despite a low erythropoietin.
    - **Presentation:** Hyperviscosity syndrome. Easy bleeding/bruising from engorged blood vessels, fatigue, hypertension, thrombosis (arterial and venous), visual disturbance, neurologic deficits, headaches, dizziness, tinnitus, pruritus after a warm bath, CHF, facial plethora, splenomegaly.
    - Commonly affects older individuals (> 60 years of age).
    - Can convert to acute myeloid leukemia in a small proportion of patients.
- Relative erythrocytosis is associated with hypovolemia and dehydration: diuresis, gastroenteritis, alcohol, burns.

DIAGNOSIS

- **PCV:** Best initial test is a CBC showing elevated RBCs/WBCs/platelets (↑ reticulocyte, ↑ Hb, ↑ Hct, ↑ PCV) with an ABG and EPO level. ↓ EPO, normal O$_2$, and Hct > 60% (key finding) suggest PCV. Most accurate test is the *JAK2* mutation (present in 95% of patients).
- Relative erythrocytosis also has an ↑ HCT, splenomegaly, but EPO is normal or increased, and O$_2$ is often low compared to PCV.

TREATMENT

- **PCV:** Target is hematocrit < 45%. Phlebotomy and aspirin provide symptom relief and prevent thrombosis. Hydroxyurea reduces cell counts. Allopurinol or rasburicase prevents ↑ in uric acid. Hydroxyurea-resistant disease is treated with ruxolitinib (inhibitor of *JAK2*).
- **Relative erythrocytosis:** Address the underlying cause and treat symptoms with phlebotomy.

KEY FACT

Mentzer index: MCV divided by RBC count (MCV/RBC). Can help distinguish between thalassemia and iron deficiency anemia. Mentzer index < 13 suggests thalassemia and > 13 suggests iron deficiency anemia.

KEY FACT

Premedication with acetaminophen and diphenhydramine is sometimes used to prevent minor transfusion reactions.

KEY FACT

Hemoglobinuria in hemolytic transfusion reaction may lead to acute tubular necrosis and subsequent renal failure.

KEY FACT

Heme is necessary for the production of hemoglobin, myoglobin, and cytochrome molecules.

KEY FACT

PCV has low erythropoietin and normal O$_2$ levels. Relative erythrocytosis has normal or increased erythropoietin with low O$_2$ levels.

A 30-year-old man from Greece comes to your office complaining of chronic fatigue. He has no significant past medical history and is on no medications. A CBC shows hemoglobin of 10.4 and MCV of 71. You start him on oral iron supplements and see him back in 4 weeks with no change in the CBC. What is the most likely diagnosis?

TABLE 2.7-5.   Transfusion Reactions

VARIABLE	ALLERGIC REACTION	ANAPHYLACTIC REACTION	FEBRILE NONHEMOLYTIC REACTION	HEMOLYTIC TRANSFUSION REACTION
Mechanism	Antibody formation against donor plasma proteins, usually after receiving plasma-containing product Type I hypersensitivity reaction	Severe allergic reaction in IgA-deficient individuals who must receive blood products without IgA	Cytokine formation during storage of blood Host antibodies against the donor HLA antigens and WBCs Type II hypersensitivity reaction	Preformed (acute) or formed (delayed) recipient antibodies against donor erythrocytes Intravascular hemolysis (ABO blood group incompatibility) or extra-vascular hemolysis (host antibody reaction against donor foreign antigen on donor RBCs) Type II hypersensitivity reaction
Presentation	Prominent urticaria, pruritus, wheezing, fever	Dyspnea, broncho-spasm, respiratory arrest, hypotension, and shock	Fever, headache, chills, flushing, rigors, and malaise 1–6 hours after transfusion	Fever, hypotension, chills, nausea, flushing, burning at the IV site, tachycardia, tachypnea, flank pain/renal failure, hemoglobinuria (intravascular hemolysis), jaundice (extravascular), during or shortly after the transfusion
Treatment	Give antihistamines If severe reaction, stop the transfusion and give epinephrine	Stop the transfusion and give epinephrine Treat anaphylactic shock as required	Stop the transfusion and give acetaminophen Leukoreduction of donor blood	Stop the transfusion immediately! Give vigorous IV fluids and maintain good urine output

BLOOD TRANSFUSION REACTIONS

Transfusions are generally safe but may result in adverse reactions (see Table 2.7-5). Febrile nonhemolytic and allergic reactions are the most common, occurring in 3–4% of all transfusions.

White Blood Cell Disorders

LEUKEMIAS

Malignant proliferations of hematopoietic cells, categorized by the type of cell involved and their level of differentiation.

Acute Leukemias

Acute myelogenous and lymphocytic leukemias are clonal disorders of early hematopoietic stem cells (blasts) resulting in unregulated growth and differentiation of WBCs in bone marrow. As the bone marrow becomes replaced by leukemia cells, patients present with signs of pancytopenia: anemia (↓ RBCs), infection (↓ mature WBCs), and hemorrhage (↓ platelets) result.

HISTORY/PE

- AML and acute lymphocytic leukemia (ALL) affect children and adults. ALL is the most common childhood malignancy.

The most likely diagnosis is β-thalassemia minor. Recognize that this patient has a microcytic anemia that did not respond to iron supplements (probably has normal iron studies) and is from the Mediterranean.

- Rapid onset and progression. Patients present with signs and symptoms of anemia (pallor, fatigue), thrombocytopenia (petechiae, purpura, bleeding), infections (ineffective and immature WBCs), and DIC (most commonly seen in acute promyelocytic leukemia [APL]). Medullary expansion into the periosteum may lead to bone pain (common in ALL).
- Exam may show hepatosplenomegaly and swollen/bleeding gums from leukemic infiltration and ↓ platelets. Leukemic cells also infiltrate the skin and CNS.

DIAGNOSIS

- **Best initial test:** CBC with smear showing blast cells.
- **Most accurate test:** Bone marrow biopsy with flow cytometry to classify leukemia type.
- Marrow that is infiltrated with blast cells is consistent with leukemia. In AML, the leukemic cells are myeloblasts; in ALL they are lymphoblasts. These cells can be distinguished by morphology (see Figure 2.7-14), cytogenetics, and immunophenotyping (see Table 2.7-6).
- WBC count can be elevated, but the cells are dysfunctional, and patients may be neutropenic with a history of frequent infection. If the WBC count is very high (> 150,000/mm³ in AML, > 400,000/mm³ in ALL), there is a risk for leukostasis (blasts occluding the microcirculation, leading to pulmonary edema, CNS symptoms, ischemic injury, and DIC).

TREATMENT

- In general, ALL and AML are treated with chemotherapy. Patients with a leukemia subtype of unfavorable cytogenetics or lack of appropriate response to chemotherapy may be candidates for bone marrow transplantation.
- All-trans-retinoic acid (ATRA) is highly effective in APL.
- To prevent tumor lysis syndrome (hyperuricemia, hyperkalemia, hypocalcemia, renal insufficiency, as blasts are destroyed by chemotherapy), patients should be well hydrated. If WBC counts are ↑, they may also be started on allopurinol or rasburicase (often used in the pediatric population) to decrease serum uric acid as renal protection. Rasburicase is contraindicated in G6PD deficiency.

TABLE 2.7-6.   Myeloblasts vs Lymphoblasts

Variable	Myeloblast	Lymphoblast
Size	Larger (2–4 times RBC)	Smaller (1.5–3.0 times RBC)
Amount of cytoplasm	More	Less
Nucleoli	Conspicuous	Inconspicuous
Granules	Common, fine	Uncommon, coarse
Auer rods	Present in 50% of cases (see Figure 2.7-13)	Absent
Myeloperoxidase	⊕	⊖
Terminal deoxynucleotidyltransferase (TdT)	⊖	⊕

KEY FACT

A characteristic sign for AML subtype M3 (APL) is the Auer rod (see Figure 2.7-13), although Auer rods can be seen in other AML subtypes.

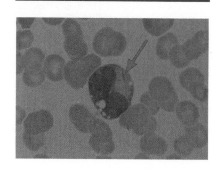

FIGURE 2.7-13.   Auer rod in AML. The red rod-shaped structure (arrow) in the cytoplasm of the myeloblast is pathognomonic. (Reproduced with permission from Dr. Peter McPhedran, Yale Department of Hematology.)

Q   1

A 35-year-old man is airlifted to the ED after a motor vehicle accident. He requires multiple transfusions, which stabilize his BP and hemoglobin. The following morning, he is transferred to his hospital room, where he begins to complain of numbness in his fingers. A prolonged QT interval is noted on an ECG. What is the most likely diagnosis?

Q   2

A 40-year-old woman sees a physician for a 6-month history of weight loss, fevers, and abdominal discomfort. Her WBC count is 56,000/mm³. The physician orders a leukocyte alkaline phosphatase (LAP) to distinguish between a leukemoid reaction and a hematologic malignancy. What is the expected result in a leukemoid reaction?

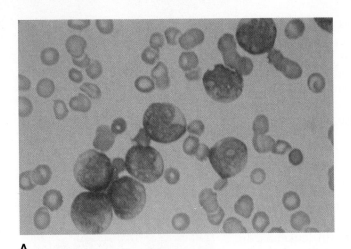
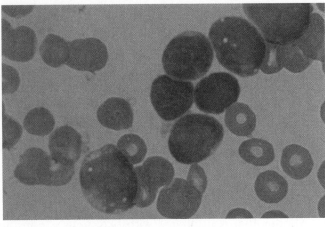

A   **B**

FIGURE 2.7-14.   AML and ALL on peripheral smear. (**A**) AML. Large, uniform myeloblasts with round or kidney-shaped nuclei and prominent nucleoli are characteristic. (**B**) ALL. Peripheral blood smear reveals numerous large, uniform lymphoblasts, which are large cells with a high nuclear-to-cytoplasmic ratio. Some lymphoblasts have visible clefts in their nuclei. (Reproduced with permission from Dr. Peter McPhedran, Yale Department of Hematology.)

- Leukostasis syndrome may be treated with hydroxyurea ± leukapheresis to ↓ WBC count.
- Indicators of poor prognosis:
  - **ALL:** Age < 1 or > 10 years; an ↑ in WBC count to > 50,000/mm³; presence of the Philadelphia chromosome t(9,22) (associated with B-cell cancer); CNS involvement at diagnosis.
  - **AML:** Age > 60 years; elevated LDH; poor-risk or complex karyotype.

Chronic Lymphocytic Leukemia

A malignant, clonal proliferation of functionally incompetent lymphocytes that accumulate in the bone marrow, peripheral blood, lymph nodes, spleen, and liver. Almost all cases involve well-differentiated B lymphocytes. Primarily affects older adults (median age 65 years); the male-to-female ratio is 2:1.

History/PE

Often asymptomatic; patients present with fatigue, malaise, and infection. Common physical findings are lymphadenopathy, hepatomegaly, and splenomegaly.

Diagnosis

- **Best initial test:** CBC with differential and smear showing mature lymphocytosis (NK cells, T cells, or B cells > 5000/mm³) and characteristic smudge cells (fragile leukemia cells crushed by the slide). See Figure 2.7-15.
- **Most accurate test:** Flow cytometry showing the CD5 marker on B cells (normally found on T cells).
- Granulocytopenia, anemia, and thrombocytopenia are common as leukemic cells infiltrate bone marrow. Abnormal function by the leukemic cells leads to hypogammaglobulinemia.
- Bone marrow biopsy is rarely required for diagnosis but may provide prognostic information.

Treatment

- Chemotherapy with fludarabine and chlorambucil.
- Treatment, however, is palliative and is often withheld until patients are symptomatic: recurrent infection, severe lymphadenopathy or splenomegaly, anemia, or thrombocytopenia (poorest prognosis).

KEY FACT

Look for smudge cells to point toward CLL. Smudge cells result from the coverslip crushing the fragile leukemia cells.

1   **A**

This patient presents with symptoms of hypocalcemia following multiple blood transfusions. Blood products often contain citrate, which binds to serum calcium, leading to hypocalcemia, which can cause prolonged QT intervals.

2   **A**

LAP would be ↑. Hematologic malignancies, in contrast, have ↓ LAP values.

- Although CLL has a low likelihood of long-term cure, extended disease-free intervals may be achieved with adequate treatment of symptoms. The clinical stage correlates with expected survival.

Chronic Myelogenous Leukemia

Clonal expansion of myeloid progenitor cells, leading to leukocytosis with excess granulocytes and basophils and sometimes ↑ erythrocytes and platelets as well. To truly be CML, the BCR-ABL translocation must be present. In > 95% of patients, this is reflected by the Philadelphia chromosome t(9,22). CML primarily affects middle-aged patients (median age 50 years).

HISTORY/PE

- Many patients are asymptomatic at diagnosis. Typical signs and symptoms are those of anemia.
- Patients can have splenomegaly with LUQ pain and early satiety. Constitutional symptoms of weight loss, anorexia, fever, and chills may also be seen.
- Patients with CML go through three disease phases:
  - **Chronic:** Without treatment, this phase typically lasts 3.5–5.0 years. Infection and bleeding complications are rare.
  - **Accelerated:** A transition toward blast crisis, with an ↑ in peripheral and bone marrow blood counts. Should be suspected when the differential shows an abrupt ↑ in basophils and thrombocytopenia (platelet count < 100,000/mm³).
  - **Blast crisis:** A large percentage of untreated CML patients will eventually reach this phase. Resembles acute leukemia; survival is 3–6 months..

DIAGNOSIS

- **Most accurate test:** Philadelphia chromosome via PCR or FISH analysis showing the t(9,22) translocation, although some cases lack the translocation.
- CBC often shows a very high WBC count—often > 100,000/mm³ at diagnosis, sometimes reaching > 500,000/mm³. The differential shows granulocytes (predominantly neutrophils) in all stages of maturation. Rarely, the WBC count will be so elevated as to cause a hyperviscosity syndrome.
- CML can be confused clinically with a leukemoid reaction (acute inflammatory response to infection with ↑ neutrophils and a left shift). LAP is low in CML and other hematologic malignancies, and LAP is high in leukemoid reactions.
- LDH, uric acid, and B₁₂ levels are also often elevated in CML.

TREATMENT

- **Chronic:** Treat with tyrosine kinase inhibitors (eg, imatinib). Young patients may be candidates for allogeneic stem cell transplantation if a matched sibling donor is available.
- **Blast crisis:** Same as that for acute leukemia, or second-generation tyrosine kinase inhibitors (eg, dasatinib, nilotinib) plus hematopoietic stem cell transplantation or a clinical trial.

Hairy Cell Leukemia

A malignant disorder of well-differentiated B lymphocytes. HCL is a rare disease that accounts for 2% of adult leukemia cases and most commonly affects older men (median age 50–55 years).

HISTORY/PE

- Typically presents with pancytopenia, bone marrow infiltration, and splenomegaly.

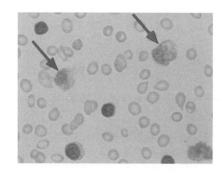

FIGURE 2.7-15.   CLL with characteristic smudge cells. The numerous small, mature lymphocytes and smudge cells (*arrows*; fragile malignant lymphocytes are disrupted during blood smear preparation) are characteristic. (Reproduced with permission from Dr. Peter McPhedran, Yale Department of Hematology.)

KEY FACT

Likely diagnosis based on age at presentation:
- **ALL:** < 13 years (but can present in any age group).
- **AML:** 13–40 years (but can present in any age group).
- **CML:** 40–60 years.
- **CLL:** > 60 years.

KEY FACT

Lymphocytosis is a common lab finding of CLL (↑ NK, T, or B cells) vs CML, which shows granulocytosis (↑ granulocytes: neutrophils, eosinophils, or basophils).

KEY FACT

Imatinib is a selective inhibitor of the BCR-ABL tyrosine kinase, the product of the t(9,22) translocation, or Philadelphia chromosome.

Q

A 41-year-old man is diagnosed with acute myelogenous leukemia (AML). Fluorescence in situ hybridization (FISH) analysis reveals that he has acute promyelocytic leukemia (APL), FAB subtype M3. What is the preferred therapy for this subtype of AML?

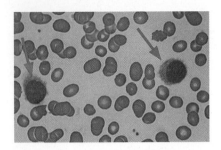

FIGURE 2.7-16. Hairy cell leukemia. Note the hairlike cytoplasmic projections from neoplastic lymphocytes. Villous lymphoma can also have this appearance. (Reproduced with permission from Dr. Peter McPhedran, Yale Department of Hematology.)

- Patients complain of weakness, fatigue, petechiae, bruising, infection (especially with atypical mycobacteria such as *Mycobacterium avium–intracellulare*), abdominal pain, early satiety, and weight loss. Presentation is similar to those of CLL except that patients rarely have lymphadenopathy.

DIAGNOSIS

- **Best initial test:** CBC with smear showing pathognomonic "hairy cells" (mononuclear cells with many cytoplasmic projections; see Figure 2.7-16) that stain with tartrate-resistant acid phosphatase (TRAP). Leukopenia can sometimes be seen as well.
- **Most accurate test:** Flow cytometry identifying the "hairy cells."

TREATMENT

- **Best initial treatment:** Cladribine.
- Alternative treatment options include pentostatin, splenectomy, and IFN-α.
- Median survival without treatment is 5 years. If left untreated, most patients will develop progressive pancytopenia and splenomegaly, eventually requiring therapy.

LYMPHOMAS

Malignant transformations of lymphoid cells residing primarily in lymphoid tissues, especially the lymph nodes. Classically organized into Hodgkin (HL) and non-Hodgkin (NHL) lymphoma (see Table 2.7-7).

Non-Hodgkin Lymphoma

NHL represents a diverse group of mature B and T cell neoplasms. Most NHLs (almost 85%) are of B-cell origin. NHL is the most common hematopoietic neoplasm and is five times more common than HL.

HISTORY/PE

The median patient age is > 50 years of age, but NHL may also be found in children, who tend to have more aggressive, higher-grade disease. Patient presentation varies with disease (see Table 2.7-8), but often includes painless peripheral lymphadenopathy, "B" symptoms (fevers, night sweats, weight loss), and masses on exam.

APL has a favorable prognosis, because it is responsive to all-*trans*-retinoic acid (ATRA) therapy. This AML subtype is also associated with an ↑ incidence of DIC and a chromosomal translocation involving chromosomes 15 and 17.

TABLE 2.7-7. Non-Hodgkin vs Hodgkin Lymphoma

NON-HODGKIN LYMPHOMA	HODGKIN LYMPHOMA
Many peripheral nodes involved; extranodal, noncontiguous spread	Single group of localized nodes, spreads contiguously and rarely involves extranodal sites
Mainly B cells, sometimes T cells	Reed-Sternberg cells: distinct CD15+ and CD30+ B cells
Peak incidence 65–75 years of age	Bimodal: young and old
HIV and autoimmune association	EBV association

Adapted with permission from Le T, et al. *First Aid for the USMLE Step 1 2018*. New York, NY: McGraw-Hill; 2018.

TABLE 2.7-8. Non-Hodgkin Lymphoma Types

Type	Occurs in	Comments
B-Cell Neoplasms		
Follicular lymphoma	Adults (mean age 55 years)	▪ Indolent course or low grade ▪ Painless waxing and waning adenopathy ▪ Localized disease (15%) may be cured with radiation therapy
Diffuse large B-cell lymphoma	Usually middle-aged and elderly	▪ Intermediate grade ▪ Most common NHL in adults ▪ Often presents with single rapidly growing mass ▪ High cure rate with R-CHOP therapy
Burkitt lymphoma	Children and adolescents	▪ High grade, "starry sky" appearance on lesion biopsy ▪ Jaw lesion in Africa, abdominal lesion in Americas ▪ Associated with EBV and t(8;14) translocation ▪ Aggressive treatment with chemotherapy
Mantle cell lymphoma	Elderly men	▪ CD5+ ▪ Rarest form of NHL
T-Cell Neoplasms		
Adult T-cell lymphoma	Adults	▪ High grade, can progress to ALL ▪ Presents with cutaneous lesions ▪ Caused by HTLV, associated with IVDA
Mycosis fungoides/ Sézary syndrome	Adults	▪ Mycosis fungoides is a T-cell lymphoma of the skin ▪ Cutaneous eczema-like lesions and pruritus are common presentations ▪ On skin biopsy see "cerebriform" lymphoid cells ▪ Can progress to Sézary syndrome (T-cell leukemia) with characteristic Sézary cells seen on blood smear

Adapted with permission from Le T, et al. *First Aid for the USMLE Step 1 2018*. New York, NY: McGraw-Hill; 2018.

DIAGNOSIS

- **Best initial test:** Excisional lymph node biopsy.
- Staging usually involves CT of the chest, abdomen, and pelvis, and bone marrow biopsy. Disease staged via Ann Arbor classification as follows:
  - Stage I, single site involved.
  - Stage II, two or more sites involved on same side of the diaphragm.
  - Stage III, multiple sites involved on both sides of the diaphragm.
  - Stage IV, diffuse disease.
  - "A" indicates no systemic symptoms; "B" indicates systemic symptoms.
- A CSF exam should be done in patients with HIV, neurologic symptoms, or 1° CNS lymphoma.

TREATMENT

- Treatment is based on histopathologic classification rather than on stage and consists of radiation, chemotherapy, or both.
- Low-grade indolent NHL treatment is generally palliative.
- High-grade aggressive NHL treatment is aggressive chemotherapy with a curative approach. A common regimen is rituximab, cyclophosphamide, doxorubicin, vincristine, and prednisone (R CHOP).

KEY FACT

The treatment of high-grade NHL may be complicated by tumor lysis syndrome, in which rapid cell death releases intracellular contents and leads to hyperkalemia, hyperphosphatemia, hyperuricemia, and hypocalcemia.

Hodgkin Lymphoma

A predominantly B-cell malignancy associated with EBV. HL has a bimodal age distribution: 30 years of age (primarily the nodular sclerosing type) and 60 years of age (mainly the lymphocyte-depleted type). It has a male predominance in childhood.

HISTORY/PE

- HL commonly presents above the diaphragm (classically as cervical adenopathy; see Figure 2.7-17A). Infradiaphragmatic involvement suggests disseminated disease.
- Patients can have systemic B symptoms, pruritus, and hepatosplenomegaly. Pel-Ebstein fevers (1–2 weeks of high fever alternating with 1–2 afebrile weeks) and alcohol-induced pain at nodal sites are rare signs specific for HL.

DIAGNOSIS

- **Best initial step:** Excisional lymph node biopsy showing the classic Reed-Sternberg cells (giant abnormal B cells with bilobar nuclei and huge, eosinophilic nucleoli, which create an "owl's-eye" appearance; see Figure 2.7-17B).
- Staging is based on the number of lymph node groups involved, the presence of B symptoms, and whether the disease involves lymph nodes on both sides of the diaphragm.

TREATMENT

- Treatment is stage-dependent, involving chemotherapy and/or radiation (in early stage disease). A common chemotherapy regimen is Adriamycin (doxorubicin), bleomycin, vinblastine, dacarbazine (ABVD).
- Radiation increases the risk for premature coronary artery disease and solid tumors (eg, breast, lung, thyroid).
- Five-year survival rates are 90% for stage I and II disease (nodal disease limited to one side of the diaphragm), 84% for stage III, and 65% for stage IV. Lymphocyte-predominant HL has the best prognosis.

KEY FACT

On physical exam, lymph nodes suspicious for malignancy are generally described as firm, fixed, nontender, circumscribed, rubbery, and > 1 cm in diameter. Benign nodes (usually from infection) are generally described as bilateral, < 1 cm, mobile, nontender (viral), or tender (bacterial).

KEY FACT

Chemotherapy and radiation can lead to 2° neoplasms such as AML, NHL, breast cancer, and thyroid cancer. Preventive measures such as mammography are warranted.

KEY FACT

Chemotherapy often induces nausea in cancer patients and should be managed with ondansetron, a serotonin 5-HT$_3$ receptor antagonist.

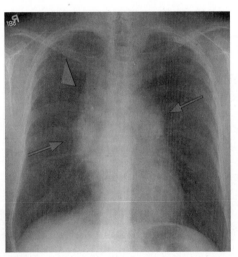

A

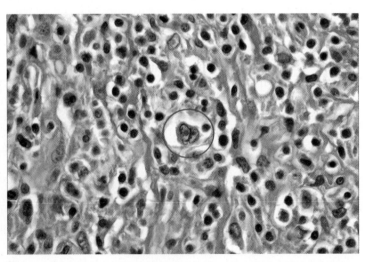

B

FIGURE 2.7-17. **Hodgkin lymphoma.** (**A**) CXR of a 27-year-old man presenting with several weeks of fevers and night sweats shows bulky bilateral hilar (*arrows*) and right paratracheal lymphadenopathy (*arrowhead*). (**B**) Lymph node sampling shows a mixed inflammatory infiltrate and a classic binucleate Reed-Sternberg cell (*circle*) consistent with Hodgkin lymphoma. (Reproduced with permission from USMLE-Rx.com.)

Plasma Cell Disorders

MULTIPLE MYELOMA

Clonal proliferation of malignant plasma cells with excessive production of monoclonal immunoglobulins (typically ineffective IgA or IgG) or immunoglobulin fragments (kappa/lambda light chains). Multiple myeloma (MM) primarily affects the elderly, peaking in the seventh decade. Risk factors include radiation and monoclonal gammopathy of undetermined significance (MGUS).

HISTORY/PE

- Patients present with bone pain or with a pathologic fracture (MM cells infiltrate bone marrow, where they activate osteoclasts, creating lytic lesions, weak bones, and hypercalcemia).
- Patients are prone to infection (IgG and IgA produced by myeloma cells are monoclonal, thus making them ineffective) and have elevated monoclonal (M) proteins in serum and/or urine.

DIAGNOSIS

- **Best initial test:** Serum protein electrophoresis showing IgG or IgA monoclonal spikes (see Figure 2.7-18).
- **Most accurate test:** Bone marrow biopsy showing > 10% monoclonal CD138+ plasma cells.
- CBC with smear may show rouleaux formation, whereas urine protein electrophoresis may show Bence-Jones protein (paraprotein). Total protein:albumin gap is often elevated.
- M protein alone is insufficient for the diagnosis of MM, as MGUS, CLL, lymphoma, Waldenström macroglobulinemia, and amyloidosis can also ↑ M protein.
- Patients should also be evaluated for anemia, hypercalcemia, and renal failure. Bone lesions are also seen with a skeletal survey (see Figure 2.7-19).

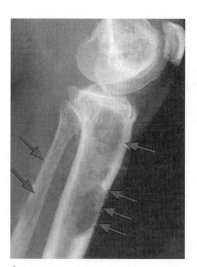
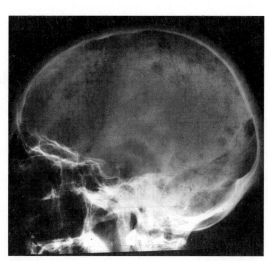

A   **B**

FIGURE 2.7-19. Multiple myeloma skeletal survey. Characteristic lytic bony lesions of multiple myeloma involving the tibia and fibula (**A**) and the skull (**B**) are seen. (Image A reproduced with permission from Lichtman MA et al. *Williams Hematology*, 8th ed. New York, NY: McGraw-Hill; 2010. Image B reproduced with permission from Kantarjian HM, Wolff RA, Koller CA. *MD Anderson Manual of Medical Oncology*, 2nd ed. New York, NY: McGraw-Hill; 2011.)

MNEMONIC

Clinical features of multiple myeloma—

CRAB—

hyper**C**alcemia
Renal involvement
Anemia
Bone lytic lesions/**B**ack pain

KEY FACT

MGUS is also a monoclonal expansion of plasma cells that is asymptomatic and may eventually lead to multiple myeloma (1–2% per year). No "CRAB" findings.

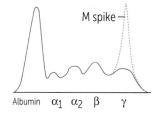

FIGURE 2.7-18. Multiple myeloma. Serum protein electrophoretic tracing showing M protein spike IgG/A (diagnostic of MM). Note that M protein spike IgM indicates Waldenström macroglobulinemia. (Reproduced with permission from Le T, et al. *First Aid for the USMLE Step 1 2018*. New York, NY: McGraw-Hill; 2018.)

KEY FACT

MM damaging renal tubules can produce an adult Fanconi syndrome.

KEY FACT

As MM is an osteoclastic process, a bone scan, which detects osteoblastic activity, may be ⊖.

TREATMENT

- Patients < 70 years of age can be treated with chemotherapy and autologous bone marrow transplant. Common chemotherapeutic agents are cyclophosphamide, bortezomib, melphalan (an oral alkylating agent), dexamethasone, and lenalidomide.
- Patients > 70 years of age are treated with melphalan and prednisone.

WALDENSTRÖM MACROGLOBULINEMIA

A clonal disorder of B cells that leads to a malignant monoclonal gammopathy. ↑ Levels of IgM result in hyperviscosity syndrome, coagulation abnormalities, cryoglobulinemia, cold agglutinin disease (leading to autoimmune hemolytic anemia), and amyloidosis. Tissue is infiltrated by IgM and neoplastic plasma cells. A chronic, indolent disease of the elderly.

HISTORY/PE

- **Presents with nonspecific symptoms:** Lethargy, weight loss, and Raynaud phenomenon from cryoglobulinemia. Organomegaly and organ dysfunction can be present.
- Neurologic problems ranging from mental status changes to sensorimotor peripheral neuropathy and blurry vision (engorged blood vessels can be noted on eye exam) are also seen.
- As with multiple myeloma, MGUS is a precursor to disease.

DIAGNOSIS

- **Most accurate test:** Bone marrow biopsy and aspirate. Marrow shows abnormal plasma cells, classically with Dutcher bodies (PAS⊕ IgM deposits around the nucleus). Serum and urine protein electrophoresis and immunofixation are also used.
- Nonspecific findings include ↑ ESR, uric acid, LDH, and alkaline phosphatase.

TREATMENT

Rituximab and chemotherapy for patients with symptomatic disease. Plasmapheresis to remove excess immunoglobulin for patients who present with signs or symptoms of hyperviscosity.

AMYLOIDOSIS

Extracellular deposition of amyloid protein fibrils resulting from a variety of causes (see Table 2.7-9). Classically a disease of the elderly.

HISTORY/PE

- Clinical presentation depends on the type, amount, and tissue distribution of amyloid. In the most common forms of systemic amyloidosis, 1° (AL) and 2° (AA), the major sites of clinically important amyloid deposition are in the kidneys, heart, and liver.
- In some disorders, amyloid deposition is limited to one organ (cerebral amyloid angiopathy in Alzheimer disease).

DIAGNOSIS

Most accurate test: Tissue biopsy with Congo red staining showing apple-green birefringence under polarized light. Immunohistochemistry can identify the amyloid protein type.

KEY FACT

Cryoglobulinemia and cold agglutinins are different disorders caused by IgM antibodies. Cryoglobulinemia is most often seen in HCV and has systemic signs such as joint pain and renal involvement. Cold agglutinins may cause finger or toe numbness and hemolytic anemia upon cold exposure and are seen with EBV, mycoplasmal infection, and Waldenström macroglobulinemia.

TABLE 2.7-9. Types of Amyloidosis

Amyloid	Cause
AL	A plasma cell dyscrasia with deposition of monoclonal light-chain fragments Associated with multiple myeloma and Waldenström macroglobulinemia
AA	Deposition of the acute-phase reactant serum amyloid A Associated with chronic inflammatory diseases (eg, rheumatoid arthritis), infections, and neoplasms
Dialysis related	Deposition of β_2-microglobulin, which accumulates in patients on long-term dialysis
Heritable	Deposition of abnormal gene products (eg, transthyretin, also known as prealbumin). A heterogeneous group of disorders
Senile-systemic	Deposition of otherwise normal transthyretin

AA, 2° amyloidosis; AL, 1° amyloidosis.

TREATMENT

- 1° Amyloidosis is treated with chemotherapy and/or autologous stem cell transplant. Chemotherapy agents are similar to that used in multiple myeloma.
- 2° Amyloidosis is treated by addressing the underlying condition.

Neutropenia

An absolute neutrophil count (ANC) < 1500/mm³, where ANC = (WBC count) × (% bands + % segmented neutrophils). Neutropenia may be caused by a combination of ↓ production, migration away from the vascular space, and ↑ destruction or utilization. It may be acquired or intrinsic. The most common causes of neutropenia in adults are infections and drugs. Other common causes include diseases that infiltrate the bone marrow such as leukemias or lymphomas, aplastic anemias, or B₁₂/folate deficiencies.

HISTORY/PE

- Patients are at ↑ risk for infection. The ↓ the neutrophil count, the ↑ the risk.
- **Acute neutropenia:** Associated with *S aureus, Pseudomonas, E coli, Proteus,* and *Klebsiella* sepsis.
- **Chronic and autoimmune neutropenia:** Presents with recurrent sinusitis, stomatitis, gingivitis, and perirectal infections rather than sepsis. Some chronic neutropenias are accompanied by splenomegaly (Felty syndrome, Gaucher disease, sarcoidosis).
- Look for drug or toxin exposure, infection, autoimmune, or neoplastic disease.

DIAGNOSIS

- **Best initial test:** CBC with smear.
- Follow neutropenia clinically with a CBC and ANC. If thrombocytopenia or anemia is present, bone marrow biopsy and aspirate should be performed.

KEY FACT

Hypothermia can be caused by fungemia.

Q **1**

A 71-year-old man seeks care for marked lethargy and constipation that are worsening. He also notes a dull back pain that is present at most times, even at night. His lab studies have been normal except for an ↑ creatinine level. What is most likely responsible for the patient's worsening renal function?

Q **2**

An 80-year-old man is seen in your clinic after an incidental finding of elevated IgG on a recent hospital admission for pneumonia. He has no signs of kidney damage, anemia, or bone lesions. The IgG level is 2100 mg/dL, and a subsequent bone marrow biopsy shows 3% plasma cells. What is the next best step?

- Serum immunologic evaluation, ANA levels, and a workup for collagen vascular disease may be merited.

TREATMENT

- **Infection management:** Neutropenic patients cannot mount an effective inflammatory response.
- Fever in the context of neutropenia (neutropenic fever) is a medical emergency; treat immediately with broad-spectrum antibiotics with pseudomonas coverage such as cefepime. Treat suspected fungal infections appropriately as well.
- Hematopoietic stem cell factors such as G-CSF can be used to shorten the duration of neutropenia. Rarely, IVIG and allogeneic bone marrow transplantation may be used.

MNEMONIC

Causes of 2° eosinophilia—

NAACP

Neoplasm
Allergies
Asthma
Collagen vascular disease
Parasites

Eosinophilia

An absolute eosinophil count ≥ 500/mm³. Eosinophilia can be triggered by the overproduction of cytokines (IL-3, IL-5, and GM-CSF) or by chemokines that stimulate the migration of eosinophils into peripheral blood and tissues. Eosinophilia may be a 1° disorder but is usually 2° to another cause. The most common cause in the developed world is allergy, whereas in the developing world it is parasitic infection.

HISTORY/PE

- Elicit a travel, medication, atopic, lymphoma/leukemia, and diet history.
- Exam varies by cause. Patients with hypereosinophilic syndrome (HES) may present with fever, anemia, and prominent cardiac findings (emboli from mural thrombi, abnormal ECGs, CHF, murmurs). Eosinophils can infiltrate and affect other organs as well.

DIAGNOSIS

- Obtain CBC with differential. CSF analysis showing eosinophilia is suggestive of a drug reaction or infection with coccidioidomycosis or a helminth.
- Hematuria with eosinophilia can be a sign of schistosomiasis.

TREATMENT

New-onset cardiac findings, eosinophilia > 100,000/mm³, or drug reactions with systemic symptoms and eosinophilia must be spotted early and should be treated with steroids (and discontinuation of offending agents).

Patients with multiple myeloma frequently have renal dysfunction 2° to urinary immunoglobulins (also known as Bence Jones protein) that have the ability to form casts, leading to cast nephropathy.

This patient has MGUS, as seen by the elevated IgG in the absence of other clinical abnormalities or symptoms. No treatment is required, but because MGUS can progress to MM, this patient should be seen regularly for signs of renal failure, anemia, or bone pain.

Transplant Medicine

- Three types of tissue transplantation are increasingly used to treat diseases:
  - **Autologous:** Transplantation from the patient to himself or herself.
  - **Allogeneic:** Transplantation from a donor to a genetically different patient.
  - **Syngeneic:** Transplantation between identical twins (from a donor to a genetically identical patient).
- With allogeneic donation, efforts are made to ABO and HLA match the donor and recipient. Despite matching and immunosuppression, however,

TABLE 2.7-10.   Types of Solid Organ Transplant Rejection

Variable	Hyperacute	Acute	Chronic
Timing after transplant	Within minutes	Between 5 days and 3 months	Months to years
Pathogenesis	Preformed antibodies	T-cell mediated	Chronic immune reaction causing fibrosis
Tissue findings	Vascular thrombi; tissue ischemia	Laboratory evidence of tissue destruction such as ↑ GGT, alkaline phosphatase, LDH, BUN, or creatinine	Gradual loss of organ function
Prevention	Check ABO compatibility	N/A	N/A
Treatment	Cytotoxic agents	Confirm with sampling of transplanted tissue; treat with corticosteroids, antilymphocyte antibodies (OKT3), tacrolimus, or MMF	No treatment; biopsy to rule out treatable acute reaction

transplants may be rejected. There are three types of solid organ rejection: hyperacute, acute, and chronic (see Table 2.7-10).

- Graft-vs-host disease (GVHD) is a complication specific to allogeneic bone marrow transplantation in which donated T cells attack host tissues, especially the skin, liver, and GI tract. It may be acute (< 100 days posttransplant) or chronic (> 100 days afterward).
  - Minor histocompatibility antigens are thought to be responsible for GVHD, which presents with skin changes, cholestatic liver dysfunction, obstructive lung disease, or GI problems.
  - Patients are treated with high-dose corticosteroids.
- Typical posttransplant immunosuppression regimens include: prednisone, mycophenolate mofetil (MMF), FK506 (tacrolimus) to suppress immune-mediated rejection, TMP-SMX, ganciclovir, and fluconazole to prevent subsequent infection in the immunosuppressed host.
- A variant of GVHD is the graft-vs-leukemia effect, in which leukemia patients who are treated with an allogeneic bone marrow transplant have significantly lower relapse rates than those treated with an autologous transplant. This difference is thought to be caused by a recognition of leukemia cells by the donor T cells.

Diseases Associated with Neoplasms

Table 2.7-11 outlines conditions that are commonly associated with neoplasms.

TABLE 2.7-11.   Disorders Associated with Neoplasms

Condition	Neoplasm
Acanthosis nigricans (hyperpigmentation and epidermal thickening) and seborrheic keratoses	Visceral malignancy (stomach, lung, breast, uterus)
Actinic keratosis	Squamous cell carcinoma of the skin
AIDS	Aggressive malignant NHLs and Kaposi sarcoma
Autoimmune diseases (eg, myasthenia gravis)	Benign and malignant thymomas
Barrett esophagus (chronic GI reflux)	Esophageal adenocarcinoma
Chronic atrophic gastritis, pernicious anemia, postsurgical gastric remnants	Gastric adenocarcinoma
Cirrhosis (eg, alcoholic, HBV, HCV, Wilson disease)	Hepatocellular carcinoma
Down syndrome	**ALL** ("We will **ALL** go **Down** together")
Immunodeficiency states	Malignant lymphomas
Multiple dysplastic nevi	Malignant melanoma
Neurofibromatosis type 1	Pheochromocytoma, neurofibroma, optic glioma
Neurofibromatosis type 2	Acoustic schwannoma
Paget disease of bone	2° Osteosarcoma and fibrosarcoma
Plummer-Vinson syndrome (atrophic glossitis, esophageal webs, anemia; all caused by iron deficiency)	Squamous cell carcinoma of the esophagus
Tuberous sclerosis (facial angiofibroma, seizures, intellectual disability)	Astrocytoma and cardiac rhabdomyoma
Ulcerative colitis	Colonic adenocarcinoma
Xeroderma pigmentosum	Squamous cell and basal cell carcinomas of the skin

INFECTIOUS DISEASE

Respiratory Infections

PNEUMONIA

Common causes of pneumonia are outlined in Tables 2.8-1 and 2.8-2.

HISTORY/PE

- May present classically or atypically.
- **Classic symptoms:** Sudden onset, fever, productive cough (purulent yellow-green sputum or hemoptysis), dyspnea, night sweats, pleuritic chest pain.

TABLE 2.8-1.   Causes of Pneumonia by Category

CATEGORY	ETIOLOGY
Atypical	*Mycoplasma, Legionella, Chlamydophila (Chlamydia) pneumoniae*
Nosocomial (health care–associated)	GNRs, *Staphylococcus*, anaerobes, *Pseudomonas* (intubated patients)
Immunocompromised	*Streptococcus pneumoniae* (most common), *Staphylococcus*, gram ⊕ rods, fungi, viruses, *Pneumocystis jirovecii* (with HIV), mycobacteria
Aspiration	Anaerobes
Alcoholics/IV drug users	*S pneumoniae, Klebsiella, Staphylococcus*
CF	*Staphylococcus, Pseudomonas, Burkholderia*, mycobacteria
COPD	*Haemophilus influenzae, Moraxella catarrhalis, S pneumoniae*
Postviral	*Staphylococcus, S pneumoniae, H influenzae*
Neonates	Group B streptococci (GBS), *Escherichia coli, Listeria*
Recurrent	Obstruction, bronchogenic carcinoma, lymphoma, Wegener granulomatosis, immunodeficiency, unusual organisms (eg, *Nocardia, Coxiella burnetii, Aspergillus, Pseudomonas*)

TABLE 2.8-2.   Common Causes of Pneumonia by Age

NEONATES	CHILDREN (6 WEEKS–18 YEARS)	ADULTS (18–40 YEARS)	ADULTS (40–65 YEARS)	ELDERLY
GBS	Viruses	*Mycoplasma*	*S pneumoniae*	*S pneumoniae*
E coli	*S pneumoniae*	*S pneumoniae*	*H influenzae*	*H influenzae*
Listeria	*Mycoplasma*	Viruses	*Mycoplasma*	Viruses
	C pneumoniae	*C pneumoniae*	Viruses	*S aureus*
	Staphylococcus aureus		Anaerobes	Gram ⊖ rods (GNRs)
				Anaerobes

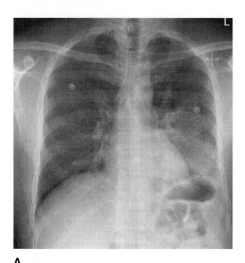
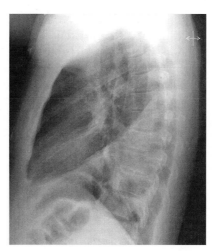

A   **B**

FIGURE 2.8-1.   Lobar pneumonia. Posteroanterior (**A**) and lateral (**B**) CXR of a 41-year-old man with cough and shortness of breath show a left lower lobe opacity consistent with lobar pneumonia. *S pneumoniae* was confirmed by sputum Gram stain and culture. (Reproduced with permission from USMLE-Rx.com.)

- **Atypical symptoms:** Gradual onset, dry cough, headache, myalgia, sore throat, GI symptoms.
- Lung exam may show ↓ or bronchial breath sounds, rales, wheezing, dullness to percussion, egophony, and/or tactile fremitus.
- Elderly patients and those with COPD, diabetes, or immune compromise may have minimal or atypical signs on physical exam.

DIAGNOSIS

- Requires two or more symptoms of acute respiratory infection plus a new infiltrate on chest x-ray (CXR) or CT (see Figure 2.8-1).
- Sputum Gram stain and culture (see Figure 2.8-2), nasopharyngeal aspirate, blood culture, and ABG are obtained in a minority of cases, mostly in hospitalized patients or outpatients with persistent symptoms.
- **Tests for specific pathogens include the following:**
  - *Legionella:* Urine *Legionella* antigen test, sputum staining with direct fluorescent antibody (DFA), culture.

> **KEY FACT**
>
> An adequate sputum Gram stain sample has many PMNs (> 25 cells/hpf) and few epithelial cells (< 10 cells/hpf).

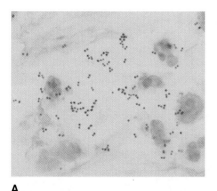
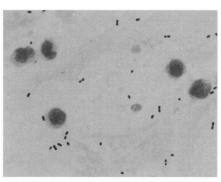

A   **B**

FIGURE 2.8-2.   Common pathogens causing pneumonia. (**A**) *S aureus*. These clusters of gram ⊕ cocci were isolated from the sputum of a patient who developed pneumonia while hospitalized. (**B**) *S pneumoniae*. Sputum sample from a patient with pneumonia. Note the characteristic lancet-shaped gram ⊕ diplococci.

MNEMONIC

Pneumonia hospitalization criteria, 2–3 = consider inpatient treatment; > 4 = admission—

CURB-65

Confusion
Uremia (BUN > 19)
Respiratory rate (> 30 breaths/min)
Blood pressure (SBP < 90 mm Hg or DBP < 60 mm Hg)
Age > **65** years

KEY FACT

The pneumococcal vaccine should be given to all children, patients > 65 years of age, patients with splenic dysfunction (eg, sickle cell) or asplenia, immunocompromised patients, and patients with chronic disease including diabetes.

- *Chlamydophila (Chlamydia) pneumoniae:* Serologic testing, polymerase chain reaction (PCR).
- *Mycoplasma:* Usually clinical. Serum cold agglutinins and serum *Mycoplasma* antigen may also be used.
- *S pneumoniae:* Urine pneumococcal antigen test, culture.
- **Viral:** Nasopharyngeal aspirate, rapid molecular tests for pathogens (eg, influenza, respiratory syncytial virus), DFA, viral culture.

TREATMENT

A summary of the recommended **best initial treatment** for pneumonia is given in Table 2.8-3.

- Outpatient treatment with oral antibiotics is recommended in uncomplicated cases.
- For patients with obstructive diseases (eg, cystic fibrosis [CF] or bronchiectasis), consider adding pseudomonas, staphylococcal, or anaerobic coverage.

COMPLICATIONS

Pleural effusion, empyema, lung abscess, necrotizing pneumonia, bacteremia. Empyema treatment requires surgical drainage and chest tube placement in addition to antibiotics.

T A B L E 2 . 8 - 3 . **Treatment of Pneumonia**

PATIENT TYPE	SUSPECTED PATHOGENS	EMPIRIC COVERAGE
Outpatient community-acquired pneumonia, ≤ 65 years of age, otherwise healthy, no antimicrobials within 3 months	*S pneumoniae, Mycoplasma pneumoniae, C pneumoniae, H influenzae,* viral	Macrolide or doxycycline
> 65 years of age or comorbidity (COPD, heart failure, renal failure, diabetes, liver disease, EtOH abuse) or antimicrobial use within 3 months	*S pneumoniae, H influenzae,* aerobic GNRs *(E coli, Enterobacter, Klebsiella), S aureus, Legionella,* viruses	Fluoroquinolone or β-lactam + macrolide
Community-acquired pneumonia requiring hospitalization	*S pneumoniae, H influenzae,* anaerobes, aerobic GNRs, *Legionella, Chlamydia*	Fluoroquinolone or antipneumococcal β-lactam + macrolide
Community-acquired pneumonia requiring ICU care	*S pneumoniae, Legionella, H influenzae,* anaerobes, aerobic GNRs, *Mycoplasma, Pseudomonas*	Antipneumococcal β-lactam + fluoroquinolone (or azithromycin)
Institution-/hospital-acquired pneumonia—hospitalized > 48 hours or in a long-term care facility > 14 days; ventilator-associated pneumonia	GNRs (including *Pseudomonas* and *Acinetobacter), S aureus, Legionella,* mixed flora	Extended-spectrum cephalosporin or carbapenem with antipseudomonal activity. Add an aminoglycoside or a fluoroquinolone for coverage of resistant organisms *(Pseudomonas)* until lab sensitivities identify the best single agent
Critically ill or worsening over 24–48 hours on initial antibiotic therapy	MRSA	Add vancomycin or linezolid; broader gram ⊖ coverage

TUBERCULOSIS

Infection caused by *Mycobacterium tuberculosis*. Roughly 2 billion people worldwide are infected with tuberculosis (TB). Initial infection usually leads to a latent infection that is asymptomatic. Most symptomatic cases (ie, active disease) are caused by reactivation of latent infection rather than to 1° exposure. Pulmonary TB is most common, but disseminated or extrapulmonary TB can occur as well. TB can infect almost any organ system, including the lungs, CNS, GU tract, bone, and GI tract.

- **Risk factors for active disease (ie, reactivation):** Immunosuppression (HIV/AIDS), alcoholism, preexisting lung disease, diabetes, advancing age.
- **Risk factors for TB exposure in the United States:** Homelessness and crowded living conditions (eg, prisons), emigration/travel from developing nations, employment in a health profession, interaction with known TB contacts.

HISTORY/PE

- Presents with cough, hemoptysis, dyspnea, weight loss, fatigue, night sweats, fever, cachexia, hypoxia, tachycardia, lymphadenopathy, an abnormal lung exam, and prolonged (> 3 weeks) symptom duration.
- HIV patients can present with atypical signs and symptoms and have higher rates of extrapulmonary TB.

DIAGNOSIS

- **Active disease:** Mycobacterial culture of sputum (or blood/tissue for extrapulmonary disease) is the **most accurate test** but can take weeks to obtain. A sputum acid-fast stain (see Figure 2.8-3) can yield rapid preliminary results and is the **best initial test** but lacks sensitivity.
  - The most common finding among typical hosts is a cavitary infiltrate in the upper lobe on CXR (see Figure 2.8-4), which may be accompanied by calcification of one or more nearby lymph nodes (Ghon complex).
  - HIV patients or those with 1° TB may show lower lobe infiltrates with or without cavitation.
  - Multiple fine nodular densities distributed throughout both lungs are typical of miliary TB, which represents hematologic or lymphatic dissemination.

KEY FACT

Interpretation and management of the Mantoux tuberculin skin test (TST or PPD) is the same for patients who have received the BCG vaccine and those who have not, although they should be tested with QuantiFERON-TB testing instead.

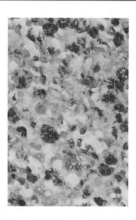

FIGURE 2.8-3. **Tuberculosis.** Note the red color ("red snappers") of tubercle bacilli on acid-fast staining. (Reproduced with permission from Milikowski C. *Color Atlas of Basic Histopathology*, 1st ed. Stamford, CT: Appleton & Lange; 1997.)

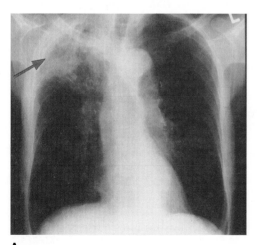

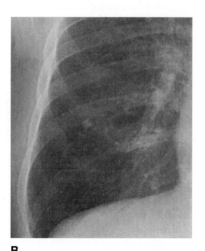

A   **B**

FIGURE 2.8-4. **Pulmonary TB.** (A) Right apical opacity with areas of cavitation (*arrow*) is seen in an elderly man with reactivation TB. (B) Coned-in view of CXR in a young man with miliary TB shows innumerable 1- to 2-mm pulmonary nodules. (Image A reproduced with permission from Halter JB, et al. *Hazzard's Geriatric Medicine and Gerontology*, 6th ed. New York, NY: McGraw-Hill; 2009. Image B reproduced with permission from USMLE-Rx.com.)

Q

A 70-year-old man presents to the ED in February with a high fever and a productive cough. He was treated for influenza 1 week ago, and his symptoms improved until 3 days ago, when they returned with greater severity. Exam now reveals cyanosis, tactile fremitus, and dullness to percussion over the left lower lobe. Against what organism should antibiotic therapy be directed?

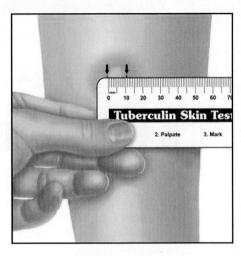

PPD is injected intradermally on the volar surface of the forearm. The diameter of induration is measured at 48–72 hours. BCG vaccination typically renders a patient PPD ⊕ but should not preclude prophylaxis as recommended for unvaccinated individuals. The size of induration that indicates a ⊕ test is interpreted as follows:

- **≥ 5 mm:** HIV or risk factors, close TB contacts, CXR evidence of TB.
- **≥ 10 mm:** Indigent/homeless, residents of developing nations, IV drug use, chronic illness, residents of health and correctional institutions, and health care workers.
- **≥ 15 mm:** Everyone else, including those with no known risk factors.

A ⊖ reaction with ⊖ controls implies anergy from immunosuppression, old age, or malnutrition and thus does not rule out TB.

FIGURE 2.8-5. Purified protein derivative (PPD) interpretation. Image on left courtesy of Centers for Disease Control and Prevention (CDC). *Core Curriculum on Tuberculosis: What the Clinician Should Know*, 6th ed. Atlanta, GA: Centers for Disease Control and Prevention; 2013.

KEY FACT

Rifampin turns body fluids orange (including tears); ethambutol can cause optic neuritis. INH may cause peripheral neuropathy and drug-induced hepatitis.

MNEMONIC

Patients with TB are RIPE for treatment—

Rifampin
Isoniazid
Pyrazinamide
Ethambutol

- **Latent disease (asymptomatic and previous exposure):** Diagnose with a ⊕ tuberculin skin test (TST; see Figure 2.8-5) or QuantiFERON-TB test.
  - Immunocompromised individuals with latent TB infection may have a ⊖ TST (anergy).
  - Evaluate all patients with a ⊕ PPD with CXR to rule out active disease.

TREATMENT

All cases (both latent and active) must be reported to local and state health departments. **Respiratory isolation** should be instituted if active TB is suspected. Treatment measures are as follows:

- **Active disease:**
  - Directly observed multidrug therapy with a four-drug regimen (INH, pyrazinamide, rifampin, ethambutol) for 2 months followed by INH and rifampin for 4 months.
  - Administer vitamin B_6 (pyridoxine) with INH to prevent peripheral neuropathy.
- **Latent disease:** For a ⊕ PPD without signs or symptoms of active disease, treat with INH for 9 months. Alternative regimens include INH for 6 months or rifampin for 4 months.

ASPERGILLOSIS

A group of diseases caused by aspergillus, typically A *fumigatus*, through infection by spores. It can be seen on silver stain as acutely (< 45°) branched septate hyphae.

Allergic Bronchopulmonary Aspergillosis

- Hypersensitivity reaction that is common in asthmatic and cystic fibrosis populations.
- **Hx/PE:** Fever, wheezing, cough, hemoptysis, mucous plugs.
- **Dx:** Pulmonary infiltrates on CXR, eosinophilia, ⊕ skin antigen test.
- **Tx:** Oral (not inhaled) corticosteroids; add itraconazole for recurrent or chronic cases.

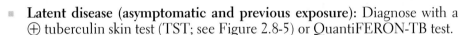

S aureus. Postviral pneumonia is an important complication of influenza, especially in the elderly. *Staphylococcus* is the most common organism responsible for early bacterial superinfection, presenting just days after the onset of influenza. Necrotizing bronchopneumonia with cavitation and abscess formation is characteristic.

Aspergilloma

- Typically discovered as an incidental radiographic finding in patients with preexisting lung disease (eg, sarcoidosis, PCP, TB).
- **Hx/PE:** May be asymptomatic or present with hemoptysis; fever and cough are less common.
- **Dx:** CXR or CT reveals a solid mass within a preexisting lung cavity; lab tests are typically normal.
- **Tx:** If symptomatic, itraconazole or curative surgical resection if the patient can tolerate the procedure.

Chronic Necrotizing Pulmonary Aspergillosis

- Rare, antibiotic-resistant pneumonia that occurs in patients with alcoholism or steroid-dependent COPD.
- **Hx/PE:** Fever, cough, hemoptysis, night sweats, fatigue.
- **Tx:** Voriconazole, surgical resection if resistant or severe.

Invasive Aspergillosis

- Severe, rapidly progressive infection that occurs exclusively in immunosuppressed patients (eg, chemotherapy, transplant).
- **Hx/PE:** Fever, cough, pleuritic chest pain, tachypnea/hypoxemia.
- **Dx:** Serum galactomannan assay is specific, but lung biopsy should be performed if negative.
- **Tx:** Voriconazole or caspofungin in addition to decreasing immunosuppressant therapy.

ACUTE PHARYNGITIS

Viral causes are more common (90% in adults), but it is important to identify streptococcal pharyngitis (group A β-hemolytic *Streptococcus pyogenes*). Etiologies are as follows:

- **Bacterial:** Group A streptococci (GAS), *Neisseria gonorrhoeae*, *Corynebacterium diphtheriae*, *M pneumoniae*.
- **Viral:** Rhinovirus, coronavirus, adenovirus, herpes simplex virus (HSV), Epstein-Barr virus (EBV), cytomegalovirus (CMV), influenza virus, coxsackievirus, acute HIV infection.

HISTORY/PE

- **Typical of streptococcal pharyngitis:** Fever, sore throat, pharyngeal erythema (see Figure 2.8-6), tonsillar exudate, cervical lymphadenopathy, soft palate petechiae, headache, vomiting, scarlatiniform rash (indicates scarlet fever).
- **Atypical of streptococcal pharyngitis:** Coryza, hoarseness, rhinorrhea, cough, conjunctivitis, anterior stomatitis, ulcerative lesions, GI symptoms.

DIAGNOSIS

Diagnosed by clinical evaluation, rapid GAS antigen detection, and throat culture. If three out of four Centor criteria are met (see Table 2.8-4), the sensitivity of rapid antigen testing is > 90%.

TREATMENT

If GAS is suspected, begin empiric antibiotic therapy with penicillin for 10 days. Cephalosporins, amoxicillin, and azithromycin are alternative options. Symptom relief can be attained with fluids, rest, antipyretics, and saltwater gargles.

> **KEY FACT**
>
> Early antibiotic treatment of streptococcal pharyngitis can prevent rheumatic fever but not glomerulonephritis.

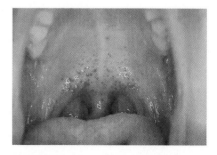

FIGURE 2.8-6. Pharyngeal erythema. *Streptococcus pyogenes* is the most common bacterial cause of pharyngitis. (Reproduced courtesy of Dr. Heinz F. Eichenwald from the Centers for Disease Control and Prevention, Atlanta, GA.)

TABLE 2.8-4. Modified Centor Criteria (Centor Criteria + Age)

CRITERIA	POINTS
Fever	1
Tonsillar exudate	1
Tender anterior cervical lymphadenopathy	1
Lack of cough	1
3–14 years of age	1
15–45 years of age	0
> 45 years of age	−1

If 4–5 points, treat empirically with antibiotics.

If 2–3 points, perform rapid antigen test. If ⊕ antigen test, treat with antibiotics; if ⊖ antigen test, perform throat culture.

If 0–1 points, no testing or antibiotics required (symptomatic treatment only).

KEY FACT

Acute necrotizing mediastinitis is a life-threatening complication of untreated retropharyngeal abscess that presents with fever, chest pain, and dyspnea. Requires urgent surgical drainage to prevent spread to the posterior mediastinum, which may cause lethal pleural and pericardial effusions.

KEY FACT

All patients with a history of rheumatic fever should be given routine penicillin prophylaxis to prevent recurrent group A strep infection.

COMPLICATIONS

- **Nonsuppurative:** Acute rheumatic fever (see the Cardiovascular chapter), poststreptococcal glomerulonephritis.
- **Suppurative:** Cervical lymphadenitis, mastoiditis, sinusitis, otitis media, retropharyngeal or peritonsillar abscess, and, rarely, thrombophlebitis of the jugular vein (Lemierre syndrome) caused by *Fusobacterium*, an oral anaerobe.
- Peritonsillar abscess may present with odynophagia, trismus ("lockjaw"), a muffled "hot potato" voice, unilateral tonsillar enlargement, and erythema, with the uvula and soft palate deviated away from the affected side. Culture abscess fluid, and localize the abscess via intraoral ultrasound or CT. Treat with antibiotics and surgical drainage.

ORAL INFECTIONS

Ludwig Angina

Rapidly progressive cellulitis of submandibular space that may cause fever and airway compromise from a rapidly expanding cellulitic edema. Usually caused by polymicrobial infection in the setting of poor oral hygiene. Intravenous (IV) broad-spectrum antibiotics and diligent airway management are necessary; surgical drainage is performed if there is abscess formation (uncommon).

Acute Lymphadenitis

Unilateral and rapid onset (< 1 week), commonly caused by *S aureus* and *S pyogenes*, typically involving the submandibular lymph nodes. Antibiotics are required if symptoms (fluctuance, fever, cellulitis) are present to prevent abscess formation.

Parotitis

Painful swelling of parotid gland caused by *S aureus* in states of dehydration, especially in the elderly and after surgery. Prevented with adequate fluid intake and oral hygiene. Treated with IV antibiotics.

SINUSITIS

Refers to inflammation of the paranasal sinuses. The maxillary sinuses are most commonly affected. Subtypes include the following:

- **Acute sinusitis (symptoms lasting < 1 month):** Most commonly associated with viruses, *S pneumoniae*, *H influenzae*, and *M catarrhalis*. Bacterial causes are rare and characterized by purulent nasal discharge, facial or tooth tenderness, hyposmia/anosmia, and symptoms lasting > 10 days.
- **Chronic sinusitis (symptoms persisting > 3 months):** A chronic inflammatory process often caused by obstruction of sinus drainage and ongoing low-grade anaerobic infections.

HISTORY/PE

- Presents with fever, facial pain/pressure, headache, nasal congestion, and discharge. Exam may reveal tenderness, erythema, and swelling over the affected area.
- High fever, leukocytosis, and a purulent nasal discharge are suggestive of acute bacterial sinusitis.

DIAGNOSIS

- A clinical diagnosis. Culture and imaging are generally not required for acute sinusitis but may guide the management of chronic cases.
- Transillumination shows opacification of the sinuses (low sensitivity).
- CT is the test of choice for sinus imaging (see Figure 2.8-7), but is usually necessary only if symptoms persist after treatment.

TREATMENT

- Most cases of acute sinusitis are viral and/or self-limited and are treated with symptomatic therapy (decongestants, antihistamines, nasal saline lavage, pain relief).
- **Acute bacterial sinusitis:** Consider amoxicillin/clavulanate for 10 days or clarithromycin, azithromycin, trimethoprim-sulfamethoxazole (TMP-SMX), a fluoroquinolone, or a second-generation cephalosporin for 10 days.
- **Chronic sinusitis:**
  - Antibiotics like those used for acute disease, although a longer course (3–6 weeks) may be necessary.
  - Adjuvant therapy with intranasal corticosteroids, decongestants, and antihistamines may be useful in combating the allergic/inflammatory component of the disease.
  - Surgical intervention may be required.

INFLUENZA

A highly contagious orthomyxovirus transmitted by droplet nuclei. There are three types of influenza: A, B, and C. Subtypes of influenza A (eg, H5N1, H1N1) are classified based on glycoproteins (hemagglutinin and neuraminidase). Relevant terms are as follows:

- **Antigenic drift:** Refers to small, gradual changes in surface proteins through point mutations. These small changes are sufficient to allow the virus to escape immune recognition, accounting for the fact that individuals can be infected with influenza multiple times.
- **Antigenic shift:** Describes an acute, major change in the influenza A subtype (significant genetic reassortment) circulating among humans; leads to pandemics.

KEY FACT

Potential complications of sinusitis include meningitis, frontal bone osteomyelitis, cavernous sinus thrombosis, and abscess formation.

KEY FACT

Beware of invasive and life-threatening fungal sinusitis (caused by *Mucor* and *Rhizopus*) in patients with poorly controlled diabetes mellitus, immune compromise, or neutropenia.

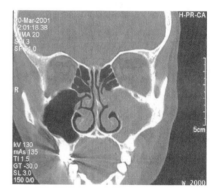

FIGURE 2.8-7. Sinusitis. Coronal CT image shows an opacified left maxillary sinus and marked associated bony thickening, consistent with chronic maxillary sinusitis. (Reproduced with permission from Lalwani AK. *Current Diagnosis & Treatment in Otolaryngology—Head and Neck Surgery*, 2nd ed. New York, NY: McGraw-Hill; 2008.)

Q

A 70-year-old man presents to the ED with 5 days of fever, productive cough, and altered mental status. He is also found to be hypotensive and tachypneic. Broad-spectrum antibiotics and fluid resuscitation are promptly administered, but the patient continues to be hypotensive. What is the next best step in treatment?

In the United States, the typical influenza season begins in November and lasts until April. Yearly vaccination with inactivated influenza virus is currently recommended for all patients ≥ 6 months of age. Children 6 months to 9 years of age require two doses of the seasonal vaccine if they are receiving the vaccine for the first time. A high-dose flu vaccine is available for people ≥ 65 years of age or those who are immunocompromised.

HISTORY/PE

Patients typically present with abrupt onset of fever, myalgia, chills, cough, coryza, and weakness. Elderly patients may have atypical presentations characterized only by confusion.

DIAGNOSIS

- **Best initial test:** Rapid influenza test of viral antigens from nasopharyngeal swab.
- **Most accurate test:** Diagnosis can be made with DFA tests, viral culture, or PCR assays. Rapid influenza tests have low sensitivity, and influenza is usually a clinical diagnosis. Leukopenia is a common finding.

TREATMENT

- Symptomatic care with analgesics and hydration.
- Antivirals such as oseltamivir or zanamivir are most effective when used within 2 days of onset and may shorten the duration of infection by 1–3 days.

COMPLICATIONS

Severe 1° viral pneumonia, 2° bacterial pneumonia (see "Postviral" in Table 2.8-1), sinusitis, bronchitis, and exacerbation of COPD and asthma can occur.

Infections of the Eyes and Ears

INFECTIOUS CONJUNCTIVITIS

Inflammation of the conjunctiva is most often bacterial or viral but can also be fungal, parasitic, allergic, or chemical. It is essential to differentiate potentially vision-threatening infectious etiologies from allergic or other causes of conjunctivitis, and to identify other vision-threatening conditions that may mimic conjunctivitis. Table 2.8-5 lists the common etiologies of infectious conjunctivitis.

ORBITAL CELLULITIS

Commonly caused by direct spread of infection from the paranasal sinuses; can lead to endophthalmitis and blindness. Usually caused by streptococci, staphylococci (including Methicillin-resistant *Staphylococcus aureus* [MRSA]), and *H influenzae* (in children). In diabetic and immunocompromised patients, the Zygomycetes *Mucor* and *Rhizopus* must be included in the differential diagnosis.

HISTORY/PE

Presents with acute-onset fever, proptosis, ↓ extraocular movement, ocular pain, and ↓ visual acuity. Look for a history of ocular trauma/surgery or sinusitis. Palatal or nasal mucosal ulceration with coexisting maxillary and/or ethmoid sinusitis suggests mucormycosis or *Rhizopus*.

KEY FACT

Orbital cellulitis can be distinguished from preseptal cellulitis by the following clinical features: restricted eye movements, ↓ visual acuity, diplopia, and proptosis.

Administration of vasopressors and ICU admission. This patient is in septic shock, probably 2° to pneumonia. Patients with pneumonia who require vasopressors or mechanical ventilation warrant admission to an ICU.

TABLE 2.8-5. Common Causes of Infectious Conjunctivitis

PATHOGEN	CHARACTERISTICS	DIAGNOSIS	TREATMENT
BACTERIAL			
Staphylococci, streptococci, *Haemophilus, Pseudomonas, Moraxella*	Foreign body sensation, purulent discharge	Gram stain and culture if severe	Antibiotic drops/ointment
N gonorrhoeae	**An emergency!** Corneal involvement can lead to perforation and blindness	Gram stain shows gram ⊖ intracellular diplococci	IM or IV ceftriaxone. Inpatient treatment if complicated
C trachomatis A–C	Neonatal infection: mucopurulent conjunctivitis Trachoma (global): recurrent epithelial keratitis in childhood; trichiasis, corneal scarring, and entropion Leading cause of preventable blindness worldwide	Neonatal infection: Giemsa stain, chlamydial cultures Trachoma: clinical (most often), PCR	Neonatal: azithromycin, tetracycline, or erythromycin for 3–4 weeks in infants Trachoma: (single oral dose) in mass treatment Surgery if needed to protect cornea from eyelashes
VIRAL			
Adenovirus (most common)	Copious watery discharge, severe ocular irritation, preauricular lymphadenopathy Occurs in epidemics		Contagious; self-limited

DIAGNOSIS

- Mostly clinical.
- **Best initial test:** Blood and tissue fluid culture. CT scan to rule out orbital abscess and intracranial involvement.

TREATMENT

- Admit and give immediate IV antibiotics; request an ophthalmologic/ENT consult.
- Abscess formation or a worsening condition may necessitate surgery.
- Diabetic and immunocompromised patients should be treated with amphotericin B and surgical debridement (often associated with cavernous sinus thrombosis) if *Mucor* or *Rhizopus* is diagnosed.

KEY FACT

Neisseria conjunctivitis is an ocular emergency often requiring inpatient parenteral antibiotic therapy.

ACUTE DACRYOCYSTITIS

- Infection of the lacrimal sac, usually by *Staphylococcus* or *Streptococcus spp.*
- **Hx/PE:** Pain and redness in the medial canthal region, less commonly fever and ↑ WBC.
- **Tx:** Most accurate treatment is immediate treatment with empiric antibiotics to prevent disastrous orbital cellulitis.

HERPES SIMPLEX KERATITIS

- Viral infection of the cornea. Common cause of blindness in the United States.

- **Hx/PE:** Presents with pain, blurred vision, tearing, and redness. Often recurrent caused by repeated exposure (outdoor occupation) or immunodeficiency.
- **Dx:** Typically clinical. However, corneal vesicles and dendritic ulcers are characteristic. Epithelial scrapings show multinucleated giant cells.
- **Tx:** Oral or topical antiviral therapy.

CONTACT LENS KERATITIS

- **Medical emergency,** often caused by *Pseudomonas* infection.
- **Hx/PE:** Typically presents with painful, red eye and opacification and ulceration of the cornea. Progressed disease can cause corneal perforation and permanent vision loss.
- **Dx:** Clinical.
- **Tx:** Immediately remove the contact lens and give topical broad-spectrum antibiotics; avoid patching.

OTITIS EXTERNA

- Inflammation of the external auditory canal, also known as "swimmer's ear." *Pseudomonas* and Enterobacteriaceae are the most common etiologic agents. Both grow in the presence of excess moisture.
- **Hx/PE:** Presents with pain, pruritus, and possible purulent discharge. Exam reveals pain with movement of the tragus/pinna (unlike otitis media) and an edematous and erythematous ear canal. See the Pediatrics chapter for a discussion of otitis media.
- **Dx:** A clinical diagnosis. Obtain a culture for severe or refractory cases. Order a CT scan if the patient appears toxic.
- **Tx: Best initial treatment** is to clean the ear and give antibiotic (ofloxacin or ciprofloxacin) and steroid eardrops. Elderly diabetics and immunocompromised individuals are at risk for necrotizing otitis externa and may require IV antibiotics (usually a fluoroquinolone or fourth-generation cephalosporin).

CNS Infections

MENINGITIS

Acute bacterial meningitis is a life-threatening emergency. Viral (also called "aseptic") meningitis is more common and clinically less morbid. Risk factors for meningitis include recent ear infection, sinusitis, immunodeficiencies, recent neurosurgical procedures, crowded living conditions (ie, college dorms, military), and sick contacts. Common causative organisms are listed in Table 2.8-6.

HISTORY/PE

About one-half of patients present with a classic triad of fever, headache, and neck stiffness. Other symptoms include malaise, photophobia, altered mental status, nausea/vomiting, seizures, or signs of meningeal irritation (⊕ Kernig and Brudzinski signs).

DIAGNOSIS

- **Best initial test:** Obtain a lumbar puncture (LP) for CSF analysis, Gram stain, and culture ideally before initiation of antibiotics; obtain glucose,

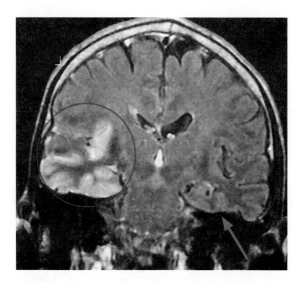

FIGURE 2.8-9. HSV encephalitis. Coronal FLAIR image of a young man with HSV encephalitis shows the characteristic MRI pattern within the cortex of the right temporal lobe *(circle)*. The left temporal lobe is also involved *(arrow)*, but to a lesser extent. (Reproduced with permission from Fauci AS, et al. *Harrison's Principles of Internal Medicine*, 17th ed. New York, NY: McGraw-Hill; 2008.)

- Give doxycycline for suspected Rocky Mountain spotted fever or ehrlichiosis. Treat Lyme encephalitis with ceftriaxone.

BRAIN ABSCESS

A focal, suppurative infection of the brain parenchyma, usually with a "ring-enhancing" appearance caused by fibrous capsule (see Figure 2.8-10). The most common pathogens are streptococci, staphylococci, and anaerobes; 80–90% are polymicrobial. Nonbacterial causes include *Toxoplasma* and *Candida*; *Aspergillus* and zygomycosis should be considered in immunocompromised hosts, and neurocysticercosis should be considered in relevant epidemiologic settings (Central and South America, sub-Saharan Africa and Asia). Modes of transmission include the following:

- **Direct spread:** Caused by paranasal sinusitis (10% of cases; frequently affects young men, and often caused by *Streptococcus milleri*), otitis media or mastoiditis (33%), or dental infection (2%).
- **Direct inoculation:** History of head trauma or neurosurgical procedures.
- **Hematogenous spread (25% of cases):** Often shows a middle cerebral artery distribution with multiple abscesses that are poorly encapsulated and located at the gray-white junction.

HISTORY/PE

Headache (most common), drowsiness, inattention, confusion, and seizures are early symptoms, followed by signs of increasing ICP and then a focal neurologic deficit (CN III and IV deficits).

DIAGNOSIS

- CT scan will show a ring-enhancing lesion with a low-density core.
- **Most accurate test:** MRI has a higher sensitivity for early abscesses and posterior fossa lesions.
- CSF analysis is not necessary and may precipitate brainstem herniation.
- Lab values may show peripheral leukocytosis, ↑ erythrocyte sedimentation rate (ESR), and ↑ C-reactive protein (CRP).

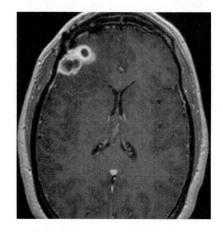

FIGURE 2.8-10. Brain abscess. Post–contrast MRI of the brain shows ring-enhancing lesions in the lateral right frontal lobe, with "daughter" lesions (smaller adjacent rings of enhancement) also noted. (Reproduced with permission from USMLE-Rx.com.)

KEY FACT

The classic clinical triad of headache, fever, and a focal neurologic deficit is present in 50% of cases of brain abscess.

Q

A 19-year-old college student is brought to the ED from her dorm room, where she was found by her roommate in a confused state. She complains of fever, nausea, vomiting, and pain in her neck and head. She has a petechial rash on her legs. CSF exam reveals a glucose level of 22 mg/dL, a protein level of 140 mg/dL, and a WBC count of 1400/mm³. What is the most likely organism responsible for her condition?

Neisseria meningitidis. Suspect meningococcal meningitis in a very ill patient with fever, headache, altered mental status, a petechial rash in the lower extremities, and a CSF profile indicative of bacterial meningitis.

TREATMENT

- **IV antibiotics:** Metronidazole + a third-generation cephalosporin ± vancomycin for 6–8 weeks. Obtain serial CT/MRIs to follow resolution. Lesions < 2 cm can often be treated medically.
- Surgical drainage (aspiration or excision) if necessary for diagnostic and/or therapeutic purposes.
- Dexamethasone with taper may be used in severe cases to ↓ cerebral edema; IV mannitol may be used to ↓ ICP. Prophylactic anticonvulsants should be given.

BOTULISM

Symmetric descending paralysis caused by ingestion of *Clostridium botulinum* spores or exposure to spores in soil of endemic regions (California, Utah). Treat with IV botulism immune-globulin and respiratory support. Consider in any infant with bulbar palsies, ptosis, constipation, or hypotonia. Avoid giving honey to young infants to avoid risk for botulism.

Human Immunodeficiency Virus

A retrovirus that targets and destroys CD4+ T lymphocytes. Infection is characterized by a high rate of viral replication that leads to a progressive decline in CD4+ count (see Figure 2.8-11).

- **CD4+ count:** Indicates the degree of immunosuppression; guides therapy and prophylaxis, and helps determine prognosis.
- **Viral load:** May predict the rate of disease progression; provides indications for treatment and gauges response to antiretroviral therapy (ART).

HISTORY/PE

- Acute HIV infection (acute infection/seroconversion, acute retroviral syndrome) occurs days to weeks after exposure. The initial infection is often asymptomatic, but patients may also present with mononucleosis-like or flulike symptoms (eg, fever, lymphadenopathy, maculopapular rash, pharyngitis, diarrhea, nausea/vomiting, weight loss, headache).
- HIV infection can later present as night sweats, weight loss, thrush (see Figure 2.8-12), recurrent infections, or opportunistic infections. Complications are inversely correlated with CD4+ count (see Figure 2.8-13).

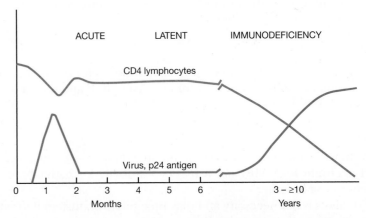

FIGURE 2.8-11. Time course of HIV infection. Note that the level of CD4 lymphocytes (*red curve*) remains normal for many years but then declines, resulting in the immunodeficiency stage, which is characterized by opportunistic infections and malignancies.

Diagnosis

- **ELISA test (high sensitivity, moderate specificity):** Detects anti-HIV antibodies in the bloodstream (can take up to 6 months to appear after exposure).
- **Western blot (low sensitivity, high specificity):** Confirmatory.
- Rapid HIV tests are now available.
- Baseline evaluation should include HIV RNA PCR (viral load), CD4+ cell count, CXR, PPD skin test or interferon-gamma release assay, Pap smear, mental status exam, VDRL/RPR, and serologies for CMV, viral hepatitis, toxoplasmosis, and VZV.
- Evaluation for acute retroviral syndrome (acute HIV) should include HIV RNA PCR (viral load); ELISA may be $\ominus$.

Treatment

- Lifelong ART for all HIV-infected patients, regardless of CD4+ count or associated symptoms/illnesses, especially benefitting those with CD4+ < 500 mm³. It is important to counsel patients about medication adherence, benefits, and risks.
- Initial regimen should generally consist of two nucleoside/nucleotide reverse transcriptase inhibitors (NRTIs) *plus* one integrase inhibitor (which can be substituted with a non-nucleoside RTI [NNRTI] or protease inhibitor if contraindicated).
- Goal of therapy is complete viral suppression (< 50 viral copies). After therapy is started, CD4+ count and viral load should be monitored monthly until suppression is achieved and every 4–6 months afterward.
- HIV genotype should be obtained before initiation of therapy and when resistance is suspected, as such testing can provide mutation information and identify resistance to specific antiretrovirals.
- In the setting of a percutaneous injury, mucous membrane exposure, or nonintact skin exposure with an HIV $\oplus$ source, begin ART as soon as

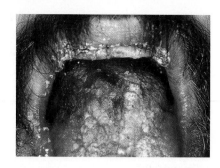

FIGURE 2.8-12. **Oral thrush in HIV-positive patient.** (Reproduced courtesy of Drs. John Molinari and Sol Silverman, Jr., Centers for Disease Control and Prevention, Atlanta, GA.)

KEY FACT

Measles, mumps, and rubella (MMR) and varicella vaccines are the only live vaccines that should be given to HIV patients (if CD4+ > 200 mm³). Do not give oral polio vaccine to HIV $\oplus$ patients or their contacts.

KEY FACT

Common AIDS-defining illnesses:
- Esophageal candidiasis.
- CMV retinitis.
- Kaposi sarcoma (human herpesvirus-8) (see Figure 2.8-14).
- CNS lymphoma, toxoplasmosis, PML.
- *P jirovecii* pneumonia or recurrent bacterial pneumonia.
- HIV encephalopathy.
- Disseminated mycobacterial or fungal infection.
- Invasive cervical cancer or anal cancer in HPV $\oplus$ patient.

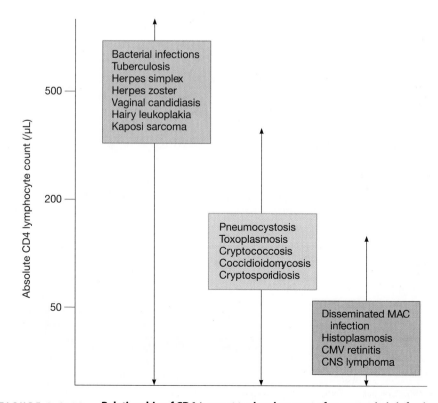

FIGURE 2.8-13. **Relationship of CD4+ count to development of opportunistic infections.** (Reproduced with permission from USMLE-Rx.com.)

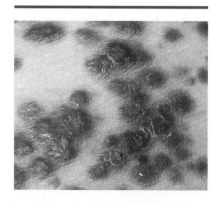

FIGURE 2.8-14. **Kaposi sarcoma (HHV-8).** A neoplasm of endothelial cells seen in HIV/AIDS and transplant patients. (Reproduced courtesy of the U.S. Department of Health and Human Services.)

TABLE 2.8-9. Prophylaxis for HIV-Related Opportunistic Infection

Pathogen	Indication for Prophylaxis	Treatment	Notes
P jirovecii pneumonia	CD4+ < 200/mm³, prior *P jirovecii* infection	High-dose IV TMP-SMX + tapered-dose steroids	Discontinue prophylaxis when CD4+ is > 200/mm³ for ≥ 3 months
Mycobacterium avium complex (MAC)	CD4+ < 50–100/mm³	Weekly azithromycin	Discontinue prophylaxis when CD4+ is > 100/mm³ for > 6 months
Toxoplasma gondii	CD4+ < 100/mm³ + ⊕ IgG serologies	Double-strength TMP-SMX	—
M tuberculosis	PPD > 5 mm or "high risk" (see TB section)	INH for 9 months (+ pyridoxine) or rifampin for 4 months	Include pyridoxine with INH-containing regimens
Candida	Multiple recurrences	Esophagitis: fluconazole Oral: fluconazole or nystatin swish and swallow	—
HSV	Multiple recurrences	Daily suppressive acyclovir, famciclovir, or valacyclovir	—
S pneumoniae	All patients	PCV13 followed by PSV23 in 2 months	Give every 5 years provided that CD4+ is > 200/mm³
Influenza	All patients	Influenza vaccine annually	—

possible with a basic two-drug regimen or an expanded regimen of three or more drugs for 4 weeks, depending on the severity of the source infection.

Table 2.8-9 outlines prophylactic measures against opportunistic infections.

Opportunistic Infections

Figure 2.8-15 illustrates the microscopic appearance of some common opportunistic organisms.

OROPHARYNGEAL CANDIDIASIS (THRUSH)

■ **Risk factors:** Xerostomia, antibiotic use, denture use, and immunosuppression (eg, HIV, leukemias, lymphomas, cancer, diabetes, corticosteroid inhaler use, immunosuppressive treatment).

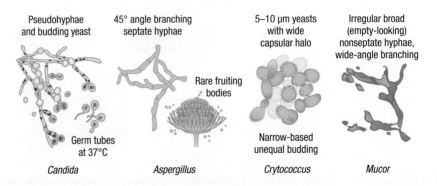

Pseudohyphae and budding yeast — Germ tubes at 37°C — *Candida*

45° angle branching septate hyphae — Rare fruiting bodies — *Aspergillus*

5–10 μm yeasts with wide capsular halo — Narrow-based unequal budding — *Crytococcus*

Irregular broad (empty-looking) nonseptate hyphae, wide-angle branching — *Mucor*

FIGURE 2.8-15. **Common opportunistic organisms.** (Reproduced with permission from USMLE-Rx.com.)

- **Hx/PE:** Presents with soft white plaques that can be rubbed off, with an erythematous base and possible mucosal burning. The differential diagnosis includes oral hairy leukoplakia (affects the lateral borders of the tongue; not easily rubbed off). Odynophagia is characteristic of candidal esophagitis.
- **Dx:** Usually clinical. KOH or Gram stain shows budding yeast and/or pseudohyphae.
- **Tx:** Treat thrush with local therapy (eg, nystatin suspension, clotrimazole tablets, or a PO azole such as fluconazole). Treat candidal esophagitis with PO azole therapy.

CRYPTOCOCCAL MENINGITIS

- **Risk factors:** AIDS, exposure to pigeon droppings.
- **Hx/PE:** Presents with headache, fever, impaired mentation, signs of increased ICP, and absent meningeal signs. The differential diagnosis includes toxoplasmosis, lymphoma, TB meningitis, AIDS dementia complex, PML, HSV encephalitis, and other fungal disease.
- **Dx:** LP (↓ CSF glucose; ↑ protein; ↑ leukocyte count with monocytic predominance, ↑↑ opening pressure); ⊕ cryptococcal antigen testing in CSF and/or blood, CSF India ink stain, and fungal culture.
- **Tx:**
  - IV amphotericin B + flucytosine for 2 weeks; then fluconazole for 8 weeks. Lifelong maintenance therapy should be administered with fluconazole until symptoms resolve and CD4+ is > 100/mm^3 for > 1 year.
  - ↑ Opening pressure may require serial LPs or a ventriculoperitoneal shunt for management.

> **KEY FACT**
>
> The CSF antigen test for cryptococcal meningitis is highly sensitive and specific.

HISTOPLASMOSIS

Risk factors include HIV/AIDS, spelunking, and exposure to bird or bat excrement, especially in the Ohio and Mississippi river valleys (see Figure 2.8-16).

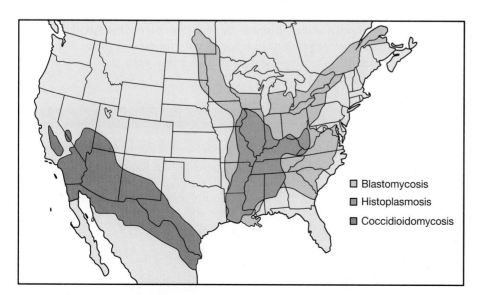

Blastomycosis
Histoplasmosis
Coccidioidomycosis

FIGURE 2.8-16. **Geographic distribution of systemic fungal infection in the United States.** (Reproduced with permission from Ryan KJ, Ray CG. *Sherris Medical Microbiology*, 5th ed. New York, NY: McGraw-Hill; 2010.)

TABLE 2.8-10. Differential Diagnosis of Opportunistic Pulmonary Fungal Infections

	HISTOPLASMOSIS	COCCIDIOIDOMYCOSIS	BLASTOMYCOSIS
Disseminated disease	Hepatosplenomegaly, lymphadenopathy, nonproductive cough	Meningitis, bone lesions, abscesses, erythema nodosum	Meningitis, bone, prostate, and skin lesions, ARDS
Diagnosis	Urine and serum polysaccharide antigens	PCR assay of bronchiolar lavage and tissue samples	Culture shows broad-budding yeast

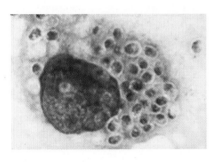

FIGURE 2.8-17. Histiocyte macrophage containing numerous yeast cells of *Histoplasma capsulatum* (Giemsa stain). (Reproduced courtesy of Dr. DT McClenan, Centers for Disease Control and Prevention, Atlanta, GA.)

 KEY FACT

Nocardia is a partially acid-fast, gram ⊕, branching rod found in soil that is a common cause of lung and CNS infection in immunocompromised hosts. TMP-SMX is the treatment of choice (see Figure 2.8-18).

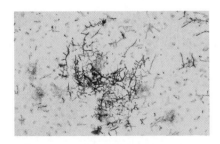

FIGURE 2.8-18. *Nocardia.* Branching filaments on acid-fast stain. (Modified with permission from Leli C, et al. Fatal *Nocardia farcinica* bacteremia diagnosed by matrix-assisted laser desorption-ionization time of flight mass spectrometry in a patient with myelodysplastic syndrome treated with corticosteroids. *Case Rep Med.* 2013;2013:368637.)

HISTORY/PE

- 1° Exposure is often asymptomatic or causes a flulike illness.
- Presentation may range from no symptoms to fulminant disease with pulmonary and/or extrapulmonary manifestations.
- Fever, weight loss, hepatosplenomegaly, lymphadenopathy, nonproductive cough, palatal ulcers, and pancytopenia indicate disseminated infection (most often within 14 days).
- The differential diagnosis includes atypical bacterial pneumonia, blastomycosis, coccidioidomycosis, TB, sarcoidosis, pneumoconiosis, and lymphoma (see Table 2.8-10).

DIAGNOSIS

- CXR shows diffuse nodular densities, focal infiltrate, cavity, or hilar lymphadenopathy (chronic infection is usually cavitary).
- Urine and serum polysaccharide antigen tests are the most sensitive for making the **initial diagnosis** of disseminated disease, monitoring response to therapy, and diagnosing relapse. Culture is also diagnostic (blood, sputum, bone marrow, CSF).
- The yeast form is seen with special stains on biopsy (bone marrow, lymph node, liver) or bronchoalveolar lavage (see Figure 2.8-17).

TREATMENT

- **Mild pulmonary disease or stable nodules:** Treat supportively in the immunocompetent host. Consider itraconazole.
- **Chronic cavitary lesions:** Give itraconazole for > 1 year.
- **Severe acute pulmonary disease or disseminated disease:** Liposomal amphotericin B **or** amphotericin B for 14 days followed by itraconazole for 1 year or longer. Lifelong maintenance therapy with daily itraconazole may be necessary.

COCCIDIOIDOMYCOSIS

A pulmonary fungal infection endemic to the southwestern United States (see Figure 2.8-16). Can present as an acute or subacute pneumonia or as a flulike illness, and may involve extrapulmonary sites, including bone, CNS, and skin (manifestations include erythema multiforme or erythema nodosum). The incubation period is 1–4 weeks after exposure. Filipino, African-American, pregnant, and HIV ⊕ patients are at ↑ risk for disseminated disease.

HISTORY/PE

Patients present with fever, anorexia, headache, chest pain, cough, dyspnea, arthralgias, and night sweats. Disseminated infection can present with meningitis, bone lesions, and soft tissue abscesses.

DIAGNOSIS

- Serology is specific but not sensitive during the first 1–2 weeks after infection. Repeat testing can increase sensitivity, and can be confirmed with immunodiffusion testing.
- PCR assays of respiratory specimens have been developed that are highly sensitive and specific.
- Obtain bronchoalveolar lavage and fungal cultures of sputum, wound exudate, or other affected tissue. Cultures are usually only obtained in hospitalized patients or patients with severe disease, and growth can take days to weeks.
- Identify *Coccidioides immitis* spherules on hematoxylin and eosin (H&E) stain or other special sputum or tissue stains.
- CXR findings may be normal or show infiltrates, nodules, cavities, mediastinal or hilar adenopathy, or pleural effusion.

TREATMENT

- **Acute:** PO fluconazole or itraconazole for mild infection. IV amphotericin B only for severe or protracted 1° pulmonary infection and disseminated disease, followed by PO azole therapy once stable.
- **Chronic:** No treatment is needed for asymptomatic chronic pulmonary nodules or cavities. Progressive cavitary or symptomatic disease usually requires surgery plus long-term azole therapy for 8–12 months.

BLASTOMYCOSIS

A fungal infection endemic to the central and southeastern United States, particularly the Mississippi and Ohio river valleys.

- **Hx/PE:** Presents similarly to coccidioidomycosis, and typically has extrapulmonary involvement in the bone, prostate, and skin.
- **Dx:** Serologic tests are not sensitive enough; culture is the only way to definitively diagnose, and a sputum smear will show broad-budding yeast.
- **Tx:** Treat symptomatic patients with itraconazole, and consider inpatient treatment with amphotericin B and ICU admission if complicated by ARDS, meningitis, or other systemic involvement.

PNEUMOCYSTIS JIROVECII PNEUMONIA

Formerly known as *Pneumocystis carinii* pneumonia, or PCP. Risk factors include impaired cellular immunity and AIDS.

HISTORY/PE

- Presents with dyspnea on exertion, fever, nonproductive cough, tachypnea, weight loss, fatigue, and impaired oxygenation. Typically, symptoms have been present for weeks.
- Can also present as disseminated disease or as local disease in other organ systems.
- The differential diagnosis includes TB, histoplasmosis, and coccidioidomycosis.

DIAGNOSIS

- Diagnosed by cytology of induced sputum or bronchoscopy specimen with silver stain and immunofluorescence (see Figure 2.8-19A). Obtain an ABG to check Pao_2.

KEY FACT

Consider coccidioidomycosis in a patient from the southwestern United States who presents with respiratory infection. HIV ⊕, Filipino, African-American, and pregnant patients are at ↑ risk for disseminated disease.

Q

A 35-year-old HIV-infected man from Ohio presents to his primary care provider with low-grade fever, dry cough, malaise, and a 5-lb weight loss over the past month. He is adherent to his HIV medications. Physical exam shows hepatosplenomegaly and palatal ulcers. His CBC reveals pancytopenia, and a CXR shows hilar lymphadenopathy. What is the next most appropriate step in management?

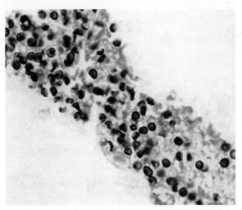

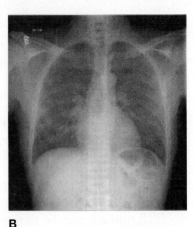

A   B

FIGURE 2.8-19. ***Pneumocystis* pneumonia. (A)** Lung tissue stained with silver uncovers folded cysts containing comma-shaped spores. **(B)** Frontal CXR shows diffuse "ground-glass" lung opacities characteristic of PCP in this patient with AIDS and a CD4+ count of 26. (Image A reproduced with permission from Ryan KJ, Ray CG. *Sherris Medical Microbiology*, 5th ed. New York, NY: McGraw-Hill; 2010. Image B reproduced with permission from USMLE-Rx.com.)

- CXR most commonly shows diffuse, bilateral interstitial infiltrates with a ground-glass appearance (see Figure 2.8-19B), but any presentation is possible.

TREATMENT

- Treat with high-dose TMP-SMX for 21 days.
- Use a prednisone taper in patients with moderate to severe hypoxemia ($Pao_2 < 70$ mm Hg or an alveolar-arterial oxygen gradient > 35).

CYTOMEGALOVIRUS

Seventy percent of adults in the United States have been infected with CMV, and most are asymptomatic; reactivation generally occurs in immunocompromised patients.

- Transmission occurs via sexual contact, vertical transmission, breast milk, respiratory droplets in nursery or day care facilities, and blood transfusions.
- Risk factors for reactivation include the first 100 days status post tissue or bone marrow transplant and HIV/AIDS (CD4+ $< 50/mm^3$ or viral load $> 10,000$ copies).

HISTORY/PE

- Systemic infection may resemble EBV mononucleosis (see the discussion of infectious mononucleosis).
- Specific manifestations include the following:
  - **CMV retinitis:** Associated with retinal detachment ("pizza pie" retinopathy); presents with floaters and visual field changes (CD4+ $< 50/mm^3$).
  - **GI and hepatobiliary involvement:** Can present with multiple nonspecific GI symptoms, including bloody diarrhea and abdominal pain. CMV, microsporidia, and cryptosporidia have been implicated in the development of AIDS cholangiopathy.
  - **CMV esophagitis:** Typically presents with odynophagia and shallow ulcers on the distal esophagus (CD4+ $< 50/mm^3$).
  - **CMV pneumonitis:** Presents with cough, fever, and sparse sputum production; associated with a high mortality rate. Much more common

in patients with hematologic malignancies and transplant patients than in those with AIDS.

- **CNS involvement:** Can include polyradiculopathy, transverse myelitis, and subacute encephalitis (CD4+ < 50/mm^3; periventricular calcifications).

DIAGNOSIS

Virus isolation, culture, tissue histopathology, serum PCR.

TREATMENT

Treat with ganciclovir, valganciclovir, or foscarnet. Treat underlying disease if the patient is immunocompromised.

MYCOBACTERIUM AVIUM COMPLEX

Ubiquitous organisms causing pulmonary and disseminated infection in several demographic groups. The 1° pulmonary form occurs in apparently healthy nonsmokers (Lady Windermere syndrome); a 2° pulmonary form affects patients with preexisting pulmonary disease such as COPD, TB, or CF. Disseminated infection occurs in AIDS patients with a CD4+ < 50/mm^3.

HISTORY/PE

- Disseminated *M avium* infection in AIDS is associated with fever, weakness, and weight loss in patients who are not on highly active ART (HAART) or chemoprophylaxis for MAC.
- Hepatosplenomegaly and lymphadenopathy are occasionally seen.
- Adrenal insufficiency is possible in the setting of adrenal infiltration.

DIAGNOSIS

- Obtain mycobacterial blood cultures (⊕ in 2–3 weeks).
- Labs show anemia, hypoalbuminemia, and ↑ serum alkaline phosphatase and LDH.
- Biopsy of lung, bone marrow, intestine, or liver reveals foamy macrophages with acid-fast bacilli. Typical granulomas may be absent in immunocompromised patients.

TREATMENT

Treat with clarithromycin + ethambutol, and consider HAART if drug-naïve. Rifabutin is second line. Continue for > 12 months and until CD4+ is > 100/mm^3 for > 6 months.

PREVENTION

Weekly azithromycin for those with a CD4+ < 50/mm^3 or AIDS-defining opportunistic infection.

TOXOPLASMOSIS

Risk factors include ingesting raw or undercooked meat and changing cat litter.

HISTORY/PE

- 1° Infection is usually asymptomatic.
- Reactivated toxoplasmosis occurs in immunosuppressed patients and may present in specific organs (brain, lung, and eye > heart, skin, GI tract, and liver).

Q

A 27-year-old man with HIV presents to his primary-care physician with fever, night sweats, weight loss, and diarrhea. Today his CD4+ count is 25 cells/mm^3. A CBC is performed and is significant for anemia (a hemoglobin level of 8 mg/dL). Other labs show hypoalbuminemia and elevated alkaline phosphatase. What could have prevented this patient's condition?

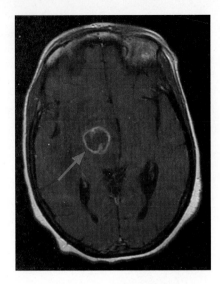

FIGURE 2.8-20. Toxoplasmosis.
(Modified with permission from Rabhi S, Amrani K, Maaroufi M, et al. Hemichorea-hemiballismus as an initial manifestation in a Moroccan patient with acquired immunodeficiency syndrome and toxoplasma infection: a case report and review of the literature. The *Pan Afr Med J.* 2011;10:9.)

KEY FACT

Ring-enhancing lesions in patients with AIDS should always prompt consideration of toxoplasmosis and CNS lymphoma.

KEY FACT

Chlamydia species cause arthritis, neonatal conjunctivitis, pneumonia, nongonococcal urethritis/PID, and LGV.

Azithromycin. The patient has signs and symptoms of disseminated *Mycobacterium avium* complex. HIV-infected patients with CD4+ counts < 50 cells/mm³ should receive prophylaxis against MAC with azithromycin once a week.

- Encephalitis is common in seropositive AIDS patients. Classically, CNS lesions present with fever, headache, altered mental status, seizures, and focal neurologic deficits.

DIAGNOSIS

- Serology, PCR (indicates exposure and risk for reactivation); tissue exam for histology, isolation of the organism in mice, or tissue culture.
- In the setting of CNS involvement, obtain a CT scan (see Figure 2.8-20) (look for multiple isodense or hypodense ring-enhancing mass lesions) or an MRI (has a predilection for the basal ganglia; more sensitive).

TREATMENT

- **Most accurate treatment:** Induction with high-dose PO pyrimethamine + sulfadiazine and leucovorin (a folic acid analog to prevent hematologic toxicity) for 4–8 weeks; maintenance with a low-dose regimen until the disease has resolved clinically and radiographically.
- TMP-SMX (Bactrim DS) or pyrimethamine + dapsone can be used for prophylaxis in patients with a CD4+ count < 100/mm³ and a ⊕ toxoplasmosis IgG.

Sexually Transmitted Diseases

CHLAMYDIA

The most common bacterial STD in the United States. Caused by *Chlamydia trachomatis*, which can infect the genital tract, urethra, anus, and eye. Risk factors include unprotected sexual intercourse and new or multiple partners. Often coexists with or mimics *N gonorrhoeae* infection (known as nongonococcal urethritis when gonorrhea is absent). Lymphogranuloma venereum (LGV) serovars of *C trachomatis* cause lymphogranuloma venereum, an emerging cause of proctocolitis.

HISTORY/PE

- Infection is often asymptomatic in men and may present with urethritis, mucopurulent cervicitis, or pelvic inflammatory disease (PID) in women.
- Exam may reveal cervical/adnexal tenderness in women or penile discharge and testicular tenderness in men.
- The differential diagnosis includes gonorrhea, endometriosis, PID, orchitis, vaginitis, and UTI.
- Lymphogranuloma venereum presents in its 1° form as a painless, transient papule or shallow ulcer. In its 2° form, it presents as painful swelling of the inguinal nodes, and in its 3° form it can present as an "anogenital syndrome" (anal pruritus with discharge, rectal strictures, rectovaginal fistula, and elephantiasis).

DIAGNOSIS

- Diagnosis is usually clinical; culture is the **gold standard**.
- Urine tests (nucleic acid amplification test) are a rapid means of detection, whereas DNA probes and immunofluorescence (for gonorrhea/chlamydia) take 48–72 hours.
- Gram stain of urethral or genital discharge may show PMNs but no bacteria (intracellular).

TREATMENT

- Doxycycline for 7 days or azithromycin once. Use azithromycin or amoxicillin in pregnant patients.

▨ Treat sexual partners, and maintain a low threshold to treat for N *gonor-rhoeae*. LGV serovars require prolonged therapy for 21 days.

COMPLICATIONS

▨ Chronic infection and pelvic pain, Reiter syndrome (urethritis, conjunctivitis, arthritis), Fitz-Hugh–Curtis syndrome (perihepatic inflammation and fibrosis). See Figures 2.8-21 and 2.8-22.

▨ Ectopic pregnancy/infertility can result from PID (in women) and epididymitis (in men).

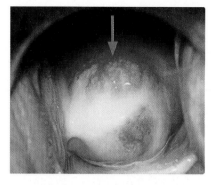

FIGURE 2.8-21. **Purulent cervical discharge in pelvic inflammatory disease.** (Adapted with permission from SOS-AIDS Amsterdam.)

GONORRHEA

A gram ⊖ intracellular diplococcus that can infect almost any site in the female reproductive tract. Infection in men tends to be limited to the urethra.

HISTORY/PE

▨ Presents with a greenish-yellow discharge, pelvic or adnexal pain, and swollen Bartholin glands. Men experience a purulent urethral discharge, dysuria, and erythema of the urethral meatus.

▨ The differential diagnosis includes chlamydia, endometriosis, pharyngitis, PID, vaginitis, UTI, salpingitis, and tubo-ovarian abscess.

DIAGNOSIS

▨ Gram stain and culture is the **gold standard** for any site (pharynx, cervix, urethra, or anus). Nucleic acid amplification tests can be sent on penile/vaginal tissue or from urine.

▨ Disseminated disease may present with monoarticular septic arthritis, rash, and/or tenosynovitis. See Figures 2.8-23 and 2.8-24.

TREATMENT

▨ Ceftriaxone IM and azithromycin PO (regardless of whether chlamydia is present). Condoms are effective prophylaxis. Treat the sexual partner or partners if possible. Fluoroquinolones should not be used because of emerging resistance.

▨ Disseminated disease requires IV ceftriaxone for at least 24 hours.

KEY FACT

Treat gonorrhea with two agents because of the high prevalence of resistance.

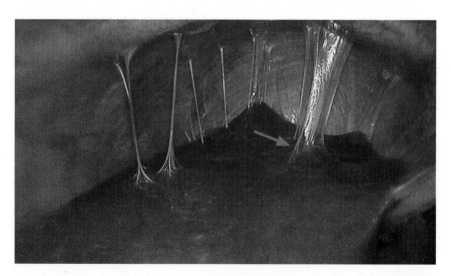

FIGURE 2.8-22. **Adhesions in Fitz-Hugh–Curtis syndrome in pelvic inflammatory disease.** Note the adhesions (*arrow*) extending from the peritoneum to the surface of the liver. (Reproduced with permission from Hic et nunc.)

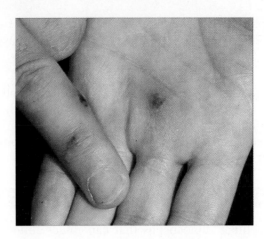

FIGURE 2.8-23. **Disseminated gonococcal infection.** Hemorrhagic, painful pustules are seen on erythematous bases. (Reproduced with permission from Wolff K, et al. *Fitzpatrick's Dermatology in General Medicine*, 7th ed. New York, NY: McGraw-Hill; 2008.)

COMPLICATIONS

Persistent infection with pain; infertility; tubo-ovarian abscess with rupture; disseminated gonococcal infection (characterized by migratory polyarthralgia, tenosynovitis, and pustular skin lesions) (see Figure 2.8-24).

SYPHILIS

Caused by *Treponema pallidum*, a spirochete. AIDS can accelerate the course of disease progression.

HISTORY/PE

- **1° (10–90 days after infection):** Presents with a painless ulcer (chancre; see Figure 2.8-25A) and local lymphadenopathy.
- **2° (4–8 weeks after chancre):** Presents with low-grade fever, headache, malaise, and generalized lymphadenopathy with a diffuse, symmetric, asymptomatic (nonpruritic) maculopapular rash on the soles and palms (see Figure 2.8-25C, D). Highly infective 2° eruptions include mucous patches called condylomata lata (see Figure 2.8-25E) and alopecia. Meningitis, hepatitis, nephropathy, and eye involvement may also be seen.
  - **Early latent (period from resolution of 1° or 2° syphilis to the end of the first year of infection):** No symptoms; ⊕ serology.

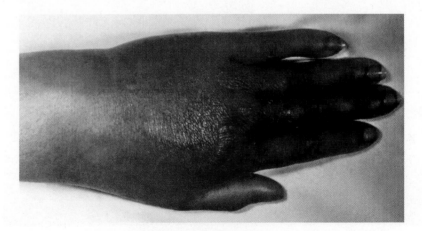

FIGURE 2.8-24. *Neisseria gonorrhoeae* **joint infection.** (Reproduced with permission from Susan Lindsley, Public Health Image Library, Centers for Disease Control and Prevention, Atlanta, GA.)

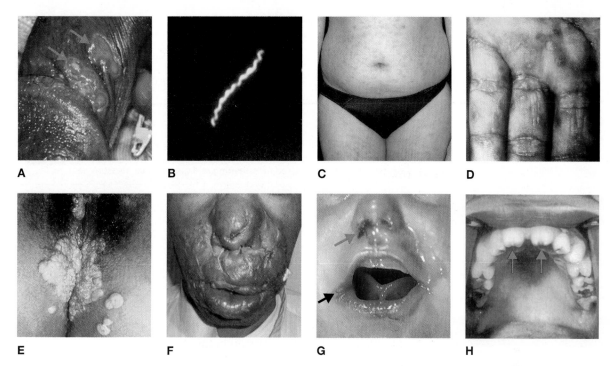

FIGURE 2.8-25. **Syphilis.** (A) Localized disease presenting with painless chancre and (B) dark-field microscopy visualizing treponemes in fluid from chancre in 1° syphilis. (C) Maculopapular rash ([D] including palms and soles) and (E) condylomata lata in 2° syphilis. (F) Gummas (chronic granulomas) in 3° syphilis. (G) Rhagades (linear scars at angle of mouth), snuffles (nasal discharge), saddle nose, and (H) notched (Hutchinson) teeth in congenital syphilis. (Image A reproduced courtesy of U.S. Department of Health and Human Services and M. Rein. Image B reproduced courtesy of U.S. Department of Health and Human Services and Renelle Woodall. Image C reproduced with permission from Dr. Richard Usatine. Image D reproduced courtesy of the U.S. Department of Health and Human Services and Robert Sumpter. Images E and H reproduced courtesy of US Department of Health and Human Services and Susan Lindsley. Image F modified with permission from Chakir K, Benchikhi H. Centro-facial granuloma revealing a tertiary syphilis. *Pan Afr Med J.* 2013;15:82. Image G reproduced courtesy of the U.S. Department of Health and Human Services and Dr. Norman Cole.)

- **Late latent (period of asymptomatic infection beyond the first year):** No symptoms; ⊕ or ⊖ serology. One-third of cases progress to 3° syphilis.
- **3° (late manifestations appearing 1–20 years after initial infection):** Presents with destructive, granulomatous gummas (see Figure 2.8-25F). Neurosyphilis includes tabes dorsalis (posterior column degeneration), meningitis, and Argyll Robertson pupil (constricts with accommodation but not reactive to light). Cardiovascular findings include dilated aortic root, aortitis, aortic root aneurysms, and aortic regurgitation.

DIAGNOSIS

- Table 2.8-11 summarizes relevant diagnostic tests.
- Venereal disease research laboratory (VDRL) test: False ⊕ results are seen with viruses (mononucleosis, HSV, HIV, hepatitis), drugs/IV drug use, rheumatic fever/rheumatoid arthritis, and SLE/leprosy.
- Neurosyphilis should be suspected and ruled out in patients with AIDS, neurologic symptoms, and a ⊕ rapid plasma reagin (RPR) test.

TREATMENT

- **1°/2°:** Benzathine penicillin IM for one dose. Tetracycline or doxycycline for 14 days may be used for patients with penicillin allergy. Pregnant patients who are penicillin allergic and have ⊕ antibody titers must be desensitized and treated with penicillin.
- **Latent infection:** Treat with benzathine penicillin. Give one dose for early latent infection; give a weekly dose for 3 weeks for late latent infection or for asymptomatic infection of unknown duration.

 KEY FACT

Syphilis is the "great imitator" because its dermatologic findings resemble those of many other diseases.

 KEY FACT

Treatment of syphilis can result in an acute flulike illness (headache, fever, chills, myalgias) known as the Jarisch-Herxheimer reaction, which results from the release of endotoxins by the killed organisms.

TABLE 2.8-11.   Diagnostic Tests for Syphilis

TEST	COMMENTS
Dark-field microscopy	Identifies motile spirochetes (only 1° and 2° lesions)
VDRL/RPR	Nontreponemal tests
	Rapid and cheap, but sensitivity is only 75–85% in 1° disease
	Many false ⊕ results
	Used for screening and quantitative measurement
FTA-ABS, TP-PA, MHA-TP, TP-EIA	Treponemal tests
	Sensitive and specific
	Used as confirmatory tests

KEY FACT

Genital lesions caused by *Haemophilus* "do cry," and herpes lesions are painful. Syphil**is** and the others are pain**less**.

KEY FACT

In a patient with a nonhealing ulcerative lesion and inguinal lymphadenopathy with a ⊖ work-up for an STI, think cancer.

- **Neurosyphilis:** Treat with penicillin IV for 10–14 days; penicillin-allergic patients should be desensitized before therapy.

GENITAL LESIONS

See Table 2.8-12 for a description of common sexually transmitted genital lesions along with an outline of their diagnosis and treatment.

TABLE 2.8-12.   Sexually Transmitted Genital Lesions

VARIABLE	KLEBSIELLA GRANULOMATIS[a] (GRANULOMA INGUINALE)	HAEMOPHILUS DUCREYI (CHANCROID)	HSV-1 OR HSV-2[B]	HPV[C]	TREPONEMA PALLIDUM (SYPHILIS)
Lesion	Papule becomes a beefy-red ulcer with a characteristic rolled edge of granulation tissue (see Image A)	Papule or pustule (chancroid) (see Image B)	Vesicle (3–7 days postexposure) (see Image C)	Papule (condylomata acuminata, warts) (see Image D)	Papule (chancre) (see Image E)
Appearance	Raised red lesions with a white border	Irregular, deep, well demarcated, necrotic	Regular, red, shallow ulcer	Irregular, pink or white, raised; cauliflower	Regular, red, round, raised
Number	One or multiple	1–3	Multiple	Multiple	Single
Size	5–10 mm	10–20 mm	1–3 mm	1–5 mm	1 cm
Pain	No	Yes	Yes	No	No
Concurrent signs and symptoms	Granulomatous ulcers	Inguinal lymphadenopathy	Malaise, myalgias, and fever with vulvar burning and pruritus	Pruritus	Regional adenopathy

(continues)

TABLE 2.8-12.   Sexually Transmitted Genital Lesions *(continued)*

Variable	*Klebsiella granulomatis*[a] (granuloma inguinale)	*Haemophilus ducreyi* (chancroid)	HSV-1 or HSV-2[b]	HPV[c]	*Treponema pallidum* (Syphilis)
Diagnosis	Clinical exam, biopsy (Donovan bodies)	Difficult to culture; diagnosis is made on clinical grounds, culture on specialized media	Tzanck smear shows multinucleated giant cells (best initial test [see Image F]); viral cultures (most accurate test); DFA or serology	Clinical exam; shave biopsy only if uncertain	Spirochetes seen under dark-field microscopy; *T pallidum* identified by serum antibody tests
Treatment[d]	Doxycycline or azithromycin	Single-dose azithromycin or ceftriaxone	Acyclovir, famciclovir, or valacyclovir for 1° infection Foscarnet if resistant	Cryotherapy, laser, or excision; topical agents such as podophyllotoxin, imiquimod, or trichloroacetic acid	Penicillin IM

A   B   C

D   E   F

[a] Previously known as *Calymmatobacterium granulomatis*.

[b] Some 85% of genital herpes lesions are caused by HSV-2.

[c] HPV serotypes 6 and 11 are associated with genital warts; types 16, 18, and 31 are associated with cervical cancer.

[d] For all, treat sexual partners.

Image A reproduced with permission from Longo DL, et al. *Harrison's Principles of Internal Medicine,* 18th ed. New York, NY: McGraw-Hill; 2012. Image B reproduced with permission from Wolff K, Johnson RA, Saavedra AP. *Fitzpatrick's Color Atlas & Synopsis of Clinical Dermatology,* 7th ed. New York, NY: McGraw-Hill; 2013. Image C reproduced with permission from Wolff K, Johnson R, Saavedra A. *Fitzpatrick's Color Atlas & Synopsis of Clinical Dermatology,* 7th ed. New York, NY: McGraw-Hill; 2013. Image D reproduced courtesy of Dr. Wiesner, Public Health Image Library, Centers for Disease Control and Prevention, Atlanta, GA. Image E reproduced courtesy of Public Health Image Library, Centers for Disease Control and Prevention, Atlanta, GA. Image F modified with permission from Yale Rosen.

Genitourinary Infections

URINARY TRACT INFECTIONS

Affect women more frequently than men caused by shorter urethral length, and ⊕ *E coli* cultures are obtained in 80% of cases. See the mnemonic SEEKS PP for other pathogens. Risk factors include the presence of catheters

Common UTI bugs—

SEEKS PP

Serratia
E coli
Enterobacter
Klebsiella pneumoniae
Staphylococcus saprophyticus
Pseudomonas
Proteus mirabilis

or other urologic instrumentation, anatomic abnormalities (eg, BPH, vesico-ureteral reflux), previous UTIs or pyelonephritis, diabetes, recent antibiotic use, sexual intercourse, immunosuppression, and pregnancy.

History/PE

- Present with dysuria, urgency, frequency, suprapubic pain, and hematuria.
- Children may present with bedwetting, poor feeding, recurrent fevers, and foul-smelling urine.
- Elderly patients may present with delirium/acute confusion and few other symptoms.
- The differential diagnosis includes vaginitis, STDs, urethritis or acute urethral syndrome, and prostatitis.

Diagnosis

- Diagnosed by clinical symptoms. In the absence of symptoms, treatment is warranted only for children, patients with anatomic GU tract anomalies, pregnant women, those with instrumented urinary tracts, patients scheduled for GU surgery, and renal transplant patients.
- **Best initial test:** Urine dipstick/urinalysis (UA); ↑ leukocyte esterase (a marker of WBCs) is 75% sensitive and up to 95% specific. ↑ Nitrites (a marker of bacteria), ↑ urine pH (*Proteus* infections), and hematuria (seen with cystitis) are also commonly seen.
- **Microscopic analysis:** Pyuria (> 5 WBCs/hpf) and bacteriuria (1 organism/hpf = 10^6 organisms/mL) are suggestive.
- **Most accurate test:** Urine culture; the gold standard is > 10^5 CFU/mL. All children with suspected UTI should undergo urinalysis and culture. Use catheterization to obtain the sample in patients who are not toilet-trained to avoid contamination.

Treatment

- **Uncomplicated UTI:** Treat on an outpatient basis with PO TMP-SMX or a fluoroquinolone for 3 days, or nitrofurantoin for 5 days. The use of fluoroquinolones should be reserved for severe symptoms in light of resistance and MRSA selection and risk for *C difficile* infection.
- **Complicated UTI** (urinary obstruction, UTI in men, renal transplant, catheters, instrumentation): Administer the same antibiotics as above, but for 7–14 days.
- **Pregnant patients:** Treat asymptomatic bacteriuria or symptomatic UTI with nitrofurantoin, oral cephalosporin, or amoxicillin for 3–7 days. Avoid fluoroquinolones, TMP-SMX, and tetracyclines. Confirm clearance with a posttreatment urine culture.
- **Urosepsis:** Patients with urosepsis should be hospitalized and initially treated with IV antibiotics. Consider broader coverage to include resistant GNRs or enterococcus.
- Prophylactic antibiotics may be given to women with uncomplicated recurrent UTIs. Check for prostatitis in men. Methenamine can also be used, which is converted to formaldehyde by acidic urine.

Prostatitis can be differentiated from a UTI by prostate tenderness on exam. Urethral catheterization and prostate massage are highly contraindicated because they increase the likelihood of bacteremia. Treat with trimethoprim/sulfamethoxazole (TMP/SMX) or ciprofloxacin for 6 weeks.

PYELONEPHRITIS

Nearly 85% of community-acquired cases of pyelonephritis result from the same pathogens that cause cystitis. Cystitis and pyelonephritis have similar risk factors.

HISTORY/PE

Signs and symptoms are similar to those of cystitis but show evidence of upper urinary tract disease: flank or costovertebral pain, fever/chills, and nausea/vomiting.

DIAGNOSIS

- **UA and culture:** Results are similar to those of cystitis, but with WBC casts. Send blood cultures to rule out urosepsis.
- **CBC:** Reveals leukocytosis.
- **Imaging:** In general, imaging is not necessary. Patients who relapse or do not respond to therapy within 48–72 hours should be evaluated by ultrasound or CT for obstruction, abscess, and other complications.

TREATMENT

- For mild cases, patients may be treated on an outpatient basis for 7–14 days.
- **Best initial treatment:** Fluoroquinolones. Encourage ↑ PO fluids, and monitor closely.
- Admit and administer IV antibiotics to patients who have serious medical complications or systemic symptoms, are pregnant, present with severe nausea and vomiting, or have suspected bacteremia. Fluoroquinolones, third- or fourth-generation cephalosporins, β-lactam/β-lactamase inhibitors, and carbapenem can be used depending on disease severity.
- Abscesses ≥ 3 cm should be drained and cultured.

Hematologic Infections

SEPSIS

The presence of systemic inflammatory response syndrome (SIRS) with a documented infection induced by microbial invasion or toxins in the bloodstream. Severe sepsis refers to sepsis with end-organ dysfunction caused by poor perfusion. Septic shock refers to sepsis with hypotension and organ dysfunction from vasodilation. Examples include the following:

- Gram ⊕ shock (eg, staphylococci and streptococci) 2° to fluid loss caused by exotoxins.
- Gram ⊖ shock (eg, *E coli*, *Klebsiella*, *Proteus*, and *Pseudomonas*) 2° to vasodilation caused by endotoxins (lipopolysaccharide).
- **Neonates:** GBS, *E coli*, *Listeria monocytogenes*, *H influenzae*.
- **Children:** *H influenzae*, pneumococcus, meningococcus.
- **Adults:** Gram ⊕ cocci, aerobic gram ⊖ bacilli, anaerobes (dependent on the presumed site of infection).
- **IV drug users/indwelling lines:** *S aureus*, coagulase ⊖ *Staphylococcus* species.
- **Asplenic patients:** Pneumococcus, *H influenzae*, meningococcus (encapsulated organisms).

HISTORY/PE

- Presents with abrupt onset of fever and chills, altered mental status, tachycardia, and tachypnea. Severe sepsis may lead to end-organ dysfunction such as renal or hepatic failure. Hypotension occurs in cases of septic shock.

KEY FACT

Pyelonephritis is the most common serious medical complication of pregnancy. Among patients with untreated bacteriuria, 20–30% will develop pyelonephritis.

KEY FACT

Urosepsis should be considered in any elderly patient with altered mental status.

- Septic shock is typically a warm shock with warm skin and extremities. This contrasts with cardiogenic shock, which typically presents with cool skin and extremities.
- Petechiae, ecchymoses, or abnormal coagulation tests suggest DIC (2–3% of cases).

DIAGNOSIS

- Make a clinical diagnosis promptly based on SIRS criteria.
- Labs show leukocytosis or leukopenia with ↑ bands, thrombocytopenia (50% of cases), evidence of ↓ tissue perfusion (↑ creatinine, ↑ LFTs, ↑ lactate), and abnormal coagulation studies (↑ INR).
- It is critical to obtain cultures of all appropriate sites (eg, blood, sputum, CSF, wound, urine).
- Imaging (CXR, CT) may aid in establishing the etiology or site of infection.

TREATMENT

- ICU admission may be required. Treat aggressively with IV fluids, empiric antibiotics (based on the likely source of infection), and vasopressors.
- Treat underlying factors (eg, remove Foley catheter or infected lines, drain abscesses).
- The 1° goal is to maintain BP and perfuse end organs.

MALARIA

A protozoal disease caused by five species of the genus *Plasmodium* (*P falciparum, P vivax, P ovale, P malariae, P knowlesi*) and transmitted by the bite of an infected female *Anopheles* mosquito. *P falciparum* has the highest morbidity and mortality, occasionally within 24 hours of symptom onset. Travelers to endemic areas should take chemoprophylaxis and use mosquito repellent and bed nets to minimize exposure.

HISTORY/PE

- Patients have a history of exposure in a malaria-endemic area, with periodic attacks of sequential chills, fever (> 41°C, or > 105.8°F), myalgias, headache, and diaphoresis occurring over 4–6 hours.
- Splenomegaly often appears 4 or more days after symptom onset. Patients are often asymptomatic between attacks, which recur every 2–3 days depending on the *Plasmodium* species involved.
- Severely ill patients may present with hyperpyrexia, prostration, impaired consciousness, pulmonary edema, acidosis, hyperventilation, and bleeding. Rash, skin ulcer, eosinophilia, lymphadenopathy, neck stiffness, or photophobia suggests a different or additional diagnosis.

DIAGNOSIS

- Timely diagnosis of the correct species is essential, because *P falciparum* can be fatal and is often resistant to standard chloroquine treatment.
- Send Giemsa- or Wright-stained thick and thin blood films for evaluation to detect plasmodium and determine the species type, respectively, and the degree of parasitemia (see Figure 2.8-26).
- CBC usually demonstrates normochromic, normocytic anemia with reticulocytosis and thrombocytopenia early in the disease.

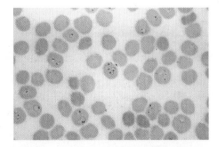

FIGURE 2.8-26. *Plasmodium falciparum* hyperparasitemia in the thin smear of a patient with cerebral malaria. (Reproduced courtesy of Steven Glenn, Public Health Image Library, Centers for Disease Control and Prevention, Atlanta, GA.)

- If resources allow, more sensitive serologic tests are available, including rapid antigen detection methods, fluorescent antibody methods, and PCR.
- In patients with altered mental status, obtain a fingerstick glucose to rule out hypoglycemia.

TREATMENT

- Uncomplicated malarial infection can be treated orally. Chloroquine has historically been the standard antimalarial medication, but high resistance rates often necessitate the use of other medications such as mefloquine, atovaquone-proguanil, or artemisinins (for severe cases).
- In cases of *P vivax*, *P ovale*, or an unknown species, primaquine is added to eradicate the hypnozoites in the liver.
- For patients traveling to endemic regions, prescribe prophylaxis consisting of atovaquone-proguanil or mefloquine given at least 2 weeks before travel and continued for 4 weeks after returning.

COMPLICATIONS

Cerebral malaria, severe hemolytic anemia, renal impairment, noncardiogenic pulmonary edema, hypoglycemia, lactic acidosis, acute hepatopathy, gram ⊖ bacteremia.

OTHER MOSQUITO-BORNE VIRUSES

The following viruses are carried by the *Aedes* mosquito and present with rash, fever, and myalgias:

- **Chikungunya:** Notably causes joint pain. Treat with supportive care.
- **Dengue:** Presents with bone pain and can be complicated by severe thrombocytopenia, bleeding, and shock. Findings of low WBC and ↑ LFTs. Treat with fluids and blood products as needed.
- **Zika:** Flavivirus that causes conjunctivitis and headache. Associated with Guillain-Barré syndrome, and can cause microcephaly if infected during pregnancy.

INFECTIOUS MONONUCLEOSIS

Most commonly occurs in young adult patients; usually caused by acute EBV infection. Transmission most often occurs through exchange of body fluids, most commonly saliva.

HISTORY/PE

- Presents with fever and pharyngitis (see Figure 2.8-27). Fatigue invariably accompanies initial illness and may persist for 3–6 months. Exam may reveal low-grade fever, generalized lymphadenopathy (especially posterior cervical), tonsillar exudate and enlargement, palatal petechiae, a generalized maculopapular rash, splenomegaly, and bilateral upper eyelid edema. Symptoms appear 2–5 weeks after infection.
- In older children/adults, it may cause mesenteric lymphadenitis, mimicking appendicitis.
- Patients who present with pharyngitis as their 1° symptom may be misdiagnosed with streptococcal pharyngitis (30% of patients with infectious mononucleosis are asymptomatic carriers of GAS in their oropharynx).
- The differential diagnosis includes CMV, toxoplasmosis, HIV, HHV-6, other causes of viral hepatitis, and lymphoma.

KEY FACT

Antimalaria contraindications:
- Primaquine: must be tested for G6PD first.
- Mefloquine: seizure, psychiatric, and cardiac conduction disorders.
- Atovaquone/proguanil: pregnant/breastfeeding, renal disease.
- Chloroquine: psoriasis.

KEY FACT

Cerebral malaria presents with headache, altered mental status, neurologic signs, retinal hemorrhages, convulsions, and delirium. If left untreated, it can rapidly progress to coma and death.

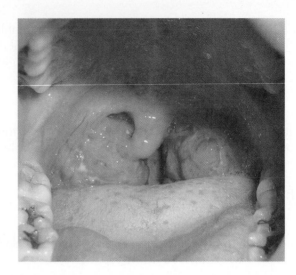

FIGURE 2.8-27. **Pharyngitis.** (Reproduced with permission from Dr. Richard Usatine.)

DIAGNOSIS

- **Best initial test:** Heterophile antibody (Monospot) test (may be ⊖ in the first few weeks after symptoms begin).
- EBV-specific antibodies can be ordered in patients with suspected mononucleosis and a ⊖ Monospot test. Monospot ⊖ and EBV-antibody ⊖ infectious mononucleosis syndromes are most often caused by CMV infection. Acute HIV and other viral etiologies should be considered.
- CBC with differential often reveals mild thrombocytopenia with relative lymphocytosis and > 10% atypical T lymphocytes.
- Comprehensive metabolic panel usually reveals mildly elevated transaminases, alkaline phosphatase, and total bilirubin.

TREATMENT

Treatment is mostly supportive, as there is no effective antiviral therapy. Corticosteroids are indicated for airway compromise caused by tonsillar enlargement, severe thrombocytopenia, or severe autoimmune hemolytic anemia.

COMPLICATIONS

- **CNS infection:** Can present as aseptic meningitis, encephalitis, meningoencephalitis, cranial nerve palsies (particularly CN VII), optic and peripheral neuritis, transverse myelitis, or Guillain-Barré syndrome.
- **Splenic rupture:** Occurs in < 0.5% of cases. More common in men, and presents with abdominal pain, referred left shoulder pain, or hemodynamic compromise. Patients should avoid contact sports for at least 4 weeks to prevent this complication.
- **Upper airway obstruction:** Treat with steroids.
- **Bacterial superinfection:** Many patients develop a 2° streptococcal pharyngitis.
- **Fulminant hepatic necrosis:** More common in men; the most common cause of death in affected men.
- **Autoimmune hemolytic anemia:** Occurs in 2% of patients during the first 2 weeks. Coombs ⊕. Mild anemia lasts 1–2 months. Treat with corticosteroids if severe.
- **Nasopharyngeal carcinoma:** Presents with epistaxis, headache and cervical lymph node spread; especially prevalent in southeast Asia.

KEY FACT

Lymphocytosis in EBV infection is predominantly caused by B-cell proliferation, but the atypical cells are T lymphocytes.

KEY FACT

Patients with mononucleosis who are given ampicillin for suspected streptococcal pharyngitis may develop a prolonged, pruritic maculopapular rash.

Fever

FEVER OF UNKNOWN ORIGIN

A temperature of $> 38.3°C$ ($> 100.9°F$) of at least 3 weeks' duration that remains undiagnosed following three outpatient visits or 3 days of hospitalization.

History/PE

Presents with fever, headache, myalgia, and malaise. The differential diagnosis includes the following:

- **Infectious:** TB, endocarditis (eg, HACEK organisms; see the discussion of infective endocarditis), occult abscess (abdominal, prostatic), osteomyelitis, catheter infections, sinusitis. In HIV patients, consider MAC, histoplasmosis, or CMV.
- **Neoplastic:** Lymphomas, leukemias, hepatic and renal cell carcinomas.
- **Autoimmune:** Still disease, SLE, cryoglobulinemia, polyarteritis nodosa, connective tissue disease, granulomatous disease (including sarcoidosis).
- **Miscellaneous:** Pulmonary emboli/DVT, IBD, alcoholic hepatitis, drug fever, familial Mediterranean fever, factitious fever.
- Idiopathic (10–15%).

Diagnosis

- Confirm the presence of fever, and take a detailed history, including family, social, sexual, occupational, dietary, exposures (pets/animals), and travel.
- **Labs:** Obtain a CBC with differential, ESR, serum protein electrophoresis, multiple blood cultures, sputum Gram stain and culture, UA and culture, and PPD. Specific tests (ANA, RF, CK, viral cultures, viral serologies/antigen tests) can be obtained if an infectious or autoimmune etiology is suspected.
- **Imaging:** Obtain an CXR. CT of the chest, abdomen, and pelvis should be done early in the work-up of a true FUO. Invasive testing (marrow/liver biopsy) is generally low yield. Laparoscopy and colonoscopy are higher yield as second-line tests (after CT).

Treatment

Stop unnecessary medications. Patients with FUO and a completely ⊖ work-up have a favorable prognosis, with fevers resolving over months to years.

NEUTROPENIC FEVER

Defined as a single oral temperature of $≥ 38.3°C$ ($≥ 101°F$) or a temperature of $≥ 38°C$ ($≥ 100.4°F$) for $≥ 1$ hour in a neutropenic patient (ie, an absolute neutrophil count < 500 cells/mm³).

History/PE

Common in cancer patients undergoing chemotherapy (neutropenic nadir 7–10 days postchemotherapy). Inflammation may be minimal or absent.

Diagnosis

- Conduct a thorough physical exam, but avoid a rectal exam in light of the bleeding risk if the patient is thrombocytopenic.

KEY FACT

Overall, infections and cancer account for the majority of cases of fever of unknown origin (FUO) ($> 60\%$). Autoimmune diseases account for $\sim 15\%$. In the elderly, rheumatic diseases account for one-third of cases.

Q **1**

A 45-year-old woman presents to the ED with fever, chills, nausea, vomiting, and severe flank pain. She has a history of multiple UTIs and was recently hospitalized for pyelonephritis. UA reveals pyuria and bacteriuria. Ultrasound performed in the ED shows what appears to be a perinephric abscess. What is the next most appropriate step in management?

Q **2**

A 17-year-old boy presents with 1 week of fever, sore throat, and progressive fatigue. Physical exam reveals palatal petechiae, large tonsils with whitish exudates, splenomegaly, and cervical and axillary lymphadenopathy. The patient says that he has been too tired to attend football practices and is concerned that he may lose his spot on the starting roster. What is the most appropriate advice to be given regarding his participation in athletics?

- Obtain a CBC with differential, serum creatinine, BUN, and transaminases; send blood, urine, lesion, sputum, and stool cultures. Consider testing for viruses, fungi, and mycobacteria.
- CXR for patients with respiratory symptoms; CT scan to evaluate for abscesses or other occult infection.

TREATMENT

Empiric antibiotic therapy with antipseudomonal agent (cefepime, piperacillin-tazobactam), and vancomycin for MRSA coverage in patients with indwelling catheters, pneumonia, or cutaneous abscess. Admission and IV antibiotics are warranted for high-risk patients (eg, hematologic malignancy, chemotherapy, neutropenia > 14 days). Routine use of colony-stimulating factors is not indicated. If fevers persist after 72 hours despite antibiotic therapy, start antifungal treatment.

1 **A**

Hospitalize the patient for empiric broad-spectrum antibiotics. This patient has complicated pyelonephritis and therefore needs to be initially managed as an inpatient. Antibiotic therapy can subsequently be narrowed and converted to PO as patient circumstances permit.

2 **A**

Tell the patient to refrain from contact sports until his physical exam normalizes. Splenomegaly 2° to infectious mononucleosis puts him at ↑ risk for splenic rupture.

Tick-Borne Infections

LYME DISEASE

A tick-borne disease caused by the spirochete *Borrelia burgdorferi*. Usually seen during the summer months, and carried by *Ixodes* ticks on white-tailed deer and white-footed mice. Endemic to the Northeast, northern Midwest, and Pacific coast.

HISTORY/PE

- Presents with the onset of rash with fever, malaise, fatigue, headache, myalgias, and/or arthralgias. Infection usually occurs after a tick feeds for > 18 hours.
- 1° (early localized disease): Erythema migrans begins as a small erythematous macule or papule that is found at the tick-feeding site and expands slowly over days to weeks. The border may be macular or raised, often with central clearing ("bull's eye"; see Figure 2.8-28).
- 2° (early disseminated disease): Presents with migratory polyarthropathies, neurologic phenomena (eg, facial nerve palsy; bilateral is classic for Lyme disease), lymphocytic meningitis and/or myocarditis, and conduction abnormalities (third-degree heart block).
- 3° (late disease): Arthritis and subacute encephalitis (memory loss and mood change).

DIAGNOSIS

- Early Lyme disease is diagnosed on clinical grounds alone (erythema migrans + endemic area). Serologic tests are not required or recommended, as IgM becomes ⊕ 1–2 weeks, and IgG 2–6 weeks after onset of erythema migrans.
- Early disseminated or late Lyme disease presenting with consistent symptoms and exposure risk factors should be diagnosed with serology. If ELISA IgM and IgG are ⊕ or equivocal, then Western blot for confirmation. Do not use for "screening" or nonspecific symptoms. Western blots sent without ELISA have high false ⊕ rates.

TREATMENT

- Treat early disease with doxycycline (or amoxicillin in children < 8 years of age and in pregnant patients); more advanced disease (eg, CNS or arthritic disease) should be treated with ceftriaxone.

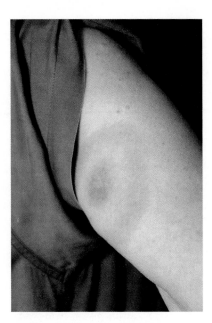

FIGURE 2.8-28. **Erythema chronicum migrans seen in Lyme disease.** Note the classic "bull's eye" lesion, which consists of an outer ring where the spirochetes are found, an inner ring of clearing, and central erythema caused by an allergic response at the site of the tick bite. (Reproduced courtesy of James Gathany, Centers for Disease Control and Prevention, Atlanta, GA.)

- Consider empiric therapy for patients with the characteristic rash, arthralgias, or a tick bite acquired in an endemic area. Prevent with tick bite avoidance.
- **Prophylaxis:** Lyme disease is not usually transmitted within the first 48 to 72 hours of tick attachment. Give one dose of doxycycline if all the following apply: tick is *Ixodes scapularis* and has been attached for ≥ 36 hours, prophylaxis is started ≤ 72 hours of removal, and local rate of infection of ticks with *Borrelia burgdorferi* is > 20%. If criteria not met, observe and treat only if erythema migrans develops.

BABESIOSIS

Tick-borne protozoal illness also transmitted by *I scapularis* (high rate of coinfection with Lyme disease). Causes flulike symptoms, intravascular hemolysis, anemia, and jaundice. Ring-shaped or "Maltese cross" organisms may be seen on blood smear. Treat with azithromycin and atovaquone.

ROCKY MOUNTAIN SPOTTED FEVER

- A disease caused by *Rickettsia rickettsii* and carried by the American dog tick (*Dermacentor variabilis*). The organism invades the endothelial lining of capillaries and causes small vessel vasculitis.
- **Hx/PE:** Presents with headache, fever, malaise, and rash. The characteristic rash is initially macular (beginning on the wrists and ankles) but becomes petechial/purpuric as it spreads centrally (see Figure 2.8-29). Altered mental status or DIC may develop in severe cases.
- **Dx:** Clinical diagnosis should be confirmed with biopsy and indirect immunofluorescence of the skin lesion.
- **Tx:** Doxycycline. The condition can be rapidly fatal if left untreated. If clinical suspicion is high, begin treatment while awaiting testing. Chloramphenicol can be used during the first two trimesters of pregnancy in

KEY FACT

"Tick testing" is a common incorrect answer choice; it has no effect on management and is not performed in a Lyme disease work-up.

KEY FACT

Rocky Mountain spotted fever starts on the wrists and ankles and then spreads centrally.

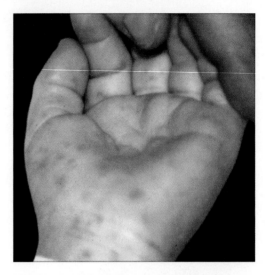

FIGURE 2.8-29. Rocky Mountain spotted fever. These erythematous macular lesions will evolve into a petechial rash that will spread centrally. (Reproduced with permission from Wolff K, Johnson RA, Saavedra AP. *Fitzpatrick's Color Atlas & Synopsis of Clinical Dermatology,* 7th ed. New York, NY: McGraw-Hill; 2013.)

uncomplicated cases, but if it is not available, doxycycline therapy should be initiated.

MNEMONIC

Presentation of endocarditis—

FROM JANE

Fever
Roth spots
Osler nodes
Murmur
Janeway lesions
Anemia
Nail hemorrhage
Emboli

Miscellaneous Infections

INFECTIVE ENDOCARDITIS

Infection of the endocardium. Most commonly affects the heart valves, especially the mitral valve. Risk factors include rheumatic, congenital, or valvular heart disease; prosthetic heart valves; IV drug use; and immunosuppression. Etiologies are as follows (see Table 2.8-13):

- *S aureus:* The causative agent in > 80% of cases of acute bacterial endocarditis in patients with a history of IV drug use.
- *Viridans* streptococci: The most common pathogens for left-sided subacute bacterial endocarditis and following dental procedures in native valves.

TABLE 2.8-13. Causes of Endocarditis

ACUTE	SUBACUTE	MARANTIC	CULTURE ⊖ (INCLUDES HACEK)	SLE
S aureus (IV drug use, prosthetic valves)	Viridans streptococci (native valve, dental procedures)	Cancer (poor prognosis)	*Haemophilus parainfluenzae*	Libman-Sacks endocarditis (autoantibody to valve)
S pneumoniae	*Enterococcus* (UTIs)	Metastases seed valves; emboli can cause cerebral infarcts	*Actinobacillus*	
N gonorrhoeae	*S epidermidis* (prosthetic valve)		*Cardiobacterium*	
	S bovis (GI insult)		*Eikenella*	
	Fungi		*Kingella*	
			Coxiella burnetii	
			Brucella	
			Bartonella	

- **Coagulase** ⊖ **Staphylococcus:** The most common infecting organism in prosthetic valve endocarditis.
- **Streptococcus bovis:** S bovis endocarditis is associated with coexisting GI malignancy. Perform colonoscopy if S bovis diagnosed.
- **Candida** and **Aspergillus** species: Account for most cases of fungal endocarditis. Predisposing factors include long-term indwelling IV catheters, malignancy, AIDS, organ transplantation, and IV drug use.

HISTORY/PE

- Constitutional symptoms are common (fever/FUO, weight loss, fatigue).
- Exam reveals a heart murmur. The mitral valve (mitral regurgitation) is more commonly affected than the aortic valve in non–IV drug users; more right-sided involvement is found in IV drug users (tricuspid valve > mitral valve > aortic valve).
- Osler nodes (small, tender nodules on the finger and toe pads), Janeway lesions (small peripheral hemorrhages; see Figure 2.8-30A), splinter hemorrhages (subungual petechiae; see Figure 2.8-30B), and Roth spots (retinal hemorrhages).

DIAGNOSIS

- Guided by risk factors, clinical symptoms, and the Duke criteria (see Table 2.8-14). The presence of two major, one major + three minor, or five minor criteria all merit the diagnosis of endocarditis. Obtain serial blood cultures from different sites before starting antibiotic therapy.
- CBC with leukocytosis and left shift; ↑ ESR and CRP.

TREATMENT

- Early empiric IV antibiotic treatment for acutely ill patients. Vancomycin + gentamicin is an appropriate choice for most patients. Tailor antibiotics once

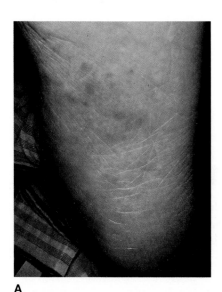

A

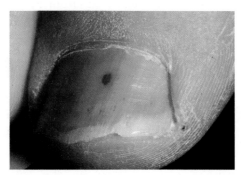

B

FIGURE 2.8-30. **Cutaneous manifestations of infective endocarditis.** (**A**) Janeway lesions. Peripheral embolization to the sole leads to a cluster of erythematous macules known as Janeway lesions. (**B**) Splinter hemorrhages. The splinter hemorrhages shown along the distal aspect of the nail plate are caused by emboli from subacute bacterial endocarditis. (Image A reproduced with permission from the Armed Forces Institute of Pathology, Bethesda, MD, as published in Knoop KJ, et al. *Atlas of Emergency Medicine*, 2nd ed. New York, NY: McGraw-Hill; 2002, Image B reproduced with permission from the Department of Dermatology, Wilford Hall USAF Medical Center and Brooke Army Medical Center, San Antonio, TX, as published in Knoop KJ, et al. *Atlas of Emergency Medicine*, 2nd ed. New York, NY: McGraw-Hill; 2002.)

KEY FACT

Otitis media should not cause pain with movement of the tragus/pinna.

Q 1

A 70-year-old woman with a history of hypertension and lymphoma presents with nausea, vomiting, and fever of 2 days' duration. She just completed her second cycle of high-dose chemotherapy. She has a temperature of 38.5°C (101.3°F). Her CXR is unchanged, and her WBC count is 900/mm³ with 25% neutrophils. After urine and blood cultures have been sent, what is the next step in management?

Q 2

A 41-year-old woman returns to the ED a week after she was discharged for diabetic ketoacidosis treatment. Today she complains of low-grade fever, tenderness and swelling over her face, and a persistent nasal discharge with occasional blood. Physical exam demonstrates necrosis in the left nasal turbinates and left eye proptosis. Specimens from the sinuses show broad, nonseptate hyphae. What is the next most appropriate step in management?

TABLE 2.8-14.　**Duke Criteria for the Diagnosis of Endocarditis**

CRITERIA	COMPONENTS
Major	1. ⊕ Blood cultures for a typical organism (either two samples drawn > 12 hours apart or three out of four drawn over the course of at least 1 hour) 2. Evidence of endocardial involvement (via transesophageal echocardiography or new murmur)
Minor	1. Predisposing risk factors/IV drug use 2. Fever ≥ 38°C (≥ 100.4°F) 3. Vascular phenomena: Septic emboli, septic infarcts, mycotic aneurysm, Janeway lesions 4. Immunologic phenomena: Glomerulonephritis, Osler nodes, Roth spots 5. Microbiologic evidence that does not meet major criteria 6. Echo findings that are consistent with IE but do not meet major criteria

the causative agent is known. Acute valve replacement is sometimes necessary if rupture occurs. The prognosis for prosthetic valve endocarditis is poor.

- **Preprocedure prophylaxis:** Endocarditis prophylaxis is only indicated in patients with the following:
  - Significant cardiac defects (prosthetic valves, unrepaired cyanotic congenital heart disease, prior history of endocarditis, transplanted heart with valvular disease).
  - Undergoing high-risk procedures (dental work involving gingival tissue or perforation of mucosa, respiratory tract surgery involving perforation of mucosa, GI or GU surgeries in patients with ongoing GI or GU infections).
- Amoxicillin is the preferred antibiotic prophylaxis. For patients who are penicillin allergic, use cephalexin, clindamycin, azithromycin, or clarithromycin.

COMPLICATIONS

Focal neurologic deficits from embolic strokes, metastatic infection (most common cause of splenic abscess), heart failure caused by valvular insufficiency, and glomerulonephritis.

ANTHRAX

Caused by the spore-forming gram ⊕ bacterium *Bacillus anthracis*. Infection is an occupational hazard for veterinarians, farmers, and individuals who handle animal wool, hair, hides, or bone meal products. Also, a biologic weapon. *B anthracis* can cause cutaneous (most common), inhalation (most deadly), or GI anthrax. There is no person-to-person spread of anthrax.

HISTORY/PE

- **Cutaneous:** Presents 1–7 days after skin exposure and penetration of spores. The lesion begins as a pruritic papule that enlarges to form an ulcer surrounded by a satellite bulbus/lesion with an edematous halo and a round, regular, raised edge. Regional lymphadenopathy is also characteristic. The lesion evolves into a black eschar within 7–10 days (see Figure 2.8-31).

1　**A**

Admit the patient and begin IV antibiotics with an antipseudomonal β-lactam (eg, cefepime, piperacillin-tazobactam, meropenem, imipenem). Febrile, neutropenic patients who are on high-dose chemotherapy, have a hematologic malignancy, or have been neutropenic for > 14 days should be admitted for empiric IV antibiotics.

2　**A**

Surgical debridement and amphotericin B. The patient has mucormycosis, a dangerous and aggressive infection found in diabetic and immunocompromised patients. Aggressive surgical debridement is warranted.

- **Inhalational:** Presents with fever, dyspnea, hypoxia, hypotension, or symptoms of pneumonia (1–3 days after exposure), classically caused by hemorrhagic mediastinitis. Patients typically do not have pulmonary infiltrates.
- **GI:** Occurs after the ingestion of poorly cooked, contaminated meat; can present with dysphagia, nausea/vomiting, bloody diarrhea, and abdominal pain.

DIAGNOSIS

Criteria for diagnosis include culture isolation or two nonculture supportive tests (PCR, immunohistochemical staining, or ELISA). CXR is the most sensitive test for inhalational disease (shows a widened mediastinum and pleural effusions).

TREATMENT

- **Best initial treatment:** Ciprofloxacin or doxycycline plus one to two additional antibiotics for at least 14 days for inhalational disease or cutaneous disease of the face, head, or neck.
- For other cutaneous disease, treat for 7–10 days. Postexposure prophylaxis (ciprofloxacin) to prevent inhalation anthrax should be continued for 60 days.

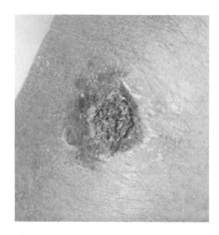

FIGURE 2.8-31. Cutaneous anthrax. Black eschar is seen on the forearm. (Reproduced courtesy of James H. Steele, Centers for Disease Control and Prevention, Atlanta, GA.)

OSTEOMYELITIS

Bone infection caused by direct spread from a soft tissue infection (80% of cases) is most common in adults, whereas infection caused by hematogenous seeding (20% of cases) is more common in children (metaphysis of the long bones) and IV drug users (vertebral bodies). Common pathogens are outlined in Table 2.8-15.

HISTORY/PE

Presents with localized bone pain and tenderness along with warmth, swelling, erythema, and limited motion of the adjacent joint. Systemic symptoms (fevers, chills) and purulent drainage may be present.

TABLE 2.8-15. Common Pathogens in Osteomyelitis

IF	THINK
No risk factors	S aureus
IV drug user	S aureus or Pseudomonas
Sickle cell disease	Salmonella
Hip replacement	S epidermidis (coagulase-negative staphylococcus)
Foot puncture wound	Pseudomonas
Chronic	S aureus, Pseudomonas, Enterobacteriaceae
Diabetic	Polymicrobial, Pseudomonas, S aureus, streptococci, anaerobes

Q

An 11-year-old African-American boy with a history of multiple hospitalizations for pain crises, all related to his sickle cell anemia, presents with fever and severe pain in his right hand. Exam shows an area of redness, tenderness, and swelling near the right second metacarpal. Labs show leukocytosis and an elevated ESR. MRI shows an area of ↑ intensity in the painful area. What pathogen is the most likely cause of his condition?

A

Salmonella. S aureus is the most common cause in patients without sickle cell disease and is the second most common organism that causes osteomyelitis in patients with sickle cell disease.

DIAGNOSIS

- **Labs:** ↑ WBC count; ↑ ESR and CRP levels in most cases. Blood cultures may be ⊕.
- **Imaging:**
  - X-rays are often ⊖ initially but may show periosteal elevation within 10–14 days. Bone scans are sensitive for osteomyelitis but lack specificity.
  - MRI (the test of choice) will show ↑ signal in the bone marrow and associated soft tissue infection (see Figure 2.8-32).
  - **Most accurate test:** Bone aspiration with Gram stain and culture. Clinical diagnosis made by probing through the soft tissue to bone is usually sufficient, as aspiration carries a risk for infection.

TREATMENT

- **Most accurate treatment:** Surgical debridement of necrotic, infected bone followed by IV antibiotics for 4–6 weeks. Empiric antibiotic selection is based on the suspected organism and Gram stain.
- Consider clindamycin plus ciprofloxacin, ampicillin/sulbactam, or oxacillin/nafcillin (for methicillin-sensitive S aureus); vancomycin (for MRSA); or ceftriaxone or ciprofloxacin (for gram ⊖ bacteria).

COMPLICATIONS

Chronic osteomyelitis, sepsis, septic arthritis. Long-standing chronic osteomyelitis with a draining sinus tract may eventually lead to squamous cell carcinoma (Marjolin ulcer).

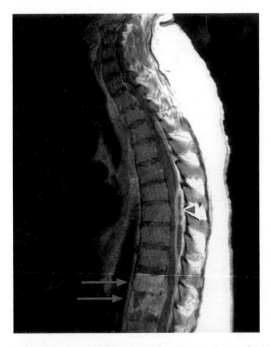

FIGURE 2.8-32. Diskitis/osteomyelitis. Sagittal contrast-enhanced MRI shows destruction of a lower thoracic intervertebral disk with abnormal enhancement throughout the adjacent vertebral bodies (*arrows*) and a posterior rim-enhancing epidural abscess (*arrowhead*) in the spinal canal. (Reproduced with permission from Tintinalli JE, et al. *Tintinalli's Emergency Medicine: A Comprehensive Study Guide,* 6th ed. New York, NY: McGraw-Hill; 2004.)

MUSCULOSKELETAL

Common Adult Orthopedic Injuries

Table 2.9-1 outlines the presentation and treatment of orthopedic injuries that commonly affect adults.

TABLE 2.9-1. Common Adult Orthopedic Injuries

UPPER EXTREMITY		
INJURY	**PRESENTATION**	**TREATMENT**
Shoulder dislocation	Anterior dislocation: Most common (95%); risk for axillary nerve injury. Patients hold arm in slight abduction and external rotation (see Images A and B) Posterior dislocation: Rare; associated with seizure and electrocution. Patients hold arm in adduction and internal rotation	Reduction followed by a sling and swath. Recurrent dislocations may need surgical treatment
Rotator cuff injury	Pain and weakness with abduction or external rotation of the humerus after fall on outstretched arm Impingement syndrome (pain caused by compression of soft tissue structures) may be present Diagnosis can be made clinically and confirmed with MRI (Do not confuse with adhesive capsulitis, characterized by significant shoulder stiffness but only mild pain with movement)	Rest and NSAIDs for minor injury Surgery for complete tear
Humerus fracture	Direct trauma. Radial nerve palsy may lead to wrist drop and loss of thumb extension	Hanging-arm cast vs coaptation splint and sling. Functional bracing
"Nightstick fracture"	Ulnar shaft fracture from direct trauma often in self-defense against a blunt object	ORIF if significantly displaced
Monteggia fracture	Diaphyseal fracture of the proximal ulna with subluxation of the radial head (see Image C). Results from fall on pronated and outstretched arm	ORIF of the shaft fracture and closed reduction of the radial head
Galeazzi fracture	Diaphyseal fracture of the radius with dislocation of the distal radioulnar joint (see Image D). Results from a direct blow to the radius	ORIF of the radius and casting of the fractured forearm in supination to reduce the distal radioulnar joint
Colles fracture	Involves the distal radius. Often results from a fall onto an outstretched hand that is in dorsiflexion, leading to a dorsally displaced, dorsally angulated fracture (see Image E). Commonly seen in the elderly (osteoporosis) and children	Closed reduction followed by application of a long-arm cast; open reduction if the fracture is intra-articular
Scaphoid fracture	Most commonly fractured carpal bone. Results from a fall onto an outstretched hand May take 2 weeks for x-rays to show fracture (see Image F). Assume a fracture if there is tenderness in anatomic snuffbox	Thumb spica cast. If displacement or scaphoid nonunion is present, treat with open reduction With proximal-third fractures, AVN may result from disruption of blood flow
Boxer's fracture	Fracture of the fifth metacarpal neck. Caused by forward trauma of a closed fist (eg, punching a wall)	Closed reduction and ulnar gutter splint; percutaneous pinning if the fracture is excessively angulated

(continues)

TABLE 2.9-1.   Common Adult Orthopedic Injuries *(continued)*

UPPER EXTREMITY		
INJURY	**PRESENTATION**	**TREATMENT**
De Quervain Tenosynovitis	New mother holding infant with outstretched thumb Pain on Finkelstein test (flexing thumb across palm and placing the wrist in ulnar deviation)	NSAIDs and casting

LOWER EXTREMITY		
INJURY	**PRESENTATION**	**TREATMENT**
Hip dislocation	Posterior dislocation: Most common (> 90%); occurs via a posteriorly directed force on an internally rotated, flexed, adducted hip ("dashboard injury"). Associated with a risk for sciatic nerve injury and AVN (see Image G) Anterior dislocation: Can injure the obturator nerve	Closed reduction followed by abduction pillow/bracing. Evaluate with CT scan after reduction
Hip fracture	↑ Risk with osteoporosis. Presents with a shortened and externally rotated leg Can be radiographically occult, so a good clinical history with ⊖ x-rays warrants further evaluation with CT or MRI Displaced femoral neck fractures associated with an ↑ risk for AVN and nonunion Associated with DVTs	ORIF. Displaced femoral neck fractures in elderly patients may require a hip hemiarthroplasty or total arthroplasty Anticoagulate to ↓ the likelihood of DVT Hip fracture involves the acetabulum and/or the proximal intracapsular femur
Femoral fracture	Direct trauma. Beware of fat emboli, which present with fever, changes in mental status, dyspnea, hypoxia, petechiae, and ↓ platelets	Intramedullary nailing of the femur. Irrigate and debride open fractures
Knee injuries	Present with knee instability and hematoma ACL: ▪ Result from a noncontact twisting mechanism, forced hyperextension, or impact to an extended knee ▪ ⊕ Anterior drawer and Lachman tests ▪ Rule out a meniscal or MCL injury (MCL injury = ⊕ valgus stress test; LCL injury = ⊕ varus stress test) PCL: ▪ Result from a posteriorly directed force on a flexed knee (eg, dashboard injury) ▪ ⊕ Posterior drawer test Meniscal tears: ▪ Result from an acute twisting injury or a degenerative tear in elderly patients ▪ Clicking or locking may be present ▪ Exam shows joint line tenderness and a ⊕ McMurray test	MRI is the diagnostic test of choice Treatment of MCL/LCL and meniscal tears can be conservative Treatment of ACL injuries in active patients is generally surgical with graft from the patellar or hamstring tendons Operative PCL reconstruction is reserved for highly competitive athletes with high-grade injuries Operative meniscal repair is for younger patients with reparable tears or older patients with mechanical symptoms who do not respond to conservative treatment
Tibial stress fracture	Direct trauma. Watch for compartment syndrome	Casting vs intramedullary nailing vs ORIF

(continues)

TABLE 2.9-1. **Common Adult Orthopedic Injuries** *(continued)*

	LOWER EXTREMITY	
INJURY	**PRESENTATION**	**TREATMENT**
Achilles tendon rupture	Presents with a sudden "pop" like a rifle shot. More likely with ↓ physical conditioning Limited plantar flexion and a ⊕ Thompson test (pressure on the gastrocnemius leading to absent foot plantar flexion)	Surgery followed by a long-leg cast for 6 weeks
Popliteal (Baker) cyst rupture	Caused by extrusion of synovial fluid into gastrocnemius or semi-membranosus bursa in patients with underlying arthritis May present with painless bulge in popliteal space, or with acute calf pain	Ultrasound to rule out DVT, then surgery if symptomatic

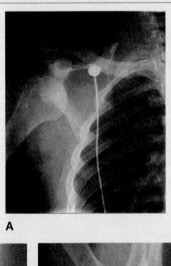
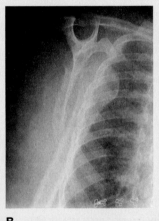
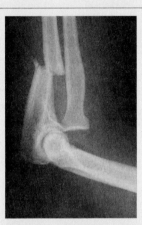

A   B   C

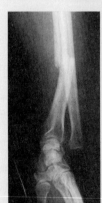
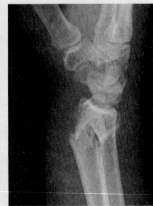
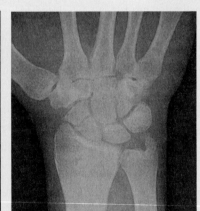
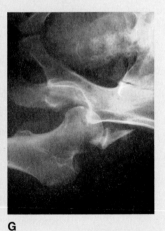

D   E   F   G

Images A, B, and F reproduced with permission from USME-Rx.com. Images C and D reproduced with permission from Knoop K, et al., editors. *The Atlas of Emergency Medicine*, 3rd ed. New York: McGraw-Hill, 2009, Figs. 11.16, 11.17. Image E reproduced with permission from Usatine RP et al., editors. *The Color Atlas of Family Medicine*, 2nd ed. New York: McGraw-Hill, 2013 Image G reproduced with permission from Doherty GM. *Current Diagnosis & Treatment: Surgery*, 13th ed. New York: McGraw-Hill, 2010.

 KEY FACT

The classic unhappy triad of knee injury involves the ACL, the MCL, and the medial meniscus. However, lateral meniscal tears are more commonly seen in acute ACL injuries.

Common Peripheral Nerve Injuries

Table 2.9-2 outlines the clinical findings of the most common peripheral nerve injuries.

TABLE 2.9-2.   Common Peripheral Nerve Injuries

Nerve	Motor Deficit	Sensory Deficit	Common Causes	Clinical Findings
Radial	Wrist extension	Dorsal forearm and hand (first 3½ fingers)	Midshaft humeral fracture. Prolonged compression at level of humerus ("Saturday night palsy")	Wrist drop
Median	Forearm pronation, thumb opposition	Palmar surface (first 3½ fingers)	Carpal tunnel	Weak wrist flexion and flat thenar eminence
Ulnar	Finger abduction	Palmar and dorsal surface (last 2 fingers)	Elbow dislocation, or entrapment at medial epicondylar groove of humerus	Claw hand
Axillary	Arm abduction	↓ Sensation over the deltoid (regimental badge area)	Anterior shoulder dislocation	
Peroneal	Dorsiflexion, eversion	Dorsal foot and lateral leg	Knee dislocation, prolonged immobilization (crossed legs), trauma to the fibula	Foot drop
Superior Gluteal	Hip adduction	None	Weakness of gluteus medius or minimus muscles	Dropping of contralateral pelvis below horizontal while walking (Trendelenburg sign)
Femoral	Hip flexion, knee extension	Anteromedial thigh and medial side of leg and foot (saphenous nerve)	Direct injury (trauma), prolonged pressure on nerve	Abnormal knee reflex
Lateral Femoral Cutaneous	None	Lateral thigh (can cause meralgia paresthetica)	Iatrogenic compression (surgeries, IVC filter placement)	

Compartment Syndrome

↑ Pressure within a confined space that compromises nerve, muscle, and soft tissue perfusion. Occurs primarily in the anterior compartment of the lower leg and in forearm 2° to trauma to the affected limb (fracture or muscle injury).

HISTORY/PE

- Presents with **p**ain **o**ut **o**f **p**roportion (**POOP**) to physical findings; **p**ain with **p**assive motion of the fingers and toes; and **p**aresthesias, **p**allor, **p**oikilothermia, **p**ulselessness, and **p**aralysis (the **6 Ps**).
- Paralysis and pulselessness occur as late signs of compartment syndrome!

DIAGNOSIS

Based on history, exam, and elevated compartment pressures (although not necessary). Calculate delta pressures (diastolic pressure − compartment pressure); ⊕ if delta pressure ≤ 30 mm Hg).

TREATMENT

Immediate fasciotomy to ↓ pressures and ↑ tissue perfusion.

Carpal Tunnel Syndrome

Entrapment of the median nerve at the wrist caused by ↓ size or space of the carpal tunnel, leading to paresthesias, pain, and occasionally paralysis. Can be precipitated by overuse of wrist flexors; associated with pregnancy, diabetes mellitus, hypothyroidism, acromegaly, and amyloidosis.

HISTORY/PE

- Presents with aching over the thenar area of the hand and proximal forearm.
- Paresthesias or numbness is seen in a median nerve distribution (first 3½ digits).
- Symptoms worsen at night and awaken patient from sleep.
- Exam shows thenar eminence atrophy (if CTS is long-standing).
- Phalen maneuver and Tinel sign are ⊕ (see Figure 2.9-1).

DIAGNOSIS

- Usually a clinical diagnosis from symptoms and signs.
- **Electrodiagnostic tests:** Nerve conduction studies and electromyography.

TREATMENT

- **Best initial treatment:** Splint the wrist in a neutral position at night and during the day if possible.
- **Medical treatment:** Corticosteroid injection of the carpal canal and NSAIDs.
- **Most definitive treatment:** Decompressing the tunnel is a widely accepted treatment, particularly for fixed sensory loss, thenar weakness, or intolerable symptoms with no improvement after splinting and/or glucocorticoids.

COMPLICATIONS

Permanent loss of sensation, hand strength, and fine motor skills.

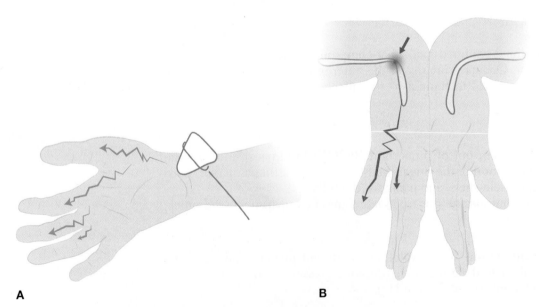

FIGURE 2.9-1. Carpal tunnel syndrome. (A) The Tinel test is performed by tapping the volar surface of the wrist over the median nerve. **(B)** The Phalen maneuver is performed by compressing the opposing dorsal surfaces of the hand with the wrists flexed together as shown. This causes tingling over the median nerve distribution. (Reproduced with permission from USMLE-Rx.com.)

Bursitis

Inflammation of the bursa by repetitive use, trauma, infection, systemic inflammatory disease (eg, autoimmune disease), or microcrystalline disorders (eg, gout). Common sites of bursitis include subacromial, olecranon, trochanteric, popliteal fossa (Baker cyst), prepatellar (housemaid's knee), and infrapatellar bursae.

PES ANSERINUS PAIN SYNDROME

Also called anserine bursitis. Presents with localized pain at the anteromedial tibia at insertion of the pes anserinus that is aggravated by overuse, obesity, knee osteoarthritis, and pressure from the opposite knee while lying on the side. Valgus stress test will not aggravate the pain, and x-rays will also be normal.

Patellofemoral Pain Syndrome

Anterior knee pain caused by overuse. Common in women, obese, and diabetics. Pain can be reproduced with knee extension. Treatment with activity modification and NSAIDs.

HISTORY/PE

Presents with localized tenderness, ↓ range of motion (ROM), edema, and erythema; patients may have a history of trauma or inflammatory disease.

DIAGNOSIS

- Mainly a clinical diagnose based on symptoms and physical exam findings.
- Needle aspiration is indicated if septic bursitis is suspected. No labs or imaging is needed.

TREATMENT

- **Best initial treatment:** Rest, heat and ice, elevation, and NSAIDs.
- Intrabursal corticosteroid injection can be considered but is contraindicated if septic bursitis is suspected.
- Septic bursitis should be treated with 7–10 days of antibiotics.

Tendinitis

An inflammatory condition characterized by pain at tendinous insertions into bone associated with swelling or impaired function. It commonly occurs in the supraspinatus, biceps, wrist extensor, patellar, iliotibial band, posterior tibial, and Achilles tendons. Overuse is the most common cause.

HISTORY/PE

- Presents with pain at a tendinous insertion that worsens with repetitive stress and resisted strength testing of the affected muscle group.
- Lateral epicondylitis (or tennis elbow) worsens with resisted extension of the wrist, and medial epicondylitis (or golfer's elbow) with resisted flexion of the wrist.

DIAGNOSIS

- Usually a clinical diagnosis.
- **Imaging:** Ultrasound or MRI may be useful in detecting tendon tears.

KEY FACT

Median nerve injury leads to the "Benediction sign" caused by an inability to close the first through third digits. Ulnar nerve injury leads to the "claw hand" caused by an inability to open the fourth to fifth digits.

KEY FACT

Volkmann contracture of the wrist and fingers is caused by compartment syndrome, which is associated with supracondylar humerus fractures. These fractures may affect the brachial artery and radial nerve. Ischemia results in fibrosis of dead muscle.

KEY FACT

Infection of the superficial bursae occurs after trauma to the skin. Infection of deep bursae is often iatrogenic following injections or aspirations.

KEY FACT

Oral fluoroquinolones are associated with an ↑ risk for tendon rupture and tendinitis.

TREATMENT

- **Best initial treatment:** Rest, NSAIDs, apply ice for the first 24–48 hours, and consider splinting, bracing, or immobilization.
- Begin strengthening exercises once pain has subsided.
- **Next best treatment:** consider corticosteroid injection. Never inject the Achilles tendon in view of the ↑ risk for rupture. Avoid repetitive injection.

Low Back Pain

Low back pain (LBP) is the second-leading symptom-related cause for office visits in the United States. Though often self-limited, it can also be a sign of more severe disease, including infection, malignancy, or AAA.

HERNIATED DISK

Causes include degenerative changes, trauma, or neck/back strain or sprain. Most common (95%) in the lumbar region, especially at L5–S1 (most common site) and L4–L5 (second most common site).

HISTORY/PE

- Presents with sudden onset of severe, electricity-like LBP, usually preceded by several months of aching, "discogenic" pain.
- Common among middle-aged and older men.
- Exacerbated by ↑ intra-abdominal pressure or Valsalva (eg, coughing).
- Associated with sciatica, paresthesias, muscle weakness, atrophy, contractions, or spasms.
- A passive straight-leg raise ↑ pain (highly sensitive but not specific).
- A contralateral (crossed) straight-leg raise ↑ pain (highly specific but not sensitive).
- Large midline herniations can cause cauda equina syndrome.

DIAGNOSIS

- Diagnosed with a ⊕ passive straight-leg raise.
- **Imaging:** MRI (see Figure 2.9-2) is the preferred test; Necessary for cauda equina syndrome or for a severe or rapidly progressing neurologic deficit.
- **Additional tests:** Obtain an ESR and a plain x-ray if other causes of back pain are suspected (eg, infection, trauma, compression fracture).

TREATMENT

- **Best initial treatment:** NSAIDs in scheduled doses, physical therapy, and local heat. Do not prescribe bed rest; continuation of regular activities is preferred.
- Epidural steroid injection or nerve block may be of benefit in those who do not respond to initial treatment.
- **Most definitive treatment:** Surgery—only in focal neurologic deficits, cauda equina syndrome, and persistent pain for at least 6 weeks.

SPINAL STENOSIS

Narrowing of the lumbar or cervical spinal canal, leading to compression of the nerve roots and spinal cord. Most commonly caused by degenerative joint disease; typically occurs in middle-aged or elderly patients.

KEY FACT

Tendinitis is a slight misnomer, as a classic cellular inflammatory response is absent or minimal in cases of overuse tendinopathy. Tendinosis is a more appropriate term referring to chronic tendinopathy without cellular inflammation.

KEY FACT

Bowel or bladder dysfunction (urinary overflow incontinence), impotence, and saddle-area anesthesia are consistent with cauda equina syndrome, a surgical emergency.

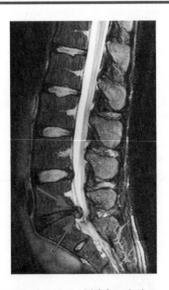

FIGURE 2.9-2. Disk herniation. Sagittal T2-weighted MRI of the lumbar spine shows posterior herniation of the L5–S1 disk. (Reproduced with permission from Fauci AS et al. *Harrison's Principles of Internal Medicine,* 17th ed. New York, NY: McGraw-Hill; 2008.)

TABLE 2.9-3. Motor and Sensory Deficits in Back Pain

NERVE ROOT	ASSOCIATED DEFICIT		
	MOTOR	**REFLEX**	**SENSORY**
L4	Foot dorsiflexion (tibialis anterior)	Patellar	Medial aspect of the lower leg
L5	Big toe dorsiflexion (extensor hallucis longus), foot eversion (peroneus muscles)	None	Dorsum of the foot and lateral aspect of the lower leg
S1	Plantarflexion (gastrocnemius/soleus), hip extension (gluteus maximus)	Achilles	Lateral aspects of the foot and little toe

HISTORY/PE

- Presents with neck pain, back pain that radiates to the arms or the buttocks and legs bilaterally, and leg numbness/weakness.
- In lumbar stenosis, leg cramping is worse with standing and with walking.
- In lumbar stenosis, symptoms improve with flexion at the hips and bending forward, which relieves pressure on the nerves.

DIAGNOSIS

MRI is the main imaging modality to use.

TREATMENT

- **Mild to moderate:** NSAIDs, weight loss, and abdominal muscle strengthening.
- **Advanced:** Epidural corticosteroid injections can provide relief.
- **Refractory:** Surgical laminectomy is needed in 75% of patients.

Table 2.9-3 outlines the motor, reflex, and sensory deficits with which LBP is associated.

Osteosarcoma

Although a rare tumor, it is the most common primary malignancy of bone in children and adolescents. It tends to occur in the metaphyseal regions of the distal femur, proximal tibia, and proximal humerus; it often metastasizes to the lungs. In adults, osteosarcoma is often a result of sarcomatous transformation of other benign tumors, including Paget disease.

HISTORY/PE

- Presents as progressive and eventually intractable pain that worsens at night.
- Constitutional symptoms such as fever, weight loss, and night sweats may be present.
- Erythema and enlargement over the site of the tumor may be seen.

See the Endocrinology chapter for a discussion of osteosarcoma vs Paget disease.

DIAGNOSIS

- **Best initial test:** Plain x-rays. These can show a Codman triangle (periosteal new-bone formation at the diaphyseal end of the lesion) or a "sunburst

KEY FACT

Most LBP is mechanical, so bed rest is contraindicated.

KEY FACT

Red flags for LBP include > 50 years of age, > 6 weeks of pain, previous cancer history, severe pain, constitutional symptoms, neurologic deficits, and loss of anal sphincter tone.

Q 1

A 23-year-old man presents to the ED with a swollen and erythematous right hand following an altercation at a bar a few days ago. The dorsum of the hand shows abrasions and x-ray films reveal a fracture of the fifth metacarpal. What is the next step in management?

Q 2

A 37-year-old man is seen after a motorcycle accident. He complains of intense leg pain, tingling in his foot, and inability to move his toes. Exam reveals pain with passive motion of his toes and palpable dorsalis pedis pulses. An x-ray film confirms a tibial fracture. What is the best treatment?

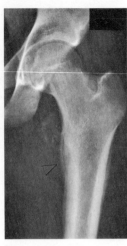
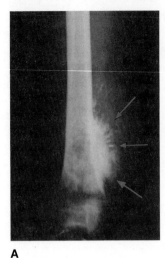

A   **B**

FIGURE 2.9-3. **Malignant bone tumors.** **(A)** Osteosarcoma. Femoral x-ray shows the typical "sunburst" appearance of osteosarcoma *(arrows)*. **(B)** Ewing sarcoma. The characteristic "onion skinning" of Ewing sarcoma *(arrowhead)* is evident in the proximal femur in this x-ray of the left hip. (Reproduced with permission from Kantarjian HM, et al. *MD Anderson Manual of Medical Oncology,* 1st ed. New York, NY: McGraw-Hill; 2006.)

pattern" of the osteosarcoma (see Figure 2.9-3)—in contrast to the multi-layered "onion skinning" that is classic for Ewing sarcoma and the "soap bubble" appearance of giant cell tumor of bone (see Figure 2.9-4).

- **Most accurate test:** Biopsy.
- CT of the chest facilitates staging (soft tissue and bony invasion) and planning for surgery.

TREATMENT

- Limb-sparing surgical procedures and pre- and postoperative chemotherapy (eg, methotrexate, doxorubicin, cisplatin, ifosfamide).
- Amputation may be necessary.

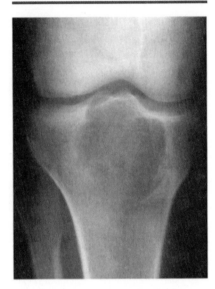

FIGURE 2.9-4. **Giant cell tumor of the bone.** Note the "soap bubble" appearance at the proximal end of the tibia. The distal end of the femur *(not shown)* is another common location. (Reproduced with permission from Skinner HB. *Current Diagnosis & Treatment in Orthopedics,* 4th ed. New York, NY: McGraw-Hill; 2006.)

Septic Arthritis

An infection of the joint space that can occur after open injury or bacteremia. Prosthetic joints greatly ↑ the risk. Rheumatoid arthritis (RA), osteoarthritis (OA), and bacteremia from endocarditis and IV drug use are also risk factors (see later).

HISTORY/PE

Presents as a warm, red, immobile joint. Palpable effusions may also be present. Fevers and chills can be seen if the patient is bacteremic.

DIAGNOSIS

- **Most accurate test:** Joint aspiration. See Table 2.9-4.
- A WBC count > 80,000 per mm³, ⊕ Gram stain, or ⊕ fluid culture.
- The most common organisms are *Staphylococcus, Streptococcus,* and gram-⊖ rods.

TREATMENT

Empirically treat with ceftriaxone and vancomycin initially until culture test results; then modify therapy for specific organisms. Septic joints are treated with joint drainage or surgical debridement.

1   **A**

If skin is broken in a boxer's fracture, assume infection by human oral pathogens and treat with surgical irrigation, debridement, and IV antibiotics to cover *Eikenella.*

2   **A**

Immediate fasciotomy for compartment syndrome (within 6 hours to prevent muscle necrosis) followed by fracture stabilization. Remember that nonpalpable pulses are a late finding.

TABLE 2.9-4 Synovial Fluid Analysis

	Normal	Noninflammatory	Inflammatory[a]	Septic
Color	Clear	Yellow	Yellow	Yellow-green
Viscosity	High	High	Low	Variable
WBC, per mm³	< 200	0–1000	1000–10,000 (up to 100,000)	10,000–100,000
PMN (%)	< 25	< 25	≥ 50	≥ 75
Glucose, mg/dL	= serum	= serum	> 25 (Crystal analysis for gout/pseudogout)	< 25

[a]A joint affected by inflammatory arthritis can become secondarily infected.

Osteoarthritis

A common, chronic, noninflammatory arthritis of the synovial joints. Characterized by deterioration of the articular cartilage and osteophyte bone formation at the joint surfaces. Risk factors include a ⊕ family history, obesity, and a history of joint trauma. Table 2.9-5 contrasts OA with RA.

HISTORY/PE

Presents with crepitus, ↓ ROM, and initially pain that worsens with activity and weight bearing but improves with rest. Morning stiffness generally lasts for < 30 minutes. Stiffness is also experienced after periods of rest ("gelling").

DIAGNOSIS

- X-rays show joint space narrowing, osteophytes, subchondral sclerosis, and subchondral bone cysts (see Figure 2.9-5). X-ray severity does not correlate with symptomatology.
- Laboratory tests, including inflammatory markers, are typically normal.

TABLE 2.9-5. Osteoarthritis vs Rheumatoid Arthritis

Variable	Osteoarthritis	Rheumatoid Arthritis
History	Affects the elderly; slow onset. Pain worsens with use	Affects the young. Prolonged morning stiffness that improves with use
Joint involvement	Affects the DIP, PIP, hips, and knees	Affects the wrists, MCP, ankles, knees, shoulders, hips, and elbows. Symmetric distribution
Synovial fluid analysis and imaging	WBC count < 2000 cells/mm³; osteophytes. X-ray shows joint space narrowing	Anti-CCP antibodies

KEY FACT

Classic findings of Ewing sarcoma: 10–20 years of age with a multilayered "onion-skinning" finding on x-ray in the diaphyseal regions of the femur. "Eat wings and onion rings."

KEY FACT

Classic findings of a giant cell tumor of bone: a woman 20–40 years of age presenting with knee pain and mass, along with a "soap bubble" appearance on x-ray in the epiphyseal/metaphyseal region of long bones.

Q 1

A 55-year-old man with a history of prostate cancer presents with LBP and bilateral leg weakness. On exam, he is found to have point tenderness on the lumbar spine and ↓ sensation in his legs. What is the best next step?

Q 2

A 15-year-old youth presents with several months' history of pain in the upper part of his thigh. The pain is worse at night. A plain film shows a small nidus of lucency. What OTC remedy is indicated?

In sexually active individuals with joint pain, consider gonococcal septic arthritis. *Neisseria gonorrhoeae* septic arthritis can present with asymmetric oligoarthritis, tenosynovitis, and skin rash.

An elevated white count in synovial fluid can be either inflammatory or infectious in etiology.

In a child with gout and inexplicable injuries, consider Lesch-Nyhan syndrome (hypoxanthine-guanine phosphoribosyltransferase [HGPRT] deficiency).

1   **A**

Give steroids to relieve spinal cord compression resulting from likely bone metastasis. MRI is the best study, but preventing permanent neurologic disability is the priority. Remember to consider multiple myeloma, which can present almost identically.

2   **A**

This adolescent patient is likely presenting with osteoid osteoma, a benign bone-forming tumor characterized by prostaglandin formation. Relief of pain is thus often achieved with NSAIDs. Tumors may self-resolve, but surgical removal of the nidus may be necessary for symptom relief.

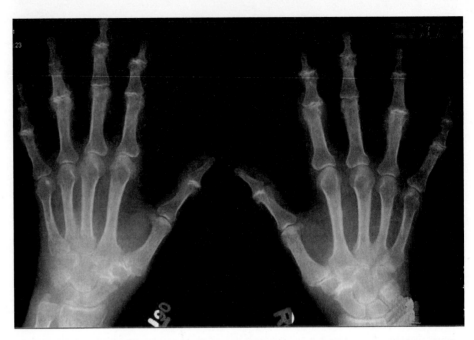

FIGURE 2.9-5. Osteoarthritis. Plain x-rays show joint space narrowing, osteophytes, and subchondral degenerative cysts involving the DIP and PIP joints, with sparing of the MCP. (Reproduced with permission from USMLE-Rx.com.)

TREATMENT

- **Best initial treatment:** Physical therapy, weight reduction, and NSAIDs. Intra-articular corticosteroid injections may provide temporary relief.
- **Most definitive treatment:** Surgery—consider joint replacement (eg, total hip/knee arthroplasty) in advanced cases. Patients are at higher risk for developing osteoporosis.

Osteoporosis

Refer to Endocrinology chapter.

Morton Neuroma

Neuropathic degeneration of nerves (most commonly between the third and fourth toes) that causes numbness, pain, and paresthesias. Often associated with a "clicking sensation" when palpating this joint space. Occurs in runners, and symptoms worsen when metatarsals are squeezed together (eg, wearing high-heeled shoes). Treatment is with padded shoe inserts.

Gout

Recurrent attacks of acute monoarticular arthritis resulting from intra-articular deposition of monosodium urate crystals caused by disorders of urate metabolism. Risk factors include male gender, obesity, postmenopausal status in women, and binge drinking.

HISTORY/PE

- Presents with excruciating joint pain of sudden onset.
- Most commonly affects the first MTP joint (podagra) and the midfoot, knees, ankles, and wrists; the hips and shoulders are generally spared.

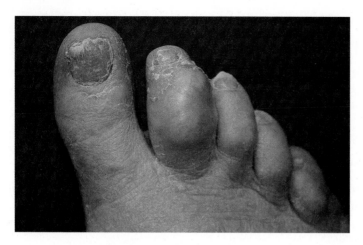

FIGURE 2.9-6. **Tophaceous gout.** Note the slowly enlarging nodule of the right second toe in a 55-year-old alcoholic, hypertensive man on hydrochlorothiazide. (Reproduced with permission from USMLE-Rx.com.)

- Joints are erythematous, swollen, and exquisitely tender.
- Tophi (urate crystal deposits in soft tissue) can be seen with chronic disease (see Figure 2.9-6). Tophi can ulcerate and discharge a chalky white substance.
- Uric acid kidney stones are seen with chronic disease.

DIAGNOSIS

- **Diagnostic tests:** Joint fluid aspirate shows needle-shaped, negatively bire-fringent crystals (vs pseudogout; see Table 2.9-6).
- **Lab tests and imaging:** Serum uric acid is usually ↑ (≥ 7.5 mg/dL), but patients may have normal levels. X-rays may show punched-out erosions with overhanging cortical bone ("rat-bite" erosions) that are seen in advanced gout.

TREATMENT

- **Acute attacks:**
  - High-dose NSAIDs (eg, indomethacin) are first line. Colchicine may also be used but is inferior to NSAIDs.
  - Steroids are used when NSAIDs are ineffective or contraindicated, as in renal disease.
- **Maintenance therapy:**
  - Allopurinol for overproducers, those with contraindications to probene-cid treatment (tophi, renal stones, chronic kidney disease), and refractory cases; probenecid for undersecretors.
  - Allopurinol can ↓ the incidence of acute urate nephropathy.
- Weight loss and avoidance of triggers of hyperuricemia will prevent recurrent attacks in many patients. Avoid alcohol consumption.

KEY FACT

Gout crystals appear yeLLow when paraLLel to the condenser.

KEY FACT

Causes of hyperuricemia:
- ↑ Cell turnover (hemolysis, blast crisis, tumor lysis, myelodysplasia, psoriasis).
- Cyclosporine.
- Dehydration.
- Diabetes insipidus.
- Diet (eg, ↑ red meat, alcohol).
- Diuretics.
- Lead poisoning.
- Lesch-Nyhan syndrome.
- Salicylates (low dose).
- Starvation.

KEY FACT

Colchicine inhibits neutrophil chemotaxis and is most effective when used early during a gout flare. However, it can cause diarrhea and bone marrow suppression (neutropenia).

TABLE 2.9-6. **Gout vs Pseudogout**

DISORDER	HISTORY	PHYSICAL FINDINGS	CRYSTAL SHAPE	CRYSTAL BIREFRINGENCE
Gout (uric acid)	Male gender, binge drinking, recent surgery	First big toe is affected	Needle shaped	⊖
Pseudogout: CPPD	Hemochromatosis or hyperparathyroidism	Wrists and knees are affected	Rhomboid	⊕

Rheumatoid Arthritis

A systemic autoimmune disorder characterized by chronic, destructive, inflammatory arthritis with symmetric joint involvement that results in synovial hypertrophy and pannus formation, ultimately leading to erosion of adjacent cartilage, bone, and tendons. Risk factors include female gender, 35–50 years of age, and HLA-DR4.

HISTORY/PE

- Insidious onset of prolonged morning stiffness (> 30 minutes) along with painful, warm swelling of multiple symmetric joints (wrists, MCP joints, PIP joints of hands, ankles, knees, shoulders, hips, and elbows) for > 6 weeks.
- Rheumatoid nodules may form at bony prominences and near joints affected by the disease.
- In late cases, ulnar deviation of the fingers is seen with MCP joint hypertrophy (see Figure 2.9-7).
- Also presents with ligament and tendon deformations (eg, swan-neck and boutonnière deformities), vasculitis, atlantoaxial subluxation (intubation risk), and keratoconjunctivitis sicca.

DIAGNOSIS

- **Diagnostic criteria** (need ≥ 6 points):
  - ↑ Rheumatoid factor (RF) (IgM antibodies against Fc IgG) or the presence of anti-CCP antibodies (1 point).
  - ↑ ESR or CRP (1 point).
  - Inflammatory arthritis of ≥ 3 or more joints (up to 5 points).
  - Symptom duration > 6 weeks (1 point).
  - Exclusion of diseases with similar clinical presentations such as psoriatic arthritis, gout, pseudogout, and systemic lupus erythematosus (SLE).
- **Labs:**
  - Anemia of chronic disease is common.
  - Synovial fluid aspirate shows turbid fluid, ↓ viscosity, and an ↑ WBC count (3000–50,000 cells/μL).

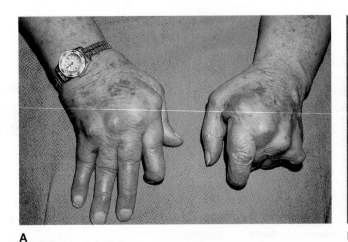

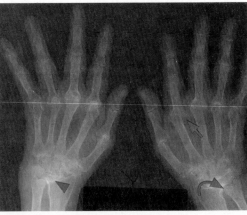

A   **B**

FIGURE 2.9-7.   Rheumatoid arthritis. (A) Note the typical ulnar deviation of the MCP joints and swelling of the MCP and PIP joints. Multiple subcutaneous rheumatoid nodules are also seen. **(B)** Hand x-ray shows symmetric erosions and joint space narrowing involving the MCP (*arrow*), carpal (*arrowhead*), and radioulnar (*curved arrow*) joints. Ulnar deviation at the MCP joint is also noted. Image A reproduced with permission from Wolff K, et al. *Fitzpatrick's Dermatology in General Medicine,* 7th ed. New York, NY: McGraw-Hill; 2008. Image B reproduced with permission from USMLE-Rx.com.)

- **X-rays** (not necessary to confirm RA):
  - **Early:** Soft tissue swelling and juxta-articular demineralization.
  - **Late:** Symmetric joint space narrowing and erosions (see Figure 2.9-7B).

TREATMENT

- **Best initial therapy:** NSAIDs. Can be ↓ or discontinued following successful treatment with disease-modifying antirheumatic drugs (DMARDs).
- DMARDs should be started early and include methotrexate (the best initial DMARD to start with), hydroxychloroquine, and sulfasalazine. Second-line agents include TNF inhibitors, rituximab (anti-CD20), and leflunomide.

COMPLICATIONS

Joint deformation, osteopenia, osteoarthritis. Extra-articular manifestations that affect several organ systems. Examples include anemia, rheumatoid nodules, scleritis, amyloidosis, cardiovascular disease, vasculitis, lung fibrosis, Caplan syndrome, carpal tunnel syndrome, Sjögren syndrome, and Felty syndrome.

Seronegative Spondyloarthropathy

ANKYLOSING SPONDYLITIS

A chronic inflammatory disease of the spine and pelvis that leads to fusion of the affected joints. Strongly associated with HLA-B27. Risk factors include male gender and a ⊕ family history.

HISTORY/PE

- Typical onset is in the late teens and early 20s. Presents with fatigue, intermittent hip pain, and LBP that worsens with inactivity and in the mornings. Pain is relieved by exercise.
- ↓ Spine flexion (⊕ Schober test), loss of lumbar lordosis, hip pain and stiffness, and ↓ chest expansion are seen as the disease progresses. Vertebral fracture may occur after minimal trauma.
- Anterior uveitis and heart block can occur.
- Associated with enthesitis (pain at insertion of tendons/ligaments) at the heel.
- Other forms of seronegative spondyloarthropathy must be ruled out, including the following:
  - **Reactive arthritis:** A disease of young men. The characteristic arthritis, uveitis, conjunctivitis, and urethritis usually follow an infection with *Campylobacter, Shigella, Salmonella, Chlamydia,* or *Ureaplasma.*
  - **Psoriatic arthritis:** An oligoarthritis that can include the DIP joints. Associated with psoriatic skin changes and sausage-shaped digits (dactylitis). X-rays show a classic "pencil in cup" deformity.
  - **Enteropathic spondylitis:** An ankylosing spondylitis–like disease characterized by sacroiliitis that is usually asymmetric and is associated with IBD.

DIAGNOSIS

- **Best initial test:** X-rays may show fused sacroiliac joints, squaring of the lumbar vertebrae, development of vertical syndesmophytes, and bamboo spine (see Figure 2.9-8).
- ⊕ HLA-B27 is found in 85–95% of cases.
- ESR or CRP is ↑ in 85% of cases.
- ⊖ RF; ⊖ antinuclear antibody (ANA).

KEY FACT

Hydroxychloroquine causes retinal toxicity.

KEY FACT

Reactive arthritis: "Can't see (uveitis), can't pee (urethritis), can't climb a tree (arthritis)."

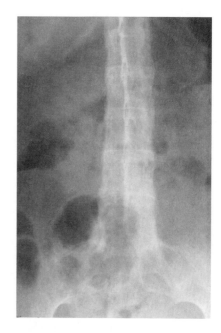

FIGURE 2.9-8. Ankylosing spondylitis. Frontal view of the thoracolumbar spine shows the classic "bamboo" appearance of the spine, which results from fusion of the vertebral bodies and posterior elements. (Reproduced with permission from Chen MY et al. *Basic Radiology,* 2nd ed. New York, NY: McGraw-Hill; 2011.)

TREATMENT

- **Best initial therapy:** NSAIDs (eg, indomethacin) for pain; exercise to improve posture and breathing.
- TNF inhibitors or sulfasalazine can be used in refractory cases.

Polymyositis and Dermatomyositis

Polymyositis is a progressive, systemic connective tissue disease characterized by immune-mediated striated muscle inflammation. Dermatomyositis presents with symptoms of polymyositis plus cutaneous involvement, although the pathogenesis is different. Most often affect patients 50–70 years of age; the male-to-female ratio is 1:2. African-American individuals are affected more often than white individuals (see Table 2.9-7).

HISTORY/PE

- See Table 2.9-7.
- Patients may also develop myocarditis and cardiac conduction deficits.
- Can be associated with an underlying malignancy, especially lung, breast, and ovarian carcinoma. Dermatomyositis is associated with ↑ rate of malignancy.

DIAGNOSIS

- Based on characteristic clinical and laboratory presentation.
- **Best initial test:** ↑ Serum creatine kinase and anti-Jo-1 antibodies can be seen (see Table 2.9-8).

TABLE 2.9-7. **Polymyositis vs Dermatomyositis**

POLYMYOSITIS	DERMATOMYOSITIS
Symmetric, progressive proximal muscle weakness and/or pain	⊕ Rash
	Heliotrope rash: A violaceous periorbital rash (see image A)
Difficulty getting up from a seat or climbing stairs	
Difficulty breathing or swallowing (advanced disease)	**A**
	"Shawl sign": A rash involving the shoulders, upper chest, and back
	Gottron papules: Papular rash with scales on the dorsa of the hands, over bony prominences (see image B)

Gottron papule

Capillary nail fold changes

B

Images reproduced with permission from Dhoble A, Puttarajappa C, Neiberg A. Dermatomyositis and supraventricular tachycardia. *Int Arch Med.* 2008;1:25.

- **Most accurate test:** Muscle biopsy can provide accurate diagnosis in atypical presentations.

TREATMENT

- **Best initial treatment:** High-dose corticosteroids with taper after 4–6 weeks to ↓ the maintenance dose.
- Azathioprine and/or methotrexate can be used in steroid-resistant or intolerant cases.

Raynaud Phenomenon

Abnormal vasoconstriction of peripheral arteries in response to cold, leading to blue or white color changes. May be primary or associated with other autoimmune conditions. Patients should be tested for antinuclear antibodies and rheumatoid factor, and can be treated with calcium channel blockers.

Systemic Sclerosis

Also called scleroderma; characterized by inflammation that leads to progressive tissue fibrosis through excessive deposition of types I and III collagen.

TABLE 2.9-8. Common Antibodies and Their Disease Associations

ANTIBODY	DISEASE ASSOCIATION
ANA	SLE
Anti-CCP	RA
Anticentromere	CREST syndrome
Anti-dsDNA	SLE
Antihistone	Drug-induced SLE
Anti-Jo-1	Polymyositis/dermatomyositis
Anti-Ro/anti-La	Sjögren syndrome
Anti-Scl-70	Systemic sclerosis
Anti-Sm	SLE
Anti–smooth muscle	Autoimmune hepatitis
c-ANCA	Vasculitis, especially granulomatosis with polyangiitis (Wegener)
p-ANCA	Vasculitis, microscopic polyangiitis
RF	RA
U1RNP antibody	Mixed connective tissue disease

A 49-year-old man presents with a painful, swollen big toe after a night of heavy drinking. His home medications are lansoprazole, ASA, sildenafil, and psyllium. Which medication should he temporarily discontinue?

CREST syndrome—

Calcinosis
Raynaud phenomenon
Esophageal dysmotility
Sclerodactyly
Telangiectasias

KEY FACT

Raynaud phenomenon may be triggered by cold temperatures and stress. It can be treated with CCBs such as nifedipine or amlodipine.

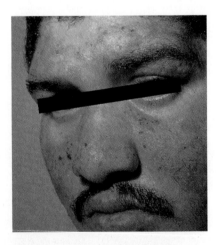

FIGURE 2.9-9. Systemic lupus erythematosus (SLE). The malar rash of SLE is a red-to-purple, continuous plaque extending across the bridge of the nose and to both cheeks. (Reproduced with permission from Bondi EE. *Dermatology: Diagnosis and Therapy*, 1st ed. Stamford, CT: Appleton & Lange; 1991.)

ASA (aspirin). This patient is having an acute gout attack, and ASA can cause ↓ excretion of uric acid by the kidney.

Commonly manifests as CREST syndrome (limited form) but can also occur in a diffuse form (20% of cases) involving the skin and the GI, GU, renal, pulmonary, and cardiovascular systems. Risk factors include female gender and 35–50 years of age.

History/PE

- Exam may reveal symmetric thickening of the skin of face and/or distal extremities.
    - **Limited cutaneous:** Head, neck, distal upper extremities.
    - **Diffuse cutaneous:** Torso, abdomen, proximal upper extremity/shoulder.
- **CREST syndrome:** Associated with limited cutaneous type.
- **Raynaud phenomenon:** Vasospasm of arteries supplying fingers causing pain and pallor (white), followed by cyanosis (blue), and finally reactive hyperemia (red).
- The diffuse form can lead to GI dysmotility, pulmonary fibrosis, cor pulmonale, acute renal failure (scleroderma renal crisis), and malignant hypertension.

Diagnosis

- Diagnosis and categorization depends on constellation of symptoms.
- RF and ANA may be ⊕.
- Anti-centromere antibodies are specific for CREST syndrome (see Table 2.9-8).
- Anti-Scl-70 (anti-topoisomerase 1) antibodies are associated with diffuse disease and a poor prognosis (see Table 2.9-8).
- Severe disease may cause microangiopathic hemolytic anemia with schistocytes.

Treatment

- Treatment is organ-based and includes frequent monitoring for progressive damage.
- Corticosteroids for acute flares (but ↑ risk for renal crisis); methotrexate for limited scleroderma.
- Calcium channel blockers (dihydropyridine) such as amlodipine for Raynaud phenomenon.
- Angiotensin-converting enzyme inhibitors for renal disease and for prevention/treatment of renal crisis.

Complications

Mortality is most commonly caused by complications of pulmonary hypertension, and resulting renal or cardiac disease.

Systemic Lupus Erythematosus

A multisystem autoimmune disorder related to antibody-mediated cellular attack and deposition of antigen-antibody complexes. African-American women are at highest risk. Usually affects women of childbearing age.

History/PE

- Presents with nonspecific symptoms such as fever, anorexia, weight loss, and symmetric joint pain.
- The mnemonic **DOPAMINE RASH** summarizes many of the key clinical manifestations of SLE (see Figure 2.9-9).

DIAGNOSIS

- The mnemonic **DOPAMINE RASH** summarizes the criteria for diagnosing SLE. Patients with four of the criteria are likely to have SLE (96% sensitive and specific).
- A ⊕ ANA is highly sensitive (present in 95–99% of cases). If ⊕ ANA, test for other antibodies, mainly anti-dsDNA and anti-Sm. Both are highly specific but not as sensitive (see Table 2.9-8).
  - **Drug-induced SLE:** ⊕ Antihistone antibodies are seen in 100% of cases but are nonspecific.
  - **Neonatal SLE:** Associated with ⊕ anti-Ro antibodies transmitted from mother to neonate.
- The following may also be seen:
  - Low complement levels.
  - Antiphospholipid antibodies (antibodies to anticardiolipin, anti–β_2-glycoprotein, or lupus "anticoagulant"). All cause hypercoagulable state and may cause recurrent spontaneous abortion.
  - Raynaud phenomenon.
  - Anemia, leukopenia, and/or thrombocytopenia.
  - Proteinuria and/or casts.

TREATMENT

- NSAIDs for mild joint symptoms.
- Corticosteroids for acute exacerbations. Be wary of Cushing syndrome and possible avascular necrosis from chronic use.
- Corticosteroids, hydroxychloroquine, cyclophosphamide, and azathioprine can be used for progressive or refractory cases. A few have specific uses:
  - **Hydroxychloroquine:** Can be used for isolated skin and joint involvement.
  - **Cyclophosphamide:** Used for severe cases of lupus nephritis. Be sure to get a renal biopsy for patients with nephritic symptoms.

Serum Sickness–like Reaction

Fever, urticarial rash, arthralgia, lymphadenopathy, and proteinuria within 1–2 weeks of exposure to a β-lactam antibiotic or sulfa drug. Symptoms resolve upon discontinuation of the drug.

Giant Cell Arteritis

Formerly temporal arteritis; caused by subacute granulomatous inflammation of the large vessels, including the aorta, external carotid (especially the temporal branch), and vertebral arteries. Risk factors include polymyalgia rheumatica (affects almost one-half of patients), > 50 years of age, and female gender.

HISTORY/PE

- Presents with new headache (unilateral or bilateral); scalp pain and temporal tenderness; and jaw claudication.
- Fever, permanent monocular blindness, aortic aneurysm, weight loss, and myalgias and/or arthralgias (especially of the shoulders and hips) are also seen.

DIAGNOSIS

- **Best initial test:** ESR > 50 mm/h (influenced by age).
- **Most accurate test:** Temporal artery biopsy. Look for thrombosis, necrosis of the media, and presence of lymphocytes, plasma cells, and giant cells.

KEY FACT

The lupus anticoagulant occurs in 5–10% of SLE cases. IgM or IgG binds proteins in clinical assay test and prolongs PTT.

KEY FACT

Libman-Sacks endocarditis: Noninfectious vegetations often seen on the mitral valve in association with SLE and antiphospholipid syndrome.

KEY FACT

SLE can cause a ⊕ VDRL or RPR test!

KEY FACT

SLE and RA both affect the MCP and PIP joints; the difference is that SLE is nondeforming.

TREATMENT

- **Best initial treatment:** High-dose prednisone immediately to prevent ocular involvement (or involvement of the remaining eye after onset of monocular blindness). If suspected contribution to vision loss, give pulse-dose steroids.
- Obtain a biopsy, but do not delay treatment. Conduct a follow-up eye exam.

COMPLICATIONS

The most feared manifestation is blindness 2° to occlusion of the central retinal artery (a branch of the internal carotid artery) that may initially present as transient vision loss.

Takayasu Arteritis

Large vessel autoimmune vasculitis common in Asian women < 40 years of age. Classic symptoms include aortic claudication, differential blood pressure in both upper extremities, and the absence of palpable pulses (pulseless disease). ESR and CRP are highly elevated. Treat with steroids.

Behçet Syndrome

Autoimmune vasculitis common in men of Turkish or Middle Eastern descent. Characterized by recurrent, painful oral ulcers, uveitis, and genital ulcers. Thrombosis is a common cause of morbidity. Treat with steroids.

Complex Regional Pain Syndrome

A pain syndrome accompanied by loss of function and autonomic dysfunction, usually occurring after trauma. The disease has three phases: acute/traumatic → dystrophic phase → atrophic phase. Not linked with true nerve injury.

HISTORY/PE

- Diffuse pain occurs out of proportion to the initial injury, often in a non-anatomic distribution.
- Pain can occur at any time relative to the initial injury.
- Loss of function of the affected limb is seen.
- Sympathetic dysfunction occurs and may be documented by skin, soft tissue, or blood flow changes.
- Skin temperature, hair growth, and nail growth may ↑ or ↓. Edema may be present.

DIAGNOSIS

A clinical diagnosis, but objective evidence of changes in skin temperature, hair growth, or nail growth may be present.

TREATMENT

- **Best initial treatment:** Trial of NSAIDs along with physical and occupational therapies.
- Other medications include corticosteroids, low-dose tricyclic antidepressants, gabapentin, pregabalin, and calcitonin (no oral medications are consistently effective).
- Chemical sympathetic blockade may relieve symptoms.
- Referral to a chronic pain specialist is appropriate for complicated cases.

Fibromyalgia

A chronic musculoskeletal pain disorder that primarily affects young women and is characterized by soft tissue and axial skeletal pain in the absence of joint pain. Inflammation is notably absent (see Table 2.9-9). May be difficult to distinguish from myofascial pain (< 11 painful areas).

- **Hx/PE:** Most common in women 30–50 years of age; associated with depression, anxiety, sleep disorders, irritable bowel syndrome (IBS), and cognitive disorders ("fibro fog").
- **Dx:** Multiple (≥ 11 of 18) painful areas over all four body quadrants and the axial skeleton must be present for diagnosis. The presence of < 11 of 18 painful areas or non–fibromyalgia-associated painful areas is known as myofascial pain syndrome.
- **Tx:** Antidepressants (tricyclic antidepressant or serotonin-norepinephrine reuptake inhibitors [SNRIs] have proven efficacy), gabapentin, pregabalin, muscle relaxants, and physical therapy (stretching, heat application, hydrotherapy). Avoid narcotics. Multidisciplinary patient education is important.

Polymyalgia Rheumatica

An inflammatory rheumatic condition characterized by aching and stiffness in the shoulders, hips, and neck. Associated with temporal arteritis. Risk factors include female gender and > 50 years of age (see Table 2.9-9).

- **Hx/PE:**
  - Presents with pain and stiffness of the shoulder and pelvic girdle musculature with difficulty getting out of a chair or lifting the arms above the head.
  - Other symptoms include fever, malaise, and weight loss. Weakness is generally not appreciated on exam.
- **Dx:** Labs reveal a markedly ↑ ESR, often associated with anemia.
- **Tx:** Low-dose prednisone (10–20 mg/day).

TABLE 2.9-9. Fibromyalgia vs Polymyalgia Rheumatica

CHARACTERISTIC	FIBROMYALGIA	POLYMYALGIA RHEUMATICA
Age and sex	Women 30–50 years of age	Women > 50 years of age
Location	Various	Shoulder and pelvic girdle
ESR	Normal	Markedly ↑ (> 100 mm/h)
Muscle biopsy	Normal	Normal
Classic findings	Anxiety, stress, point tenderness, ⊖ workup	Temporal arteritis; response to steroids
Treatment	Antidepressants, NSAIDs, rest	Low-dose prednisone

Q

A 55-year-old woman presents to the clinic with a chief complaint of "blindness." She states that she experienced a temporary loss of vision in her left eye. She has also been experiencing new headaches and soreness in her jaw. Her vision exam is unremarkable. What diagnostic exam should be ordered?

NOTES

A

Monocular amaurosis fugax is associated with giant cell (temporal) arteritis and may progress to complete vision loss. A temporal artery biopsy should be obtained.

NEUROLOGY

Clinical Neuroanatomy

Tables 2.10-1 to 2.10-4 highlight critical aspects of clinical neuroanatomy, including the clinical presentation of common spinal cord lesions; facial nerve lesions; and pertinent clinical reflexes.

TABLE 2.10-1. Spinal Tract Functions

TRACT	FUNCTION	CLINICAL EFFECTS OF LESION
Lateral corticospinal	Movement of ipsilateral limbs and body	Ipsilateral paresis at and below level of lesion
Dorsal column medial lemniscus	Fine touch, vibration, conscious proprioception	Ipsilateral loss of fine touch, vibration, and proprioception at and below level of lesion
Spinothalamic	Pain, temperature	Contralateral loss of pain and temperature at and below level of lesion

TABLE 2.10-2. Spinal Cord Lesions

AREA AFFECTED	DISEASE	CHARACTERISTICS
	Poliomyelitis and spinal muscular atrophy	LMN lesions only, caused by destruction of anterior horns; flaccid paralysis
	Multiple sclerosis	Caused by demyelination; random and asymmetric lesions; white matter of spinal cord, mostly cervical region
	Brown-Séquard hemisection	Contralateral loss of pain and temperature sensation one to two levels below lesion Ipsilateral hemiparesis and diminished dorsal column sensation below level of lesion
	Amyotrophic lateral sclerosis	Combined UMN and LMN deficits with no sensory or oculomotor deficits; both UMN and LMN signs Commonly presents as fasciculations with eventual atrophy and weakness of hands; fatal Riluzole treatment modestly ↑ survival by ↓ presynaptic glutamate release Commonly known as Lou Gehrig disease in the United States and motor neuron disease in the United Kingdom. For **Lou** Gehrig disease, give ri**lou**zole
Posterior spinal arteries / Anterior spinal artery	Complete occlusion of anterior spinal artery	Spares dorsal columns. Sensory-motor dissociation Associated with abdominal aortic surgery

(continues)

TABLE 2.10-2. Spinal Cord Lesions *(continued)*

AREA AFFECTED	DISEASE	CHARACTERISTICS
	Central cord syndrome	Weakness more pronounced in upper extremities than lower extremities Caused by hyperextension injuries in individuals > 50 years of age
	Tabes dorsalis	Caused by 3° syphilis. Results from degeneration (demyelination) of dorsal columns and roots → impaired sensation and proprioception, progressive sensory ataxia (inability to sense or feel the legs) → poor coordination Associated with Charcot joints (repeated unknowing trauma to joint caused by lack of pain), shooting pain, Argyll Robertson pupils Exam will demonstrate absence of deep tendon reflex and ⊕ Romberg sign
	Syringomyelia	Syrinx (CSF-filled cavity within spinal cord) expands and damages anterior white commissure of spinothalamic tract. Can arise from trauma or tumors; seen in 35% of Chiari malformations. Results in a capelike, bilateral loss of pain and temperature in upper extremities
	Vitamin B$_{12}$ deficiency	Subacute combined degeneration—demyelination of dorsal columns, lateral corticospinal tracts, and spinocerebellar tracts; ataxic gait, paresthesia, impaired position and vibration sense
	Cauda equina syndrome	Compression of spinal roots L2 and below, most likely caused by disc herniation; saddle anesthesia, loss of bladder and anal sphincter control, and absent knee and ankle jerk reflexes

Modified with permission from Le T, et al. *First Aid for the USMLE Step 1 2018.* New York, NY: McGraw-Hill Education; 2018.

TABLE 2.10-3. Facial Nerve Lesions

TYPE	DESCRIPTION	COMMENTS
UMN lesion	Lesion of the motor cortex: contralateral paralysis of the lower face only	**AL**exander **Bell** with **STD: A**IDS, **L**yme, **S**arcoid, **S**urgery, **T**umors, **D**iabetes
LMN lesion	Peripheral ipsilateral facial paralysis with inability to close the eye on the involved side. If it occurs idiopathically, it is Bell palsy. Gradual recovery is seen in most cases	
Facial nerve palsy	Seen as a complication in **A**IDS, **L**yme disease, **S**arcoidosis, Parotid **S**urgery, **T**umors, and **D**iabetes	

Face area of motor cortex
Corticobulbar tract (UMN lesion—central)
Upper division
Lower division
Facial nucleus
CN VII (LMN lesion—peripheral; cannot wrinkle forehead)

Adapted with permission from Le T, et al. *First Aid for the USMLE Step 1 2018.* New York, NY: McGraw-Hill Education; 2018. Image reproduced with permission from USMLE-Rx.com.

TABLE 2.10-4. Commonly Tested Reflexes

DISTRIBUTION	LOCATION	MNEMONIC
C5, 6 / C7, 8 / L3, 4 / S1, 2	Biceps = C5 nerve root	1–2, tie your shoe
	Triceps = C7 nerve root	3–4, kick the door
	Patella = L4 nerve root	5–6, pick up sticks
	Achilles = S1 nerve root	7–8, close the gate
	Babinski—dorsiflexion of the big toe and fanning of other toes; sign of UMN lesion, but normal reflex in the first year of life	

Adapted with permission from Le T et al. *First Aid for the USMLE Step 1 2018.* New York, NY: McGraw-Hill; 2018.

HIGH-YIELD PERIPHERAL NERVES

- **Femoral nerve:** Innervates anterior thigh muscles and controls knee extension and hip flexion.
- **Lateral femoral cutaneous nerve:** Sensation to lateral thigh. Can be compressed as a result of surgeries or procedures (IVC filter placement) and can cause paresthesias (meralgia paresthetica).

TRIGEMINAL NEURALGIA

Recurrent, severe pain along distributions of the trigeminal nerve (CN V), often triggered by cold or minor trauma. Treat with carbamazepine. If bilateral, suspect multiple sclerosis.

CAUDA EQUINA SYNDROME

Compression of lumbar and sacral nerve roots. May be caused by epidural abscess, trauma, or metastatic cancer.

- **Dx:** Presents with saddle anesthesia, bowel or bladder incontinence, hyporeflexia, and asymmetric muscle weakness.
- **Tx:** MRI, and surgical evaluation (in that order).

Conus medullaris syndrome presents similarly with robust parasympathetic dysfunction, but has symmetric weakness. Treatment is the same as for cauda equina.

Vascular Disorders

STROKE

Disruption of cerebral blood flow leads to death of brain cells, resulting in acute onset of focal neurologic deficits. Can be ischemic (80%) or hemorrhagic (20%). Table 2.10-5 contrasts modifiable and nonmodifiable risk factors associated with stroke. Common etiologies are listed later.

- Atherosclerosis of the extracranial (carotid and vertebral) and intracranial vessels (internal carotid, cerebral, basilar, and vertebral arteries).
- Chronic hypertension, hypercholesterolemia, and diabetes can damage perforating vessels supplying deep regions of brain, leading to lacunar infarcts.
- Cardiac or aortic emboli.

KEY FACT

Cerebrovascular accident is the fifth most common cause of death and a leading cause of major disability in the United States.

T A B L E   2 . 1 0 - 5 .   **Modifiable and Nonmodifiable Risk Factors for Stroke**

MODIFIABLE RISK FACTORS	NONMODIFIABLE RISK FACTORS
"Live the way a **COACH SH**oul**DD**": **C**AD **O**besity **A**trial fibrillation **C**arotid stenosis **H**ypercholesterolemia **S**moking **H**ypertension (highest risk factor) **D**iabetes **D**rug use (cocaine, IV drugs)	**FAME:** **F**amily history of MI or stroke **A**ge > 60 **M**ale gender **E**thnicity (African-American, Hispanic, Asian)

- **Other causes:** Hypercoagulable states, craniocervical dissection, venous sinus thrombosis, sickle cell anemia, vasculitis (eg, giant cell arteritis).

HISTORY/PE

Symptoms are dependent on the vascular territory affected (see Table 2.10-6).

Q

A 82-year-old woman presents to the ED with a 2-day history of difficulty speaking and weakness in her right face and arm. During the interview, she speaks in two- to three-word choppy sentences but can follow commands. She cannot repeat what you say. Where is her lesion?

T A B L E   2 . 1 0 - 6 .   **Common Stroke Symptoms by Vessel Territory**

VESSEL TERRITORY	DISTINGUISHING SYMPTOMS
Middle cerebral artery	Contralateral paresis and sensory loss in the face and arm; gaze; homonymous hemianopsia preference toward the side of the lesion Nondominant hemisphere—neglect Dominant hemisphere (90% left side)—aphasia
Anterior cerebral artery	Contralateral paresis and sensory loss in the leg; cognitive or personality changes; urinary incontinence
Posterior cerebral artery	Vertigo; homonymous hemianopsia; ipsilateral sensory loss of face, CN IX and CN X; contralateral sensory loss of limbs; limb ataxia
Lacunar	Symptoms are pure motor, pure sensory, ataxic hemiparesis, dysarthria, or clumsy hand Strokes affecting the thalamus may cause thalamic pain syndrome several weeks after the event, with hypersensitive pain response over the affected area of the body
Small penetrating arteries of basal ganglia and internal capsule	Eye deviation toward lesion (putamen injury), contralateral hemiparesis and sensory loss
Transient ischemic attack	Any of the symptoms above, depending on location of vascular lesion Neurologic deficit lasts < 24 hours (most last < 1 hour) Often without findings on MRI
PICA/vertebral (Wallenberg syndrome)	Loss of pain and temperature sensation on ipsilateral face and contralateral body Ipsilateral bulbar weakness Ipsilateral Horner syndrome Vertigo, nystagmus
Carotid artery dissection	Sudden headache, neck pain, Horner syndrome Caused by oropharyngeal injury

MNEMONIC

MCA stroke can cause CHANGes—

Contralateral paresis and sensory loss in the face and arm
Hemiparesis
Aphasia (dominant)
Neglect (nondominant)
Gaze preference toward the side of the lesion

MNEMONIC

Contraindications to tPA therapy (major ones italicized)—

SAMPLE STaGES

Stroke or head trauma within the last 3 months
***A**nticoagulation with INR > 1.7 or prolonged PTT*
MI in past 3 months
Prior intracranial hemorrhage
Low platelet count (< 100,000/mm³)
***E**levated BP: Systolic > 185 mm Hg or diastolic > 110 mm Hg*
*Major **S**urgery in the past 14 days*
TIA (mild symptoms or rapid improvement of symptoms) within 6 months
Gl or urinary bleeding in the past 21 days or Glucose < 50
***E**levated (> 400 mg/dL) or ↓ (< 50 mg/dL) blood glucose*
Seizures present at onset of stroke

*If values can be corrected using appropriate treatment before the 3–4.5-hour period, consider tPA treatment.

A

This patient presents with Broca aphasia. In Broca aphasia, the lesion is in the posterior frontal cortex of the dominant side of the brain, in this case the left.

DIAGNOSIS

- **Best initial step:** Head CT without contrast (see Figure 2.10-1A) to differentiate ischemic from hemorrhagic stroke and identify potential candidates for thrombolytic therapy. Ischemic strokes < 6 hours old are usually not visible on CT scan.
- Labs to draw immediately, in case thrombolytic therapy or intervention may be required, include CBC, PT/PTT, cardiac enzymes and troponin, and BUN/creatinine.
- Diffusion-weighted MRI (follow-up to CT) (see Figure 2.10-1B) to identify early ischemic changes not detected on CT.
- **Determine underlying cause of stroke:**
  - **Cardioembolic:** ECG; echocardiogram; Holter monitor if initial ECG normal.
  - **Thrombotic:** Carotid ultrasonography; MRA; CTA; transcranial Doppler; conventional angiography (see Figure 2.10-1C).
  - **Other potential causes that should be worked up if there is a high index of suspicion:** hypercoagulable states; sickle cell disease; vasculitis.

TREATMENT

Acute treatment measures are as follows:

- **Hemorrhagic stroke:** See intracerebral hemorrhage discussion.
- **Ischemic stroke:**
  - Thrombolytics (tPA) if < 3–4.5 hours since onset of stroke and no bleeding or absolute contraindications. Permissive hypertension allowed in stroke for perfusion of ischemic area, but patient's systolic BP must be < 185 and diastolic BP < 110 mm Hg for tPA. Note: Because of uncertainties within this 3–4.5-hour window, the USMLE exam will make it very clear how long it has been since onset of symptoms.
  - ASA if > 3 hours since onset of stroke/TIA.
  - Treat fever and hyperglycemia as both are associated with poorer prognoses in the setting of acute stroke.
  - Monitor for signs and symptoms of brain swelling, ↑ intracranial pressure (ICP), and herniation. Treat acutely with mannitol and hyperventilation.
  - Prevent and treat poststroke complications, such as aspiration pneumonia, urinary tract infection (UTI), and deep vein thrombosis (DVT).

Preventive and long-term treatment measures are as follows:

- Hypertension management (diastolic BP < 80 mm Hg).
- Diabetes management (blood sugar level approximately 100 mg/dL).
- Blood lipids management with a statin.
- Acetylsalicylic acid (ASA) or clopidogrel.
- Diet, exercise, and a reasonable BMI.
- For cardioembolic strokes, anticoagulation. In new atrial fibrillation (AF) or hypercoagulable states, the target 0 is 2–3. In cases involving a prosthetic valve, the target INR is 2.5–3.5.
- For vascular pathology (pipe failure), antiplatelet medication.
- **Carotid endarterectomy:** If stenosis is > 60% in symptomatic patients or > 70% in asymptomatic patients (contraindicated in 100% occlusion; see Figure 2.10-2). Benefits may also occur in lower absolute percent stenosis; use clinical judgment when answering these questions.

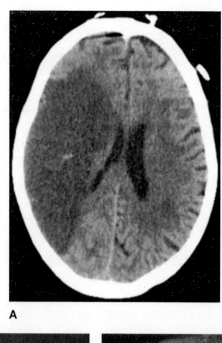

A

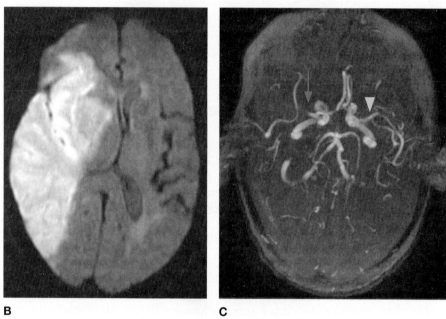

B   C

FIGURE 2.10-1. **Acute ischemic stroke.** Acute left hemiparesis in a 62-year-old woman. **(A)** Noncontrast head CT with loss of gray and white matter differentiation and asymmetrically decreased size of the right lateral ventricle in a right MCA distribution (indicating mass effect). **(B)** Diffusion-weighted MRI with reduced diffusion in the same distribution, consistent with an acute infarct; diffusion-weighted sequences are the most sensitive modality for diagnosing an acute ischemic infarct. **(C)** MRA shows the cause: an abrupt occlusion of the proximal right MCA (red arrow). Compare with the normal left MCA (yellow arrowhead). (Reproduced with permission from USMLE-Rx.com.)

SUBARACHNOID HEMORRHAGE

Etiologies of SAH include ruptured saccular aneurysms (berry aneurysms), arteriovenous malformation (AVM), and trauma; usually the bleed is located in the convexity of hemisphere to the circle of Willis.

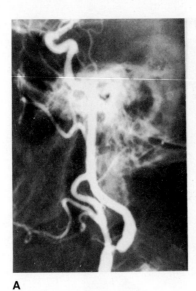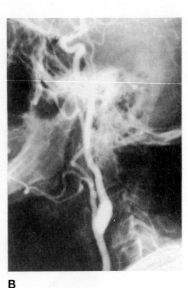

A   **B**

FIGURE 2.10-2. **Vascular studies pre- and postendarterectomy.** (**A**) Carotid arteriogram showing stenosis of the proximal internal carotid artery. (**B**) Postoperative arteriogram with restoration of the normal luminal size following endarterectomy. (Reproduced with permission from Way LW. *Current Surgical Diagnosis & Treatment,* 10th ed. Stamford, CT: Appleton & Lange; 1994.)

KEY FACT

SAH = "the worst headache of my life" with sudden onset.

Migraine = a gradually worsening headache (peak intensity > 30 minutes)

MNEMONIC

Conditions associated with berry aneurysms that can MAKE an SAH more likely—

Marfan syndrome
Aortic coarctation
Kidney disease (autosomal dominant, polycystic)
Ehlers-Danlos syndrome
Sickle cell anemia; **S**moking tobacco
Atherosclerosis
History (familial); **H**ypertension; **H**yperlipidemia

HISTORY/PE

- Aneurysmal SAH presents with an abrupt-onset, intensely painful "thunderclap" headache, often followed by neck stiffness (caused by meningeal irritation). Other signs of meningeal irritation, including photophobia, nausea/vomiting, and meningeal stretch signs (Kernig and Brudzinski signs), can also be seen.
- More than one-third of patients will give a history of a "sentinel bleed" ("warning leak") days to weeks before presentation.
- In the absence of neurosurgical intervention, rapid development of obstructive hydrocephalus or seizures often leads to ↓ arousal or frank coma and death.

DIAGNOSIS

- Immediate head CT without contrast (see Figure 2.10-3A) to look for blood in the subarachnoid space.
- Lumbar puncture (LP) if CT is ⊖ to look for RBCs, xanthochromia (yellowish cerebrospinal fluid [CSF] caused by breakdown of RBCs), ↑ protein (from the RBCs), and ↑ intracranial pressure (ICP) a few hours after onset of thunderclap headache.
- Four-vessel angiography (or equivalent noninvasive angiography such as CT angiography with three-dimensional reconstructions) should be performed once SAH has been confirmed (see Figure 2.10-3B–D) to identify source of bleeding. Noninvasive angiography is warranted in high-risk cases and in those with high clinical suspicion even if CT and LP are unrevealing.

TREATMENT

- **Most definitive treatment:** Neurosurgery. May perform angiographic coiling and/or stenting to stabilize aneurysm.
- Prevent rebleeding (most likely to occur in the first 24 hours) by maintaining systolic BP < 150 mm Hg until the aneurysm has been clipped or coiled.

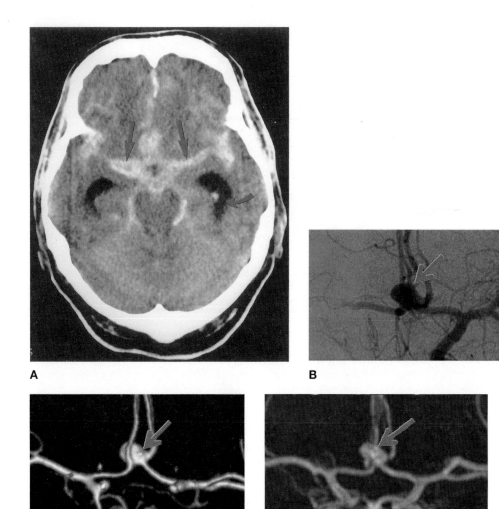

FIGURE 2.10-3.   Subarachnoid hemorrhage. Noncontrast CT (**A**) showing SAH filling the basilar cisterns and sylvian fissures (*straight arrows*). The curved arrow shows the dilated temporal horns of the lateral ventricles/hydrocephalus. Coned-down images (*right*) from a catheter angiogram (**B**), a CT angiogram (**C**), and an MRA (**D**) show a saccular aneurysm arising from the anterior communicating artery (*arrow*). (Image A reproduced with permission from Tintinalli JE, et al. *Tintinalli's Emergency Medicine: A Comprehensive Study Guide*, 6th ed. New York, NY: McGraw-Hill; 2004. Images B, C, and D reproduced with permission from Doherty GM. *Current Diagnosis & Treatment: Surgery*, 13th ed. New York, NY: McGraw-Hill; 2010.)

- Prevent vasospasm and subsequent ischemic stroke (most likely to occur 4–10 days after SAH) by administering calcium channel blockers (CCBs), such as nimodipine.
- Vasospasm is a major cause of delayed morbidity and mortality in patients with SAH.
- ↓ ICP by raising the head of the bed and instituting hyperventilation in an acute setting (< 30 minutes after onset).
- Treat hydrocephalus through a lumbar drain, serial LPs, or ventriculoperitoneal shunt.

INTRACEREBRAL HEMORRHAGE

Bleeding within brain parenchyma. Commonly affects deep brain regions such as basal ganglia, thalamus, pons, and cerebellum. Some risk factors

Q   **1**

A 68-year-old man presents to the ED with numbness and droop on the right side of the face, difficulty talking, and numbness and weakness in the right arm that began 2 hours ago. Where is this lesion, and what is the next best step in management?

Q   **2**

A 59-year-old man with prior medical history of polycystic kidney disease was admitted for treatment of subarachnoid hemorrhage (SAH). Four days after admission, he developed weakness in his right arm. What could have prevented this?

Q   **3**

A 59-year-old man with prior medical history of polycystic kidney disease is admitted for treatment of SAH. Four hours after admission, he develops weakness in his left arm. What is the cause of this new finding?

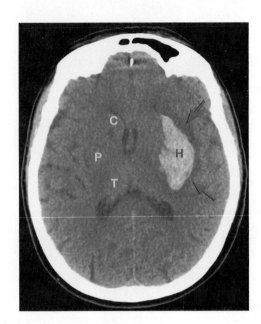

FIGURE 2.10-4. **Intracerebral hemorrhage.** Noncontrast head CT shows an intraparenchymal hemorrhage (H) and surrounding edema (arrows) centered in the left putamen, a common location for hypertensive hemorrhage. C, P, and T denote the normal contralateral caudate, putamen, and thalamus. (Reproduced with permission from Fauci AS, et al. *Harrison's Principles of Internal Medicine,* 17th ed. New York, NY: McGraw-Hill; 2008.)

KEY FACT

A "blown pupil" suggests ipsilateral third nerve compression.

---

1   **A**

Left MCA occlusion is the location, as aphasia and contralateral sensory loss and weakness are part of the description. CT of brain without contrast should be done to rule out hemorrhage and assess whether tPA should be initiated.

2   **A**

This patient's focal weakness is probably caused by ischemia secondary to vasospasm.

3   **A**

New onset of neurologic symptoms within 24 hours following a SAH is most likely caused by rebleeding of the aneurysm (as opposed to bleeding days after, which is caused by vasospasm).

---

include hypertension, tumor, and illicit drug use. Hypertension is the most common cause of intracerebral hemorrhage.

HISTORY/PE

- **Early symptoms/signs:** Focal motor or sensory deficits that often worsen as the hematoma expands.
- **Late symptoms/signs:** Features of increased intracranial pressure (eg, vomiting and headache, bradycardia, reduced alertness).

DIAGNOSIS

Immediate noncontrast head CT (see Figure 2.10-4). Look for hyperdense areas, mass effect, or edema that may predict herniation.

TREATMENT

- Monitor for signs of rebleed, shift, and possible herniation.
  - Suspect herniation if patient develops Cushing triad (hypertension, bradycardia, irregular respirations), fixed pupils, or loss of consciousness.
  - Herniation is a medical emergency. Treat with craniectomy to allow edema to expand outward.

SUBDURAL AND EPIDURAL HEMATOMA

See Table 2.10-7.

CAVERNOUS SINUS THROMBOSIS

A common etiology involves an uncontrolled infection of central facial skin, the orbit, or nasal sinuses that leads to septic thrombosis of the cavernous sinus. *Staphylococcus aureus* is the most common causative agent. Current antimicrobials have greatly ↓ both incidence and mortality.

TABLE 2.10-7. **Subdural Hematoma vs Epidural Hematoma**

	SUBDURAL	EPIDURAL
Common etiology	Head trauma → rupture of bridging veins → accumulation of blood between dura and arachnoid membranes	Head trauma → lateral skull fracture → tear of middle meningeal artery → accumulation of blood between skull and dura mater
Epidemiology	Elderly, alcoholics	Severe trauma
History/PE	Headache; altered mental status; contralateral hemiparesis; focal neurologic findings; altered mental status in elderly Onset: subacute or chronic	Immediate loss of consciousness followed by a lucid interval (minutes to hours)
Diagnosis	CT findings: crescent-shaped, concave hyperdensity acutely (isodense subacutely; hypodense chronically)	CT findings: lens-shaped, biconvex hyperdensity
Treatment	Neurosurgical evacuation if symptomatic Subdural hematomas may regress spontaneously	Emergent neurosurgical evacuation Can quickly evolve to brain herniation and death 2° to the arterial source of bleeding
Note:	In the setting of mild traumatic brain injury without vomiting, headache, and loss of consciousness but normal head CT, observe for 4–6 hours. If observation period is unremarkable, the patient can be sent home with extensive return precautions.	

Images reproduced with permission from Aminoff MJ. *Clinical Neurology*, 3rd ed. Stamford, CT: Appleton & Lange; 1996.

HISTORY/PE

- Headache is the most common presenting symptom.
- Patients may present with orbital pain, edema, visual disturbances (2° to oculomotor, abducens, or trochlear nerve involvement). On exam, they typically appear ill and have a fever.
- **Late findings:** Altered mental status such as confusion, drowsiness, or coma suggest spread to the CNS or sepsis.

DIAGNOSIS

- MRI (with gadolinium and MR venography) is the main method for diagnosis, but CT angiography and CT venography are also often used for diagnosis.

 KEY FACT

Altered mental status associated with an expanding epidural hematoma occurs within minutes to hours and classically includes: acute loss of consciousness → lucid interval → gradual loss of consciousness. With a subdural hematoma, such changes can occur within days to weeks.

- Lab studies show ↑ WBC count.
- Blood cultures reveal the causative agent in up to 50% of cases.

TREATMENT

- Treat aggressively and empirically with broad-spectrum antibiotics:
    - Vancomycin + third- or fourth-generation cephalosporin (eg, ceftriaxone or cefepime).
    - Metronidazole to cover anaerobic infection from sinus or dental sources.
    - Antifungal therapy is required for fungal cases.
- IV antibiotics are recommended for at least 3–4 weeks.
- Surgical drainage may be necessary if there is no response to antibiotics within 24 hours.

Headaches

Headaches can either be primary/idiopathic (ie, migraine, cluster, tension-type) or secondary (resulting from underlying disease, such as tumor or intracranial hemorrhage).

COMMON PRIMARY HEADACHES

Migraine Headache

Recurrent headache disorder with attacks that last 4–72 hours. Headache is typically unilateral, pulsating, moderate or severe in intensity, and aggravated by routine physical activity. Affects women more than men; often familial; onset is usually by the teens to early 20s. Linked to changes in vascular tone and neurotransmitters (serotonin, dopamine). Triggers include certain foods (eg, red wine, cheese), fasting, stress, menses, OCPs, bright light, and disruptions in normal sleep patterns.

HISTORY/PE

- Presents with a throbbing headache (> 2 hours, but usually < 24 hours) that is associated with nausea, vomiting, photophobia, and noise sensitivity. Headache is usually relieved by sleep and darkness. Migraine can occur with or without aura.
    - **Classic presentation of migraine with aura:** Unilateral pulsating HA, preceded by a visual aura in the form of either scintillating scotomas (bright or flashing lights) or visual field cuts.

DIAGNOSIS

Based on the history and an otherwise ⊖ work-up.

TREATMENT

- Avoid known triggers.
- Abortive therapy includes triptans (after OTC NSAIDs have failed), alone or in addition to other analgesics such as naproxen. Consider symptomatic treatment for nausea.
- Prophylaxis for frequent or severe migraines includes anticonvulsants (eg, valproate, gabapentin, topiramate), TCAs (eg, amitriptyline), β-blockers (propranolol), and CCBs.
- Routine aerobic exercise and good sleep hygiene.

Cluster Headache

Men are affected more often than women; average age of onset is 25 years.

HISTORY/PE

- Presents as a brief, excruciating, unilateral periorbital headache that lasts from 30 minutes to 3 hours, during which time the patient tends to be extremely restless.
- Attacks tend to occur in clusters of time, affecting the same part of the head at the same time of day (commonly during sleep) during a certain season of the year.
- Associated symptoms include ipsilateral lacrimation of the eye, conjunctival injection, Horner syndrome, and nasal stuffiness.

DIAGNOSIS

Classic presentations with a history of repeated attacks over an extended period do not need imaging. First episodes require a work-up (ie, MRI, carotid artery ultrasound) to exclude structural brain lesion or disorders associated with Horner syndrome (ie, carotid artery dissection, cavernous sinus infection).

TREATMENT

- **Acute therapy:** High-flow O_2 or sumatriptan injection.
- **Prophylactic therapy:** Verapamil is first line. Alternatives include lithium, valproic acid, and topiramate.

Tension-Type Headache

- **Hx:** Presents with tight, bandlike pain around the head that is triggered by fatigue or stress. Nonspecific symptoms (eg, anxiety, poor concentration, difficulty sleeping) may also be seen. Usually occurs at the end of the day.
- **Dx:** Must have at least two of the following characteristics: bilateral location, pressing/tightening quality; mild-moderate intensity; not aggravated by routine physical activity. Rule out giant cell arteritis in patients > 50 years of age with new headaches by obtaining an ESR, even if headaches are mild with no associated constitutional or vascular symptoms.
- **Tx:** Relaxation, massage, hot baths, and avoidance of exacerbating factors. NSAIDs and acetaminophen are first-line abortive therapy, but triptans can also be considered.

SECONDARY HEADACHES

Consider secondary headaches when "red flags" are present.

HISTORY/PE

- Significant findings include fever or rash (consider meningitis or other infectious causes), jaw claudication (specific for temporal arteritis), or constitutional symptoms such as weight loss (associated with neoplastic, inflammatory, or infectious conditions).
- Photophobia, nausea, vomiting, and neck stiffness can be associated with aneurysmal SAH and meningitis caused by meningeal irritation.
- Conduct full general and neurologic exams, including a funduscopic exam.

KEY FACT

If a 30-year-old woman complains of headaches at the end of the day that worsen with stress and improve with relaxation or massage, think tension-type headache.

KEY FACT

Tension-type headaches are the most common type of headache diagnosed in adults.

Q **1**

A 28-year-old woman with no prior medical history presents with throbbing, unilateral headache that is exacerbated by menstruation and minimally relieved by acetaminophen and lying in a dark room. She would like something that would provide more symptomatic relief. What abortive therapy would you prescribe?

Q **2**

A 24-year-old woman with a BMI of 33 presents with a 3-week history of constant retro-orbital headache with occasional nausea, vomiting, and tinnitus. She also developed new-onset diplopia 2 hours before presentation. On physical exam, she is noted to have papilledema. What is the most likely diagnosis, and what are the risk factors for this condition?

1   **A**

This patient's symptoms are consistent with migraine headaches. You would prescribe a triptan for abortive therapy.

2   **A**

Given this patient's symptoms and risk factors, she probably has pseudotumor cerebri, also known as idiopathic intracranial hypertension (IIH). In IIH, symptoms are suggestive of a brain tumor, and CSF pressure will be ↑; however, neuroimaging will be normal. Obesity, tetracycline, growth hormone, and excess vitamin A are risk factors for the disease. Treatment is with acetazolamide, frequent lumbar punctures, and ventriculoperitoneal shunt if needed.

- **Neurologic sequelae:** Look for diplopia, altered mental status or associated symptoms (numbness, weakness, dizziness, ataxia, visual disturbances), papilledema, or pupillary abnormalities (partial CN III palsy or Horner syndrome).

DIAGNOSIS

- If SAH is suspected, obtain a head CT without contrast.
- Obtain a CBC to rule out systemic infections.
- If temporal arteritis is suspected, obtain an ESR.

TREATMENT

- Directed toward underlying cause of headaches.
- Analgesics for pain relief.

Seizure Disorders

Sudden changes in neurologic activity caused by abnormal electrical activity in the brain that can often be detected on EEG. See Table 2.10-8 for common etiologies by age. Etiologies of seizures, and their distinguishing features, include the following:

- **Idiopathic epilepsy (recurrent, unprovoked seizures):** May be caused by genetics, developmental factors, early life brain injuries, and so on.
- **Acquired epilepsy could be caused by the following:**
  - Structural brain lesion (tumor, stroke, AVM hemorrhage, or developmental abnormality). Tend to have focal onset or focal postictal deficit, suggesting focal CNS pathology.
  - **Non-neurologic etiologies:** Hypoglycemia, hyponatremia, hypocalcemia, hyperosmolar states, hepatic encephalopathy, uremia, porphyria, drug overdose (cocaine, antidepressants, neuroleptics, methylxanthines, lidocaine), drug withdrawal (alcohol and other sedatives), eclampsia, hyperthermia, hypertensive encephalopathy, head trauma, and cerebral hypoperfusion.

HISTORY/PE

- **Partial:** Abnormal electrical activity arises from a discrete region (or multiple discrete regions) of the brain. Can involve motor features caused by sensory, autonomic, or psychic features (eg, fear, déjà vu, hallucinations). Aura is common (auditory, visual, olfactory, or tactile hallucinations). A postictal focal neurologic deficit (eg, hemiplegia/hemiparesis, or Todd paralysis) is possible and usually resolves within 24 hours. Can be simple or complex.
  - **Simple:** No impaired level of consciousness.

TABLE 2.10-8.   Causes of Seizure by Age Group

INFANTS (< 2 YEARS)	CHILDREN (2–10 YEARS)	ADOLESCENTS (10–18 YEARS)	ADULTS (18–35 YEARS)	ADULTS (> 35 YEARS)
Perinatal injury	Idiopathic	Idiopathic	Trauma	Trauma
Infection	Infection	Trauma	Alcoholism	Stroke
Metabolic	Trauma	Drug withdrawal	Brain tumor	Metabolic disorders
Congenital	Febrile	Arteriovenous malformations (AVM)		Alcoholism
				Brain tumor

- **Complex:** Typically involve the temporal lobe (70–80%) with bilateral spread of the aberrant electrical discharge, leading to impaired level of consciousness. Postictal confusion/disorientation/amnesia are characteristic.
- **Generalized seizures:** Seizure activity that involves both cerebral hemispheres resulting in impaired level of consciousness. Examples include tonic-clonic, absence, myoclonic, clonic, tonic, and atonic.
  - **Tonic-clonic:** Sudden loss of consciousness with extension of the back and contraction of muscles (chest and extremities), repetitive, symmetric clonic (alternation between muscle contraction and relaxation) movements. Etiology often idiopathic. Simple and complex partial seizures may evolve into secondary generalized tonic-clonic seizures.
    - Marked by incontinence and tongue biting.
    - Patients may appear cyanotic during the ictal period.
    - Postictal confusion and drowsiness. Muscle aches and headaches may also be present.
  - **Childhood absence epilepsy:** Is a form of generalized seizure. Presents with brief (5- to 10-second), often unnoticeable episodes of impaired consciousness (petit mal seizures) occurring up to hundreds of times per day. Can appear to be daydreaming or staring. Symptoms may include sudden stop in motion, lip smacking, eyelid flutter, and chewing motions. Can be triggered by hyperventilation. No postictal phase. Begins in childhood; subsides before adulthood. Often familial.

Diagnosis

- Clinical history by a bystander and physical exam are always clues to the diagnosis and differentiating among similarly appearing clinical symptoms—history of brain trauma, infection, neoplasm, stroke, or developmental issues.
- **Best initial step:** Obtain an EEG.
  - **Partial seizures:** Look for epileptogenic focus.
  - **Childhood absence epilepsy:** EEG shows 3-per-second spike-and-wave discharges (remember classic EEG findings, but do not worry about learning how to read them!). EEG changes can be triggered by hyperventilation.
  - **Tonic-clonic:** EEG typically shows 10-Hz activity during the tonic phase and slow waves during the clonic phase.
  - If EEG is normal during event concerning for seizure, think of pseudoseizures.
- Serum prolactin levels may be elevated in the immediate postictal period of generalized and complex-partial seizures.
- **Rule out:** Systemic causes with a CBC, electrolytes, calcium, fasting glucose, LFTs, a renal panel, RPR, ESR, and a toxicology screen.
- A focal seizure implies a focal brain lesion. Evaluate by CT or MRI with contrast.

Treatment

- Secure airway when appropriate.
- For acute seizures lasting longer than 5 minutes, see treatment of status epilepticus later.
- In cases of systemic 2° seizures, treat the underlying cause.
- Anticonvulsants for partial and tonic-clonic seizures, levetiracetam, phenytoin, carbamazepine, phenobarbital, and valproic acid have similar efficacy and can be used as chronic monotherapy.
  - In children, phenobarbital is the first-line anticonvulsant.
  - If a certain antiepileptic is ineffective as monotherapy, try an alternative. If alternative is ineffective, try a regimen of multiple antiepileptics.

KEY FACT

If an adult patient presents with an episode of lip smacking associated with an impaired level of consciousness and followed by confusion, think complex partial seizures.

KEY FACT

If a patient presents with uncontrollable twitching of his thumb and is fully aware of his symptoms, think simple partial seizures.

KEY FACT

If a patient presents with clonic movements associated with loss of consciousness and incontinence, think tonic-clonic (grand mal) seizures.

KEY FACT

If a child is brought from school to her pediatrician after experiencing multiple intermittent 5-second episodes of staring into space, think childhood absence epilepsy.

KEY FACT

Petit mal seizures may be described with the classic EEG finding of 3-per-second spike-and-wave discharges.

Q

A 40-year-old man presents to the ED with a single simple partial seizure of 1 minute but is no longer symptomatic. He also complains of 2 months of morning headaches and one episode of vomiting in the past week. What is the next step in management?

- Other treatment options include gabapentin, topiramate, and oxcarbazepine.
- **Absence seizures:** First-line is ethosuximide; second-line is valproic acid.
- **Intractable temporal lobe seizures:** Consider anterior temporal lobectomy.
- Treatment is not necessary for a single episode of seizure.

STATUS EPILEPTICUS

A **medical emergency** consisting of prolonged seizures (use > 5 minutes) or two or more seizures that occur without a return to baseline consciousness within 30 minutes.

- Common causes include anticonvulsant withdrawal/noncompliance, anoxic brain injury, EtOH/sedative withdrawal or other drug intoxication, metabolic disturbances (eg, hyponatremia), head trauma, and infection.
- Mortality is 10–20%.

DIAGNOSIS

- Treatment and diagnostic work-up should be initiated simultaneously.
- Determine the underlying cause with collateral history, physical exam, CBC, electrolytes, calcium, glucose, ABGs, LFTs, BUN/creatinine, ESR, antiepileptic drug levels, and a toxicology screen.
- Continuous EEG monitoring if nonconvulsive status epilepticus is suspected or if patient is not waking up after clinically obvious seizures stop.
- If intracranial pathology is suspected, obtain a stat head CT.
- Obtain an LP in the setting of fever or meningeal signs, but only after a CT scan has been obtained to assess the safety of the LP.

TREATMENT

- Maintain airway, breathing, circulation (ABCs); consider rapid intubation for airway protection.
- To rapidly treat potential etiologies, administer thiamine, followed by glucose.
- SE treatment strategies vary greatly among different institutions. Following is an example guide:
  - Give an IV benzodiazepine (lorazepam or diazepam) within 0–5 minutes.
  - Give another dose of IV benzodiazepine at 5–10 minutes.
  - If patient is still seizing at 20 minutes, give fosphenytoin, valproate sodium, phenobarbital (if severe), levetiracetam, or continuous infusion of midazolam.
  - For refractory status epilepticus (RSE), give continuous antiepileptic drugs (AEDs) with bolus for breakthrough SE. Early intubation is advisable when giving continuous AEDs.

Vertigo

Before discussing conditions that cause vertigo, it is worth defining vertigo and differentiating it from lightheadedness. "Dizziness" is often used to describe vertigo and lightheadedness. Vertigo feels as if one or one's surroundings are moving when there is no actual movement. Lightheadedness feels as if one is about to faint or "pass out." Conscious sensation of vertigo occurs in the cerebral cortex as a result of an error signal of observed over expected from the lower centers.

BENIGN PAROXYSMAL POSITIONAL VERTIGO

A common cause of recurrent peripheral vertigo resulting from displacement of an otolith ("earstone") that leads to disturbances in the semicircular canals.

HISTORY/PE

Patients present with transient, episodic vertigo (lasting < 1 minute) and nystagmus triggered by changes in head position (eg, while turning in bed, getting in and out of bed, or reaching overhead). Patients may complain of vertiginous or nonvertiginous dizziness or lightheadedness.

DIAGNOSIS

- **Dix-Hallpike maneuver:** Have the patient turn his or her head 45 degrees right or left and go from a sitting to a supine position. If vertigo and the typical nystagmus (fast phase toward the affected side) are reproduced, benign paroxysmal positional vertigo is the likely diagnosis.
- Nystagmus that persists for > 1 minute, gait disturbance, or vomiting should raise concern for a central lesion.

TREATMENT

- Epley maneuver (an extended version of the Dix Hallpike maneuver used as treatment) resolves 80% of cases.
- The condition usually subsides spontaneously in weeks to months, but 30% recur within 1 year. Long-term use of antivertigo medications (eg, meclizine) are generally contraindicated, as they have limited efficacy, they are sedating, and they inhibit vestibular compensation, which may lead to chronic unsteadiness.

ACUTE PERIPHERAL VESTIBULOPATHY (LABYRINTHITIS OR VESTIBULAR NEURITIS)

HISTORY/PE

- Presents with acute onset of severe vertigo, head motion intolerance, and gait unsteadiness accompanied by nausea, vomiting, and nystagmus.
- **Labyrinthitis:** Auditory or aural symptoms (tinnitus, ear fullness, or hearing loss). Lateral pontine/cerebellar stroke (anterior inferior cerebellar artery territory) may present with similar symptoms, but may have additional occipital headache, ataxia, nystagmus.
- **Vestibular neuritis:** Lacks auditory or aural symptoms. Lateral medullary/cerebellar stroke (posterior inferior cerebellar artery territory) can present with similar symptoms.

DIAGNOSIS

- A diagnosis of exclusion once the more serious causes of vertigo (eg, cerebellar/brain stem stroke) have been ruled out.
- Acute peripheral vestibulopathy demonstrates the following:
  - An abnormal vestibulo-ocular reflex as determined by a bedside head impulse test (ie, rapid head rotation from lateral to center while staring at the examiner's nose).
  - A predominantly horizontal nystagmus that always beats in one direction, opposite the lesion.
  - No vertical eye misalignment by alternate cover testing.
- If patients are "high risk" (ie, if they have atypical eye findings or neurologic symptoms or signs, cannot stand independently, have head or neck

KEY FACT

Progressive bilateral (high-frequency) sensorineural hearing loss and occasional tinnitus is normal (presbycusis). It is typically noticed by 60 years of age.

KEY FACT

If a patient complains of vertigo and vomiting for 1 week after having been diagnosed with a viral infection, think acute vestibular neuritis.

pain, are > 50 years of age, or have one or more stroke risk factors), MRI with diffusion-weighted imaging is indicated.

TREATMENT

Acute treatment consists of corticosteroids given < 72 hours after symptom onset and antivertigo agents (eg, meclizine). The condition usually subsides spontaneously within weeks to months.

MÉNIÈRE DISEASE

A cause of recurrent vertigo with unilateral auditory symptoms that affects at least 1 in 500 individuals in the United States. More common among women. This disorder of the inner ear is characterized by ↑ volume of endolymph.

HISTORY/PE

- Presents with recurrent episodes of severe vertigo, hearing loss, tinnitus, and ear fullness, episodes often lasting minutes to hours. Nausea and vomiting are typical. Patients progressively lose low-frequency hearing over years and may become deaf on the affected side.
- Rule out cerebellopontine angle tumors by MRI.

DIAGNOSIS

The diagnosis is made clinically and is based on a thorough history and physical exam. Two episodes lasting ≥ 20 minutes with remission of symptoms between episodes, hearing loss documented at least once with audiometry, and tinnitus or aural fullness are needed to make the diagnosis once other causes (eg, TIA, otosyphilis) have been ruled out.

TREATMENT

- **Acute:** Meclizine or benzodiazepines to control spinning sensation during acute attacks; antiemetics for nausea/vomiting.
- **Chronic:** Dietary changes that limit salt intake to avoid fluid retention; diuretics.
- For severe unilateral cases, intratympanic injection of gentamicin into the middle ear (absorbed by the inner ear) has been shown to reduce the frequency and severity of vertigo attacks.

SYNCOPE

One of the most common causes of loss of consciousness 2° to a sudden drop in cerebral perfusion. Etiologies can be cardiac or noncardiac. Presyncope can be associated with noncardiac causes and is described as a feeling of imminent loss of consciousness without actual fainting. Commonly confused with seizures.

HISTORY/PE

- Patients may report a trigger (eg, orthostatics, standing for a long period of time, fear/sight of blood, Valsalva maneuver).
- **Noncardiac:** Typically involves prodromal symptoms that lead to loss of consciousness and muscle tone for < 30 seconds and recovery within seconds. Screen for the following potential etiologies:
  - **Orthostatic hypotension:** Symptoms triggered by postural changes. Common causes include dehydration and autonomic neuropathy (commonly seen in patients with diabetes).

- **Vasovagal:** Sudden increase in vagal tone triggered by prolonged standing, emotional distress, painful stimuli. Patient may experience prodromal symptoms of nausea, warmth, and diaphoresis before syncope.
- **Cardiac:** Does not typically involve prodromal/postdromal symptoms; patient may have history of arrhythmia, valvular disease, or structural heart disease. Screen for the following potential etiologies:
  - Left ventricular outflow tract obstruction (LVOTO) (eg, aortic stenosis, hypertrophic obstructive cardiomyopathy); syncope with exertion or during exercise.
  - **Arrhythmia:** History of CAD, MI, cardiomyopathy, Wolff-Parkinson-White syndrome, or reduced EF.
  - **Torsades de pointes:** Triggered by electrolyte abnormalities (K+; Mg+) or any medications that can prolong QT interval.

DIAGNOSIS

- Unless there is a clear vasovagal syncope in a young patient with no history of cardiac disease or risk factors, place all patients on telemetry or Holter monitoring to evaluate for arrhythmia, and rule out myocardial ischemia with an ECG and cardiac enzymes.
- Consider an echocardiogram, a tilt-table test, or neuroimaging, especially vascular imaging.
- Consider seizure and rule out with EEG if the following occur:
  - Patient experiences limb jerking that is unilateral or lasts > 30 seconds.
  - Patient has prolonged confusion after the episode.
  - Patient bites the lateral aspect of his or her tongue.

TREATMENT

Treat the underlying cause; avoid triggers.

Disorders of the Neuromuscular Junction

MYASTHENIA GRAVIS

An autoimmune disorder caused by antibodies that bind to postsynaptic acetylcholine (ACh) receptors located at the neuromuscular junction. Most often affects young adult women and older men, and can be associated with thymoma, thyrotoxicosis, and other autoimmune disorders.

HISTORY/PE

- Presents with fluctuating ptosis or double vision, bulbar symptoms (eg, dysarthria, dysphagia), and proximal muscle weakness. Symptoms typically worsen with fatigue at the end of the day.
- Patients may report difficulty in climbing stairs, rising from a chair, brushing hair, and swallowing.
- Myasthenic crisis is rare but includes the potentially lethal complications of respiratory compromise and aspiration. It may be precipitated by medications (fluoroquinolones), trauma, or surgery. Treatment is with airway management, IVIG or plasmapheresis, and IV steroids.

DIAGNOSIS

- **Best initial diagnostic test:** Acetylcholine receptor antibody. Edrophonium (Tensilon test) is an anticholinesterase inhibitor that can be used as a diagnostic tool because it rapidly reverses symptoms.

- Application of an ice pack over the eyelids may improve symptoms. (This test is a board favorite.)
- An abnormal single-fiber EMG and/or a decremental response to repetitive nerve stimulation can yield additional confirmation.
- Chest CT is used to evaluate for thymoma.

TREATMENT

- Anticholinesterase inhibitors (pyridostigmine) are used for symptomatic treatment.
- Prednisone, other immunosuppressants (eg, azathioprine, cyclosporine, mycophenolate mofetil), plasmapheresis, or IVIG can also be used for treatment.
- Resection of thymoma can be curative.
- Avoid giving certain antibiotics (eg, aminoglycosides, fluoroquinolones) and drugs (eg, β-blockers) to patients with myasthenia gravis because of their direct/indirect effects on the neuromuscular junction.

LAMBERT-EATON MYASTHENIC SYNDROME

A paraneoplastic autoimmune disorder caused by antibodies directed toward presynaptic calcium channels in the neuromuscular junction. Small cell lung carcinoma is a significant risk factor (60% of cases).

HISTORY/PE

Presents with weakness of proximal muscles along with depressed or absent deep tendon reflexes. Extraocular, respiratory, and bulbar muscles are typically spared. Weakness will improve with ↑ activity.

DIAGNOSIS

Repetitive nerve stimulation reveals a characteristic incremental response. Also diagnosed by autoantibodies to presynaptic calcium channels and a chest CT indicative of a lung neoplasm.

TREATMENT

- Treat small cell lung carcinoma.
- 3,4-diaminopyridine or guanidine can be given; acetylcholinesterase inhibitors (eg, pyridostigmine) can be added to either regimen.
- Corticosteroids and azathioprine can be combined or used alone for immunosuppression in cases where a neoplasm cannot be identified and an autoimmune cause is suspected.

Demyelinating Lesions

MULTIPLE SCLEROSIS

Multiple sclerosis (MS) is a demyelinating disorder of central nervous system of unclear etiology, but it is thought to be immune mediated. The female-to-male ratio is 3:2, and it is typically diagnosed between 20 and 40 years of age. MS becomes more common with increasing distance from the equator during childhood. Subtypes are relapsing-remitting (most common), 1° progressive, 2° progressive, and progressive relapsing.

HISTORY/PE

- Presents with multiple neurologic complaints that are separate in time and space and are not explained by a single lesion. As the disease progresses, permanent deficits can accumulate.

KEY FACT

Repetitive nerve stimulation reveals a characteristic incremental response in Lambert-Eaton myasthenic syndrome but shows a decremental response in myasthenia gravis.

KEY FACT

Anterior mediastinal mass with clinical weakness = thymoma (in a patient with myasthenia gravis) until proven otherwise

KEY FACT

Lung mass with weakness = Eaton-Lambert syndrome (in a patient with SCLC) until proven otherwise

KEY FACT

The classic triad (Charcot triad) in MS is scanning speech, intranuclear ophthalmoplegia, and nystagmus.

- Limb weakness, gait unsteadiness, paresthesias, optic neuritis, ophthalmoplegia (caused by involvement of the medial longitudinal fasciculus), diplopia, vertigo, nystagmus, urinary retention, sexual and bowel dysfunction, depression, and cognitive impairment are also seen. Symptoms classically worsen transiently with hot showers.
- Attacks are unpredictable but on average occur every 1.5 years, lasting for 2–8 weeks.
- Neurologic symptoms can come and go or be progressive. Those with a relapsing and remitting history have the best prognosis.

DIAGNOSIS

- **Most accurate tests:** Use MRI and LP as outlined by McDonald Diagnostic Criteria for definitive diagnosis.
- MRI (diagnostic test of choice for MS) shows multiple, asymmetric, often periventricular white matter lesions (Dawson fingers), especially in the corpus callosum. Active lesions enhance with gadolinium.
- CSF reveals ↑ IgG index, or at least two oligoclonal bands not found in the serum (nonspecific).

TREATMENT

- **Acute exacerbations:** High-dose, IV corticosteroids. Plasma exchange in patients who do not respond to corticosteroids.
- **Disease-modifying medications:** Ocrelizumab for progressive MS. Immunomodulators for relapsing—remitting MS can ↓ the number of relapses. Treat with injectable "ABCs": Interferon-β_{1a} (**A**vonex/Rebif), interferon-β_{1b} (**B**etaseron), and copolymer-1 (**C**opaxone). Now, a number of oral small molecules and infusions of monoclonal antibodies are more common.
- Symptomatic therapy is crucial and includes baclofen for spasticity, cholinergics for urinary retention, anticholinergics for urinary incontinence, carbamazepine or amitriptyline for painful paresthesias, and antidepressants for clinical depression.

GUILLAIN-BARRÉ SYNDROME

An acute, rapidly progressive demyelinating autoimmune disorder of the peripheral nerves that results in weakness. Also known as acute inflammatory demyelinating polyneuropathy. Associated with recent *Campylobacter jejuni* infection, viral infection, or influenza vaccine (in extremely rare cases). Approximately 85% of patients make a complete or near-complete recovery (may take up to 1 year). The mortality rate is < 5%.

HISTORY/PE

- Classically presents with progressive (over days), symmetric, ascending paralysis (distal to proximal), and areflexia. In severe cases, paralysis can progress to involve the trunk, diaphragm, and cranial nerves.
- Autonomic and sensory nerves may also be affected, leading to glove-and-stocking distribution paresthesias and autonomic dysregulation.

DIAGNOSIS

- Evidence of diffuse demyelination is seen on nerve conduction studies, which show ↓ nerve conduction velocity.
- Supported by a CSF protein level > 55 mg/dL with little or no pleocytosis (albuminocytologic dissociation).
- Remember that ascending paralysis with normal CSF findings and without autonomic dysfunction is characteristic of tick-borne paralysis, not Guillain-Barré syndrome.

KEY FACT

Pregnancy may be associated with a ↓ in MS symptoms.

KEY FACT

For optic neuritis, give IV, not oral, corticosteroids.

MNEMONIC

The 4 "A's" of Guillain-Barré syndrome—

Acute inflammatory demyelinating polyradiculopathy
Ascending paralysis
Autonomic neuropathy
Albuminocytologic dissociation (increased albumin in CSF)

TREATMENT

- Frequently monitor maximal negative inspiratory force (NIF) inspiratory force (NIF) and vital capacity to determine whether patient should be admitted to ICU for impending respiratory failure.
- Plasmapheresis and IVIG are first-line treatments. Corticosteroids are not indicated.
- Aggressive physical rehabilitation is imperative.

KEY FACT

If a 55-year-old man presents with slowly progressive weakness with increased reflexes in his left upper extremity and later in his right (upper motor neuron signs), associated with fasciculations and atrophy (lower motor neuron signs), but without bladder disturbance and with a normal cervical MRI, think amyotrophic lateral sclerosis.

KEY FACT

Some 25% of people have "bulbar onset" ALS, which presents with difficulty swallowing, loss of tongue motility, and difficulty speaking (slurred or nasal quality).

KEY FACT

Bulbar involvement suggests pathology above the foramen magnum, which distinguishes ALS from cervical spondylosis with compressive myelopathy as the cause of symptoms.

AMYOTROPHIC LATERAL SCLEROSIS

A chronic, progressive degenerative disease, usually of unknown etiology, that is characterized by loss of upper and lower motor neurons. Also known as Lou Gehrig disease in the United States and motor neuron disease in the United Kingdom. ALS has an unrelenting course and almost always progresses to respiratory failure and death, usually within 5 years of diagnosis. Men are more commonly affected than women, and onset is generally between 40 and 80 years of age.

HISTORY/PE

- Presents with asymmetric, slowly progressive weakness (over months to years) affecting the arms, legs, diaphragm, and lower cranial nerves. Some patients initially present with fasciculations (muscle twitching). Weight loss is common.
- Associated with UMN and/or LMN signs (see Table 2.10-9).
- Sensation, eye movements, and sphincter tone are generally spared.
- Emotional lability is a common feature.

DIAGNOSIS

- The clinical presentation is usually diagnostic. "Bulbar involvement" (involvement of the tongue [CN XII] or oropharyngeal muscles [CN IX, X]) suggests pathology above the foramen magnum and generally excludes the most common differential diagnosis, cervical spondylosis with compressive myelopathy, as a cause.
- EMG/nerve conduction studies reveal widespread denervation and spontaneous action potentials (fibrillation potentials). Such studies are principally performed to exclude other demyelinating motor neuropathies.
- CT/MRI of the cervical spine is done to exclude structural lesions, such as cervical spondylosis with compressive myelopathy. Especially useful in those without bulbar involvement.

TABLE 2.10-9. UMN vs LMN Signs

CLINICAL FEATURES	UMN	LMN
Pattern of weakness	Pyramidal (arm extensor and leg flexor weaknesses)	Variable
Tone	Spastic ($\uparrow$)	Flaccid ($\downarrow$)
Deep tendon reflex (DTR)	$\uparrow$ (hyperreflexia)	$\downarrow$ (hyporeflexia)
Miscellaneous signs	Babinski reflex, pronator drift	Atrophy, fasciculations

TREATMENT

Supportive measures and patient education. Riluzole may delay disease progression by ↓ glutamate. Edaravone, while new, is a medication used for advanced ALS.

Dementia

Table 2.10-10 and the sections below contrast the time course, diagnostic criteria, and treatment of common types of dementia.

ALZHEIMER DISEASE

Risk factors include age, female gender, family history, Down syndrome, and low educational status. Pathology involves neurofibrillary tangles, neuritic plaques with amyloid deposition, amyloid angiopathy (↑ risk for spontaneous lobar hemorrhage), and neuronal loss.

HISTORY/PE

- Usually presents first with amnesia for newly acquired information (distant memory is usually intact), followed by visuospatial deficits (difficulty performing ADLs, getting lost in familiar places), language deficits, and cognitive decline that can be accompanied by depression and agitation.
- Mild cognitive impairment may precede Alzheimer disease by 10 years.
- **Early stages:** Physical exam is generally normal except for mental status.
- **Late findings:** May include noncognitive neurologic deficits, dyspraxia (difficulty with learned motor tasks), and urinary incontinence.

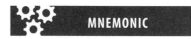

MNEMONIC

Differential diagnosis—

DEMENTIAS

Neuro**D**egenerative diseases
Endocrine
Metabolic
Exogenous
Neoplasm
Trauma
Infection (eg, HIV-associated dementia)
Affective disorders
Stroke/**S**tructural

TABLE 2.10-10. **Types of Dementia**

TYPE	TIME COURSE	PATHOLOGY	IMAGING/STUDIES
Alzheimer disease	Gradual	Diffuse atrophy with enlarged ventricles, senile plaques, and neurofibrillary tangles, initially temporal lobe	Definitive diagnosis cannot be made with neuroimaging at this time MRI/CT may show diffuse cortical atrophy, especially in the temporal and parietal lobes
Vascular dementia	Stepwise	Strokes in multiple areas of cerebral cortex	Brain imaging reveals evidence of old infarctions or extensive deep white-matter changes 2° to chronic ischemia
Frontotemporal dementia (Pick disease)	Gradual	Pick bodies (round intraneuronal inclusions). In frontal lobes	MRI/CT show frontotemporal atrophy
Normal pressure hydrocephalus	Gradual/abrupt	—	CT/MRI reveal ventricular enlargement
Creutzfeldt-Jakob disease	Abrupt	Prion proteins on biopsy Spongiform degeneration	MRI with diffusion-weighted imaging may show ↑ T2 and FLAIR intensity in the putamen and the head of the caudate and is also used to exclude structural brain lesions EEG shows periodic sharp wave complexes
Lewy Body dementia	Gradual	Lewy bodies (clumps of α- synuclein proteins)	MRI/CT to rule out other diagnoses

DIAGNOSIS

- A diagnosis of exclusion suggested by clinical features and by an insidiously progressive cognitive decline without substantial motor impairment.
- Definitively diagnosed on autopsy.
- MRI or CT may show atrophy, especially in temporal/parietal lobes, and can rule out other causes, particularly vascular dementia, normal-pressure hydrocephalus (NPH), and chronic subdural hematoma.
- CSF is normal.
- Neuropsychological testing can help distinguish dementia from depression.
- Hypothyroidism, vitamin B_{12} deficiency, and neurosyphilis should be ruled out.

TREATMENT

- **Prevention of disease progression:** No treatment has yet been proven effective.
- Cholinesterase inhibitors (ie, donepezil) are first-line therapy for treatment of symptoms in mild to moderate disease but do not affect outcome. Memantine, an NMDA receptor antagonist, may slow decline in moderate to severe disease.
- **Treatment of associated symptoms:**
    - Provide supportive therapy for the patient and family. Make the environment adapt to the patient.
    - Treat depression, agitation, sleep disorders, hallucinations, and delusions.

VASCULAR DEMENTIA

Dementia associated with a history of stroke and cerebrovascular disease (vascular dementia) is the second most common type of dementia.

HISTORY/PE

- Stepwise decline in cognitive functioning.
- May be associated with other symptoms of stroke, such as sensory or motor deficits.
- Risk factors include age, hypertension, diabetes, embolic sources, and a history of stroke.

DIAGNOSIS

Criteria for the diagnosis of vascular dementia include the presence of dementia and two or more of the following:

- Focal neurologic signs on exam.
- Symptom onset that was abrupt, stepwise, or related to stroke.
- MRI shows large lacunar infarct burden in cortical and subcortical areas.

TREATMENT

Protocols for the prevention and treatment of vascular dementia are the same as those for stroke.

FRONTOTEMPORAL DEMENTIA (PICK DISEASE)

A rare, progressive form of dementia characterized by atrophy of the frontal and temporal lobes.

HISTORY/PE

- Patients present with disinhibition and significant changes in behavior and personality early in the disease. Other symptoms include speech

KEY FACT

If a patient shows abrupt changes in symptoms over time rather than a steady decline, think vascular dementia.

disturbance, inattentiveness, impulsive behaviors, and, occasionally, extrapyramidal signs.
- Frontotemporal dementia rarely begins > 75 years of age.

DIAGNOSIS

Suggested by clinical features and by evidence of frontotemporal atrophy seen on MRI or CT.

TREATMENT

Symptomatic.

NORMAL PRESSURE HYDROCEPHALUS

A potentially treatable form of dementia that is thought to arise from impaired reabsorption of CSF.

HISTORY/PE

Symptoms include the classic triad of dementia, gait apraxia, and urinary incontinence. Headaches and other signs of ↑ ICP (eg, papilledema) typically do not appear, although continuous ICP monitoring may reveal spikes of elevated pressure.

DIAGNOSIS

- Suggested by clinical features; gait is classically described as "magnetic" or with "feet glued to the floor."
- CT or MRI shows ventricular enlargement out of proportion to sulcal atrophy (see Figure 2.10-5).
- LP reveals normal CSF pressures and can be therapeutic.

> **KEY FACT**
>
> NPH = "**W**et (incontinence), **W**obbly (gait apraxia), and **W**acky (dementia)."

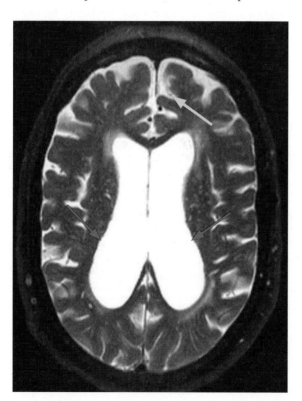

FIGURE 2.10-5.   Normal pressure hydrocephalus. T2-weighted MRI from a 60-year-old woman with slowly developing urinary incontinence, gait instability, and early dementia shows marked dilation of the lateral ventricles (*red arrows*). This is out of proportion to the sulci (*yellow arrow*), which appear normal. (Reproduced with permission from USMLE-Rx.com.)

Q

A 71-year-old woman is brought to her primary care physician's office by her son, who is concerned that she has had worsening recent memory, difficulty participating in her daily activities, restlessness, and difficulty sleeping for the past year. She scores a 22 on the Mini-Mental State Exam (MMSE). What is the most likely diagnosis?

TREATMENT

LP or continuous lumbar CSF drainage for several days may cause clinically significant improvement of the patient's symptoms. If so, surgical ventriculo-peritoneal shunting is the treatment of choice.

CREUTZFELDT-JAKOB DISEASE

Although it is the most common prion disease, Creutzfeldt-Jakob disease (CJD) remains an extremely rare form of dementia. CJD is a member of the transmissible spongiform encephalopathies, all of which are characterized by spongy degeneration, neuronal loss, and astrocytic proliferation. In CJD, an abnormal protease-resistant prion protein accumulates in the brain.

HISTORY/PE

- CJD causes a subacute dementia with ataxia and/or startle-induced myoclonic jerks with rapid clinical progression that is noted weeks to months after symptom onset.
- New-variant CJD (mad cow disease) is a more slowly progressive prion disease seen in younger people with a history of eating contaminated beef or contaminated human brains (kuru).

DIAGNOSIS

- Suggested by clinical features.
- Differential diagnosis includes limbic encephalitis, Hashimoto (steroid-responsive) encephalopathy, and toxic encephalopathy (eg, lithium or bismuth).
- ↑ Levels of CSF 14-3-3 and tau protein are seen, indicating rapid destruction of neurons.
- Definitive diagnosis can be made only by brain biopsy or autopsy, but MRI or EEG (for detection of periodic sharp wave complexes) may be helpful. Specimens must be handled with special precautions to prevent transmission.

TREATMENT

Currently, there is no effective treatment. Most patients die within 1 year of symptom onset.

LEWY BODY DEMENTIA

Dementia of unclear etiology in persons 50–85 years of age characterized by progressive cognitive changes, visual hallucinations, and Parkinson-like movement abnormalities such as bradykinesia.

HISTORY/PE

- **Physical and cognitive symptoms** may present around the same time and include the following:
  - **Physical:** Bradykinesia, rigidity, tremor, and shuffling gait with narrow-leg stance.
  - **Cognitive:** Progressive problems with visual-spatial processing, attention, executive dysfunction and memory.
- Psychiatric symptoms are common and can include hallucinations, delusions, depression, and anxiety.

DIAGNOSIS

- Usually clinical.
- Imaging and/or neuropsychological evaluation to rule out other diagnoses.

KEY FACT

CJD's rapid progression and presence of myoclonus distinguish it from other dementias.

Alzheimer disease is the likely diagnosis. The key differences between Alzheimer disease and normal aging is that in normal aging, patients can perform their activities of daily living, complain of memory loss yet provide detailed information about their forgetfulness, and have a score > 24 on the MMSE.

- Definitive diagnosis via brain biopsy or autopsy. Specimens will reveal abnormal clumps of α-synuclein proteins within neurons (Lewy bodies).

TREATMENT

Symptomatic treatment; no disease-modifying agents are available.

Movement Disorders

HUNTINGTON DISEASE

A rare, hyperkinetic, autosomal dominant disease involving CAG triplet repeat sequences in the *HD* gene on chromosome 4. The number of repeats typically expands in subsequent generations, leading to earlier expression and more severe disease (anticipation). Life expectancy is 20 years from the time of diagnosis.

HISTORY/PE

- Presents at 30–50 years of age with gradual onset of chorea (purposeless, involuntary dancelike movements), altered behavior, and dementia (begins as irritability, clumsiness, fidgetiness, moodiness, and antisocial behavior).
- Weight loss and depression may also be seen.

DIAGNOSIS

- Clinical diagnosis confirmed by genetic testing.
- CT/MRI show cerebral atrophy (especially of the caudate and putamen; see Figure 2.10-6).

TREATMENT

- There is no cure and disease progression cannot be halted. Treat symptomatically.

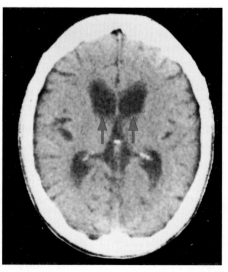 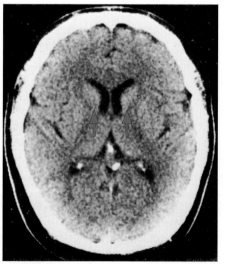

A   B

FIGURE 2.10-6. Atrophy of the cerebral and caudate nuclei in Huntington disease. (A) Noncontrast CT in a 54-year-old patient with Huntington disease shows atrophy of the caudate nuclei (arrows) and diffuse cerebral atrophy with dilation of the lateral ventricles. (B) A normal 54-year-old subject (arrows on caudate nuclei). (Reproduced with permission from Ropper AH, Samuels MA. *Adams & Victor's Principles of Neurology,* 9th ed. New York, NY: McGraw-Hill; 2009.)

 KEY FACT

If a 43-year-old man presents with gradual onset of chorea, irritability, and behavioral disturbances and his father experienced these symptoms at a slightly older age, think Huntington disease.

Q

A 65-year-old man presents to his internist with 10 years of bilateral hand tremors. His mother and older brother have similar tremors. He denies difficulty concentrating, trouble with rising from seated positions, or recent falls. What is the most likely diagnosis?

A

Essential tremor is the most likely diagnosis. Unlike the resting tremor in Parkinson disease, essential tremors are suppressed at rest and exacerbated with movements. Remember that bilateral tremors are less common in early Parkinson disease, and patients with Parkinson disease are more likely to present with multiple symptoms. Treat essential tremors with propranolol, primidone, and topiramate.

- Reserpine or tetrabenazine can be given to minimize unwanted movements. Psychosis should preferably be treated with atypical antipsychotics to ↓ the risk for extrapyramidal side effects or tardive dyskinesia. SSRIs are first-line therapy for depression.
- New gene therapy trials to reduce or eliminate triple repeats are underway.
- Genetic counseling should be offered to offspring.

PARKINSON DISEASE

A primarily motor disorder that usually begins after 50 years of age and is caused by loss of dopaminergic cells, initially in the substantia nigra. Parkinsonism (nonidiopathic) has symptoms similar to Parkinson disease and can be caused by antipsychotic use, multiple subcortical infarcts ("vascular parkinsonism"), toxin ingestion, and trauma.

HISTORY/PE

- "Parkinson tetrad" consists of the following:
  - **Resting tremor** (eg, "pill rolling"): A frequency of 4–6 Hz that ↓ with voluntary movement.
  - **Rigidity:** "Cogwheeling."
  - **Akinesia/bradykinesia:** Slowed movements caused by difficulty initiating movements. Festinating gait (small, shuffling steps) without arm swing is also seen.
  - **Postural instability:** Stooped posture, impaired righting reflexes, falls. Can often be a very early finding in Parkinson disease.
  - See TRAP mnemonic.
- **Other manifestations:** Masked facies, memory loss, and micrographia.

TREATMENT

- **Best initial treatment:**
  - Levodopa/carbidopa combination therapy is the mainstay of treatment. Levodopa is a dopamine precursor that can cross the blood-brain barrier. Carbidopa blocks the peripheral conversion of levodopa to prevent the side effects of levodopa (nausea and vomiting).
    - Early side effects: Hallucinations, dizziness, headache, and agitation.
    - Late side effects: Involuntary movements.
  - Dopamine agonists (ropinirole, pramipexole, bromocriptine) can be used for treatment in early disease.
    - Side effects: Hypotension, somnolence, confusion, hallucinations, and compulsive gambling.
- **Next best treatment:**
  - Selegiline (an MAO-B inhibitor) may be neuroprotective and may ↓ the need for levodopa.
    - Side effects: Confusion and insomnia.
  - Catechol-O-methyltransferase (COMT) inhibitors (entacapone or tolcapone) are not given alone but ↑ the availability of levodopa to the brain and may ↓ motor fluctuations.
  - Anticholinergics (trihexyphenidyl or benztropine)—generally used in younger patients whose primary symptom is tremor.
    - Side effects: Dry mouth, blurred vision, constipation, nausea, urinary retention, ankle edema, and livedo reticularis.
- If medical therapy is insufficient, surgical pallidotomy or deep brain stimulators may produce clinical benefit.

RESTLESS LEGS SYNDROME

Urge to move legs (more prominent at night) and associated dysesthesias that are relieved with movement. Associated with neuropathy, iron deficiency anemia. Treat with dopamine agonists (ropinirole, pramipexole) or gabapentin.

Neoplasms

Intracranial neoplasms may be 1° (30%) or metastatic (70%).

- Of all 1° brain tumors, 40% are benign, and these rarely spread beyond the CNS.
- Metastatic tumors are most often from 1° lung, breast, kidney, and GI tract neoplasms and melanoma. They occur at the gray-white junction; may be multiple discrete nodules; and are characterized by rapid growth, invasiveness, necrosis, and neovascularization.
- More common in men than in women, except for meningiomas.

HISTORY/PE

- Symptoms depend on tumor type and location (see Tables 2.10-11 and 2.10-12), local growth and resulting mass effect, cerebral edema, or ↑ ICP 2° to ventricular obstruction. Although headaches are often thought of as the main presenting symptom, only 31% of patients present with headache at diagnosis, and only 8% have headache as the sole presenting feature.
- Seizures or slowly progressive focal motor deficits are the most common presenting features.
- When ↑ ICP is the presenting feature, symptoms include headache, nausea/vomiting, and diplopia (false localizing CN VI palsies). In the era of neuroimaging, it is relatively rare for patients to present with ↑ ICP.
- **Other presenting symptoms:** Visual field abnormalities, neurologic deficits, psychiatric symptoms.

DIAGNOSIS

- **Best initial test:** CT and MRI with and without contrast to localize and determine the extent of the lesion.
  - Gadolinium-enhanced MRI is generally better for visualizing soft tissue tumors and vascularity.
  - CT is preferred for evaluating skull base lesions and for emergencies (eg, obstructive hydrocephalus) when an MRI cannot be rapidly acquired.
- Histologic diagnosis via CT-guided biopsy or surgical biopsy.

TREATMENT

- Consider resection (if possible), radiation, and chemotherapy after appropriate consultation with medical and surgical oncology teams.
- Therapy is highly dependent on tumor type, histology, progression, and site (see Tables 2.10-11 and 2.10-12).
- If ICP is ↑, manage ICP with the following:
  - Head elevation (↑ venous outflow from brain).
  - Hyperventilation (↓ CO_2 leads to cerebral vasoconstriction resulting in ↓ vasogenic edema).
  - Corticosteroids (↓ vasogenic edema).
  - Mannitol (extraction of free water from brain via osmotic diuresis).
  - Removal of CSF.
- AEDs can be used in patients who have had a seizure.

KEY FACT

Lesions to the superior colliculus can result in Parinaud syndrome, paralysis of conjugate vertical gaze.

KEY FACT

Most CNS tumors are metastatic. The most common 1° CNS tumors in adults are glioblastoma multiforme and meningiomas. The most common 1° CNS tumors in children are astrocytomas followed by medulloblastomas.

MNEMONIC

Most common cancers that metastasize to brain—

Lung and Skin Go to the BRain

Lung
Skin
GI
Breast
Renal

KEY FACT

Two-thirds of 1° brain tumors in adults are supratentorial. One-third of those in children are supratentorial.

KEY FACT

Symptoms of ↑ ICP:
- Nausea.
- Vomiting.
- Diplopia.
- Headache that is worse in the morning, with bending over, or with recumbency.

TABLE 2.10-11. **Common 1° Neoplasms in Adults**

TUMOR	BENIGN VS MALIGNANT	PRESENTATION	TREATMENT
Astrocytoma (diffuse, anaplastic, grade IV/glioblastoma) 	Low grade: diffuse— benign, or high grade Anaplastic: malignant Glioblastoma: malignant	Presentation of astrocytomas depends on location of tumor. Some symptoms include headache, seizures, or focal deficits Glioblastoma is the most common malignant 1° brain tumor. Progresses rapidly and has a poor prognosis (< 1 year from time of diagnosis)	Surgical removal/resection Radiation and chemotherapy have variable results
Meningioma	Generally benign	Presentation depends on location; often related to cranial neuropathy or is an incidental finding	Surgical resection; radiation for unresectable tumors
Vestibular schwannoma (also known as acoustic neuroma)	Generally benign	Unilateral hearing loss, tinnitus, vertigo, and loss of balance Bilateral in NF2	Surgical resection, focal radiation, or monitoring

Glioblastoma multiforme and meningioma images reproduced courtesy of the US Department of Health and Human Services and Armed Forces Institute of Pathology. Schwannoma image reproduced courtesy of MRT-Bild.

Neurocutaneous Disorders

NEUROFIBROMATOSIS

The most common neurocutaneous disorder. There are two major types: neurofibromatosis 1 (NF1, or von Recklinghausen syndrome) and neurofibromatosis 2 (NF2). Both are autosomal dominant diseases.

TABLE 2.10-12. Common 1° Neoplasms in Children

TUMOR	PATHOLOGY	PRESENTATION	TREATMENT
Pilocytic astrocytoma	Generally benign, well circumscribed, stain ⊕ for GFAP Posterior fossa/infratentorial tumor	Presents with drowsiness, headache, ataxia, nausea, vomiting, cranial neuropathy Slow-growing with protracted course	Resection if possible; radiation
Medulloblastoma	A primitive neuroectodermal tumor Arises from the fourth ventricle or cerebellar vermis and causes ↑ ICP Posterior fossa/infratentorial tumor	Highly malignant but radiosensitive; may seed the subarachnoid space May cause obstructive hydrocephalus Truncal ataxia caused by involvement of cerebellar vermis	Surgical resection coupled with radiation and chemotherapy
Craniopharyngioma	The most common suprasellar tumor in children Calcification is common (distinguishes it from pituitary adenoma)	Benign Most commonly causes bitemporal hemianopsia caused by compression of the optic chiasm	Surgical resection

MRI of pilocytic astrocytoma reproduced with permission from Hafez RFA. Stereotaxic gamma knife surgery in treatment of critically located pilocytic astrocytoma: preliminary result. *World J Surg Oncol* 2007;5:39. CT of medulloblastoma reproduced with permission from US Department of Health and Human Services and Armed Forces Institute of Pathology. CT of craniopharyngioma reproduced with permission from Garnet MR, Puget S, Grill J, et al. Craniopharyngioma. *Orphanet J Rare Dis.* 2007;2:18.

HISTORY/PE

- Diagnostic criteria for NF1 include two or more of the following:
    - Six café-au-lait spots (flat, uniformly hyperpigmented macules).
    - Two neurofibromas (benign peripheral nerve sheath tumors) of any type (see Figure 2.10-7).
    - Freckling in the axillary or inguinal area.
    - Optic glioma.
    - Two Lisch nodules (pigmented iris hamartomas).
    - Bone abnormality (eg, kyphoscoliosis).
    - A first-degree relative with NF1.

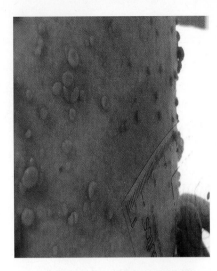

FIGURE 2.10-7. Neurofibromas associated with neurofibromatosis.
(Reproduced with permission from USMLE-Rx.com.)

KEY FACT

NF1 and NF2 are clinically evident by 15 and 20 years of age, respectively.

KEY FACT

Vestibular schwannomas (also known as acoustic neuromas) present with ipsilateral tinnitus, hearing loss, and vertigo. The treatment of choice is surgical resection.

- **Diagnostic criteria for NF2 are as follows:**
  - Bilateral vestibular schwannomas (also known as acoustic neuromas).
  - First-degree relative with NF2 and either:
    - Unilateral acoustic neuromas.
    - Two of any of the following tumor types: neurofibroma, meningioma, glioma, or schwannoma.
  - Other features include seizures, skin nodules, and café au lait spots.

DIAGNOSIS

- MRI of the brain, brainstem, and spine with gadolinium.
- Conduct a complete dermatologic exam, ophthalmologic exam, and family history. Auditory testing is recommended.

TREATMENT

- There is **no cure;** treatment is symptomatic (eg, surgery for kyphoscoliosis or debulking of tumors).
- Vestibular schwannomas (see Table 2.10-11) and optic gliomas can be treated with surgery or radiosurgery. Meningiomas can be resected.
- Drugs affecting the mTOR pathway can be used to reduce tumor growth.

TUBEROUS SCLEROSIS

Autosomal dominant disorder that affects many organ systems, including the CNS, skin, heart, retina, and kidneys.

HISTORY/PE

- Presents with infantile spasms or seizures, "ash-leaf" hypopigmented lesions (Figure 2.10-8A) on the trunk and extremities, and mental disability (↑ likelihood with early age of onset).
- Other skin manifestations include sebaceous adenomas (small red nodules on the nose and cheeks in the distribution of a butterfly; Figure 2.10-8B) and a shagreen patch (a rough papule in the lumbosacral region with an orange-peel consistency).

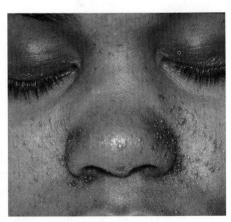

A   **B**

FIGURE 2.10-8. Tuberous sclerosis. (A) "Ash-leaf" macules on a patient with tuberous sclerosis and **(B)** sebaceous adenomas in a butterfly distribution. (Image A reproduced with permission from Tonekaboni SH, Tousi P, Ebrahimi A, et al. Clinical and para clinical manifestations of tuberous sclerosis: a cross sectional study on 81 pediatric patients. *Iran J Child Neurol* 2012;6(3):25-31. Image B adapted with permission from Fred H, van Dijk H. Images of memorable cases: case 143. Connexions Web site. December 4, 2008. Available at: http://cnx.org/content/m14923/1.3/.)

- Other symptoms are 2° to small benign tumors that grow on the face, eyes, brain, kidney, and other organs. For example:
  - CHF from cardiac rhabdomyoma; renal disease from renal cysts, angiolipomas, or carcinomas.
  - Developmental disability from brain lesions.

DIAGNOSIS

- Usually clinical.
- Ash-leaf lesions are enhanced by a Wood UV lamp.
- Imaging:
  - **MRI of brain:** Evaluate for subependymal giant cell astrocytoma and calcified tubers (potato-like nodules) within the cerebrum in the periventricular area. If lesions obstruct CSF outflow, obstructive hydrocephalus can develop.
  - **Echocardiography:** Evaluate for rhabdomyoma of the heart, especially in the apex of the left ventricle (affects > 50% of patients).
  - **MRI of abdomen:** Evaluate for renal disease (cysts, angiolipoma, and/or carcinoma).
- **EEG:** Evaluate for seizure activity.

TREATMENT

- Treatment should be based on symptoms (eg, cosmetic surgery for facial sebaceous adenomas).
- Treat seizures if present. If infantile spasms are present, treat with ACTH or vigabatrin.
- Surgical intervention may be indicated in the setting of ↑ ICP from obstructive hydrocephalus or for seizures associated with an epileptogenic focus or severe developmental delay.

STURGE-WEBER SYNDROME

Neurocutaneous condition characterized by port-wine stain (cavernous hemangioma) in the trigeminal nerve distribution, and intracranial calcifications that resemble a "tram-line." Hemianopia, glaucoma, and hemiparesis may also be seen.

Aphasia

A general term for speech and language disorders. Usually results from lesions (eg, strokes, tumors, abscesses) in the "dominant hemisphere." The left hemisphere is dominant in > 95% of right-handed people and in 60–80% of left-handed people.

BROCA APHASIA

A disorder of spoken and/or written language production, with intact comprehension. Caused by an insult to the Broca area in the posterior inferior frontal cortex (see Figure 2.10-9). Often 2° to a left superior MCA stroke. Also known as motor aphasia.

HISTORY/PE

Presents with impaired speech production, frustration with awareness of deficits, arm and facial hemiparesis, hemisensory loss, and apraxia of the oral muscles. Speech is described as "telegraphic" with few words and frequent pauses.

KEY FACT

Infantile spasms occur in children < 3 years of age and can consist of head bobbing, flexor spasms, extensor spasms, or movements that mimic the startle response. They may be associated with psychomotor regression or behavioral changes.

KEY FACT

Broca aphasia = motor aphasia, expressive aphasia, or nonfluent aphasia

Wernicke aphasia = sensory aphasia, receptive aphasia, or fluent aphasia

Q

A 61-year-old man presents to the ED with a 6-month history of progressively worsening nausea and morning headache. The patient is in no apparent acute distress. What is the preferred diagnostic study?

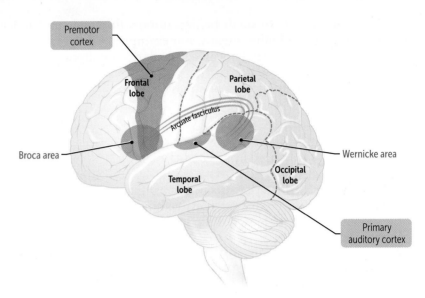

FIGURE 2.10-9. **Cerebral cortex with Broca and Wernicke areas highlighted.** (Reproduced with permission from USMLE-Rx.com.)

KEY FACT

In true Broca and Wernicke aphasia, repetition is impaired. If repetition is intact, the deficit is called transcortical motor aphasia (TMA) or transcortical sensory aphasia (TSA), which is caused by a lesion around the Broca and Wernicke areas, respectively. Also, called secondary aphasia.

MNEMONIC

BROca is **BRO**ken and **W**ernicke is **W**ordy.

TREATMENT

Speech therapy (varying outcomes with intermediate prognosis).

WERNICKE APHASIA

A disorder of language comprehension with intact yet nonsensical production. Caused by an insult to the Wernicke area in the left posterior superior temporal (perisylvian) lobe. Often 2° to left inferior/posterior MCA embolic stroke (see Figure 2.10-9).

HISTORY/PE

Presents with preserved fluency of language with impaired repetition and comprehension, leading to "word salad." Patients are unable to follow commands; make frequent use of neologisms (made-up words) and paraphasic errors (word substitutions); and show lack of awareness of deficits.

TREATMENT

Treat the underlying etiology, and institute speech therapy.

Coma

Unconsciousness marked by limited to no response to stimuli (ie, a state of unarousable unresponsiveness). Lesser states of impaired arousal are known as "obtundation" or "stupor." Coma is caused by dysfunction of both cerebral hemispheres or the brainstem (pons or higher) caused by structural or toxic-metabolic insults. Causes include the following:

- Diffuse hypoxic/ischemic encephalopathy (eg, post–cardiac arrest).
- Diffuse axonal injury from high-acceleration trauma (eg, motor vehicle accidents).
- Brain herniation (eg, cerebral mass lesion, SAH with obstructive hydrocephalus).

This patient presents with symptoms that are concerning for increased ICP. As he is not in acute distress, MRI is the preferred study because it is better for visualizing soft tissue and vascularity.

- Widespread infection (eg, viral encephalitis or advanced bacterial meningitis).
- Massive brainstem hemorrhage or infarction.
- Central pontine myelinolysis.
- Electrolyte disturbances (eg, hypoglycemia).
- Exogenous toxins (eg, opiates, benzodiazepines, EtOH, other drugs).
- Generalized seizure activity or postictal states.
- Endocrine (eg, severe hypothyroidism) or metabolic dysfunction (eg, thiamine deficiency).

HISTORY/PE

- Obtain a complete medical history from witnesses, including current medications (eg, sedatives).
- Conduct thorough medical and neurologic exams, including assessments of mental status, spontaneous motor activity, muscle tone, breathing pattern, funduscopy, pupillary response, eye movements, corneal reflex, gag reflex, and motor or autonomic responses to noxious stimuli applied to the limbs, trunk, and face (eg, retromandibular pressure, nasal tickle).

DIAGNOSIS

- Typically made by a combination of the history/physical and laboratory tests or neuroimaging.
- **Best initial step:** Check glucose, electrolytes, calcium; perform renal panel, LFTs, ABGs, a toxicology screen, and blood and CSF cultures. Other metabolic tests (eg, TSH) may be performed based on the clinical index of suspicion.
- Obtain a head CT without contrast before other imaging to evaluate for hemorrhage or structural changes. Imaging should precede LP in light of the risk for herniation.
- Obtain an MRI to exclude structural changes and ischemia (eg, brainstem).
- Rule out catatonia, conversion unresponsiveness, "locked-in" syndrome, or persistent vegetative state (PVS), all of which can be confused with true coma (see Table 2.10-13).

TREATMENT

Initial treatment should consist of the following measures:

- **Stabilize the patient:** Attend to **ABCs**.
- **Reverse the reversible:** Administer **DONT**—Dextrose, Oxygen, Naloxone, and Thiamine.

KEY FACT

Artificial life support can be discontinued only after two physicians have declared the patient legally brain dead.

TABLE 2.10-13. Differential Diagnosis of Minimally Conscious State

VARIABLE	"LOCKED-IN" SYNDROME	PERSISTENT VEGETATIVE STATE	COMA	BRAIN DEATH
Alertness	Wakeful and aware with retained cognitive abilities	Awake but not aware; Eyes open and closed—sleep-wake cycles present	Unconscious, eyes closed; no sleep-wake cycles	Unconscious; no sleep-wake cycles
Most common causes	Central pontine myelinolysis, brainstem stroke, advanced ALS	Diffuse cortical injury or hypoxic ischemic injury	Diffuse hypoxic encephalopathy, widespread infection, electrolyte disturbances, toxins	Same as coma
Voluntary motor ability	Eyes and eyelids	None	None	None
Respiratory drive	Yes	Yes	Yes	None

Identify and treat the underlying cause and associated complications.

 Prevent further damage.

Nutritional Deficiencies

Table 2.10-14 describes neurologic syndromes commonly associated with nutritional deficiencies.

Ophthalmology

VISUAL FIELD DEFECTS

Figure 2.10-10 illustrates common visual field defects and the anatomic areas with which they are associated.

GLAUCOMA

In the eye, aqueous humor produced by the ciliary body on the iris travels through the pupil into the anterior chamber and is then drained back into

TABLE 2.10-14. **Neurologic Syndromes Associated with Nutritional Deficiencies**

Vitamin	Syndrome	Signs/Symptoms	Classic Patients	Treatment
Thiamine (vitamin B₁)	Wernicke encephalopathy	The classic triad consists of encephalopathy, ophthalmoplegia, and ataxia	Alcoholics (toxin effect on cerebellar Purkinje fibers), hyperemesis, starvation, renal dialysis, AIDS. Can be brought on or exacerbated by high-dose glucose administration	Reversible almost immediately with thiamine administration Always give thiamine before glucose
	Korsakoff dementia	Above plus anterograde and retrograde amnesia, horizontal nystagmus, and confabulations	Same as above. Usually occurs in Wernicke syndrome that was treated too late or inadequately	Irreversible
Cyanocobalamin (vitamin B₁₂)ᵃ	Peripheral neuropathy; subacute combined degeneration (SCD)	Gradual, progressive onset. Symmetric paresthesias, stocking-glove sensory neuropathy, leg stiffness, spasticity, paraplegia, bowel and bladder dysfunction, sore tongue, and dementia Associated with elevated methylmalonic acid levels	Patients with pernicious anemia; strict vegetarians; status post–gastric or ileal resection; ileal disease (eg, Crohn); alcoholics or others with malnutrition	B₁₂ injections or large oral doses
Folateᵃ	Folate deficiency	Irritability; personality changes without the neurologic symptoms of CSD	Alcoholics	Reversible if corrected early

ᵃAssociated with ↑ homocysteine and an ↑ risk for vascular events.

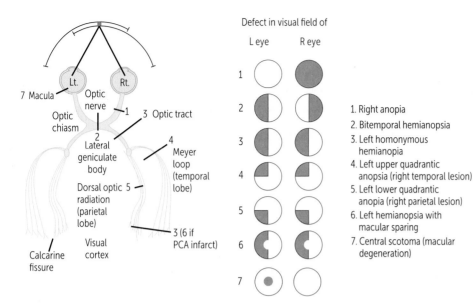

Defect in visual field of

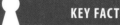

1. Right anopia
2. Bitemporal hemianopsia
3. Left homonymous hemianopsia
4. Left upper quadrantic anopsia (right temporal lesion)
5. Left lower quadrantic anopsia (right parietal lesion)
6. Left hemianopsia with macular sparing
7. Central scotoma (macular degeneration)

FIGURE 2.10-10. Visual field defects. (Reproduced with permission from Le T, et al. First Aid for the USMLE Step 1 2018. New York, NY: McGraw-Hill, 2018.)

the bloodstream via the trabecular meshwork in the angle of the anterior chamber.

- Any process that disrupts this natural flow can ↑ intraocular pressure (IOP), damaging the optic nerve and causing visual field deficits. Glaucoma is the result of such damage to the nerve.
- Open-angle glaucoma is much more common in the United States than closed-angle glaucoma (see Figure 2.10-11 and Table 2.10-15).

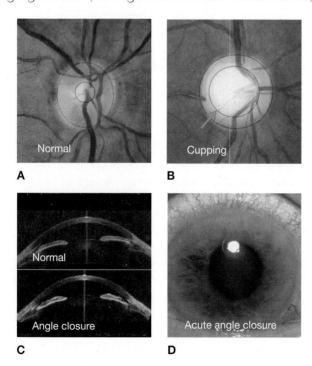

FIGURE 2.10-11. Findings in open- and closed-angle glaucoma. (A) Normal optic disk. (B) Cupping (increased cup-to-disk ratio) seen in open-angle glaucoma. (C) Iris, pupil, and cornea in normal eye compared with eye with closed-angle glaucoma. (D) Fixed, dilated pupil seen in closed-angle glaucoma. (Images A and B reproduced with permission from EyeRounds. Image C reproduced with permission from Low S, Davidson AE, Holder GE, et al. Autosomal dominant Best disease with an unusual electrooculographic light rise and risk for angle-closure glaucoma: a clinical and molecular genetic study. Mol Vis. 2011;17:2272–2282. Image D reproduced with permission from Dr. Jonathan Trobe.)

KEY FACT

Closed-angle glaucoma headaches are triggered by darkness (caused by pupillary dilation). Migraine headaches are triggered by bright lights.

KEY FACT

Open-angle glaucoma generally occurs bilaterally, but closed-angle glaucoma occurs unilaterally.

Q 1

A 39-year-old man presents to the ED with severe eye pain, photophobia, and a persistent sensation that something is in his eye. You are suspicious of a corneal abrasion. What are the risk factors for this condition, and what diagnostic test can you do to confirm your suspicion?

Q 2

A 45-year-old white man presents to the ED with sudden-onset headache and a dilated pupil in his right eye that is nonreactive to light. His right eye is hard to the touch. What is the most likely diagnosis, and what medications should be avoided in this patient?

TABLE 2.10-15.   Closed-Angle vs Open-Angle Glaucoma

	CLOSED-ANGLE GLAUCOMA	OPEN-ANGLE GLAUCOMA
Etiology	Disrupted flow of aqueous humor into the anterior chamber results in ↑ pressure in the posterior chamber, leading to angle closure that ↓ drainage	Diseased trabecular meshwork results in ↓ drainage leading to gradual ↑ in IOP and progressive vision loss
Risk factors	Family history, older age (55–70 years), Asian, hyperopia, prolonged pupillary dilation (prolonged time in a dark area, stress, medications), anterior uveitis, and lens dislocation	Risk factors include > 40 years of age, African-American ethnicity, diabetes, and myopia
History/PE	Extreme, sudden-onset eye pain, blurred vision, headache, nausea, and vomiting A hard, red eye is seen; the pupil is dilated and nonreactive to light	Should be suspected in patients > 35 years of age who need frequent lens changes and have mild headaches, visual disturbances, and impaired adaptation to darkness; usually asymptomatic until late in the clinical course Characterized by gradual loss of peripheral vision Cupping of the optic nerve head is seen on funduscopic exam (see Figure 2.10-11)
Diagnosis	Best initial test: Ocular tonometry (to measure intraocular pressure) can quickly provide additional information. Gonioscopy is the gold standard Fixed pupil and hard, red eye	Best initial test: Tonometry, ophthalmoscopic visualization of the optic nerve and cupping of optic disk, and visual field testing are most important
Treatment	A medical emergency that can cause blindness. Treatment to ↓ IOP is as follows: Eyedrops (timolol, pilocarpine) Systemic medications (oral or IV acetazolamide, IV mannitol) Laser peripheral iridotomy, which creates a hole in the peripheral iris, is curative and can be performed prophylactically Do not give any medications that cause pupillary dilation (atropine)	Treat with topical β-blockers (timolol, betaxolol) to ↓ aqueous humor production Pilocarpine to ↑ aqueous outflow Carbonic anhydrase inhibitors (acetazolamide) can also be used If medication fails, lser trabeculoplasty or a trabeculectomy can improve aqueous drainage

1 **A**

Risk factors of corneal abrasion include trauma, foreign body, and contact lens use. Use a penlight to document pupillary function and the presence/absence of a foreign body. A fluorescein exam can be diagnostic and will show a corneal staining defect.

2 **A**

This patient presentation is consistent with closed-angle glaucoma. Avoid pupil-dilating medications such as atropine, which will ↑ IOP and prevent drainage of aqueous humor.

CATARACTS

- Lens opacification resulting in obstructed passage of light. Associated with diabetes, hypertension, advanced age, and exposure to radiation.
- **Hx/PE:** Presents with loss of visual acuity and difficulty with night vision.
- **Tx:** Surgical lens removal and replacement.

AGE-RELATED MACULAR DEGENERATION

More common among white individuals, women, smokers, and those with a family history.

HISTORY/PE

- Presents with painless loss of central vision. Early signs include distortion of straight lines and loss of other aspects of fine visual acuity.
- **Atrophic ("dry") macular degeneration:** Responsible for 80% of cases. Causes gradual vision loss.
- **Exudative or neovascular ("wet") macular degeneration:** Much less common, but associated with more rapid and severe vision damage.

DIAGNOSIS

- **Atrophic ("dry") macular degeneration:** Funduscopy reveals drusen (accumulation of white/yellow extracellular material) and/or pigmentary changes.
- **Exudative or neovascular ("wet") macular degeneration:** Hemorrhage and subretinal fluid are present (see Figure 2.10-12).

TREATMENT

- **Atrophic AMD:** No treatment is currently available, although a combination of vitamins (vitamin C, vitamin E, beta-carotene, and zinc) has been found to slow disease progression. Be cautious giving high doses of vitamin E and beta-carotene to patients who smoke as there is an association of ↑ mortality rate from lung cancer in people taking high doses of these supplements.
- **Exudative AMD:**
    - VEGF inhibitors have been shown to improve vision (ranibizumab, bevacizumab) or slow visual loss (pegaptanib) in patients with exudative AMD.
    - Photodynamic therapy using a laser to selectively target retinal vessels for coagulation. May be useful in conjunction with VEGF inhibitors.

RETINAL VASCULAR OCCLUSION

Occurs in elderly patients and is often idiopathic (see Table 2.10-16).

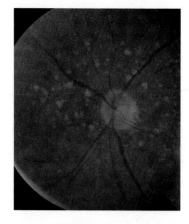

FIGURE 2.10-12. Macular degeneration with evidence of drusen and fibrosis in the macula. (Reproduced with permission from USMLE-Rx.com.)

> ### KEY FACT
>
> In the United States, macular degeneration is the leading cause of permanent bilateral visual loss in the elderly.

> ### KEY FACT
>
> Retinal detachment presents with sudden onset flashing lights and blurred vision. Patients typically describe a curtain coming down over their eye. Ophthalmoscopy shows a gray, elevated retina.

TABLE 2.10-16. Central Retinal Artery vs Central Retinal Vein Occlusion

	CENTRAL RETINAL ARTERY OCCLUSION	CENTRAL RETINAL VEIN FUNDOSCOPY
History/PE	Presents with sudden, painless, unilateral blindness; pupil is sluggishly reactive to direct light Patients present with a cherry-red spot on the fovea (blue arrow), retinal swelling (whitish appearance to the nerve fiber layer), and retinal arteries that may appear bloodless Transient occlusion is comparable to transient ischemic attack and is known as amaurosis fugax	Presents with rapid, painless vision loss of variable severity; associated with hypertension A swollen optic disc with hemorrhages, venous stasis retinal hemorrhages, cotton-wool spots, and macular edema may be seen on funduscopic exam
Treatment	Ocular massage with high-flow oxygen administration; intra-arterial thrombolysis within 8 hours	Laser photocoagulation (variable results)

Image A reproduced with permission from USMLE-Rx.com. Image B reproduced with permission from Alasil T, Rauser ME. Intravitreal bevacizumab in the treatment of neovascular glaucoma secondary to central retinal vein occlusion: a case report. *Cases J* 2009;2:176.

NOTES

OBSTETRICS

Physiology of Normal Pregnancy

THE BASICS OF PREGNANCY

The terms and concepts that follow are central to an understanding of the physiologic processes of pregnancy.

- **Gravidity:** Number of times a woman has been pregnant.
- **Parity:**
  - Number of pregnancies that led to a birth beyond 20 weeks' gestational age or an infant weighing > 500 g.
  - In prenatal assessment, TPAL expresses the number of term deliveries (T), the number of preterm deliveries (P), the number of abortuses (A), and the number of living children (L).
- **Developmental age (DA):** Number of weeks and days since fertilization; usually unknown.
- **Gestational age (GA):** The number of weeks and days measured from the first day of the last menstrual period (LMP). GA can also be determined by the following:
  - **Fundal height:** Umbilicus – 20 weeks + 1 cm/week thereafter.
  - **Fetal heart tones (Doppler):** Typically 10–12 weeks.
  - **Quickening or appreciation of fetal movement:** Occurs at 17–18 weeks at the earliest.
  - **Ultrasonography:**
    - Measures fetal crown-rump length (CRL) at 6–12 weeks.
    - Measures biparietal diameter (BPD), femur length (FL), and abdominal circumference (AC) from 13 weeks.
    - Ultrasound measurement of GA is most reliable during the first trimester.

DIAGNOSIS OF PREGNANCY

β-hCG

- The standard for diagnosing pregnancy. Can be detected in serum or urine.
- Serum hCG is more sensitive and preferred if menstrual period is < 1 week late.
- Produced by the placenta; peaks at 100,000 mIU/mL by 10 weeks' GA.
- ↓ Throughout the second trimester; levels off in the third trimester.
- hCG levels double approximately every 48 hours during early pregnancy. This is often used to diagnose ectopic pregnancy when doubling is abnormal.

Ultrasonography

- Used to confirm an intrauterine pregnancy.
- Gestational sac is visible on transvaginal ultrasonography by:
  - Five weeks' GA.
  - A β-hCG in the range of 1000–1500 mIU/mL.

NORMAL PHYSIOLOGY OF PREGNANCY

The normal physiologic changes that occur during pregnancy are graphically illustrated according to system in Figures 2.11-1 and 2.11-2.

- Low back pain is common in the third trimester, caused by ↑ pressure from the uterus and laxity of muscles and joints.

KEY FACT

A G3P1 woman is one who has had three pregnancies but only one birth beyond 20 weeks' GA and/or an infant who weighs at least 500 g.

KEY FACT

Get a quantitative serum β-hCG:
- To diagnose ectopic pregnancy and follow for resolution after treatment.
- To monitor trophoblastic disease.
- To screen for fetal aneuploidy.

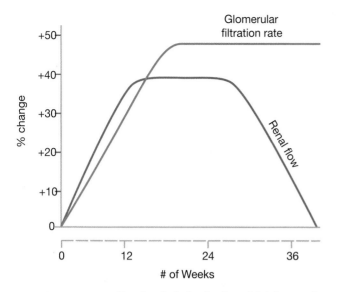

SYSTEM	PARAMETER	PATTERN
Renal	Renal Flow	Increases 25-50%
	Glomerular filtration rate	Increases early, then plateaus
Weight	Uterine weight	Increases from about 60-70g to about 900-1200g
	Body weight	Average 11-kg (25-lb) increase

FIGURE 2.11-1. **Renal and uterine/body weight changes in normal pregnancy.** (Reproduced with permission from USMLE-Rx.com.)

- Maternal failure to gain appropriate weight is associated with intrauterine growth restriction (IUGR), while excess weight gain is associated with diabetes.
- Pregnancy causes a hypercoagulable state.

Prenatal Care

The goal of prenatal care is to prevent, diagnose, and treat conditions that can lead to adverse outcomes in pregnancy. Expected weight gain, nutrition, and exercise recommendations are outlined in Table 2.11-1. See Table 2.11-2 for some important factors that can cross the placenta.

TABLE 2.11-1. **Recommendations for Standard Prenatal Care**

CATEGORY	RECOMMENDATIONS
Weight gain	Guidelines for weight gain according to prepregnancy BMI: ■ Underweight (BMI < 19.8): 12–18 kg ■ Acceptable (BMI 19.8–26.0): 11–16 kg ■ Overweight (BMI 26.1–29.0): 7–11 kg ■ Severely overweight (BMI > 29.0): 5–9 kg
Nutrition	Guidelines for nutritional supplementation: ■ An additional 100–300 kcal/day; 500 kcal/day during breastfeeding ■ Folic acid supplements ($\downarrow$ neural tube defects for all reproductive-age women) ■ Iron ■ Calcium Additional guidelines for complete vegetarians: ■ Vitamin D ■ Vitamin B$_{12}$
Exercise	Thirty minutes of moderate exercise daily, while avoiding contact sports

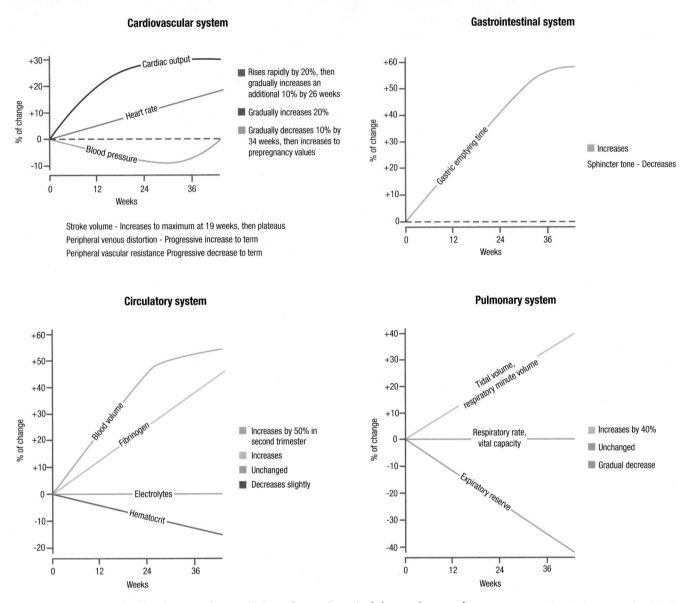

FIGURE 2.11-2. **Cardiopulmonary, hematologic, and gastrointestinal changes in normal pregnancy.** (Reproduced with permission from USMLE-Rx.com.)

TABLE 2.11-2. **Factors That Can Cross the Placenta**

IMMUNOGLOBULINS	ORGANISMS	DRUGS
IgG	*Toxoplasma gondii*	See the teratology discussion later
	Rubella	
	HIV	
	Varicella-zoster virus	
	CMV	
	Enteroviruses	
	Treponema pallidum	
	Listeria monocytogenes	
	Parvovirus B19	

Prenatal Diagnostic Testing

Table 2.11-3 outlines a typical prenatal diagnostic testing schedule by week. The sections that follow describe each recommended screening modality.

QUAD SCREENING

Quad screening consists of four elements (see Table 2.11-4): maternal serum α-fetoprotein (MSAFP), inhibin A, estriol, and β-hCG.

- **MSAFP:** Produced by the fetus and enters the maternal circulation. Results are reported as multiples of the median (MoMs).
    - Measurement results depend on accurate gestational dating. Multiple gestations and uterine leiomyomata (fibroids) may cause size/date discrepancy.
    - MSAFP is rarely tested alone, as quad screening has ↑ sensitivity for detecting chromosomal abnormalities.

TABLE 2.11-3. Prenatal Diagnostic Testing Schedule

WEEKS	PRENATAL DIAGNOSTIC TESTING
Prenatal visits	Weeks 0–28: Every 4 weeks Weeks 29–35: Every 2 weeks Weeks 36–birth: Every week
Initial visit	Heme: CBC, Rh factor, type and screen Infectious disease: UA and culture, rubella antibody titer, HBsAg, RPR/VDRL, cervical gonorrhea and chlamydia, PPD, HIV, TB testing (or MTB), Pap smear (to check for dysplasia); consider HCV and varicella based on history If indicated: HbA$_{1c}$, sickle cell screening Discuss genetic screening: Tay-Sachs disease, cystic fibrosis, Spinal muscular atrophy
9–14 weeks	Offer PAPP-A + nuchal translucency (NT) or NIPT (noninvasive prenatal testing) or ± Chorionic villus sampling (CVS)
15–22 weeks	Offer maternal serum α-fetoprotein (MSAFP) or quad screen (AFP, estriol, β-hCG, and inhibin A) ± amniocentesis
18–20 weeks	Ultrasonography for full anatomic screen
24–28 weeks	One-hour glucose challenge test for gestational diabetes screen
28–30 weeks	RhoGAM for Rh⊖ women (after antibody screen) RhoGAM should be administered to any unsensitized Rh⊖ woman during any occasion of fetal-maternal blood mixing (eg, spontaneous abortion (SAB), placental abruption) even if < 28 weeks' gestation
35–37 weeks	GBS culture; repeat CBC
34–40 weeks	In high-risk patients, cervical chlamydia and gonorrhea cultures, HIV, RPR

TABLE 2.11-4. Quad Screening

	MSAFP	ESTRIOL	INHIBIN A	β-HCG
Trisomy 18	↓	↓	↓	↓
Trisomy 21	↓	↓	↑	↑

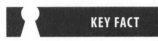

- ↑ **MSAFP** (> 2.5 MoMs) is associated with the following:
  - Open neural tube defects (anencephaly, spina bifida).
  - Abdominal wall defects (gastroschisis, omphalocele).
  - Multiple gestation.
  - Incorrect gestational dating.
  - Fetal death.
  - Placental abnormalities (eg, placental abruption).
- ↓ **MSAFP** (< 0.5 MoM) is associated with the following:
  - Trisomy 21 and 18.
  - Fetal demise.
  - Incorrect gestational dating.

KEY FACT

Still **UNDER**age at 18: trisomy **18** = ↓ AFP, ↓ estriol, ↓ β-hCG, ↓ inhibin A.

NUCHAL TRANSLUCENCY

- Recommended at weeks 9–14.
- PAPP-A + nuchal translucency + free β-hCG can detect ~ 91% of cases of Down syndrome and ~ 95% of cases of trisomy 18.
- Advantages:
  - A screen of pregnant women (> 35 years of age).
  - Available earlier than CVS and less invasive than CVS (see later).

KEY FACT

2 up, 2 down: trisomy **21** = ↓ AFP, ↓ estriol, ↑ β-hCG, ↑ inhibin A.

CHORIONIC VILLUS SAMPLING

Table 2.11-5 outlines the relative advantages and disadvantages of CVS and amniocentesis (see Figure 2.11-3).

TABLE 2.11-5. Prenatal Screening for Fetal Genetic Abnormalities

VARIABLE	CELL-FREE FETAL DNA	CVS	AMNIOCENTESIS
GA	10 weeks	10–12 weeks	15–20 weeks
Procedure	Isolation of fetal DNA from blood sample obtained from mother	Transcervical or transabdominal aspiration of placental tissue	Transabdominal aspiration of amniotic fluid using an ultrasound-guided needle
Advantages	Noninvasive	Genetically diagnostic Available at an earlier GA	Genetically diagnostic
Disadvantages	May be limited because of low concentration of fetal DNA in maternal circulation	Risk for fetal loss is relatively high (1%) Cannot detect open neural tube defects Limb defects are associated with CVS at < 9 weeks	Premature rupture of membranes (PROM), chorioamnionitis, fetal-maternal hemorrhage

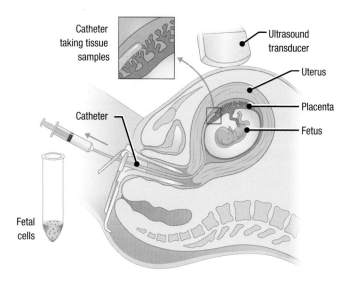

FIGURE 2.11-3. **Chorionic villus sampling.** (Reproduced with permission from USMLE-Rx.com.)

AMNIOCENTESIS

Indicated for the following:

- Women > 35 years of age at the time of delivery.
- Abnormal nuchal translucency, abnormal quad screen, or abnormal non-invasive prenatal testing.
- Rh-sensitized pregnancy to obtain fetal blood type or to detect fetal hemolysis.
- Evaluation of fetal lung maturity. Lecithin-to-sphingomyelin ratio ≥ 2.5 or to presence of phosphatidylglycerol (performed during the third trimester) indicates lung maturity.

Teratology

Major defects are apparent in about 3% of births and in roughly 4.5% of children by 5 years of age. Table 2.11-6 outlines common teratogenic agents.

Maternal-Fetal Infections

Can occur at any time during pregnancy, labor, and delivery. Common sequela include the following:

- Premature delivery.
- CNS abnormalities.
- Anemia.
- Jaundice.
- Hepatosplenomegaly.
- Growth restriction.

The most common pathogens involved can be remembered through use of the **ToRCHeS** mnemonic (see Table 2.11-7).

MNEMONIC

TORCHeS *pathogens—*

Toxoplasmosis
Other[a]
Rubella
CMV
Herpes simplex virus
HIV
Syphilis
[a]Parvovirus, varicella, *Listeria,* TB, malaria, fungi.

KEY FACT

Pregnant women should not change a cat's litterbox to prevent exposure to toxoplasmosis.

TABLE 2.11-6. **Common Teratogenic Agents and Their Associated Defects**

Drugs and Chemicals	Defects
ACEIs	Fetal renal tubular dysplasia and neonatal renal failure, oligohydramnios, IUGR, lack of cranial ossification
Alcohol	Fetal alcohol syndrome (growth restriction before and after birth, mental retardation, midfacial hypoplasia, smooth philtrum, renal and cardiac defects) Consumption of > 6 drinks per day is associated with a 40% risk for fetal alcohol syndrome
Amphetamines	Preterm delivery, placental abruption, preeclampsia, IUGR, fetal demise
Androgens	Virilization of female fetuses; advanced genital development in male fetuses. Most commonly caused by maternal luteomas
Carbamazepine	Neural tube defects, fingernail hypoplasia, microcephaly, developmental delay, IUGR
Cocaine	Bowel atresias; congenital malformations of the heart, limbs, face, and GU tract; microcephaly; IUGR; cerebral infarctions
DES	Clear cell adenocarcinoma of the vagina or cervix, vaginal adenosis, abnormalities of the cervix and uterus or testes, possible infertility
Lead	↑ SAB rate; stillbirth
Lithium	Congenital heart disease (Ebstein anomaly)
Methotrexate	↑ SAB rate
Organic mercury	Cerebral atrophy, microcephaly, mental retardation, spasticity, seizures, blindness
Phenytoin	IUGR, mental retardation, microcephaly, dysmorphic craniofacial features, cardiac defects, fingernail hypoplasia
Radiation	Microcephaly, mental retardation Medical diagnostic radiation delivering < 0.05 Gy to the fetus has no teratogenic risk
Streptomycin and kanamycin	Hearing loss; CN VIII damage
Tetracycline	Permanent yellow-brown discoloration of deciduous teeth; hypoplasia of tooth enamel
Thalidomide	Bilateral limb deficiencies, anotia and microtia, cardiac and GI anomalies
Trimethadione and paramethadione	Cleft lip or cleft palate, cardiac defects, microcephaly, mental retardation
Valproic acid	Neural tube defects (spina bifida); minor craniofacial defects
Vitamin A and derivatives	↑ SAB rate, microtia, thymic agenesis, cardiovascular defects, craniofacial dysmorphism, microphthalmia, cleft lip or cleft palate, mental retardation
Warfarin (wages war on the fetus)	Nasal hypoplasia and stippled bone epiphyses, developmental delay, IUGR, ophthalmologic abnormalities

TABLE 2.11-7.   **Diagnosis and Treatment of Common Congenital Infections**

Disease	Transmission	Symptoms	Diagnosis	Treatment	Prevention
Toxoplasmosis	Transplacental; 1° infection via consumption of raw meat or contact with cat feces	Hydrocephalus Intracranial calcifications Chorioretinitis Ring-enhancing lesions on MRI	Serologic testing	Pyrimethamine + sulfadiazine	Avoid exposure to cat feces or uncooked meat during pregnancy; spiramycin prophylaxis for the third trimester
Rubella	Transplacental in the first trimester	Purpuric "blueberry muffin" rash Cataracts Mental retardation Hearing loss PDA	Serologic testing	Symptomatic	Immunize before pregnancy; vaccinate the mother after delivery if serologic titers remain ⊖
CMV	Primarily transplacental	Petechial rash Periventricular calcifications	Urine culture; PCR of amniotic fluid	Postpartum ganciclovir	N/A
HSV	Intrapartum transmission if the mother has active lesions; transplacental transmission is rare	Skin, eye, and mouth infections Life-threatening CNS/systemic infection	Serologic testing	Acyclovir	Perform a C-section if lesions are present at delivery
HIV	In utero, at delivery, or via breast milk	Often asymptomatic Failure to thrive Bacterial infections ↑ Incidence of upper and lower respiratory diseases	ELISA, Western blot	HAART	AZT or nevirapine in pregnant women with HIV; perform elective C-section if viral load is > 1000 Treat infants with prophylactic AZT; avoid breastfeeding
Syphilis	Intrapartum; transplacental transmission is possible	Maculopapular skin rash Lymphadenopathy Hepatomegaly "Snuffles": mucopurulent rhinitis Osteitis Late congenital syphilis: Saber shins Saddle nose CNS involvement Hutchinson triad: peg-shaped central incisors, deafness, interstitial keratitis	Dark-field microscopy, VDRL/RPR, FTA-ABS	Penicillin (if allergic, should desensitize and give penicillin)	Penicillin in pregnant women who test ⊕

Spontaneous Abortion

The loss of products of conception (POC) before the 20th week of pregnancy. More than 80% of cases occur in the first trimester. Risk factors are as follows:

- **Chromosomal abnormalities:** A factor in approximately 50% of SABs in the first trimester, 20–30% in second-trimester losses, and 5–10% in third-trimester losses.
- **Maternal factors:**
  - **Inherited thrombophilias:** Factor V Leiden, prothrombin, antithrombin, proteins C and S, methylene tetrahydrofolate reductase (hyperhomocysteinemia).
  - **Immunologic issues:** Antiphospholipid antibodies; alloimmune factors.
  - **Anatomic issues:** Uterine and cervical abnormalities, incompetent cervix, cervical conization or loop electrosurgical excision procedure (LEEP), cervical injury, DES exposure.
  - **Endocrinologic issues:** Diabetes mellitus (DM), hypothyroidism, progesterone deficiency.
  - **Genetics:** Osteogenesis imperfecta type II, aneuploidy incompatible with life (most common Trisomy 16).
    - Osteogenesis imperfecta type II is severe and lethal. Infants present with multiple fractures and die in utero or shortly after birth.
  - **Other:** Maternal trauma, ↑ maternal age, infection, dietary deficiencies.
- **Environmental factors:** Tobacco, alcohol, excessive caffeine (> 500 mg/day), toxins, drugs, radiation.
- **Fetal factors:** Anatomic malformation.
- **Recurrent SAB:** Two or more consecutive SABs or three SABs in 1 year, causes dependent on timing. To determine possible causes, karyotype both parents, perform work-up on mother for hypercoagulability, evaluate uterine anatomy.
  - **Early (< 12 weeks):** Chromosomal abnormalities likely cause.
  - **Late (12–20 weeks):** Hypercoagulable states (eg, antiphospholipid syndrome, SLE, factor V Leiden, protein S deficiency).

If antiphospholipid antibodies are detected, false-positive VDRL and falsely prolonged PTT may be seen. Provide low-molecular-weight heparin and low-dose aspirin for prophylaxis against recurrent SAB.

HISTORY/PE
See Table 2.11-8 for types of SAB.

DIAGNOSIS

- Diagnosis by clinical presentation and physical exam.
- **Nonviable pregnancy:** Gestational sac > 25 mm without a fetal pole or absence of fetal cardiac activity when CRL > 7 mm on transvaginal ultrasonography.
- **Best initial test:** Ultrasonography can identify the following:
  - Gestational sac 5–6 weeks from the LMP.
  - Fetal pole at 6 weeks.
  - Fetal cardiac activity at 6–7 weeks.
- **Next best test:** Serum β-hCG.

TREATMENT

- See Table 2.11-8 for treatment specific to the type of SAB.
- Administer RhoGAM if the mother is Rh ⊖.

KEY FACT

To remember the cervical exam during Inevitable and Incomplete SABs:

- The **I's** (Inevitable and Incomplete) are **Open**.

TABLE 2.11-8. Types of SAB

Type	Symptoms/Signs	Diagnosis	Treatment
Complete	Bleeding and cramping stopped. POC expulsion	Closed os Ultrasonography shows no POC	None
Threatened	Uterine bleeding ± abdominal pain (often painless) No POC expulsion	Closed os + intact membranes + fetal cardiac motion on ultrasonography	Pelvic rest for 24–48 hours and follow-up ultrasonography to assess viability of fetus
Incomplete	Partial POC expulsion; bleeding/mild cramping Visible tissue on exam	Open os. POC present on ultrasonography	Manual uterine aspiration (MUA) if < 12 weeks or D&C; may also use misoprostol or expectant management in inevitable and missed SAB
Inevitable	Uterine bleeding and cramps No POC expulsion	Open os ± rupture of membranes (ROM) POC present on ultrasonography	
Missed	Asymptomatic ± cramping No bleeding	Closed os No fetal cardiac activity; POC present on ultrasonography	
Septic	Foul-smelling discharge, abdominal pain, fever, and cervical motion tenderness; ± POC expulsion Maternal mortality is 10–15%	Hypotension, hypothermia, ↑ WBC count Blood cultures	MUA or D&C and IV antibiotics
Intrauterine fetal demise	Absence of fetal cardiac activity > 20 weeks GA	Uterus small for GA; no fetal heart tones or movement on ultrasonography	If < 24 weeks, perform D&E If > 24 weeks, induce labor within 1–2 weeks based on patient preference Do NOT perform C-section, even for breech presentation Offer autopsy to attempt to determine cause of death

Elective Termination of Pregnancy

It has been estimated that 50% of all pregnancies in the United States are unintended. Some 25% of all pregnancies end in elective abortion. Options for elective abortion depend on GA and patient preference (see Table 2.11-9).

If fever, vomiting, purulent discharge, and/or hemodynamic instability are seen after an elective abortion, septic abortion should be suspected. This is a medical emergency that requires broad-spectrum antibiotics and immediate surgery to remove infected tissue.

Q

A 23-year-old G1P0 woman at 15 weeks' GA presents with abdominal pain and mild bleeding from the cervix. On pelvic exam, some POC are found to be present in the vaginal vault. What test is necessary to determine the next step in management?

TABLE 2.11-9. **Elective Termination of Pregnancy**

TRIMESTER	PROCEDURE	TIMING
First (90% ABs)	Medical management:	Up to:
	▪ Oral mifepristone (low dose) + oral/vaginal misoprostol	49 days' GA
	▪ IM/oral methotrexate + oral/vaginal misoprostol	49 days' GA
	▪ Vaginal or sublingual or buccal misoprostol (high dose), repeated up to three times	59 days' GA
	Surgical management:	13 weeks' GA
	▪ Manual uterine aspiration	
	▪ D&C with vacuum aspiration	
Second (10% ABs)	Obstetric management: Induction of labor (typically with prostaglandins, amniotomy, and oxytocin)	13–24 weeks' GA (depending on state laws)
	Surgical management: D&C	Same as above

Normal Labor and Delivery

OBSTETRIC EXAM

- Leopold maneuvers are used to determine fetal lie (longitudinal or transverse) and, if possible, fetal presentation (breech or cephalic).
- **Cervical exam:**
  - Evaluate dilation, effacement, station, cervical position, and cervical consistency.
  - Confirm or determine fetal presentation.
  - Determine fetal position through palpation of the fetal sutures and fontanelles.
  - Conduct a sterile speculum exam if rupture of membranes (ROM) is suspected.
  - Determine station, or engagement of the fetal head relative to a line through the ischial spines of the maternal pelvis. $\ominus$ Station = fetal head superior to this line; $\oplus$ station = fetal head inferior to this line.
- **Labor:** Uterine contractions plus cervical change.
- Table 2.11-10 depicts the normal stages of labor.
- **Braxton-Hicks contractions:**
  - Also known as "false labor."
  - Mild, irregular contractions without cervical change.
  - Management involves reassurance and normal surveillance after ruling out true labor.
- **Oxytocin side effects:**
  - Hyponatremia.
  - Tachysystole.
  - Hypotension.

FETAL HEART RATE MONITORING

- Monitoring can be performed with an electrode attached to the fetal scalp (a method that yields more precise results), or external monitoring can be conducted using Doppler ultrasound (a less invasive option).

A

Ultrasonography should be performed to determine if all the POC have been expelled (ie, if the uterus is empty). If so, it is a complete abortion and the POC should be sent to pathology to confirm fetal tissue with no other treatment. If POC are retained, it is an incomplete abortion, and manual uterine aspiration or D&C is indicated. Medical management with misoprostol may also be appropriate.

TABLE 2.11-10.   Stages of Labor

STAGE		STARTS/ENDS	DURATION		COMMENTS
			NULLIPAROUS	MULTIPAROUS	
First					
	Latent	Onset of labor to 6 cm dilation	≤ 20 h	≤ 14 h	Prolongation seen with excessive sedation/hypotonic uterine contractions
	Active	6 cm to complete cervical dilation (10 cm)	4–6 h (1.2 cm/hour)	2–3 h (1.5 cm/h)	Prolongation seen with cephalopelvic disproportion
Second		Complete cervical dilation to delivery of infant	0.5–3.0 h	5–30 minutes	Neonate goes through all cardinal movements of delivery
Third		Delivery of infant to delivery of placenta	0–0.5 h	0–0.5 h	Uterus contracts and placenta separates to establish hemostasis

- Continuous electronic fetal heart rate (FHR) monitoring has not been shown to be more effective than appropriate intermittent monitoring in low-risk patients.

Recommendations for FHR Monitoring

- **In low-risk pregnancies,** review FHR tracings:
  - First stage of labor—every 30 minutes.
  - Second stage of labor—every 15 minutes.
- **In high-risk pregnancies,** review FHR tracings:
  - First stage of labor—every 15 minutes.
  - Second stage of labor—every 5 minutes.

Components of FHR Evaluation

- **Rate (normal = 110–160 bpm):**
  - **FHR < 110 bpm:** Bradycardia. Can be caused by congenital heart malformations or by severe hypoxia (2° to uterine hyperstimulation, cord prolapse, or rapid fetal descent).
  - **FHR > 160 bpm:** Tachycardia. Causes include hypoxia, maternal fever, and fetal anemia.
- **Variability:** See Figures 2.11-4 and 2.11-5.
  - **Absent variability:** Indicates severe fetal acidemia.
  - **Minimal variability:** < 6 bpm. Indicates fetal hypoxia or the effects of opioids, magnesium, or sleep cycle.
  - **Normal variability:** 6–25 bpm.
  - **Marked variability:** > 25 bpm. May indicate fetal hypoxia; may occur before a ↓ in variability.
  - **Sinusoidal variability:** Points to serious fetal anemia; a pseudosinusoidal pattern may also occur during maternal meperidine use.
- **Accelerations:** Onset of an ↑ in FHR > 15 beats above baseline to a peak in < 30 seconds. Reassuring because they indicate proper function fetal autonomic nervous system.
- **Decelerations:** See Table 2.11-11.

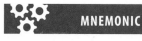

MNEMONIC

VEaL CHoP

Variable deceleration = **C**ord compression
Early deceleration = **H**ead compression
Late deceleration = **P**lacental insufficiency

A 17-year-old G1P0 girl with a history of genital HSV presents at 37 weeks in labor. What is the appropriate management of the patient at delivery?

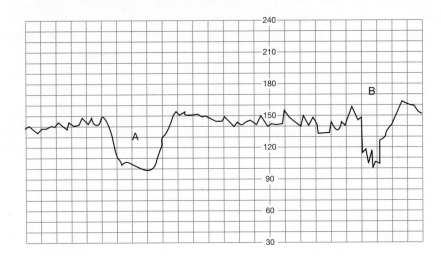

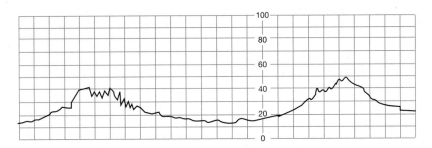

FIGURE 2.11-4. **Varying (variable) fetal heart rate decelerations.**

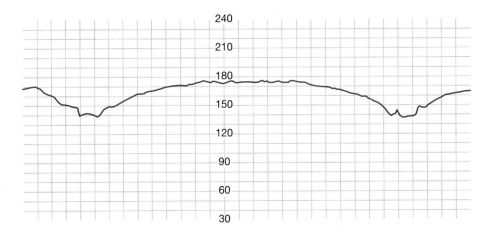

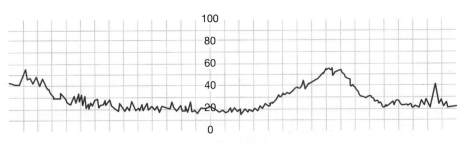

FIGURE 2.11-5. **Late fetal heart rate decelerations.** Late decelerations caused by utero-placental insufficiency resulting from placental abruption. Immediate C-section delivery was performed. Umbilical artery pH was 7.05, and Po$_2$ was 11 mm Hg. (Reproduced with permission from USMLE-Rx.com.)

A

If the patient has any active lesions at the time of delivery, perform a C-section.

TABLE 2.11-11. **Types of Fetal Deceleration**

TYPE	DESCRIPTION	ETIOLOGY	SCHEMATIC
Early	A visually apparent, gradual (onset to nadir in > 30 seconds) ↓ in FHR with a return to baseline that mirrors the uterine contraction	Head compression from the uterine contraction (normal)	
Late	A visually apparent, gradual (onset to nadir in > 30 seconds) ↓ in FHR with return to baseline whose onset, nadir, and recovery occur after the beginning, peak, and end of uterine contraction, respectively	Uteroplacental insufficiency and fetal hypoxemia	
Variable	An abrupt (onset to nadir in < 30 seconds), visually apparent ↓ in FHR 15 bpm below baseline lasting ≥ 15 seconds but < 2 minutes	Umbilical cord compression	

Reproduced with permission from Cunningham FC, et al. *Williams Obstetrics,* 23rd ed. New York, NY: McGraw-Hill; 2010.

ANTEPARTUM FETAL SURVEILLANCE

In general, antepartum fetal surveillance is used in pregnancies in which the risk for antepartum fetal demise is ↑. Testing is initiated in most at-risk patients at 32–34 weeks (or 26–28 weeks if there are multiple worrisome risk factors present). The following assessments are made:

- **Fetal movement assessment:**
  - Assessed by the mother as the number of fetal movements over 1 hour.
  - On average, it takes 2 hours for a mother to obtain 10 fetal movements.

TABLE 2.11-12. **Nonstress Test Interpretation**

Reactive NST (normal response)	Two accelerations lasting at least 15 seconds over 20-minute period (see Figure 2.11-6): ■ ≥ 15 bpm above baseline if > 32 weeks GA ■ ≥ 10 bpm above baseline if < 32 weeks GA
Nonreactive NST	Insufficient accelerations over a 40-minute period Perform further tests (eg, a biophysical profile, or BPP) Lack of FHR accelerations may occur with any of the following: ■ Fetal sleeping (most common) ■ GA < 32 weeks ■ Fetal CNS anomalies ■ Maternal sedative or narcotic administration

- Maternal reports of ↓ fetal movements should be evaluated by means of the following tests:
- **Nonstress test (NST):**
  - Performed with the mother resting in the lateral tilt position (to prevent supine hypotension).
  - FHR is monitored externally by Doppler along with a tocodynamometer to detect uterine contractions. Acoustic stimulation may be used.
  - See Table 2.11-12 for NST interpretation.
- **Contraction stress test (CST):**
  - Performed in the lateral recumbent position.
  - FHR is monitored during spontaneous or induced (via nipple stimulation or oxytocin) contractions.
  - Reactivity is determined from fetal heart monitoring, as with the NST.
  - Contraindicated in women with preterm membrane rupture or known placenta previa; those with a history of uterine surgery; and those who are at high risk for preterm labor.
  - See Table 2.11-13 for CST interpretation.

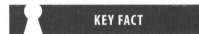

KEY FACT

A ⊖ CST is good; a ⊕ one is bad.

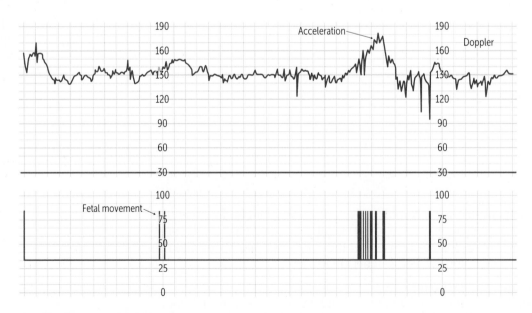

FIGURE 2.11-6. **Reactive nonstress test.** (Reproduced with permission from USMLE-Rx.com.)

TABLE 2.11-13. **Contraction Stress Test Interpretation**

Positive CST	Late decelerations following 50% or more of contractions in a 10-minute window. Raises concerns about fetal compromise. Delivery is warranted
Negative CST	No late or significant variable decelerations within 10 minutes and at least three contractions
Equivocal CST	Intermittent late decelerations or significant variable decelerations

- **Biophysical profile (BPP):** Uses real-time ultrasonography to assign a score of 2 (normal) or 0 (abnormal) to five parameters: fetal tone, breathing, movement, amniotic fluid volume, and NST. Scoring is as follows:
  - **8–10:** Reassuring for fetal well-being.
  - **6:** Considered equivocal. Term pregnancies are usually delivered with this profile.
  - **0–4:** Extremely worrisome for fetal asphyxia; strong consideration should be given to immediate delivery if no other explanation is found.
  - Pregnancies > 41 weeks are at risk for uteroplacental insufficiency and oligohydramnios. Perform biophysical profile at 41 weeks to screen for fetal hypoxia.
- **Amniotic fluid index (AFI):** Sum of the measurements of the deepest cord-free amniotic fluid measured in each of the abdominal quadrants.
- **Modified biophysical profile (mBPP):**
  - NST + AFI.
  - A normal test consists of a reactive NST and an AFI > 5 cm.
- **Umbilical artery Doppler velocimetry:**
  - Used only when IUGR is suspected.
  - With IUGR, there is a reduction and even a reversal of umbilical artery diastolic flow.
- Oligohydramnios (AFI < 5 cm) always warrants further work-up.

MNEMONIC

When performing a BPP—

Test the Baby, MAN!

Fetal **T**one
Fetal **B**reathing
Fetal **M**ovement
Amniotic fluid volume
Nonstress test

OBSTETRIC ANALGESIA AND ANESTHESIA

- Uterine contractions and cervical dilation result in visceral pain (T10–L1).
- Descent of the fetal head and pressure on the vagina and perineum result in somatic pain (pudendal nerve, S2–S4).
- In the absence of a medical contraindication, maternal request is a sufficient medical indication for pain relief during labor.
  - Transient hypotension is a common complication and does not require treatment unless there are signs of vasomotor shock (caused by inadvertent injection of medication into dural space).
  - Epidural anesthesia can cause postpartum urinary retention. Urethral catheterization is diagnostic and therapeutic.
- Absolute contraindications to regional anesthesia (epidural, spinal, or combination) include the following:
  - Refractory maternal hypotension.
  - Maternal coagulopathy.
  - Maternal use of a once-daily dose of low-molecular-weight heparin within 12 hours.
  - Untreated maternal bacteremia.
  - Skin infection over the site of needle placement.
  - ↑ ICP caused by a mass lesion.

KEY FACT

If "morning sickness" persists after the first trimester, think hyperemesis gravidarum.

KEY FACT

Important to rule out trophoblastic disease with ultrasound in a pregnant patient who presents with severe nausea and vomiting.

Medical Complications of Pregnancy

HYPEREMESIS GRAVIDARUM

Persistent vomiting not related to other causes, acute starvation (usually large ketonuria), and weight loss (usually at least a 5% ↓ from prepregnancy weight).

- More common in first pregnancies, multiple gestations, and molar pregnancies.
- ↑ β-hCG and ↑ estradiol have been implicated in its pathophysiology.

HISTORY/PE

Distinguish from "morning sickness" (which usually starts 4–7 weeks of pregnancy and resolves < 16 weeks, but can occur throughout pregnancy), acid reflux, gastroenteritis, hyperthyroidism, and neurologic conditions.

DIAGNOSIS

- Clinical diagnosis.
- **Best initial test:** Ultrasonography; evaluate for trophoblastic disease or multiple gestation.
- Evaluate for electrolyte abnormalities, abnormal liver enzymes, amylase, and lipase.
- Wernicke encephalopathy from B_1 deficiency may be present in severe cases. Look for gait ataxia and oculomotor dysfunction.

TREATMENT

- **Best initial treatment:**
  - Dietary changes and doxylamine-pyridoxine.
  - If no response, discontinue doxylamine-pyridoxine and add metoclopramide, promethazine, or prochlorperazine.
  - Further add ondansetron if vomiting is not resolved.
- If dehydrated, administer IV fluids, IV nutritional supplementation, and ondansetron IV.

DIABETES IN PREGNANCY

Diabetes in pregnancy is divided into the following two categories:

- **Gestational diabetes mellitus (GDM):** Onset occurs during pregnancy.
- **Pregestational diabetes mellitus:** Onset occurs before pregnancy. If the woman has risk factors for DM, screen with fasting glucose or HbA_{1c}; eg, BMI > 25 kg/m² (> 23 kg/m² for Asians), first-degree relative with DM, high-risk ethnicity (African-American, Asian, Hispanic, Pacific Islander, Native American), polycystic ovarian syndrome, prior delivery of baby > 4.1 kg (9 lb) or diagnosis of GDM, hypertension or on treatment for hypertension, previous HbA_{1c} > 5.7% or impaired glucose tolerance or impaired fasting glucose, or HDL-C < 35 mg/dL or triglycerides > 250 mg/dL.

Gestational Diabetes Mellitus

Carbohydrate intolerance of variable severity that is first diagnosed during pregnancy. Occurs in 3–5% of all pregnancies, and is usually diagnosed in the third trimester (24–28 weeks).

HISTORY/PE

- Typically asymptomatic.
- May present with edema, polyhydramnios, or a large-for-gestational-age infant (> 90th percentile).

DIAGNOSIS

- **Best initial test:** Screen with a 1-hour 50-g glucose challenge test.
    - Venous plasma glucose is measured 1 hour later.
    - Performed at 24–28 weeks.
    - Values ≥ 140 mg/dL are considered abnormal.
- Confirm with an oral 3-hour (100-g) glucose tolerance test (**next test if ⊕ screening test**) showing any two of the following:
    - Fasting: > 95 mg/dL.
    - 1 hour: > 180 mg/dL.
    - 2 hours: > 155 mg/dL.
    - 3 hours: > 140 mg/dL.

TREATMENT

- **Mother:**
    - **Best initial treatment:** American Diabetes Association (ADA) diet, regular exercise, and strict glucose monitoring (four times per day).
    - Add insulin if dietary control is insufficient. Tight maternal glucose control (fasting ≤ 95 mg/dL; 1 hour postprandial ≤ 140 mg/dL; 2-hour postprandial ≤ 120 mg/dL) improves outcomes.
    - Give intrapartum insulin and dextrose to maintain tight control during delivery.
- **Fetus:**
    - Obtain periodic ultrasonography and NSTs to assess fetal growth and well-being.
    - It is recommended to induce labor at 39–40 weeks in patients with gestational diabetes controlled on insulin or an oral hypoglycemic agent.

KEY FACT

Keys to the management of gestational diabetes: (1) ADA diet; (2) insulin if needed; (3) ultrasonography for fetal growth; and (4) NST beginning at 34 weeks if requiring insulin or an oral hypoglycemic.

COMPLICATIONS

More than 50% of patients go on to develop glucose intolerance and/or type 2 DM later in life. At 6–12 weeks postpartum, screen for DM (75 g 2-hour GTT) and repeat testing every 3 years if normal results.

Pregestational Diabetes and Pregnancy

Observed in 1% of all pregnancies. Insulin requirements may ↑ as much as threefold. Poorly controlled DM is associated with an ↑ risk for congenital malformations, fetal loss, and maternal/fetal morbidity during labor and delivery.

KEY FACT

Greater than 8, investigate! If HbA$_{1c}$ is > 8%, look for congenital abnormalities.

TREATMENT

- **Mother:**
    - Renal, ophthalmologic, neural tube, and cardiac evaluation to assess for end-organ damage.
    - **Best initial treatment:** Lifestyle modification with diet and exercise. Add insulin therapy if poor response.
    - Strict glucose control is important to minimize fetal defects.
        - Fasting morning: ≤ 95 mg/dL.
        - 1-hour postprandial: < 140 mg/dL.
        - 2-hour postprandial: < 120 mg/dL.
        - Overnight glucose: 60–99 mg/dL.

KEY FACT

If UA before 20 weeks reveals glycosuria, think pregestational diabetes.

KEY FACT

Hyperglycemia in the first trimester suggests preexisting diabetes and should be managed as pregestational diabetes.

- **Delivery and postpartum:**
  - Maintain normoglycemia (80–100 mg/dL) during labor with an IV insulin drip and hourly glucose measurements.
  - Consider delivery in the setting of poor maternal glucose control, preeclampsia, macrosomia, or evidence of fetal lung maturity.
  - Consider C-section delivery in the setting of an estimated fetal weight (EFW) > 4500 g.
  - Encourage breastfeeding with an appropriate ↑ in caloric intake.
- **Fetus:**
  - **16–24 weeks:**
    - Quad screen for developmental anomalies (16–18 weeks).
    - Ultrasonography to determine fetal age and growth (18–20 weeks).
    - Fetal echo to evaluate for cardiac anomalies (22–24 weeks).
  - **32–34 weeks:**
    - Close fetal surveillance (eg, NST, CST, BPP). (If poor glucose control or small vessel disease, start at 26 weeks).
    - Admit if maternal DM has been poorly controlled or fetal parameters are a concern.
    - Serial ultrasonograms for fetal growth.

COMPLICATIONS

See Table 2.11-14.

GESTATIONAL AND CHRONIC HYPERTENSION

Defined as follows:

- **Gestational hypertension:**
  - Idiopathic hypertension (systolic BP > 140 mmHg or diastolic BP > 90 mmHg measured twice > 4 hours apart) without significant proteinuria (< 300 mg/L).
  - Develops at > 20 weeks GA.
  - As many as 25% of patients may go on to develop preeclampsia.
  - Must normalize within 12 weeks after pregnancy.
- **Chronic hypertension:**
  - Presents before conception or at < 20 weeks GA.
  - If increased BP persists for > 12 weeks postpartum.
  - Up to one-third of patients may develop superimposed preeclampsia.

TABLE 2.11-14. Complications of Pregestational Diabetes Mellitus

MATERNAL COMPLICATIONS	FETAL COMPLICATIONS
DKA (type 1) or hyperglycemic hyperosmolar nonketotic coma (type 2)	Macrosomia or IUGR
	Cardiac and renal defects
Preeclampsia/eclampsia	Neural tube defects (eg, sacral agenesis)
Cephalopelvic disproportion (from macrosomia) and need for C-section	Hypocalcemia
	Polycythemia
Preterm labor	Hyperbilirubinemia
Infection	Hypoglycemia from hyperinsulinemia
Polyhydramnios	RDS
Postpartum hemorrhage	Birth injury (eg, shoulder dystocia)
Maternal mortality	Perinatal mortality

TREATMENT

- Monitor BP closely.
- **Best initial treatment:** Treat with appropriate antihypertensives (eg, methyldopa, labetalol, nifedipine).
- If systolic BP > 160 mm Hg or diastolic BP > 110 mm Hg, this is a hypertensive crisis. Treat with labetalol or hydralazine or nifedipine because of short onset of action.
- Do not give angiotensin-converting enzyme inhibitors (ACEIs) or diuretics.
  - ACEIs are known to lead to uterine ischemia.
  - Diuretics can aggravate low plasma volume to the point of uterine ischemia.

COMPLICATIONS

Similar to those of preeclampsia (see later).

PREECLAMPSIA

- New-onset hypertension (systolic BP ≥ 140 mm Hg or diastolic BP ≥ 90 mm Hg) and proteinuria (> 300 mg of protein in a 24-hour period or elevated urine or protein/creatinine ratio of 0.3 or more) occurring at > 20 weeks GA.
- Or new-onset hypertension with new onset of any of the following (with or without proteinuria):
  - Platelet count < 100,000/μL.
  - Serum creatinine > 1.1 mg/dL or doubling of creatinine concentration in the absence of other renal disease.
  - Liver transaminases at least twice the upper limit of normal.
  - Pulmonary edema.
  - Cerebral or visual symptoms.
- **HELLP syndrome:** A variant of preeclampsia with a poor prognosis.
  - Consists of hemolytic anemia, elevated liver enzymes, and low platelets (see mnemonic).
  - The etiology is unknown, but clinical manifestations are explained by vasospasm leading to distention of hepatic capsule, hemorrhage, and organ necrosis.
  - Risk factors include nulliparity, African-American ethnicity, extremes of age (< 20 or > 35 years), multiple gestation, molar pregnancy, renal disease (caused by SLE or type 1 DM), a family history of preeclampsia, and chronic hypertension.

HISTORY/PE

See Table 2.11-15 for the signs and symptoms of preeclampsia.

TREATMENT

- Delivery of the fetus is the only cure for preeclampsia.
- **Close to term or worsening preeclampsia:** Induce delivery with IV oxytocin, prostaglandin, or amniotomy.
  - Deliver no later than 37 weeks.
- **Far from term (< 34 weeks):** Treat with modified bed rest and expectant management.
- Prevent intrapartum seizures with a continuous magnesium sulfate drip.
  - Watch for signs of magnesium toxicity (loss of DTRs, respiratory paralysis, coma).
  - Continue seizure prophylaxis for 24 hours postpartum.
  - Treat magnesium toxicity with IV calcium gluconate.

MNEMONIC

Preeclampsia classic triad—

It's not just HyPE

Hypertension
Proteinuria
Edema

MNEMONIC

HELLP *syndrome—*

Hemolysis
Elevated **LF**Ts
Low *Platelets*

KEY FACT

Signs of severe preeclampsia are persistent headache or other cerebral or visual disturbances, persistent epigastric pain, and hyperreactive reflexes.

A 36-year-old G1P0 woman with a history of SLE at 36 weeks GA presents with headache and RUQ pain. She is admitted and found to have a BP of 165/100 and 170/105 mm Hg when tested twice 6 hours apart, and 3+ protein on urine dipstick. Once her BP has been controlled with labetalol, what are the next steps in management?

TABLE 2.11-15. **Presentation of Preeclampsia and Eclampsia**

DISEASE SEVERITY	SIGNS AND SYMPTOMS
Mild preeclampsia	Usually asymptomatic BP $\geq$ 140/90 mm Hg on two occasions > 4 hours apart Proteinuria (> 300 mg/24 hours or 1 to 2 $\oplus$ urine dipsticks) Edema
Severe preeclampsia	Any one of the following: ▪ BP > 160/110 mm Hg on two occasions > 4 hours apart ▪ Renal: proteinuria (> 5 g/24 hours or 3 to 4 $\oplus$ urine dipsticks) or oliguria (< 500 mL/24 h) ▪ Cerebral changes: severe headache, somnolence ▪ Visual changes: blurred vision, scotomata ▪ Other: progressive renal insufficiency, pulmonary edema; RUQ pain, hemolysis, elevated liver enzymes, thrombocytopenia (HELLP syndrome)
Eclampsia	Most common signs preceding an eclamptic attack are headache, visual changes, and RUQ/epigastric pain Seizures are severe if not controlled with anticonvulsant therapy

- **Severe preeclampsia:**
  - Control BP with labetalol and/or hydralazine (goal < 160/110 mm Hg with a diastolic BP of 90–100 mm Hg to maintain fetal blood flow).
  - Continuous magnesium sulfate drip.
  - Deliver by induction or C-section when the mother is stable.

COMPLICATIONS

Prematurity, fetal distress, stillbirth, placental abruption, seizure, DIC, cerebral hemorrhage, serous retinal detachment, fetal/maternal death.

ECLAMPSIA

New-onset grand mal seizures in women with preeclampsia.

HISTORY/PE

See Table 2.11-15 for the signs and symptoms of eclampsia.

TREATMENT

- Delivery of the fetus is the only cure for eclampsia.
- ABCs with supplemental O_2.
- Seizure control/prophylaxis with magnesium.
  - If seizures recur, give IV diazepam.
  - Monitor for clinical magnesium toxicity; no need to routinely monitor magnesium blood levels if renal function is normal.
  - Monitor fetal status.
  - Control BP (labetalol and/or hydralazine).
  - Limit fluids; Foley catheter for strict I/Os.
- Initiate emergent delivery once the patient is stable and convulsions are controlled.
- Postpartum management is the same as that for preeclampsia.

A

The patient has severe preeclampsia. Start a magnesium sulfate drip for seizure prophylaxis and deliver by induction or C-section.

- Seizures may occur antepartum (25%), intrapartum (50%), or postpartum (25%); most occur within 48 hours after delivery.

COMPLICATIONS

Cerebral hemorrhage, aspiration pneumonia, hypoxic encephalopathy, thromboembolic events, fetal/maternal death.

URINARY TRACT INFECTION AND PYELONEPHRITIS DURING PREGNANCY

Asymptomatic bacteriuria occurs in up to 7% of pregnant women, and 30–40% will subsequently develop a UTI or pyelonephritis if untreated. Persistent untreated bacteriuria places the patient at a higher risk for preterm labor, low birth weight, and perinatal mortality. *Escherichia coli* is responsible for 70–90% of infections.

HISTORY/PE

- **Asymptomatic bacteriuria:** $\oplus$ Urine culture on first-trimester screen ($\geq 10^5$ colonies).
- **UTI:** Dysuria, urinary urgency and frequency.
- **Pyelonephritis:** Same as UTI, + fever and costovertebral angle tenderness.

DIAGNOSIS

Best initial test: Urinalysis and $\oplus$ urine culture.

TREATMENT

- **Asymptomatic bacteriuria and UTI:** 3–7 days nitrofurantoin (avoid in first trimester if possible), cephalexin, or amoxicillin-clavulanate. Follow-up culture at 1 week as test of cure.
- **Pyelonephritis:** Admit to hospital, IV fluids, IV third-generation cephalosporins; Suppressive antibiotics with agent culture susceptible for remainder of pregnancy and follow-up culture.

ANTEPARTUM HEMORRHAGE

- Any bleeding that occurs after 20 weeks' gestation.
- Complicates 3–5% of pregnancies.
- Most common causes are placental abruption and placenta previa (see Table 2.11-16 and Figure 2.11-7).
- Other causes include other forms of abnormal placentation (eg, placenta accreta), ruptured uterus, genital tract lesions, and trauma.

Obstetric Complications of Pregnancy

ECTOPIC PREGNANCY

Most often tubal (95%), but can be abdominal, ovarian, or cervical.

HISTORY/PE

- Presents with unilateral lower abdominal pain and vaginal spotting/bleeding, although some patients are asymptomatic.
- Associated with etiologies that cause scarring to the fallopian tubes, including a history of PID, pelvic surgery, DES use, or endometriosis.
- Differential diagnosis includes surgical abdomen, abortion, ovarian torsion, PID, and ruptured ovarian cyst.

KEY FACT

It may be necessary to adjust the doses of antiepileptic drugs in patients with seizure disorders, excluding pre-eclampsia and eclampsia, that worsen in pregnancy. The risks and benefits must be weighed in doing so.

KEY FACT

With third-trimester bleeding, think anatomically:
- Vagina: Bloody show, trauma.
- Cervix: Cervical cancer, cervical/vaginal lesion.
- Placenta: Placental abruption, placenta previa.
- Fetus: Fetal bleeding.

TABLE 2.11-16.   **Placental Abruption vs Placenta Previa vs Vasa Previa**

VARIABLE	PLACENTAL ABRUPTION	PLACENTA PREVIA	VASA PREVIA
Pathophysiology	Premature (before delivery) separation of normally implanted placenta	Abnormal placental implantation: ▪ Total: Placenta covers the cervical os ▪ Marginal: Placenta extends to the margin of the os ▪ Low lying: Placenta is in close proximity to the os	Velamentous umbilical cord insertion and/or bilobed placenta causing vessels to pass over the internal os
Incidence	1 in 100	1 in 200	1 in 2500
Risk factors	Hypertension, abdominal/pelvic trauma, tobacco or cocaine use, previous abruption, rapid decompression of an overdistended uterus, excessive stimulation	Prior C-sections, grand multiparity, advanced maternal age, multiple gestation, prior placenta previa	Multiple gestation, IVF, accessory placental lobes, single umbilical artery, placenta previa, low-lying placenta
Symptoms	Painful, dark vaginal bleeding that does not spontaneously cease Abdominal pain; uterine hypertonicity Fetal distress	Painless, bright red bleeding that often ceases in 1–2 hours with or without uterine contractions Usually no fetal distress	Painless bleeding at rupture of membranes with fetal bradycardia
Diagnosis	Primarily clinical Transabdominal/transvaginal ultrasonography sensitivity is only 50%; look for a retroplacental clot Most useful for ruling out previa	Transabdominal/transvaginal ultrasonography sensitivity is > 95%; look for an abnormally positioned placenta	Transvaginal ultrasonography with color Dopplers showing vessels passing over the internal os
Management	Stabilize patients with mild abruption and a premature fetus; manage expectantly (hospitalize; start IV and fetal monitoring; type and cross-match blood; bed rest) Moderate to severe abruption: Immediate delivery is indicated (vaginal delivery with amniotomy if mother and fetus are stable and delivery is expected soon; C-section for maternal or fetal distress)	Do not perform a vaginal exam! Stabilize patients with a premature fetus; manage expectantly Give tocolytics Serial ultrasonograms to assess fetal growth; resolution of partial previa Betamethasone 28–32 weeks to help with fetal lung maturity if may need early delivery Deliver by C-section. Indications for delivery include labor, life-threatening bleeding, fetal distress, documented fetal lung maturity, and 36 weeks GA	Acute bleeding = emergency C-section delivery Diagnosis before bleeding: Steroids at 28–32 weeks to help with fetal lung maturity, hospitalization at 30–32 weeks for close monitoring and scheduled C-section delivery at 35 weeks
Complications	Hemorrhagic shock DIC occurs in 10% of patients Recurrence risk is 5–16% and ↑ to 25% after two previous abruptions Fetal hypoxia	↑ Risk for placenta accreta Vasa previa (fetal vessels crossing the internal os) Preterm delivery, PROM, IUGR, congenital anomalies Recurrence risk is 4–8%	Fetal exsanguination

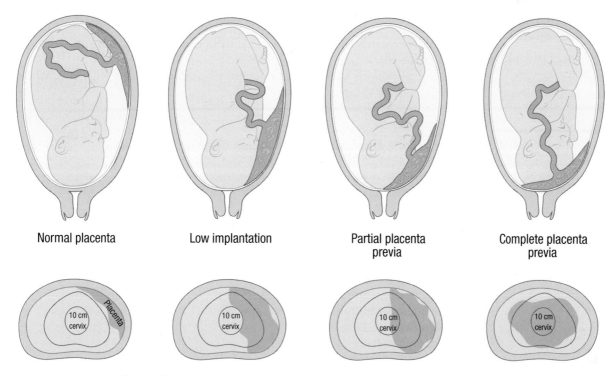

Normal placenta   Low implantation   Partial placenta previa   Complete placenta previa

FIGURE 2.11-7. **Placental implantation.** (Reproduced with permission from USMLE-Rx.com.)

DIAGNOSIS

- Approach a woman of reproductive age presenting with abdominal pain as a ruptured ectopic pregnancy until proven otherwise.
- **Best initial test:** Transvaginal ultrasonogram showing an empty uterus (see Figure 2.11-8).
- **Next best test:** Serial serum β-hCG stratifies patients where transvaginal ultrasound is nondiagnostic:
  - >1500 IU/L → repeat β-hCG and ultrasound in 2 days.
  - <1500 IU/L → serial β-HCG until levels reach 1500 IU/L (which is when an intrauterine pregnancy should be seen).

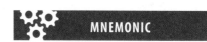

MNEMONIC

The classic triad of ectopic pregnancy PAVEs the way for diagnosis—

Pain (abdominal)
Amenorrhea
Vaginal bleeding
Ectopic pregnancy

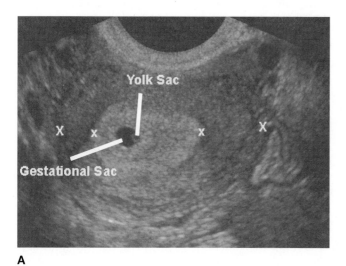

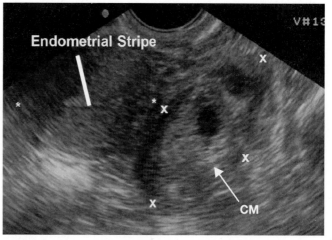

A

B

FIGURE 2.11-8. **Normal intrauterine pregnancy and ectopic pregnancy.** Transvaginal ultrasonogram showing (**A**) a normal intrauterine pregnancy with a gestational sac containing a yolk sac within the uterine cavity, and (**B**) a complex mass (CM)/ectopic pregnancy adjacent to an empty uterus. (Reproduced with permission from Tintinalli JE, et al. *Tintinalli's Emergency Medicine: A Comprehensive Study Guide*, 6th ed. New York, NY: McGraw-Hill; 2004.)

TREATMENT

- Medical treatment (methotrexate) is sufficient for small, unruptured tubal pregnancies.
- Surgical options include salpingectomy or salpingostomy with evacuation (laparoscopy vs laparotomy).

COMPLICATIONS

Tubal rupture and hemoperitoneum (an obstetric emergency).

INTRAUTERINE GROWTH RESTRICTION

An EFW less than the 10th percentile for GA.

HISTORY/PE

Risk factors include the following:

- Maternal systemic disease leading to uteroplacental insufficiency (intrauterine infection, hypertension, anemia).
- Maternal substance abuse.
- Placenta previa.
- Multiple gestation.
- Symmetric IUGR results from aneuploidy, congenital anomalies, and intrauterine infection.
- Asymmetric IUGR results from maternal hypertension or other maternal chronic disease.

DIAGNOSIS

- **Best initial test:** Ultrasound to confirm gestational age and fetal weight.
- Confirm serial fundal height measurements with ultrasonography.
- Perform ultrasonography for EFW.
- Umbilical artery Doppler velocimetry shows flow reversal.

TREATMENT

- Explore the underlying etiology, and correct if possible.
- If the patient is near due date, administer steroids (eg, betamethasone) to accelerate fetal lung maturity; requires 48 hours before delivery.
- Perform fetal monitoring with NST, CST, BPP, and umbilical artery Doppler velocimetry.
- A nonreassuring status near term may prompt delivery.

COMPLICATIONS

↑ Perinatal morbidity and mortality.

FETAL MACROSOMIA

A birth weight > 95th percentile. A common sequela of gestational diabetes.

- **Dx:**
  - **Best initial test:** Ultrasound to estimate fetal size.
  - **Most accurate test:** Weigh the newborn at birth (prenatal diagnosis is imprecise).
- **Tx:** Planned C-section delivery may be considered for an EFW > 5000 g in women without diabetes and for an EFW > 4500 g in women with diabetes.
- **Complications:** ↑ Risk for shoulder dystocia (leading to brachial plexus injury and Erb-Duchenne palsy) as birth weight ↑.

POLYHYDRAMNIOS

An AFI ≥ 25 on ultrasonography. May be present in normal pregnancies, but fetal chromosomal developmental abnormalities must be considered.

- **Etiologies:**
  - Maternal DM.
  - Multiple gestation.
  - Isoimmunization.
  - Pulmonary abnormalities (eg, cystic lung malformations).
  - Fetal GI tract anomalies (eg, duodenal atresia, tracheoesophageal fistula, anencephaly).
  - Twin-twin transfusion syndrome.
- **Hx/PE:** Usually asymptomatic.
- **Dx:** Fundal height greater than expected.
  - Evaluation includes ultrasonography for fetal anomalies, glucose testing for DM, and Rh screen.
- **Tx:** Planned C-section is etiology specific.
- **Complications:** Preterm labor, fetal malpresentation, cord prolapse.

OLIGOHYDRAMNIOS

An AFI < 5 on ultrasonography. Usually asymptomatic, but IUGR or fetal distress may be present.

- **Etiologies:**
  - Fetal urinary tract abnormalities (eg, renal agenesis, GU obstruction).
  - Chronic uteroplacental insufficiency.
  - Postterm pregnancy (> 41 weeks).
  - ROM.
- **Dx:** The sum of the deepest amniotic fluid pocket in all four abdominal quadrants on ultrasonography.
- **Tx:** Rule out inaccurate gestational dates. Treat the underlying cause if possible.
- **Complications:**
  - Associated with a 40-fold ↑ in perinatal mortality.
  - Other complications include musculoskeletal abnormalities (eg, clubfoot, facial distortion), pulmonary hypoplasia, umbilical cord compression, and IUGR.

RH ISOIMMUNIZATION

Fetal RBCs leak into the maternal circulation, and maternal anti-Rh IgG antibodies form that can cross the placenta, leading to hemolysis of fetal Rh RBCs (erythroblastosis fetalis; see Figure 2.11-9). Occurs only in Rh⊖ women; ↑ risk with previous SAB or TAB or previous delivery with no RhoGAM given.

DIAGNOSIS

Sensitized Rh⊖ mothers with titers > 1:16 should be closely monitored with serial ultrasonograms and amniocentesis for evidence of fetal hemolysis.

TREATMENT

In severe cases, initiate preterm delivery when fetal lungs are mature. Before delivery, intrauterine blood transfusions can be given to correct a low fetal hematocrit.

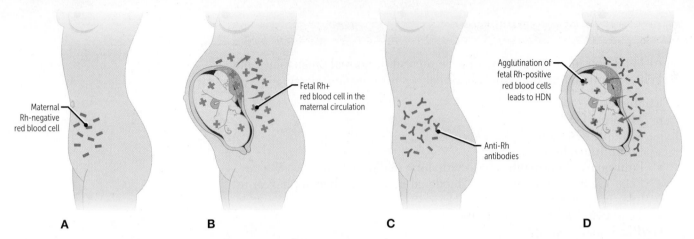

FIGURE 2.11-9. (A) Rh ⊖ mother before pregnancy. (B) Rh ⊕ fetus in Rh ⊖ mother. (C) After delivery, the mother develops antibodies to Rh antigen. (D) Rh ⊕ fetus in the next pregnancy. Maternal antibodies, from Rh isoimmunization at the time of the previous delivery, cross the placenta and cause hemolysis of RBCs in the fetus. HDN, hemolytic disease of the newborn. (Reproduced with permission from USMLE-Rx.com.)

PREVENTION

- If the mother is Rh⊖ and the father is Rh⊕ or unknown, give RhoGAM at 28 weeks (Rh immune globulin).
- If the baby is Rh⊕, give the mother RhoGAM postpartum. The dose is based on the Kleihauer-Betke test. Inadequate dosing can lead to alloimmunization.
- Give RhoGAM to Rh⊖ mothers who undergo abortion or who have had an ectopic pregnancy, amniocentesis, vaginal bleeding, or placenta previa/placental abruption. Type and screen is critical; follow β-hCG closely, and prevent pregnancy for 1 year.

COMPLICATIONS

- Hydrops fetalis when fetal hemoglobin is < 7 g/dL.
- Fetal hypoxia and acidosis, kernicterus, prematurity, death.

GESTATIONAL TROPHOBLASTIC DISEASE

A range of proliferative trophoblastic abnormalities that can be benign or malignant.

- **Benign GTD:** Includes complete and incomplete molar pregnancies (see Table 2.11-17).
- **Malignant GTD:** Molar pregnancy may progress to malignant GTD, including the following:
  - Invasive hydatidiform moles (10–15%).
  - Choriocarcinoma (2–5%).
- Complications of malignant GTD include pulmonary or CNS metastases and trophoblastic pulmonary emboli.

HISTORY/PE

- Presents with first-trimester uterine bleeding, hyperemesis gravidarum, preeclampsia/eclampsia at < 24 weeks, and uterine size greater than dates.
- Risk factors include extremes of age (< 20 or > 40 years) and a diet deficient in folate or β-carotene.

DIAGNOSIS

- **Best initial test:** Pelvic exam may reveal enlarged ovaries (bilateral theca-lutein cysts) or expulsion of grapelike molar clusters into the vagina.
- **Next best/most accurate test:** Pelvic ultrasonography reveals a "snowstorm" appearance with no gestational sac or fetus present (see Figure 2.11-10).
- Labs show markedly ↑ serum β-hCG (usually > 100,000 mIU/mL).

TABLE 2.11-17. **Complete vs Incomplete Moles**

Variable	Complete	Incomplete
Mechanism	Sperm fertilization of an empty ovum	Normal ovum fertilized by two sperm
Karyotype	46,XX	69,XXY
Fetal tissue	No fetal tissue	Contains fetal tissue

- Chest x-ray (CXR) may show lung metastases.
- D&C reveals "cluster-of-grapes" tissue.

TREATMENT

- **Best initial treatment:** Evacuate the uterus with D&C.
- Follow with weekly β-hCG.
- Treat malignant disease with chemotherapy (methotrexate or dactinomycin).
- Treat residual uterine disease with hysterectomy.
- Chemotherapy and irradiation are highly effective for metastases.

MULTIPLE GESTATION

Affect 3% of all live births. Since 1980, the incidence of monozygotic (identical) twins has remained steady, whereas the incidence of dizygotic (fraternal) and higher order births has ↑.

HISTORY/PE

Characterized by rapid uterine growth, excessive maternal weight gain, and palpation of three or more large fetal parts on Leopold maneuvers.

DIAGNOSIS

- Ultrasonography.
- β-hCG, human placental lactogen, and MSAFP are elevated for GA.

TREATMENT

- Multifetal reduction and selective fetal termination is an option for higher-order multiple pregnancies.

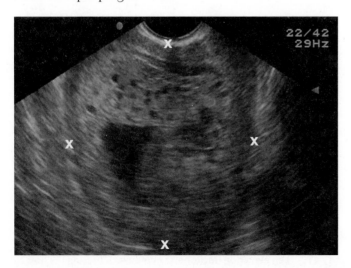

FIGURE 2.11-10. **Molar pregnancy.** Transvaginal ultrasonogram shows a large, complex intrauterine mass with cystic regions that have the characteristic appearance of grapes. (Reproduced with permission from Tintinalli JE, et al. *Tintinalli's Emergency Medicine: A Comprehensive Study Guide,* 6th ed. New York, NY: McGraw-Hill; 2004.)

- Antepartum fetal surveillance for IUGR.
- Management by a high-risk specialist is recommended.

Complications

- **Maternal:** Patients are six times more likely to be hospitalized with complications of pregnancy. ↑ Incidence of placenta previa and need for C-section delivery.
- **Fetal:** Twin-to-twin transfusion syndrome, IUGR, preterm labor, and ↑ incidence of congenital malformations.

Abnormal Labor and Delivery

SHOULDER DYSTOCIA

Affects 0.6%–1.4% of all deliveries in the United States. Risk factors include obesity, diabetes, a history of a macrosomic infant, and a history of prior shoulder dystocia.

Diagnosis

Diagnosed by a prolonged second stage of labor, recoil of the perineum ("turtle sign"), and lack of spontaneous restitution.

Treatment

- In the event of dystocia, the following maneuvers may be attempted:
  - McRoberts maneuver; see Figure 2.11-11.
  - Apply suprapubic pressure.

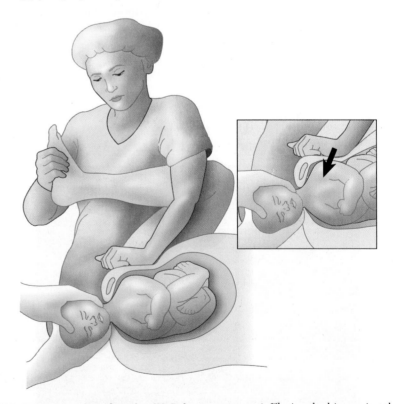

FIGURE 2.11-11.   Leg elevation (McRoberts maneuver). Flexing the hips against the abdomen. The leg positioning illustrated here can be used to assist in a delivery where the infant is at risk for shoulder dystocia. (Reproduced with permission from Cunningham FG, et al. *Williams Obstetrics,* 23rd ed. New York, NY: McGraw-Hill; 2010.)

- Woods screw maneuver (Enter the vagina and attempt rotation.)
- Passing fetal arm.
- Episiotomy.

Clavicular fractures may result in C8-T1 brachial plexus injury that may cause Horner syndrome, Erb-Duchenne palsy, or Klumpke palsy. These brachial plexus injuries usually resolve spontaneously.

FAILURE TO PROGRESS

Associated with chorioamnionitis, occiput posterior position, nulliparity, and elevated birth weight.

DIAGNOSIS

- **First-stage protraction or arrest:** Labor that fails to produce adequate rates of progressive cervical change.
- **Prolonged second-stage arrest:** Arrest of fetal descent. Most commonly caused by fetal malposition. See Table 2.11-18 for definitions based on parity and anesthesia.

TREATMENT

See Table 2.11-18.

COMPLICATIONS

- Chorioamnionitis leads to fetal infection, pneumonia, and bacteremia.
- Permanent injury occurs in 10%.
- The risk for postpartum hemorrhage is 11%; that of fourth-degree laceration is 3.8%.

TABLE 2.11-18. Failure to Progress

STAGE	DEFINITION	TREATMENT[a]
FIRST STAGE: FAILURE TO HAVE PROGRESSIVE CERVICAL CHANGE		
Latent	▪ Primi: > 20 h ▪ Multi: > 14 h	Therapeutic rest via parenteral analgesia; oxytocin; amniotomy; cervical ripening
Active	Dilation of at least 6 cm and either: ▪ No change in dilation with 4 h of adequate contractions or ▪ No change in dilation with 6 h of inadequate contractions	Amniotomy; oxytocin; C-section if the previous interventions are ineffective
SECOND STAGE: ARREST OF FETAL DESCENT		
	▪ Primi: > 2 h; > 3 h with epidural ▪ Multi: > 1 h; > 2 h with epidural	Close observation with a ↓ in epidural rate and continued oxytocin Assisted vaginal delivery (forceps or vacuum) C-section

[a]Augmentation with oxytocin should be considered when contraction frequency is < 3 in a 10-minute period or intensity of contraction is < 25 mm Hg above baseline.

RUPTURE OF MEMBRANES

Distinguished as follows:

- **Spontaneous ROM:** Occurs after or at the onset of labor.
- **Premature ROM:** Occurs > 1 hour before onset of labor. May be precipitated by vaginal or cervical infections, abnormal membrane physiology, or cervical incompetence.
- **Preterm PROM (PPROM):** ROM occurring at < 37 weeks' gestation.
- **Prolonged ROM:** ROM occurring > 18 hours before delivery. Risk factors include low socioeconomic status, young maternal age, smoking, and STDs.

HISTORY/PE

Patients often report a "gush" of clear or blood-tinged amniotic fluid. Uterine contractions may be present.

DIAGNOSIS

- Sterile speculum exam reveals pooling of amniotic fluid in the vaginal vault.
- Nitrazine paper test is ⊕ (paper turns blue, indicating alkaline pH of amniotic fluid).
- Fern test is ⊕ (a ferning pattern is seen under a microscope after amniotic fluid dries on a glass slide).
- Ultrasonography to assess amniotic fluid volume.
- If diagnosis is uncertain, ultrasonography-guided transabdominal instillation of indigo carmine dye can be used to check for leakage (unequivocal test).
- Minimize infection risk; do not perform digital vaginal exams on women who are not in labor or for whom labor is not planned immediately.
- Check fetal heart tracing, maternal temperature, WBC count, and uterine tenderness for evidence of chorioamnionitis.

TREATMENT

- **Depends on GA and fetal lung maturity:**
  - **Term:** First check GBS status and fetal presentation; then labor may be induced or the patient can be observed for 6 hours.
  - **34–36 weeks GA:** Labor induction may be considered.
  - **< 32 weeks GA:** Expectant management with bed rest and pelvic rest.
- **Antibiotics:** To prevent infection and to prolong the latency period in the absence of infection.
- **Antenatal corticosteroids:**
  - Give betamethasone or dexamethasone for 48 hours.
  - Promotes fetal lung maturity in the absence of intra-amniotic infection before 32–36 weeks GA.
- If signs of infection or fetal distress develop, give antibiotics (ampicillin and gentamicin) and induce labor.

COMPLICATIONS

Preterm labor and delivery, chorioamnionitis, placental abruption, cord prolapse.

PRETERM LABOR

Onset of labor between 20 and 37 weeks' gestation. The 1° cause of neonatal morbidity and mortality.

- Risk factors include previous preterm delivery (highest risk factor), multiple gestation, infection, PROM, uterine anomalies (eg, prior surgery),

KEY FACT

To minimize the risk for infection, do not perform digital vaginal exams on women with PROM.

polyhydramnios, placental abruption, poor maternal nutrition, and low SES.
- Patients found to have a short cervix at < 24 weeks' gestation are at high risk for preterm labor. Progesterone administration ↓ risk in these patients.
- Most patients have no identifiable risk factors.

HISTORY/PE

Presents with menstrual-like cramps, onset of low back pain, pelvic pressure, and new vaginal discharge or bleeding.

DIAGNOSIS

- Requires the following:
  - Regular uterine contractions (three or more contractions of 30 seconds each over a 30-minute period).
  - Concurrent cervical change at < 37 weeks' gestation.
- Assess for contraindications to tocolysis such as infection, nonreassuring fetal testing, or placental abruption.
- Sterile speculum exam to rule out PROM.
- Ultrasonography to rule out fetal or uterine anomalies, verify GA, and assess fetal presentation and amniotic fluid volume.
- Obtain cultures for chlamydia, gonorrhea, and GBS; obtain a UA and urine culture.

TREATMENT

- Hydration and bed rest.
- Tocolytic therapy (β-mimetics, $MgSO_4$, CCBs, prostaglandin inhibitors) if < 34 weeks' gestation, unless contraindicated.
- Magnesium for cerebral palsy prophylaxis if < 32 weeks' gestation.
- Steroids to accelerate fetal lung maturity.
- Penicillin or ampicillin for GBS prophylaxis if preterm delivery is likely.

COMPLICATIONS

RDS, intraventricular hemorrhage, PDA, necrotizing enterocolitis, retinopathy of prematurity, bronchopulmonary dysplasia, death.

FETAL MALPRESENTATION

Any presentation other than vertex (ie, head closest to birth canal, chin to chest, occiput anterior). Risk factors include prematurity, prior breech delivery, uterine anomalies, polyhydramnios or oligohydramnios, multiple gestation, PPROM, hydrocephalus, anencephaly, and placenta previa.

HISTORY/PE

- Breech presentations are the most common form and involve presentation of the fetal lower extremities or buttocks into the maternal pelvis (see Figure 2.11-12). Subtypes include the following:
  - **Frank breech (50–75%):** The thighs are flexed, and the knees are extended.
  - **Footling breech (20%):** One or both legs are extended below the buttocks.
  - **Complete breech (5–10%):** The thighs and knees are flexed.

TREATMENT

- **Follow:** Up to 75% spontaneously change to vertex by week 38.
- **External cephalic version:** If the fetus has not reverted spontaneously, a version may be attempted by applying directed pressure to the maternal

KEY FACT

Preterm labor = regular uterine contractions + concurrent cervical change at < 37 weeks' gestation.

KEY FACT

Breech presentation is the most common fetal malpresentation.

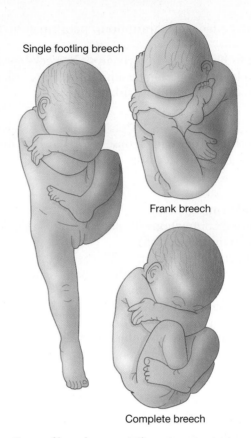

Single footling breech

Frank breech

Complete breech

FIGURE 2.11-12. **Types of breech presentations.** (Reproduced with permission from DeCherney AH. *Current Obstetric & Gynecologic Diagnosis & Treatment,* 8th ed. Stamford, CT: Appleton & Lange; 1994.)

abdomen to turn the infant to vertex. The success rate is roughly 50%. Risks of version are placental abruption and cord compression, so be prepared for an emergency C-section if needed.

■ **Trial of breech vaginal delivery:** Attempt only if delivery is imminent. Complications include cord prolapse and/or head entrapment.

■ **Elective C-section:** Recommended given the lower risk for fetal morbidity.

INDICATIONS FOR C-SECTION

See Table 2.11-19 for indications. For both elective and indicated C-section delivery, sodium citrate should be used in the mother to ↓ gastric acidity and prevent acid aspiration syndrome.

TABLE 2.11-19. **Indications for C-section**

MATERNAL FACTORS	FETAL AND MATERNAL FACTORS	FETAL FACTORS
Prior classical C-section (vertical incision predisposes to uterine rupture with vaginal delivery)	Cephalopelvic disproportion (the most common cause of 1° C-section)	Fetal malposition (eg, posterior chin, transverse lie, shoulder presentation)
Active genital herpes infection	Placenta previa/placental abruption	Fetal distress
Cervical carcinoma	Failed operative vaginal delivery	Cord compression/prolapse
Maternal trauma/demise	Postterm pregnancy (relative indication)	Erythroblastosis fetalis (Rh incompatibility)
HIV infection		
Prior transverse C-section (relative indication)		

EPISIOTOMY

Surgical extension of the vaginal opening into the perineum. Can be median (midline) or mediolateral.

COMPLICATIONS

- **Extension to the anal sphincter (third degree) or rectum (fourth degree):** More common with midline episiotomy.
- **Other:** Bleeding, infection, dyspareunia, rectovaginal fistula formation, or maternal death (rare).
- Routine use of episiotomy is not recommended.

Puerperium

Normal changes after delivery include transient fevers and chills, lochia (vaginal discharge), uterine contraction, and uterine involution.

Postpartum urinary retention is also common and caused by bladder atony. This can be managed with catheterization and encouragement of ambulation, and usually resolves spontaneously.

Radiating suprapubic pain exacerbated by weight bearing may occur because of diastasis of the pubic symphysis. This is more common following a traumatic delivery, and treatment is with supportive care.

POSTPARTUM HEMORRHAGE

A loss of > 1000 mL irrespective of the type of delivery. May occur before, during, or after delivery of the placenta. Table 2.11-20 summarizes common causes.

TABLE 2.11-20. Common Causes of Postpartum Hemorrhage

VARIABLE	UTERINE ATONY	GENITAL TRACT TRAUMA	RETAINED PLACENTAL TISSUE
Risk factors	Uterine overdistention (multiple gestation, macrosomia, polyhydramnios) Exhausted myometrium (rapid or prolonged labor, oxytocin stimulation) Uterine infection Conditions interfering with contractions (anesthesia, myomas, $MgSO_4$)	Precipitous labor Operative vaginal delivery (forceps, vacuum extraction) Large infant Inadequate episiotomy repair	Placenta accreta/increta/percreta Placenta previa Uterine leiomyomas Preterm delivery Previous C-section/curettage
Diagnosis	Palpation of a soft, enlarged, "boggy" uterus Most common cause of postpartum hemorrhage (90%)	Manual and visual inspection of the lower genital tract for any laceration > 2 cm long	Manual and visual inspection of the placenta and uterine cavity for missing cotyledons Ultrasound may also be used to inspect the uterus
Treatment[a]	Bimanual uterine massage (usually successful) Oxytocin infusion Methergine (methylergonovine) if not hypertensive $PGF_{2\alpha}$	Surgical correction of the physical defect	Manual removal of remaining placental tissue Curettage with suctioning (carries risk for uterine perforation)

[a]For all uterine causes, when bleeding persists after conventional therapy, uterine/internal iliac artery ligation, uterine artery embolization, or hysterectomy can be lifesaving.

COMPLICATIONS

- Acute blood loss (potentially fatal).
- Anemia caused by chronic blood loss (predisposes to puerperal infection).
- Sheehan syndrome.

Uterine Inversion

An uncommon cause of postpartum hemorrhage. This occurs when the uterine fundus prolapses through the cervix and vagina and can often be visible as a smooth mass protruding from the vagina. Treatment involves manually replacing the uterus and monitoring hemodynamic status.

Uterine Rupture

Very rare but life-threatening complication that may occur in women with a history of multiple uterine surgeries. Loss of fetal station is pathognomonic for this condition, and fetal parts may be palpable in the abdomen but not in the vagina. Treatment involves emergent laparotomy.

POSTPARTUM INFECTION

A temperature $\geq$ 38°C for at least 2 of the first 10 postpartum days (not including the first 24 hours).

Risk factors for postpartum endometritis include emergent C-section, PROM, prolonged labor, multiple intrapartum vaginal exams, intrauterine manipulations, delivery, low SES, young age, prolonged ruptured membranes, bacterial colonization, and corticosteroid use.

TREATMENT

Broad-spectrum empiric IV antibiotics (eg, clindamycin and gentamicin) until patients have been afebrile for 48 hours (24 hours for chorioamnionitis). Add ampicillin for complicated cases.

COMPLICATIONS

- Septic pelvic thrombophlebitis:
  - Pelvic infection leads to infection of the vein wall and intimal damage, leading in turn to thrombogenesis. The clot is then invaded by microorganisms.
  - Suppuration follows, with liquefaction, fragmentation, and, finally, septic embolization.
  - Presents with abdominal and back pain and a "picket-fence" fever curve ("hectic" fevers) with wide swings from normal to as high as 41°C (105.8°F) that is unresponsive to antibiotics.
  - Diagnose with blood cultures and CT looking for a pelvic abscess.
  - Treat with broad-spectrum antibiotics and anticoagulation with heparin for 7–10 days.

SHEEHAN SYNDROME (POSTPARTUM PITUITARY NECROSIS)

Pituitary ischemia and necrosis that lead to anterior pituitary insufficiency 2° to massive obstetric hemorrhage and shock.

- Hx/PE:
  - The 1° cause of anterior pituitary insufficiency in adult females.
  - The most common presenting syndrome is failure to lactate (caused by ↓ prolactin levels).

KEY FACT

Postpartum endometritis:
- Fever > 38°C within 36 hours.
- Uterine tenderness.
- Malodorous lochi.

MNEMONIC

The 7 W's of postpartum fever (10 days postdelivery)—

Womb (endomyometritis)
Wind (atelectasis, pneumonia)
Water (UTI)
Walk (DVT, pulmonary embolism)
Wound (incision, episiotomy)
Weaning (breast engorgement, abscess, mastitis)
Wonder drugs (drug fever)

- Other symptoms include weakness, lethargy, cold intolerance, genital atrophy, and menstrual disorders.
- **Dx:**
  - **Best initial test:** Provocative hormonal testing.
  - **Most accurate test:** MRI of the pituitary gland and hypothalamus to rule out tumor or other pathology.
- **Tx:** Replacement of all deficient hormones. Some patients may recover TSH and even gonadotropin function after cortisol replacement alone.

LACTATION AND BREASTFEEDING

- During pregnancy, ↑ estrogen and progesterone result in breast hypertrophy and inhibition of the action of prolactin on the breast.
- After delivery of the placenta, hormone levels ↓ markedly, and prolactin stimulates the alveolar epithelial cells, activating milk production. ↑ Prolactin will ↓ LH and FSH, causing anovulation and amenorrhea during breastfeeding.
- Periodic infant suckling leads to further release of prolactin and oxytocin, which stimulate myoepithelial cell contraction and milk ejection ("letdown reflex").
- Colostrum ("early breast milk") contains protein, fat, secretory IgA, and minerals.
- Within 1 week postpartum, mature milk with protein, fat, lactose, and water is produced.
- High IgA levels in colostrum provide passive immunity for the infant and protect against enteric bacteria.
- Other potential benefits include the following:
  - ↓ Incidence of infant allergies.
  - ↓ Incidence of early URIs and GI infections.
  - Facilitation of mother-child bonding.
  - Maternal weight loss.
- Contraindications to breastfeeding include HIV infection, active drug use (including marijuana), and use of certain medications (eg, tetracycline, chloramphenicol).
- Women who desire to suppress lactation should wear a supportive bra, avoid nipple stimulation, apply ice packs to the breasts, and use NSAIDs to reduce pain. Breast binding should be avoided as it ↑ risk for mastitis.

MASTITIS

Cellulitis of the periglandular tissue caused by nipple trauma from breastfeeding coupled with the introduction of bacteria, usually *Staphylococcus aureus*, from the infant's pharynx into the nipple ducts.

HISTORY/PE

- Symptoms often begin 2–4 weeks postpartum, are usually unilateral, and include the following:
  - Breast tenderness.
  - Erythema, edema, warmth, and possible purulent nipple drainage.
- Significant fever, chills, and malaise can also be seen.

DIAGNOSIS

- Differentiate from simple breast swelling.
- Infection is suggested by focal symptoms, an ↑ WBC count, and fever.

TREATMENT

- Continued breastfeeding to prevent the accumulation of infected material (or use of a breast pump in patients who are no longer breastfeeding).
- PO antibiotics (dicloxacillin, cephalexin, amoxicillin/clavulanate, azithromycin, clindamycin).
- If no clinical improvement within 48–72 hours, evaluate with breast ultrasonography to assess for abscess. If present, treat with incision and drainage.

GYNECOLOGY

Menarche and Normal Female Development

- In order: Thelarche (breast development, onset 8–13 years) → pubarche (pubic hair growth) → growth acceleration → menarche (onset 10–16 years).
  - Ages for these stages of development vary by race/ethnicity.

Figure 2.12-1 graphically illustrates the stages of normal female development.

Normal Menstrual Cycle

The progression of a normal menstrual cycle is detailed below and illustrated in Figure 2.12-2.

Menstruation and follicular phase (days 0–13):
- Starts with menstruation and ends at luteinizing hormone (LH) surge/ovulation.
- May vary, but typically lasts ~ 13 days.
- ↑ Frequency of GnRH pulse → ↑ follicle-stimulating hormone (FSH) → growth of follicles → ↑ estrogen production.
- Results in the development of straight glands and thin secretions of the uterine lining (proliferative phase).
- **By late follicular phase:** Dominant follicle is selected and ↑ in size, uterine endometrium thickens, and cervical mucus becomes stringy.

Ovulation (day 14):
- Estradiol reaches a peak → positive feedback to the pituitary gland → LH surge (smaller FSH rise) → rupture of the ovarian follicle and release of a mature ovum → travels to oviduct/uterus.
- Ruptured follicular cells differentiate into the corpus luteum.

Luteal phase (days 15–28):
- Length of time (10–14 days) that the corpus luteum can survive without further LH or hCG stimulation.
- Change from estrogen to progesterone predominance: Corpus luteum produces progesterone and some estradiol, allowing the endometrial lining to develop thick and tortuous endometrial glands with thick secretions (secretory phase).
- In the absence of fertilization and implantation, ↓ LH → ↓ progesterone and estradiol by the corpus luteum → results in sloughing of the endometrial lining.
- With ↓ estrogen and progesterone, there is no longer negative feedback to FSH, which then increases and restarts menstruation/follicular phase.

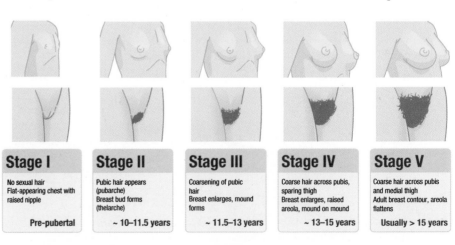

FIGURE 2.12-1. **Normal female development.** (Reproduced with permission from USMLE-Rx.com.)

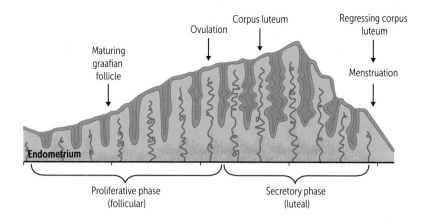

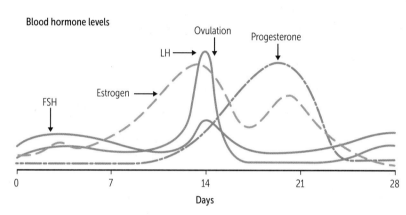

F I G U R E 2 . 1 2 - 2 . **Normal menstrual cycle.** (Reproduced with permission from USMLE-Rx.com.)

Menopause

Cessation of menses for a minimum of 12 months as a result of follicular depletion.

HISTORY/PE

- The average age of onset is 51 years.
- Symptoms include hot flashes, pruritus and vaginal dryness caused by vaginal atrophy, insomnia, anxiety/irritability, poor concentration, mood changes, dyspareunia, and loss of libido.
- "Premature menopause" (also known as premature ovarian failure) is cessation of menses before 40 years of age.

DIAGNOSIS

- A clinical diagnosis. The following studies are not routine but may be helpful:
  - **Labs:** ↑ FSH; then ↑ LH.
  - Serum TSH should be measured because of overlap of symptoms and common age of presentation of hypothyroidism and menopause.

TREATMENT

- **Best initial treatment:** Hormone replacement therapy ([HRT], combination estrogen and progestin):
  - If moderate to severe vasomotor symptoms → lowest dose for short duration to manage symptoms.
  - May ↑ the incidence of breast cancer with long-term use at high doses.

- May ↑ cardiovascular morbidity and mortality with long-term use at high doses.
  - **Contraindications:** Vaginal bleeding, breast cancer (known or suspected), untreated endometrial cancer, history of thromboembolism, chronic liver disease, and hypertriglyceridemia.
- **Non-HRT:** SSRI/SNRIs, clonidine, and/or gabapentin to ↓ the frequency of hot flashes.
- **Topical estrogen preparation:** For vaginal atrophy. Does NOT have the same contraindications as systemic HRT.
- **Calcium supplements ± bisphosphonates:** For osteoporosis. DEXA scan is used to measure bone mineral density (BMD). Supplemental treatment includes daily calcium/vitamin D and weight-bearing exercise.

Contraception

Eighty-five percent of sexually active women with no contraception will become pregnant within 1 year. Table 2.12-1 describes the effectiveness of contraceptive methods along with their relative advantages and disadvantages. See Table 2.12-2 for contraindications to common methods of contraception. Emergency contraception (EC) methods prevent pregnancy after unprotected sex or contraceptive failure. Table 2.12-3 describes the various methods of EC.

Abnormalities of the Menstrual Cycle

1° AMENORRHEA/DELAYED PUBERTY

The absence of menses by 15 years of age with 2° sexual development present, or the absence of 2° sexual characteristics by 13 years of age.

HISTORY/PE

- **Absence of 2° sexual characteristics** (no estrogen production).
  - **1° Ovarian insufficiency:** Most common cause (~ 50%). Depletion of ovarian follicles and oocytes most commonly from Turner syndrome (45, XO). Also consider history of radiation therapy and chemotherapy or gonadal dysgenesis.
  - **Central hypogonadism:** Can be caused by a variety of factors, including the following:
    - Undernourishment, stress, hyperprolactinemia, or exercise.
    - CNS tumor (consider prolactin-secreting pituitary adenoma if galactorrhea) or cranial irradiation.
    - Kallmann syndrome (isolated gonadotropin deficiency) associated with anosmia.
    - Constitutional growth delay.
- **Presence of 2° sexual characteristics** (estrogen production but other anatomic or genetic problems): Etiologies include the following:
  - **Müllerian agenesis:** Absence of upper two-thirds of the vagina; uterine abnormalities.
  - **Imperforate hymen:** Presents with hematocolpos (blood in the vagina) that cannot escape, along with a bulging hymen.
  - **Complete androgen insensitivity:** Patients present with breast development (aromatization of testosterone to estrogen) but are amenorrheic and lack pubic hair.

TABLE 2.12-1. Contraceptive Methods

METHOD	MECHANISM	ADVANTAGES	DISADVANTAGES
MOST EFFECTIVE: > 99%			
Implant (progestin-only implant)	Inhibits ovulation; ↑ cervical mucus viscosity	Effective for up to 3 years Immediate fertility once removed Safe with breastfeeding Lighter periods	Irregular periods, scarring at site of insertion (upper arm)
Intrauterine device (IUD) with progestin	Progesterone leads to cervical mucus thickening and endometrial decidualization	Effective for up to 5 years Immediate fertility once removed Safe with breastfeeding Lighter periods; less cramping	Spotting (up to 6 months), acne Risk for uterine perforation (1/1000) ↑ Risk for ectopic pregnancy (rare)
Copper T IUD	Foreign body results in inflammation; copper has a spermicidal effect	Effective for up to 10 years Immediate fertility once removed No hormonal exposure Safe with breastfeeding	↑ Cramping and heavier bleeding (5–10%) Risk for uterine perforation (1/1000) ↑ Risk for ectopic pregnancy (rare)
Surgical sterilization (vasectomy, tubal ligation)		Permanently effective; safe with breastfeeding	Tubal ligation: Irreversible; ↑ risk for ectopic pregnancy (rare) Vasectomy: Most failures are a result of not waiting for 2 ⊖ semen samples
VERY EFFECTIVE: 90–99%			
Medroxyprogesterone	IM injection (progestin) Suppresses ovulation and decidualizes endometrium	Lighter or no periods Each shot works for 3 months	Irregular bleeding, weight gain Decreases in BMD (reversible) Delayed fertility after discontinuation (up to 10 months)
Transdermal patch ("the patch")	Combined weekly estrogen and progestin dermal patch	Predictable, lighter, less painful menses Weekly administration	Thromboembolism risk (especially in smokers > 35 years of age, patients with chronic HTN)
Vaginal ring	Combined low-dose progestin and estrogen vaginal ring	Can make periods more regular Can be placed intravaginally for 3 weeks; remove for 1 week (menses will occur during this time) Safe to use continuously	May ↑ vaginal discharge Spotting (first 1–2 months) Thromboembolism risk (especially in smokers > 35 years of age, patients with chronic HTN)
OCPs (combination estrogen and progestin)	Inhibit FSH/LH, suppressing ovulation; thicken cervical mucus; decidualize endometrium	↓ Risk for ovarian and endometrial cancers[a] Predictable, lighter, less painful menses Can improve acne Varied fertility upon cessation	Requires daily compliance Breakthrough bleeding (10–30%) Thromboembolism risk (especially in smokers > 35 years of age) Cannot be used in patients of any age who have migraines with aura Hypertension GERD (progesterone relaxes the lower esophageal sphincter)
Progestin-only "minipills"	Thicken cervical mucus	Safe with breastfeeding	Requires strict compliance with daily timing

(continues)

TABLE 2.12-1.   Contraceptive Methods *(continued)*

METHOD	MECHANISM	ADVANTAGES	DISADVANTAGES
MODERATELY EFFECTIVE: 75–90%			
Male condoms	A latex sheath covers the penis	The only method that effectively protects against pregnancy and STDs, including HIV	Possible allergy to latex or spermicides
Diaphragm with spermicide	A barrier is inserted over the cervix to prevent entry of sperm	Some protection against STDs	Must be fitted by the provider
Female condom	A barrier sheath is inserted into the vagina	Some protection against STDs	Can be difficult to use
Fertility awareness methods (natural family planning)	Sexual intercourse is avoided on days in the menstrual cycle on which conception is likely (near the time of ovulation)	No side effects	Requires the partner's participation No STD/HIV protection
LESS EFFECTIVE: 68–74%			
Withdrawal	The penis is removed before ejaculation	No side effects	No STD/HIV protection Not recommended as a 1° method
Spermicide	A substance that inhibits sperm motility	May be used as a 2° method	Not recommended as a 1° method

aOther combined hormonal methods (eg, patch, ring) may also protect against endometrial and ovarian cancer; however, data are still lacking given their relatively recent introduction.

TABLE 2.12-2.   Contraindications to Common Methods of Contraception

ESTROGEN-CONTAINING HORMONAL METHODSa	IUDs (PROGESTERONE AND COPPER)
Pregnancy	Severe uterine structural abnormality (bicornuate, septate)
History of stroke, hypertension, deep venous thrombosis/pulmonary embolism	Known or suspected pregnancy
Breast cancer	Active gynecologic infection (within 3 months)
Undiagnosed abnormal vaginal bleeding	Unexplained vaginal/uterine bleeding
Estrogen-dependent cancer	Suspected gynecologic malignancy
Benign or malignant liver neoplasm	Copper T alone:
Abnormal liver function	▪ Copper intolerance (allergy, Wilson disease)
Current tobacco use and > 35 years of age	▪ Severe dysmenorrhea and/or menorrhagia
Migraine with aura	Progestin IUD alone:
	▪ Levonorgestrel allergy
	▪ Breast cancer
	▪ Acute liver disease or liver tumor

aIncludes OCPs, vaginal ring, and transdermal patch.

TABLE 2.12-3.   Emergency Contraceptive Methods

METHOD	ADVANTAGES	DISADVANTAGES
"Morning-after pill"[a] (progesterone agonist/ antagonist)	Does not disrupt embryo postimplantation Safe for all women VERY effective	Expensive Not over the counter
Oral contraceptive taper	Useful for women who have OCPs at home	Nausea, vomiting, fatigue, headache, dizziness, breast tenderness Not over the counter
Progestin only (80% effective)	Same as above Fewer nausea/vomiting side effects	
Copper T IUD (99% effective)[b]	The most effective emergency contraceptive method Can be used as emergency contraceptive and continued for up to 10 years of contraception	High initial cost of insertion Must be inserted by the provider No protection against STDs Must test for pregnancy and STDs before insertion

[a]Used within 120 hours of unprotected sex.
[b]Used within 7 days of unprotected sex.

- ■ **Congenital adrenal hyperplasia:** Can present as virilization with amenorrhea or oligomenorrhea; often presents in infancy with ambiguous genitalia.
- ■ **PE:** Pubertal development, genital exam, signs of androgen excess, physical features of Turner syndrome.

DIAGNOSIS

- ■ **Perform pregnancy test.**
- ■ **Assess for anatomic abnormalities** (imperforate hymen): Physical exam, ultrasonography.
  - ■ **Uterus absent:** Karyotype and serum testosterone to assess if abnormal müllerian development (46,XX, normal female testosterone levels), and androgen insensitivity (46,XY, normal male testosterone levels).
  - ■ **Uterus present:** FSH, LH levels.
    - ■ ↑ FSH: Primary ovarian insufficiency. Obtain karyotype for Turner syndrome (45,X).
    - ■ Normal/↓ FSH: Central hypogonadism, constitutional growth delay. Measure serum prolactin, thyrotropin especially if galactorrhea.
- ■ **If signs of hyperandrogenism:** Consider androgen-secreting neoplasm. Check serum testosterone, dehydroepiandrosterone-sulphate (DHEAS).
- ■ **If hypertensive:** Evaluate for congenital adrenal hyperplasia (CAH; 17-hydroxylase and 21-hydroxylase deficiencies).

See Table 2.12-4 for etiologies and Figure 2.12-3 for work-up of 1° amenorrhea.

TREATMENT

- ■ **Constitutional growth delay:** No treatment is necessary.
- ■ **Hypogonadism:** Begin HRT with estrogen alone at the lowest dose. Begin cyclic estrogen/progesterone therapy 12–18 months later (if the uterus is present).
- ■ **Anatomic:** Requires surgical intervention.

KEY FACT

For Turner syndrome, think streak gonads, shield chest, amenorrhea, webbed neck, aortic coarctation, and bicuspid aortic valve.

KEY FACT

The first step in the work-up of 1° or 2° amenorrhea is a pregnancy test!

TABLE 2.12-4. Etiologies of 1° Amenorrhea

	GnRH	LH/FSH	Estrogen/ Progesterone	Etiology
Constitutional growth delay	↓	↓	↓ (prepuberty levels)	Puberty has not started
Hypogonadotropic hypogonadism	↓	↓ or normal	↓	Hypothalamic or pituitary problem, low caloric intake, excessive exercise
Hypergonadotropic hypogonadism	↑	↑	↓	Ovaries have failed to produce estrogen
Anovulatory problem	↑ or ↓	Normal	↑ Estrogen/ ↓ Progesterone	Problem with estrogen receptors, immature hypothalamic-pituitary-ovarian axis (adolescents only)
Anatomic problem	Normal	Normal	Normal	Menstrual blood cannot get out

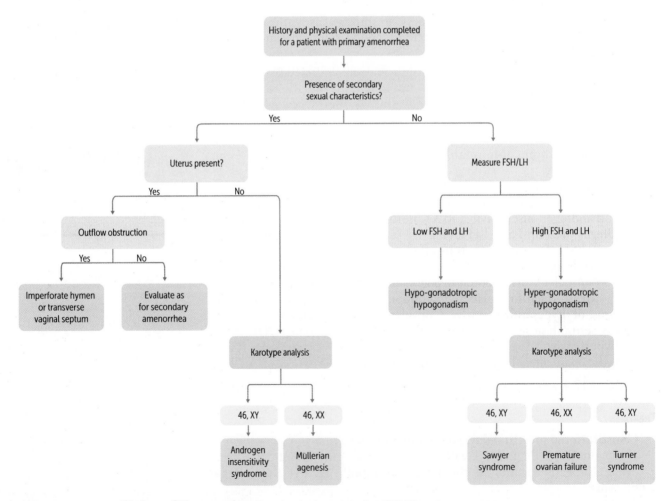

FIGURE 2.12-3. **Work-up of 1° amenorrhea.** (Reproduced with permission from USMLE-Rx.com)

2° AMENORRHEA

The absence of menses for 6 consecutive months in women who have passed menarche. Etiology includes:

- Pregnancy.
- Obesity.
- **Ovary:** Polycystic ovarian syndrome (PCOS), premature ovarian insufficiency, chemotherapy.
- **Hypothalamus:** Neoplasm, functional hypothalamic amenorrhea (nutrition, exercise, and stress), systemic illness (diabetes mellitus type 1 [DM1], celiac disease).
- **Pituitary gland:** Adenoma (eg, prolactin secreting), sellar masses, Sheehan syndrome.
- **Thyroid gland:** Hypothyroidism.
- **Uterus:** Asherman syndrome, cervical stenosis.

DIAGNOSIS

- History and physical exam.
- Give patient a pregnancy test.
- If ⊖, measure FSH, TSH and prolactin.
  - ↑ FSH indicates primary ovarian insufficiency.
  - ↑ TSH indicates hypothyroidism.
  - ↑ Prolactin (inhibits the release of GnRH and thus LH and FSH); points to a pituitary pathology. Order an MRI of the pituitary gland to look for a prolactin-secreting pituitary adenoma.
- Initiate a progestin challenge (10 days of progestin). See Figure 2.12-4 for an algorithm of the diagnostic work-up.
  - ⊕ **Progestin challenge (withdrawal bleed):** Indicates anovulation that is probably caused by noncyclic gonadotropin secretion, pointing to PCOS or idiopathic anovulation.
  - ⊖ **Progestin challenge (no bleed):** Indicates uterine abnormality or estrogen deficiency.
- **Signs of hyperglycemia (polydipsia, polyuria) or hypotension:** Conduct a 1-mg overnight dexamethasone suppression test to distinguish CAH (21-hydroxylase deficiency), Cushing syndrome, and Addison disease.
- **Clinical virilization:** If present, measure testosterone, DHEA-S, and 17-hydroxyprogesterone.
- **Mild pattern:** PCOS, CAH, or Cushing syndrome.
- **Moderate to severe pattern:** Look for an ovarian or adrenal tumor.

TREATMENT

- **Hypothalamic:** Reverse the underlying cause and induce ovulation with gonadotropins if trying to conceive. If not, oral contraceptives.
- **Tumors:** Excision; medical therapy for prolactinomas (eg, cabergoline, bromocriptine).
- **Premature ovarian failure** (< 40 years of age): If the uterus is present, treat with combined oral contraceptives or estrogen plus progestin replacement therapy.

1° DYSMENORRHEA

Menstrual pain associated with ovulatory cycles in the absence of pathologic findings. Caused by uterine vasoconstriction, anoxia, and sustained contractions mediated by an excess of prostaglandin (PGF2α).

Q 1

A 56-year-old woman presents with complaints of insomnia, vaginal dryness, and lack of menses for 13 months. What is the most likely diagnosis?

Q 2

A 16-year-old girl presents with ↓ appetite, insomnia, and amenorrhea for 3 months. What is the most likely diagnosis, and how will you confirm it?

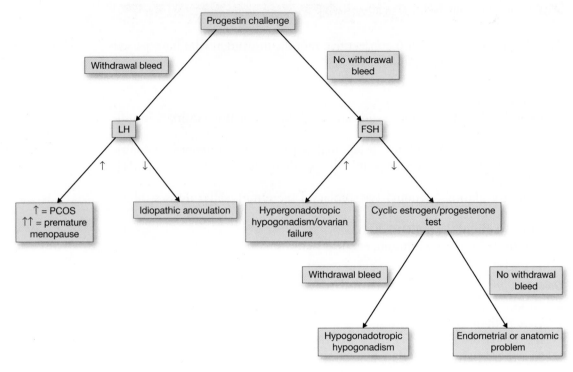

FIGURE 2.12-4. Work-up of 2° amenorrhea.

History/PE

- Presents with low, midline, spasmodic pelvic pain that often radiates to the back or inner thighs.
- Cramps occur in the first 1–3 days of menstruation and may be associated with nausea, diarrhea, headache, and flushing.
- No pathologic findings on pelvic exam.

Diagnosis

A diagnosis of exclusion. Rule out 2° dysmenorrhea (see later).

Treatment

NSAIDs; topical heat therapy; combined hormonal contraception, progestin intrauterine device (IUD).

2° DYSMENORRHEA

Menstrual pain for which an organic cause exists. Common causes include endometriosis, adenomyosis, fibroids, adhesions, and PID.

History/PE

- Patients may have a palpable uterine mass, cervical motion tenderness, adnexal tenderness, or vaginal or cervical discharge. However, normal abdominal and pelvic exams do not rule out pathology.
- See Table 2.12-5 for distinguishing features of endometriosis vs adenomyosis.

1 **A**

The most likely diagnosis is menopause. As a clinical diagnosis, menopause does not require the ordering of any tests. However, if you are trying to rule it out as a cause of 2° amenorrhea, you may consider ordering an FSH level. Elevation is suggestive of menopause.

2 **A**

The most likely diagnosis is pregnancy. Confirm with a β-hCG test.

TABLE 2.12-5.   Endometriosis vs Adenomyosis

VARIABLE	ENDOMETRIOSIS	ADENOMYOSIS
Definition	Functional endometrial glands and stroma outside the uterus	Endometrial tissue in the myometrium of the uterus
History/PE	Cyclic pelvic and/or rectal pain and dyspareunia Uterus not enlarged but painful nodules, restricted range of motion	Classic triad of pain, menorrhagia, and an enlarged, boggy, symmetric uterus
Diagnosis	Requires direct visualization by laparoscopy or laparotomy Classic lesions have a blue-black ("raspberry") or dark brown ("powder-burned") appearance The ovaries may have endometriomas ("chocolate cysts")	MRI can aid in diagnosis but is costly Ultrasonography is useful but cannot always distinguish between leiomyoma and adenomyosis Ultimately a pathologic diagnosis
Treatment	Pharmacologic: Inhibit ovulation. Combination hormonal contraception (first line), GnRH analogues (leuprolide), danazol, NSAIDs, or progestins Conservative surgical treatment: Excision, cauterization, or ablation of the lesions and lysis of adhesions Twenty percent of patients can become pregnant subsequent to treatment Definitive surgical treatment: TAH/BSO ± lysis of adhesions	Pharmacologic: Largely symptomatic relief. NSAIDs (first line) plus combined hormonal contraception or progestins Conservative surgical treatment: Endometrial ablation or resection using hysteroscopy; complete eradication of deep adenomyosis is difficult and results in ↑ treatment failure Definitive surgical treatment: Hysterectomy is the only definitive treatment
Complications	Infertility (the most common cause among menstruating women > 30 years of age)	May very rarely progress to endometrial carcinoma

DIAGNOSIS

- Obtain a β-hCG test to exclude ectopic pregnancy.
- Perform a pelvic exam to assess uterine size, tenderness, and consistency, and to evaluate for ovarian masses.
- Order the following:
    - CBC with differential to rule out infection.
    - UA to rule out UTI.
    - Gonococcal/chlamydial swabs to rule out STDs/PID.
- Consider ultrasound to assess endometrium, uterus, and ovaries (look for pelvic pathology causing pain [see Table 2.12-5]).

TREATMENT

Treatment is etiology specific.

ABNORMAL UTERINE BLEEDING

- Normal menstrual bleeding ranges from 2 to 7 days. Abnormal uterine bleeding refers to alterations in quantity, duration, or frequency. Classified by acronym PALM-COEIN.
- **PALM** refers to structural causes—**P**olyp, **A**denomyosis, **L**eiomyoma, and **M**alignancy/hyperplasia.
- **COEIN** refers to nonstructural causes—**C**oagulopathy, **O**vulatory dysfunction, **E**ndometrial, **I**atrogenic, and **N**ot yet classified.

KEY FACT

Polyps are not associated with pain.

KEY FACT

Postmenopausal vaginal bleeding is cancer until proven otherwise.

HISTORY/PE

- **Assess the extent of bleeding:**
    - **Oligomenorrhea:** An ↑ length of time between menses (35–90 days between cycles).
    - **Polymenorrhea:** Frequent menstruation (< 21-day cycle).
    - **Menorrhagia:** ↑ Amount of flow (> 80 mL of blood loss per cycle) or prolonged bleeding (flow lasting > 8 days); may lead to anemia.
    - **Metrorrhagia:** Bleeding between periods.
    - **Menometrorrhagia:** Excessive and irregular bleeding.
    - On pelvic exam, look for an enlarged uterus, a cervical mass, or polyps to assess for myomas, pregnancy, or cervical cancer.

DIAGNOSIS

- β-hCG test to rule out pregnancy.
- CBC to evaluate for anemia.
- Pap smear to rule out cervical cancer.
- Gonorrhea/chlamydia probe to rule out cervical bleeding from cervicitis.
- TFTs and prolactin to rule out hyper-/hypothyroidism and hyperprolactinemia.
- Platelet count, PT/PTT to rule out von Willebrand disease and factor XI deficiency, primarily in adolescent patients.
- Ultrasonography to look for uterine masses, polycystic ovaries, and thickness of the endometrium.
- **Perform endometrial biopsy:**
    - If the endometrium is ≥ 4 mm in a postmenopausal woman, or if the patient is > 45 years of age.
    - If the patient is > 35 years of age with risk factors for endometrial hyperplasia (eg, obesity, diabetes).

TREATMENT

- **Acute heavy bleeding:**
    - High-dose estrogen IV stabilizes the endometrial lining and typically stops bleeding within 1 hour. Transition to combined oral contraceptive or add progestin when bleeding stabilized.
    - If estrogen is contraindicated, can give high-dose progestin therapy alone.
    - If bleeding is not controlled within 12–24 hours, a D&C is often indicated.
- **Ovulatory bleeding (menorrhagia):**
    - NSAIDs to ↓ blood loss.
    - Tranexamic acid can be given for 5 days during menses.
    - If the patient is hemodynamically stable, give OCPs, oral or injectable progestin, or insert a progestin IUD.
- **Anovulatory bleeding:**
    - Goal is to convert proliferative endometrium to secretory endometrium (to ↓ the risk for endometrial hyperplasia/cancer).
    - Progestins for 10 days to stimulate withdrawal bleeding.
    - Combined hormonal contraception.
    - Progestin IUD.
- **If medical management fails:**
    - D&C.
    - Hysteroscopy to identify endometrial polyps or to perform directed uterine biopsies.
    - Uterine artery embolization if fibroids are the cause of menorrhagia.

KEY FACT

Best initial treatment of abnormal uterine bleeding consists of NSAIDs to ↓ blood loss!

KEY FACT

Combined hormonal contraception and the progesterone containing IUD are highly effective treatment options for menorrhagia.

- Hysterectomy or endometrial ablation appropriate for the following:
  - Women for whom hormonal treatment fails.
  - Women who no longer desire fertility.
  - Women who have symptomatic anemia and/or who experience a disruption in their quality of life from persistent, unscheduled bleeding.

Reproductive Endocrinology

CONGENITAL ADRENAL HYPERPLASIA

A deficiency of at least one enzyme required for the biochemical synthesis of cortisol from cholesterol (see Figure 2.12-5 and Table 2.12-6). Includes the following:

- **21-hydroxylase deficiency:** Accounts for ∼ 90% of CAH cases; "classic" form is most severe and presents as a newborn infant girl with ambiguous genitalia and adrenal insufficiency (with or without life-threatening salt wasting). "Nonclassic" is a late-onset form that presents with androgen excess or could be asymptomatic. Cannot convert 17-hydroxyprogesterone to 11-deoxycortisol → ↓ cortisol synthesis → ↑ adrenal stimulation → ↑ ACTH and androgens.
- **11β-hydroxylase deficiency:** Second most common cause of adrenal hyperplasia. Cannot convert 11-deoxycortisol to cortisol or 11-deoxycorticosterone to corticosterone, also leading to ↑ ACTH and androgens.

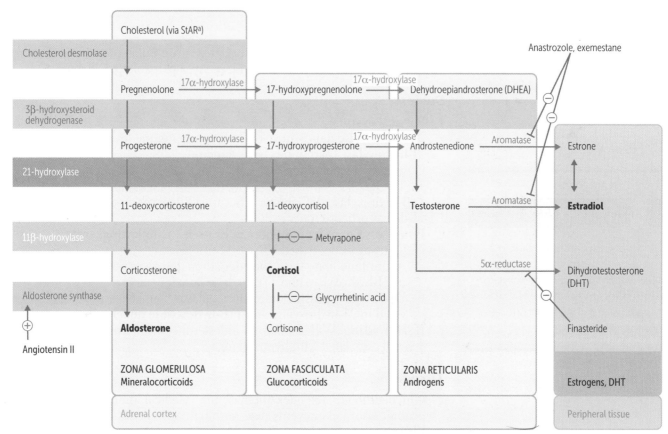

ᵃRate-limiting step.

FIGURE 2.12-5. **Glucocorticoid biosynthesis pathway.** (Modified with permission from USMLE-Rx.com.)

TABLE 2.12-6.   Overview of Congenital Adrenal Hyperplasia

Enzyme Deficiency	Mineralocorticoids	Cortisol	Sex Hormones	BP	[K⁺]	Labs	Presentation
17α-hydroxylase[a]	↑	↓	↓	↑	↓	↓ Androstenedione	XY: ambiguous genitalia, undescended testes XX: lacks secondary sexual development
21-hydroxylase[a]	↓	↓	↑	↓	↑	↑ Renin activity ↑ 17-hydroxypro-gesterone	Most common Presents in infancy (salt wasting) or childhood (precocious puberty) XX: virilization
11β-hydroxylase[a]	↓ Aldosterone ↑ 11-deoxycorticosterone (results in ↑ BP)	↓	↑	↑	↓	↓ Renin activity	XX: virilization

[a]All congenital adrenal enzyme deficiencies are characterized by an enlargement of both adrenal glands caused by ↑ ACTH stimulation (caused by ↓ cortisol).

Modified with permission from Le T, et al. *First Aid for the USMLE Step 1 2018.* New York, NY: McGraw-Hill; 2018.

KEY FACT

- Hirsutism = male hair pattern.
- Virilization = frontal balding, muscularity, clitoromegaly, and deepening of the voice.
- Defeminization = ↓ breast size; loss of feminine adipose tissue.

KEY FACT

21-hydroxylase deficiency can present with hypotension, whereas 11β-hydroxylase and 17-hydroxylase deficiencies can present with hypertension caused by accumulation of deoxycorticosterone.

History/PE

Androgen excess: Genital ambiguity, premature pubarche, menstrual irregularity, infertility, hirsutism, acne, and, rarely, a palpable pelvic mass.

Diagnosis

- Physical exam.
- **21-hydroxylase deficiency:** ↑ 17-OH progesterone levels: substrate for 21-hydroxylase (part of newborn screen).
- Cosyntropin stimulation test is gold standard, but not necessary if ↑↑ 17-OH.
- **11β-hydroxylase deficiency:** ↑ Serum 11-deoxycortisol and 11-deoxycorticosterone.
- **Both:** Next, in order of importance, assess the following levels:
  - Cortisol → decreased.
  - Androstenedione (also consider adrenal/ovarian neoplasm) → elevated in 21-hydroxylase and 11β-hydroxylase deficiency.
  - DHEA (also consider adrenal neoplasm, Cushing syndrome) → elevated in 21-hydroxylase and 11β-hydroxylase deficiency.
- **If salt wasting:** Will also have ↓ aldosterone, ↓ sodium, ↑ potassium, and ↑ renin associated with hypovolemia.

Treatment

- Glucocorticoids (eg, dexamethasone). Medical therapy for adrenal and ovarian disorders prevents new terminal hair growth but does not resolve hirsutism.
- Add mineralocorticoid therapy (eg, fludrocortisone) if salt wasting.
- Laser ablation, electrolysis, or conventional hair removal techniques must be used to remove unwanted hair.

POLYCYSTIC OVARIAN SYNDROME

A syndrome of excess testosterone and excess estrogen, PCOS has a prevalence of 6–10% among US women of reproductive age and is the most common cause of infertility in women. Diagnosis requires fulfillment of two of the following three (Rotterdam criteria):

- Polycystic ovaries (via ultrasonography).
- Oligo- and/or anovulation.
- Clinical and/or biochemical evidence of hyperandrogenism.

HISTORY/PE

- **Common presentation:** Obesity (BMI > 30 kg/m^2), menstrual cycle disturbances, infertility, acne, androgenic alopecia, and hirsutism from hyperandrogenism.
- **Women with PCOS are also at ↑ risk for the following:**
    - **DM type 2:** Acanthosis nigricans.
    - **Metabolic syndrome:** Insulin resistance, atherogenic dyslipidemia, and hypertension.

DIAGNOSIS

- **Biochemical testing of hyperandrogenemia:** ↑ Testosterone.
    - ↑ Free testosterone is more sensitive than total testosterone (total can be normal) because of low sex hormone–binding globulin.
    - Exclude other causes of hyperandrogenism: DHEA-S to rule out adrenal tumor.
    - Pelvic ultrasound to rule out androgen-secreting ovarian tumor.
    - 17-OH progesterone to rule out nonclassical CAH.
    - Consider screening in the setting of clinical signs of Cushing syndrome (eg, moon facies, buffalo hump, abdominal striae) or acromegaly (eg, ↑ head size).
- **Evaluate for metabolic abnormalities:**
    - Two-hour oral glucose tolerance test.
    - Fasting lipid and lipoprotein levels (total cholesterol, HDL, LDL, triglycerides).
- **Optional tests:** Not necessary if both oligomenorrhea and signs of hyperandrogenism are present.
    - **Transvaginal ultrasonography:** Look for more than 11 small (2–9 mm), subcapsular follicles forming a "pearl necklace" sign (see Figure 2.12-6). Seen in roughly two-thirds of women with PCOS.
    - **Gonadotropins:** ↑ LH/FSH ratio (> 2:1).
    - **24-hour urine for free cortisol:** Adult-onset CAH or Cushing syndrome.

TREATMENT

- **Women who are not attempting to conceive:** Treat with a combination of combined hormonal contraception or progestin ± metformin (or other insulin-sensitizing agents).
- **Women who are attempting to conceive:** Clomiphene (selective estrogen receptor modulator) ± metformin is first-line treatment for ovulatory stimulation.
- **Symptom-specific treatment:**
    - **Hirsutism:** Combination OCPs are first line; antiandrogens (spironolactone, finasteride) and metformin may also be used.
    - **Obesity, cardiovascular risk factors, lipid levels:** Diet, weight loss (can also help regulate ovulation), and exercise plus potentially lipid-controlling medication (eg, statins).

KEY FACT

The most severe form of PCOS is **HAIR-AN** syndrome: **H**yper**A**ndrogenism, **I**nsulin **R**esistance, and **A**canthosis **N**igricans.

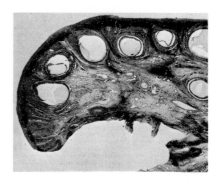

FIGURE 2.12-6. Polycystic ovary with prominent multiple cysts. (Reproduced with permission from DeCherney AH, Nathan R. *Current Diagnosis & Treatment: Obstetrics & Gynecology*, 10th ed. New York, NY: McGraw-Hill; 2007.)

KEY FACT

Combined hormonal contraception or progestin ↓ the risk for endometrial hyperplasia/carcinoma among women with PCOS.

Q   1

A 28-year-old woman comes to clinic for a wellness exam. She describes that approximately 2 weeks after her menses, she experiences intense, sharp lower quadrant abdominal pain that lasts a couple of hours. The pain varies from the right to the left side each cycle. What is the name of this phenomenon?

Q   2

A 23-year-old woman presents with fever and abdominal pain of 2 days' duration. She has a ⊕ chandelier sign. Antibiotics are started. What is the next step in management?

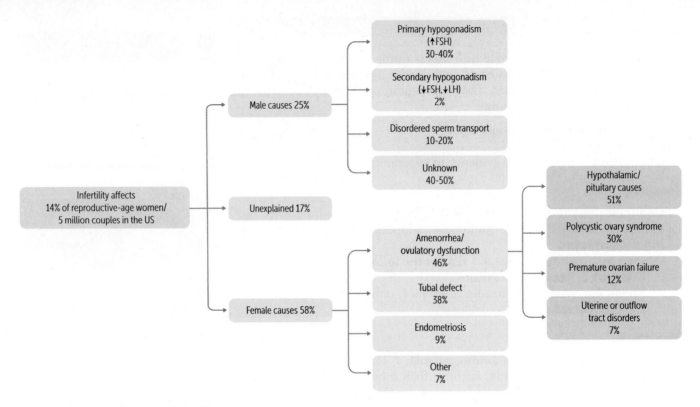

FIGURE 2.12-7. **Causes of infertility.** (Reproduced with permission from USMLE-Rx.com.)

COMPLICATIONS

↑ Risk for early-onset DM type 2; ↑ risk for miscarriages; ↑ long-term risk for breast and endometrial cancer because of unopposed estrogen secretion.

INFERTILITY

- The inability to conceive after 12 months of normal, regular, unprotected sexual activity in women < 35 years of age; and after 6 months of regular, unprotected intercourse in women ≥ 35 years of age.
- 1° Infertility is characterized by no prior pregnancies; 2° infertility occurs in the setting of at least one prior pregnancy. Etiologies are shown in Figure 2.12-7 and Table 2.12-7.

Gynecologic Infections

CYST AND ABSCESS OF THE BARTHOLIN DUCT

Obstruction of the Bartholin duct may lead to cyst formation, as mucus continues to accumulate behind the obstruction, causing cystic dilation. An obstructed Bartholin duct that becomes infected can develop a polymicrobial abscess.

HISTORY/PE

- **Cysts:** 1–3 cm in size, unilateral, and often asymptomatic. If larger, lead to periodic, painful swelling and dyspareunia.
- **Diagnosis is clinical:** Mass at medial labia majora or lower vestibular area on physical exam.
- **Abscess:** Extremely painful, warm, fluctuant mass in same location as above, possible cellulitis.

1 **A**

This is called mittelschmerz, pain at ovulation caused by progesterone production. It can switch sides depending on which ovary ovulates in a given cycle.

2 **A**

Pelvic ultrasonography to rule out tubo-ovarian abscess.

TABLE 2.12-7.   Infertility Work-up

ETIOLOGY	HISTORY/PE	DIAGNOSIS	TREATMENT
Male factors	Testicular injury or infection Medications (corticosteroids, cimetidine, spironolactone) Pituitary, thyroid, or liver disease Signs of hypogonadism Varicocele	Semen analysis TSH Prolactin Karyotype (to rule out Klinefelter syndrome)	Treatment of hormonal deficiency Intrauterine insemination (IUI) Donor insemination IVF Intracytoplasmic sperm injection
Ovulatory factors	Age (incidence ↑ with age) Symptoms of hyper-/hypothyroidism Galactorrhea Menstrual cycle abnormalities Pituitary tumors	Menstrual history Basal body temperature Ovulation predictor Midluteal progesterone Early follicular FSH ± estradiol level (ovarian reserve) TSH, prolactin, androgens Ovarian sonography (antral follicle count) Endometrial biopsy (luteal-phase defect)	Treatment depends on the etiology (eg, levothyroxine, dopamine) Induction of ovulation with clomiphene, gonadotropins, and pulsatile GnRH IUI IVF
Tubal/pelvic factors	History of PID, appendicitis, endometriosis, pelvic adhesions, tubal surgery	Hysterosalpingogram Endometrial biopsy	Laparoscopic resection or ablation of endometriomas or fibroids IVF
Cervical factors	Cryotherapy, conization, or DES exposure in utero	Pap smear Physical exam Antisperm antibodies	IUI with washed sperm IVF
Uterine factors	Polyps Fibroids Congenital anomalies	Ultrasound Sonohysterogram Hysterosalpingogram	Surgical treatment

TREATMENT

- **Asymptomatic cysts:** No therapy ± warm soaks. Consider drainage and biopsy if > 40 years of age to exclude carcinoma.
- **Abscess:** Aspiration or incision and drainage to prevent reaccumulation; test for gonorrhea and *Chlamydia* and other pathogens.
- Antibiotics are unnecessary unless cellulitis or STI present.

VAGINITIS

A spectrum of conditions that cause vulvovaginal symptoms such as itching, burning, irritation, and abnormal discharge. The most common causes are bacterial vaginosis, vulvovaginal candidiasis, and trichomoniasis (see Table 2.12-8).

HISTORY/PE

- Presents with a change in discharge, malodor, pruritus, irritation, burning, swelling, dyspareunia, and dysuria.
- Normal secretions are as follows:
  - Midcycle estrogen surge: Clear, elastic, mucoid secretions.
  - Luteal phase/pregnancy: Thick and white secretions; adhere to the vaginal wall.

A 20-year-old woman is diagnosed with trichomonas and prescribed an antibiotic. She calls her physician complaining of flushing, nausea, and emesis. What antibiotic was the patient prescribed and what should she have been warned of?

She was prescribed metronidazole. She should have been warned to stay away from alcohol while taking it, as it causes a disulfiram-like reaction.

- Conduct a thorough exam of the vulva, vaginal walls, and cervix.
- If there are many WBCs and no organism on saline smear, suspect *Chlamydia*.

DIAGNOSIS/TREATMENT

- Vaginal fluid for vaginal pH, amine (whiff) test, wet mount (with saline), and 10% potassium hydroxide (KOH) microscopy.
- If purulent discharge, numerous leukocytes on wet prep, cervical friability, and any symptoms of PID, order DNA tests or cultures for *Neisseria gonorrhoeae* or *Chlamydia trachomatis* to rule out cervicitis.
- Treatment is etiology specific (see Table 2.12-8).

CERVICITIS

- Inflammation of the uterine cervix. Etiologies are as follows:
  - **Infectious (most common):** *Chlamydia*, gonococcus, *Trichomonas*, HSV. *Chlamydia trachomatis* is more common than gonococcus in mucopurulent cervicitis.
  - **Noninfectious:** Trauma, radiation exposure, malignancy.
- All sexually active women < 25 years of age should undergo yearly screening for *Chlamydia* and *Neisseria* because of ↑ rates of asymptomatic infection and ↑ risk for infertility in untreated infections.
- **Hx/PE:** Yellow-green mucopurulent discharge; ⊕ cervical motion tenderness; absence of other signs of PID.
- **Dx/Tx:** See the discussion of STDs in the Infectious Disease chapter. If mucopurulent. Empiric treatment for both *C trachomatis* and *N gonorrhoeae*.

PELVIC INFLAMMATORY DISEASE

A polymicrobial infection of the upper genital tract. Associated with *N gonorrhoeae* (one-third of cases), *C trachomatis* (one-third of cases), and endogenous aerobes/anaerobes. Risk factors include non-white ethnicity, douching, smoking, multiple sex partners, and prior STDs and/or PID.

HISTORY/PE

- Presents with lower abdominal pain, fever, chills, menstrual disturbances, and purulent cervical discharge.
- Cervical motion tenderness (chandelier sign) and adnexal tenderness.
- Orogenital contact can cause gonococcal pharyngitis along with PID.

DIAGNOSIS

- Diagnosed by the presence of acute lower abdominal or pelvic pain plus one of the following:
  - Uterine tenderness.
  - Adnexal tenderness.
  - Cervical motion tenderness.
- First, order a β-hCG test to rule out pregnancy.
- A WBC count > 10,000 cells/μL has poor positive and negative predictive value for PID.
- Ultrasonography may show thickening or dilation of the fallopian tubes, fluid in the cul-de-sac, a multicystic ovary, or tubo-ovarian abscess.

TREATMENT

- Antibiotic treatment should not be delayed while awaiting culture results. All sexual partners should be examined and treated appropriately.
- **Outpatient regimens:**
  - **Regimen A:** Ceftriaxone IM for one dose + azithromycin PO for one dose or ceftriaxone IM + doxycycline (if allergic to azithromycin).

TABLE 2.12-8. **Causes of Vaginitis**

VARIABLE	BACTERIAL VAGINOSIS	TRICHOMONAS	YEAST
Incidence	15–50% (most common)	5–50%	15–30%
Etiology	Not an infection: shift in vaginal flora (↑ anaerobes such as *Gardnerella vaginalis*, ↓ lactobacilli)	Protozoal flagellates (an STD)	Usually *Candida albicans*
Risk factors	Pregnancy, multiple sexual partners, female sexual partner, frequent douching	Unprotected sex with multiple partners	DM, antibiotic use, pregnancy, corticosteroids, HIV, OCP use, ↑ frequency of intercourse, tight-fitting clothing
History	Odor, ↑ discharge	↑ Discharge, odor, pruritus, dysuria	Pruritus, dysuria, burning, ↑ discharge
Exam	Mild vulvar irritation	"Strawberry petechiae" in the upper vagina/cervix	Erythematous, excoriated vulva/vagina
Discharge	Homogeneous, grayish-white, fishy/stale odor	Profuse, malodorous, yellow-green, frothy	Thick, white, curdy texture without odor
Wet mount[a]	"Clue cells" (epithelial cells coated with bacteria [see Image A]); "No clue why I smell fish in the vagina garden"	Motile trichomonads (flagellated organisms that are slightly larger than WBCs [see Image B])	Budding yeast or hyphae
KOH prep	⊕ "Whiff" test (fishy smell)		Pseudohyphae (see Image C)
Treatment	PO or vaginal metronidazole or vaginal clindamycin	Single-dose PO metronidazole or tinidazole Treat partners, otherwise a "ping-pong effect"; test for other STDs	Topical azole or PO fluconazole
Complications	Chorioamnionitis/endometritis, infection, preterm delivery, PID	Same as for bacterial vaginosis	

A

B

C

[a]If there are many WBCs and no organism on saline smear, suspect *Chlamydia*.

Image A reproduced with permission from USMLE-Rx.com. Image B reproduced courtesy of the US Department of Health and Human Services. Image C reproduced with permission from Wolff K, et al. *Fitzpatrick's Color Atlas & Synopsis of Clinical Dermatology*, 5th ed. New York, NY: McGraw-Hill; 2005.

- **Regimen B:** Ofloxacin or levofloxacin for 14 days ± metronidazole for 14 days. This is only in special cases since there is an increase in quinolone-resistant *N gonorrhoeae*.
- If nucleic acid amplification testing for either *N gonorrhoeae* or *Chlamydia* is ⊖, treatment is not indicated. However, treatment should not be delayed for NAAT.
- **Inpatient antibiotic regimens:**
  - Cefoxitin or cefotetan plus doxycycline for 14 days.
  - Clindamycin plus gentamicin for 14 days.

- Surgery:
  - Drainage of a tubo-ovarian/pelvic abscess is appropriate if:
    - Mass persists after antibiotic treatment.
    - Abscess is > 4–6 cm.
    - Mass is in the cul-de-sac in the midline and drainable through the vagina.
  - If the patient's condition deteriorates, perform exploratory laparoscopy or laparotomy.
  - Surgery may range from TAH/BSO with lysis of adhesions in severe cases to conservative surgery for women who desire to maintain fertility.

COMPLICATIONS

- Repeated episodes of infection, chronic pelvic pain, dyspareunia, and ectopic pregnancy.
- Infertility (10% after the first episode, 25% after the second episode, and 50% after a third episode).
- Fitz-Hugh–Curtis syndrome (presents with associated perihepatitis, RUQ pain, abnormal liver function, and referred right shoulder pain).

TOXIC SHOCK SYNDROME

Caused by preformed *Staphylococcus aureus* toxin (TSST-1); can occur within 5 days of using tampons. The incidence in menstruating women is now 6–7/100,000 annually. Nonmenstrual cases are nearly as common as menstrual cases (eg, surgical, burns).

HISTORY/PE

- Presents with abrupt onset of fever, vomiting, and watery diarrhea.
- A diffuse macular erythematous rash involving the palms and soles is seen.
- Nonpurulent conjunctivitis is common.
- Desquamation, especially of the palms and soles, generally occurs during recovery within 1–2 weeks of illness.

DIAGNOSIS

- Based on clinical presentation. Fever > 38.9°C, hypotension, skin findings, involvement of three or more organ systems.
- Blood cultures are ⊖, given that it is caused by a preformed toxin and not invasive properties of the organism.

TREATMENT

- Rapid rehydration, exam for foreign objects in vaginal canal, drainage if localized infection found.
- Empiric antibiotics: Clindamycin + vancomycin.
- If methicillin-sensitive *S aureus* isolated in wound, clindamycin + oxacillin OR nafcillin.
- If methicillin-resistant *S aureus* isolated, clindamycin + vancomycin OR linezolid.

COMPLICATIONS

- Mortality rate associated with TSS is 3–6%.
- Causes of death include cardiac arrhythmias, cardiomyopathy, respiratory failure caused by ARDS, and coagulopathy caused by DIC.

Gynecologic Neoplasms

Gynecologic cancers include uterine, endometrial, ovarian, cervical, and vulvar neoplasms. Ovarian cancer carries the highest mortality.

UTERINE LEIOMYOMA (FIBROIDS)

The most common benign neoplasm of the female genital tract. They present as discrete, round, firm, and often multiple tumors composed of smooth muscle and connective tissue and may cause infertility or menorrhagia.

- Fibroids are hormone sensitive; size will ↑ in pregnancy and ↓ after menopause.
- Malignant transformation to leiomyosarcoma is rare (0.1%–0.5%).
- **Prevalence:** More common in African-American women (50%) than in white women (25%).

HISTORY/PE

- Majority of cases are asymptomatic.
- Symptomatic patients may present with the following:
  - **Bleeding:** Longer, heavier periods; anemia.
  - **Mass effect:** Pelvic/rectal pressure constipation, and urinary frequency or retention.
  - **Pain:** 2° Dysmenorrhea, dyspareunia.
  - **Pelvic symptoms:** A firm, nontender, irregular enlarged ("lumpy-bumpy"), or cobblestone uterus may be felt on physical exam.

DIAGNOSIS

- **Physical exam.**
- **Ultrasonography (transvaginal):** To look for uterine myomas; can also exclude ovarian masses. Calcification indicates necrosis.
- **MRI:** Can delineate intramural, subserosal, and submucous myomas. Best modality for visualization, usually reserved in preparation for surgery, or if concerned for leiomyosarcoma (new or growing mass in postmenopausal woman).
- **CBC:** To assess for anemia.

TREATMENT

- If asymptomatic, expectant management with annual pelvic exams and CBCs as needed.
- **Pharmacologic:**
  - Combined hormonal contraception.
  - Medroxyprogesterone acetate or danazol to slow or stop bleeding.
  - GnRH analogues (leuprolide or nafarelin) to ↓ the size of myomas, suppress further growth, and ↓ surrounding vascularity. Also used before surgery.
  - NSAIDs for pain.
- **Surgery:**
  - **Women of childbearing years:** Abdominal or hysteroscopic myomectomy.
  - **Women who have completed childbearing:** Total or subtotal abdominal or vaginal hysterectomy.
  - **Uterine artery embolization** (~ 25% will need further invasive treatment).
  - Emergent surgery may be required if torsion of a pedunculated myoma occurs.

KEY FACT

An irregular and mobile uterus is the key physical exam finding for fibroids.

KEY FACT

If a uterine mass continues to grow after menopause, suspect malignancy.

COMPLICATIONS

Infertility may be caused by a myoma that distorts the uterine cavity and plays a role similar to that of an IUD.

ENDOMETRIAL CANCER

Type I endometrioid adenocarcinomas derive from atypical endometrial hyperplasia and are the most common female reproductive cancer in the United States. Type II cancers derive from serous or clear cell histology (see Table 2.12-9). Although type II cancers tend to be more aggressive, diagnosis and management are similar for both types. Type 1 is the most curable gynecologic cancer.

HISTORY/PE

- Vaginal bleeding (early finding).
- Pain (late finding).
- Metabolic syndrome.

DIAGNOSIS

- First, physical exam and pregnancy test if premenopausal.
- Second, ultrasonography. If postmenopausal, can do transvaginal and evaluate endometrial stripe (< 4 mm unlikely to be endometrial cancer). Shows thickened endometrium with hypertrophy and neoplastic change in very advanced cases (Figure 2.12-8).
- Finally, endometrial biopsy. If postmenopausal and any bleeding, must perform a biopsy regardless of ultrasonography results.

TREATMENT

- High-dose progestins for women who desire future fertility.
- Hysterectomy and BSO ± radiation for postmenopausal women.
- Hysterectomy and BSO with adjuvant chemotherapy and/or radiation for advanced-stage cancer.

CERVICAL CANCER

The endocervix lies proximal to the external os, is nonvisible, and is composed of columnar cells (similar to the lower uterine segment). The ectocervix is visible and composed of squamous cells (similar to the vagina). The

TABLE 2.12-9. Types of Endometrial Cancer

VARIABLE	TYPE I: ENDOMETRIOID	TYPE II: SEROUS
Epidemiology	75% of endometrial cancers	25% of endometrial cancers
Etiology	Unopposed estrogen stimulation (eg, obesity, tamoxifen use, exogenous estrogen-only therapy)	Unrelated to estrogen; the p53 mutation is present in 90% of cases
Precursor lesion	Hyperplasia and atypical hyperplasia	None
Mean age at diagnosis	55 years	67 years
Prognosis	Favorable	Poor

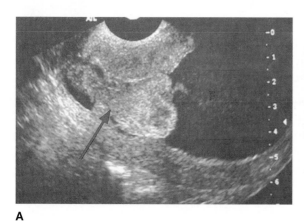

A

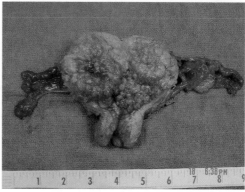

B

FIGURE 2.12-8.   Endometrial cancer. **(A)** Sagittal endovaginal ultrasonogram demonstrates a mass (*arrow*) in the lower uterine segment endometrial canal, with fluid (*F*) distending the canal in the fundus. **(B)** Gross specimen from a different patient shows a large mass filling the endometrial canal and invading the myometrium. (Image A reproduced with permission from USMLE-Rx.com. Image B reproduced with permission from Schorge JO, et al. *Williams Gynecology*. New York, NY: McGraw-Hill; 2008.)

exposure of columnar cells to an acidic vaginal pH results in metaplasia to squamous cells. The normal squamocolumnar junction (transformation zone) is in the ectocervix and can be exposed to carcinogens, resulting in cervical intraepithelial neoplasia (CIN), an abnormal proliferation or overgrowth of the basal cell layer.

- Human papillomavirus (HPV) DNA is found in 99.7% of all cervical carcinomas. HPV 16 is the most prevalent type in squamous cell carcinoma; HPV 18 is most prevalent in adenocarcinoma.
- Additional risk factors include immunosuppression, infection with HIV or a history of STDs, tobacco use, high parity.
- HPV vaccine may protect against HPV types 6, 11 (cause 90% of genital warts) and 16, 18 (cause 70% of cervical cancer). Can be given to both males and females from 11 to 27 years of age.

HISTORY/PE

- Metrorrhagia, postcoital spotting, and cervical ulceration are the most common signs.
- Bloody or purulent, malodorous, nonpruritic discharge may appear after invasion.

SCREENING

- American Congress of Obstetricians and Gynecologists (ACOG) currently recommends that screening for cervical cancer begin at 21 years of age regardless of onset of sexual activity.
- Screening recommendations for women with previously normal exams:
  - < 21 years of age: No screening.
  - 21–29 years of age: Perform Pap smear (cytology) every 3 years.
  - 30–65 years of age: Perform Pap smear every 3 years, or perform cotesting (Pap smear + HPV test) every 5 years.
  - 65 years of age: Stop screening if prior tests were negative.
  - See Table 2.12-10 for classification systems of Pap smears.
- Women with DES exposure (risk for clear cell cancer) and/or immunocompromised status (including HIV positivity) should continue to be screened as long as they do not have a life-limiting condition.
- Women with HIV should be screened with cytology twice in their first year after diagnosis, and then annually.

TABLE 2.12-10.   Classification of Pap Smears

CIN	BETHESDA SYSTEM
Benign	Negative
Benign with inflammation	ASC-US ASC-H
CIN I	LSIL
CIN II	HSIL
CIN III	HSIL
Invasive cancer	Invasive cancer

Cervical intraepithelial neoplasia (CIN) is the histologic classification. The Bethesda system is used for reporting cytological diagnoses.

KEY FACT

Fifty percent of women with cervical cancer had not had a Pap smear in the 3 years preceding their diagnosis, and another 10% had not been screened in 5 years.

DIAGNOSIS

Diagnosis and follow-up of specific subtypes of cervical lesions is outlined here (these guidelines do not apply to adolescents and pregnant women). Cotesting (HPV test and Pap smear) is routinely done starting at 30 years of age.

1. **Women 21–24 years of age with cervical cytology showing atypical squamous cells of undetermined significance (ASC-US) or low-grade squamous intraepithelial lesion (LSIL):**
   - Repeat cytology at 12 months (preferred):
     - If ⊖, ASC-US, or LSIL: Repeat cytology at 12 months and if ⊖ x 2 and then routine screening, but if ASC or higher then colposcopy.
     - If ASC-H, HSIL, atypical glandular cells: Colposcopy.

   Or
   - Reflex HPV DNA testing (only if ASC-US):
     - If ⊖: Routine screening.
     - If ⊕: Follow algorithm above.
2. **ASC-US and > 24 years:**
   - Reflex HPV DNA testing (preferred):
     - If ⊖: Cotesting in 3 years.
     - If ⊕: Colposcopy.

   Or
   - Repeat cytology at 12 months:
     - If ⊖: Routine screening.
     - If ASC-US or higher: Colposcopy.
3. **ASC-H: Colposcopy regardless of HPV status**
4. **LSIL (21–24 years and above):**
   - If HPV ⊖ (≥ 30 years): Repeat cotesting at 12 months (preferred).
     - If ⊖: Repeat cotesting in 3 years.
     - If HPV ⊕ or ASC or higher: Colposcopy.
   - If no HPV test (24–30 years): Colposcopy.
   - If HPV ⊕ (≥ 30 years): Colposcopy.
   - If unsatisfactory or no visible lesion: Endocervical sampling.
   - If CIN II, III: See the management of CIN below.
   - Pregnant women: Colposcopy preferred but can defer until 6 weeks postpartum.
5. **AGC:**
   - All women with cervical cytology showing AGC should have colposcopy with endocervical sampling for biopsy.
   - Women > 35 years of age or those with abnormal bleeding raising concern for endometrial neoplasia should have colposcopy with endocervical and endometrial sampling.
6. **ASC-H and HSIL in 21–24 years:** Colposcopy, and then proceed as follows:
   - If CIN II, III: Treatment as below.
   - If no CIN II, III: Colposcopy and cytology at 6-month intervals for 2 years.
     - If ⊖ twice in a row, then can continue to routine screening.
     - If HSIL for 1 year: Biopsy.
7. **HSIL and > 24 years:** Immediate loop electrosurgical excision (not if pregnant) or colposcopy.

TREATMENT

For noninvasive disease, treatment based on biopsy results for noninvasive lesions (stage 0 disease) is as follows:

- **CIN I preceded by ASC-US, LSIL, or HPV ⊕.**
  - Follow-up is the mainstay of treatment.
  - Cotesting at 12 months (or cytology if < 30 years of age).
    - If ASC or higher or HPV ⊕: Colposcopy.
    - If two ⊖ tests: Resume routine screening.

KEY FACT

Pregnancy is not a contraindication for colposcopy or cervical biopsy. However, endocervical curettage is deferred during pregnancy because of risk for preterm delivery.

KEY FACT

Subtypes of cervical lesions:
- ASC-US: Atypical squamous cells of undetermined significance.
- ASC-H: Atypical squamous cells—cannot exclude HSIL.
- LSIL: Low-grade intraepithelial lesion.
- AGC: Atypical glandular cells of undetermined significance.
- HSIL: High-grade squamous intraepithelial lesion.

- CIN I preceded by ASC-H or HSIL.
- Cotesting (or cytology if < 30 years of age) at 12 and 24 months.
  - If HPV and cytology ⊖: Resume routine screening.
  - If HPV ⊕ or abnormal cytology other than HSIL: Colposcopy.
  - If HSIL: Diagnostic excision procedure (unless 21–24 years of age or pregnant).
  Or
- Diagnostic excision procedure (unless 21–24 years of age or pregnant).
- CIN I, 21–24 years of age:
  - After ASC-US, LSIL: Repeat cytology at 12 months.
  - If < ASC-H or HSIL: Repeat cytology at 12 months.
  - If ASC-H or higher: Colposcopy.
- CIN II and III:
  - Ablation: Cryotherapy or laser ablation.
  - Excision: LEEP; laser and cold-knife conization.
  - In young women: Can observe with colposcopy and cytology at 6 and 12 months.
- Postablative or excisional therapy follow-up is as follows:
  - CIN I, II, or III with ⊖ margins: Pap smear at 12 months and/or HPV testing.
  - CIN II or III with ⊕ margins: Pap smear at 6 months; consider a repeat endocervical curettage.
- Treatment based on biopsy results for invasive disease is as follows (for staging, see Figure 2.12-9):
  - Microinvasive carcinoma (stage IA1): Treat with cone biopsy and close follow-up or simple hysterectomy.
  - Stages IA2, IB1, IB2, IIA: May be treated either with radical hysterectomy or with radiation therapy plus chemotherapy alone.
  - Stages IIB, III, IV: Treat with radiation therapy plus concurrent cisplatin-based chemotherapy.

	STAGE 0	STAGE 1	STAGE 2	STAGE 3	STAGE 4
Extent of turmor	Carcinoma in-situ	Confined to cervix and/or uterus	Spreads beyond uterus but not to pelvic wall or lower 1/3 of vagina	Spreads to pelvic sidewall or lower 1/3 of vagina	Invades bladder, rectum, or distant metastasis beyond true pelvis
5-year survival	93%	IA 93% IB 80%	IIA 63% IIB 58%	IIIA 35% IIIB 32%	16% IVA 15% IVB
Stage at presentation		47%	28%	21%	4%

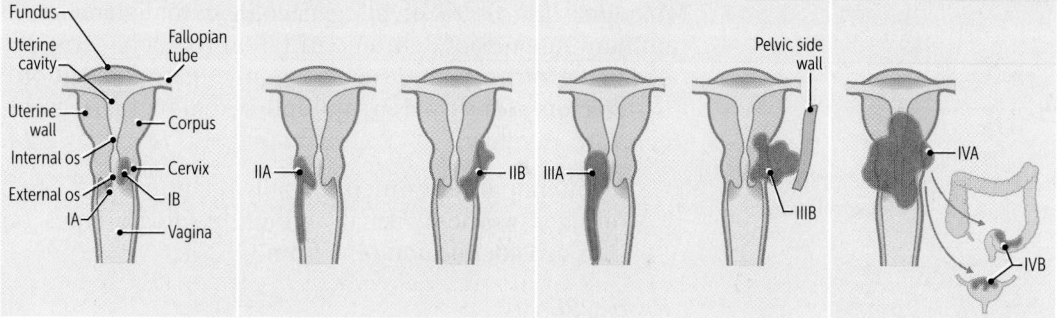

FIGURE 2.12-9.   **Staging of cervical cancer.** Anatomic display of the stages of cervix cancer, defined by location, extent of tumor, frequency of presentation, and 5-year survival. (Reproduced with permission from USMLE-Rx.com.)

PROGNOSIS

- Overall 5-year relative survival rate for carcinoma of the cervix is 68% in white women and 55% in African-American women.
- **5-year survival rates are inversely proportionate to the stage of cancer:**
  - Stage 0: 99–100%.
  - Stage IA: > 95%.
  - Stage IB–IIA: 80–90%.
  - Stage IIB: 65%.
  - Stage III: 40%.
  - Stage IV: < 20%.
- Almost two-thirds of patients with untreated carcinoma of the cervix die of uremia when ureteral obstruction is bilateral.

VULVAR CANCER

Risk factors include HPV (types 16, 18, and 31), lichen sclerosus, infrequent medical exams, diabetes, obesity, hypertension, cardiovascular disease, smoking, high-risk sexual behavior, and immunosuppression. Vulvar intraepithelial neoplasia (VIN) is precancerous and is more commonly found in premenopausal women.

HISTORY/PE

- Presents with pruritus, pain, or ulceration of the mass.
- Additional symptoms include the following:
  - Early: Lesions can appear white, pigmented, raised, thickened, nodular, or ulcerative.
  - Late: Presents with a large, cauliflower-like or hard ulcerated area in the vulva.

DIAGNOSIS

Vulvar punch biopsy for any suspicious lesions or persistent vulvar pruritus, especially in postmenopausal women.

TREATMENT

- **Lichen sclerosus:** High-potency topical steroids (may not prevent progression to cancer).
- **High-grade VIN:** Topical chemotherapy, laser ablation, wide local excision, skinning vulvectomy, and simple vulvectomy.
- **Invasive:**
  - Radical vulvectomy and regional lymphadenectomy.
  - Wide local excision of the 1° tumor with inguinal lymph node dissection ± preoperative radiation, chemotherapy, or both.

VAGINAL CANCER

Accounts for 1–2% of all gynecologic malignancies. Risk factors include immunosuppression, chronic irritation (eg, long-term pessary use or prolapse of female organs), low socioeconomic status, radiation for cervical cancer, hysterectomy for dysplasia, multiple sexual partners, and DES exposure. Etiologies are as follows:

- **Postmenopausal women:** Usually squamous cell carcinoma.
- **Younger women:** Usually other histologic types (eg, adenocarcinoma, clear cell adenocarcinoma from DES).

HISTORY/PE

- Presents with abnormal vaginal bleeding, an abnormal discharge, or postcoital bleeding.
- Found in the upper third of the vagina in 75% of patients.

KEY FACT

Lichen sclerosus key words are "atrophic" and "paperlike" skin.

DIAGNOSIS

Definitive diagnosis is with biopsy and staging.

TREATMENT

- Local excision of involved areas when they are few and small.
- Extensive involvement of the vaginal mucosa may require partial or complete vaginectomy.
- Invasive disease requires radiation therapy or radical surgery.

OVARIAN CANCER

Most ovarian tumors are benign, but malignant tumors are the leading cause of death from reproductive tract cancer. There is no screening test for ovarian cancer. Risk factors include the following:

- Age, low parity, ↓ fertility, or delayed childbearing.
- ⊕ Family history. Patients with one affected first-degree relative have a 5% lifetime risk. With two or more affected first-degree relatives, the risk is 7%.
- The *BRCA1* mutation carries a 45% lifetime risk for ovarian cancer. The *BRCA2* mutation is associated with a 25% lifetime risk.
- Lynch II syndrome, or hereditary nonpolyposis colorectal cancer (HNPCC), is associated with an ↑ risk for colon, ovarian, endometrial, and breast cancer.
- OCPs taken for 5 years or more ↓ risk by 29%.

HISTORY/PE

- Both benign and malignant ovarian neoplasms are generally asymptomatic.
- Mild, nonspecific GI symptoms or pelvic pressure/pain may be seen.
- Early disease is typically not detected on routine pelvic exam.
- Some 75% of woman present with advanced malignant disease, as evidenced by abdominal pain and bloating, a palpable abdominal mass, and ascites.
- Table 2.12-11 differentiates the benign and malignant characteristics of pelvic masses.

KEY FACT

Frequency of female genital tract cancers: endometrial > ovarian > cervical
Number of deaths: ovarian > endometrial > cervical

TABLE 2.12-11.   Benign vs Malignant Pelvic Masses

FINDING	BENIGN	MALIGNANT
EXAM: PELVIC MASS		
Mobility	Mobile	Fixed
Consistency	Cystic	Solid or firm
Location	Unilateral	Bilateral
Cul-de-sac	Smooth	Nodular
TRANSVAGINAL ULTRASONOGRAPHY: ADNEXAL MASS		
Size	< 8 cm	> 8 cm
Consistency	Cystic	Solid or cystic and solid
Septations	Unilocular	Multilocular
Location	Unilateral	Bilateral
Other	Calcifications	Ascites

DIAGNOSIS

- **Tumor markers** (see Table 2.12-12): ↑ CA-125 is associated with epithelial cell cancer (90% of ovarian cancers) but is used only as a marker for progression and recurrence.
    - **Premenopausal women:** ↑ CA-125 may point to benign disease such as endometriosis or TOA.
    - **Postmenopausal women:** ↑ CA-125 (> 35 units) indicates an ↑ likelihood that the ovarian tumor is malignant.
- **Transvaginal ultrasonography:** Used to screen high-risk women and as the first step in the work-up of symptomatic women (eg, pelvic fullness, pelvic pain). A solid mass with thick septations +/− ascites on ultrasound is highly suggestive of neoplasm.

TREATMENT

- **Ovarian masses in premenarchal women:** Masses > 2 cm in diameter require close clinical follow-up and often surgical removal.
- **Ovarian masses in premenopausal women:**
    - Observation is appropriate for asymptomatic, mobile, unilateral, simple cystic masses < 8–10 cm in diameter. Most resolve spontaneously.
    - Surgically evaluate masses > 8–10 cm in diameter and those that are complex and/or unchanged on repeat pelvic exam and ultrasonography.
- **Ovarian masses in postmenopausal women:**
    - Closely follow with ultrasonography asymptomatic, unilateral simple cysts < 5 cm in diameter with a normal CA-125.
    - Surgically evaluate palpable masses.

TABLE 2.12-12. Ovarian Tumor Characteristics

TUMOR	MARKER	CHARACTERISTICS
Epithelial	CA-125	Serous adenocarcinoma is the most common; may present with abdominal distension, bowel obstruction, adnexal mass
Endodermal sinus (yolk sac)	AFP	Very aggressive, may be seen in ovaries and/or sacrococcygeal area in young children; gross exam shows yellow, friable, solid mass
Embryonal carcinoma	AFP, β-hCG	Very rare, may be seen in adolescents; may present with precocious puberty and abnormal uterine bleeding
Choriocarcinoma	β-hCG	Can develop during or after pregnancy in mother or baby; malignancy of trophoblastic tissue; may be associated with bilateral theca-lutein cysts; spreads hematogenously
Dysgerminoma	LDH	Most commonly seen in adolescents; sheets of uniform "fried egg" cells
Granulosa cell	Inhibin	Most common malignant stromal tumor, often seen in women in their 50s, produces estrogen and/or progesterone → may lead to postmenopausal bleeding, Call-Exner bodies on histology

- Ovarian cancer treatment:
  - Surgery:
    - Surgical staging: Hysterectomy/BSO with omentectomy and pelvic and paraaortic lymphadenectomy.
    - Benign neoplasms warrant tumor removal or unilateral oophorectomy.
  - **Postoperative chemotherapy:** Routine except for women with early-stage or low-grade ovarian cancer.
  - **Radiation therapy:** Effective for dysgerminomas.

PREVENTION

- Women with the BRCA1 gene mutation should be screened annually with ultrasonography and CA-125 testing. Prophylactic oophorectomy is recommended by 40 years of age or whenever childbearing is completed.
- OCP use ↓ the risk for ovarian cancer.
- There is no routine screening for ovarian cancer.

Pelvic Organ Prolapse

Risk factors for pelvic organ prolapse include vaginal birth, genetic predisposition, advancing age, prior pelvic surgery (hysterectomy), connective tissue disorders, and ↑ intra-abdominal pressure associated with obesity or straining with chronic constipation.

HISTORY/PE

- Presents with the sensation of a bulge or protrusion in the vagina (see Figure 2.12-10).
- Urinary or fecal incontinence, a sense of incomplete bladder emptying, and/or dyspareunia are also seen.

DIAGNOSIS

The degree of prolapse can be evaluated by having the woman perform the Valsalva maneuver while in the lithotomy position.

Normal  Uterine prolapse

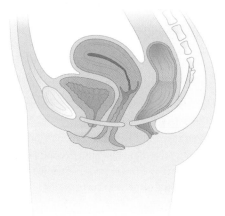
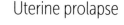
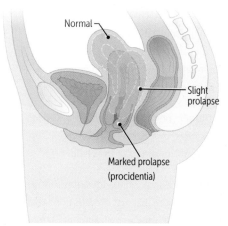

FIGURE 2.12-10. **Uterine prolapse.** Diagram on the right illustrates different degrees of uterine prolapse. (Reproduced with permission from USMLE-Rx.com.)

MNEMONIC

Causes of urinary incontinence without specific urogenital pathology—

DIAPPERS

Delirium/confusional state
Infection
Atrophic urethritis/vaginitis
Pharmaceutical
Psychiatric causes (especially depression)
Excessive urinary output (hyperglycemia, hypercalcemia, CHF)
Restricted mobility
Stool impaction

TREATMENT

- Supportive measures include a high-fiber diet and weight reduction in obese patients and limitation of straining and lifting.
- Pessaries may reduce prolapse and are helpful in women who do not wish to undergo surgery or who are chronically ill.
- Surgical procedure depends on where the prolapse is located:
  - Vaginal vault prolapse is treated with hysterectomy with vaginal vault suspension.
  - Anterior/posterior vaginal wall: Repair the anterior or posterior wall (colporrhaphy).

Urinary Incontinence

The involuntary loss of urine caused by either bladder or sphincter dysfunction.

HISTORY/PE

- Table 2.12-13 outlines the types of incontinence along with their distinguishing features and treatment (see also the **DIAPPERS** mnemonic).
- Exclude fistula in cases of total incontinence.
- Look for neurologic abnormalities in cases of urge incontinence (spasticity, flaccidity, rectal sphincter tone) or distended bladder in overflow incontinence.

DIAGNOSIS/TREATMENT

- Obtain a UA and urine culture to exclude UTI.
- Voiding diary.
- Consider urodynamic testing.
- Serum creatinine to exclude renal dysfunction.

TABLE 2.12-13. Types of Incontinence

TYPE	HISTORY OF URINE LOSS	MECHANISM	TREATMENT
Total	Uncontrolled loss at all times and in all positions	Loss of sphincteric efficiency (previous surgery, nerve damage, cancer infiltration) Abnormal connection between the urinary tract and the skin (fistula)	Surgery
Stress	After ↑ intra-abdominal pressure (coughing, sneezing, lifting)	Urethral sphincteric insufficiency caused by laxity of pelvic floor musculature Common in multiparous women or after pelvic surgery	Kegel exercises and pessary Urethral sling procedure
Urge[a]	Strong, unexpected urge to void that is unrelated to position or activity	Detrusor hyperreflexia or sphincter dysfunction caused by inflammatory conditions or neurogenic disorders of the bladder	Pelvic floor exercises, bladder training Pharmacologic interventions: anticholinergics (first-line), β-agonists such as mirabegron (second-line)
Overflow[b]	Chronic urinary retention	Chronically distended bladder with ↑ intravesical pressure that just exceeds the outlet resistance, allowing a small amount of urine to dribble out	Placement of urethral catheter in acute settings Treat underlying diseases Timed voiding

[a]Etiologies include inhibited contractions, local irritation (cystitis, stone, tumor), and CNS causes.
[b]Etiologies include physical agents (tumor, stricture), neurologic factors (lesions), and medications.

- Obtain a cystogram to demonstrate fistula sites and descensus of the bladder neck.
- Table 2.12-13 outlines treatment options according to subtype.

Pediatric Gynecology

PEDIATRIC VAGINAL DISCHARGE

Etiologies of vaginal discharge in pediatric patients include the following:

- **Infectious vulvovaginitis:** May present with a malodorous, yellow-green, purulent discharge. Causes include the following:
    - **Group A streptococcus:** The most common infectious cause.
    - *Candida:* Recent antibiotic therapy, immunosuppressed (eg, diabetes). Rare in children.
    - **STDs:** Typically from sexual abuse.
- Foreign objects.
- **Noninfectious vulvovaginitis:** Causes include contact dermatitis and eczema.
- **Sarcoma botryoides (rhabdomyosarcoma):** A malignancy with lesions that have the appearance of "bunches of grapes" within the vagina.

PRECOCIOUS PUBERTY

Onset of 2° sexual characteristics in a child < 8 years of age. Subtypes are as follows (see Table 2.12-14):

- **Central precocious puberty:** Early activation of hypothalamic GnRH production.
- **Peripheral precocious puberty:** Results from GnRH-independent mechanisms.

HISTORY/PE

- Signs of estrogen excess (breast development and possibly vaginal bleeding) suggest ovarian cysts or tumors.
- Signs of androgen excess (pubic and/or axillary hair, enlarged clitoris, and/or acne) suggest adrenal tumors or CAH.

DIAGNOSIS

Figure 2.12-11 illustrates an algorithm for the work-up of precocious puberty.

TABLE 2.12-14. Causes of Precocious Pubertal Development

CENTRAL (GnRH DEPENDENT)	PERIPHERAL (GnRH INDEPENDENT)
Constitutional (idiopathic)	Congenital adrenal hyperplasia
Hypothalamic lesions (hamartomas, tumors, congenital malformations)	Adrenal tumors
Dysgerminomas	McCune-Albright syndrome (polyostotic fibrous dysplasia)
Hydrocephalus	Gonadal tumors (especially granulosa cell tumor, which secretes estrogen)
CNS infections	Exogenous estrogen, oral (OCPs) or topical
CNS trauma/irradiation	Ovarian cysts (females)
Pineal tumors (rare)	
Neurofibromatosis with CNS involvement	
Tuberous sclerosis	

KEY FACT

Pediatric vaginal discharge may be normal, but STDs resulting from sexual abuse must be ruled out and, if found, reported to Child Protective Services.

KEY FACT

If onset of 2° sexual characteristics is seen by 8 years of age, work up for precocious puberty by determining bone age and conducting a GnRH stimulation test to distinguish central from peripheral precocious puberty.

KEY FACT

A patient with McCune-Albright syndrome presents with precocious puberty, café au lait spots, and bony abnormalities (polyostotic fibrous dysplasia).

KEY FACT

Central precocious puberty: ↑ Estradiol, ↑ LH, ↑ FSH
Peripheral precocious puberty: ↑ Estradiol, ↓ LH, ↓ FSH

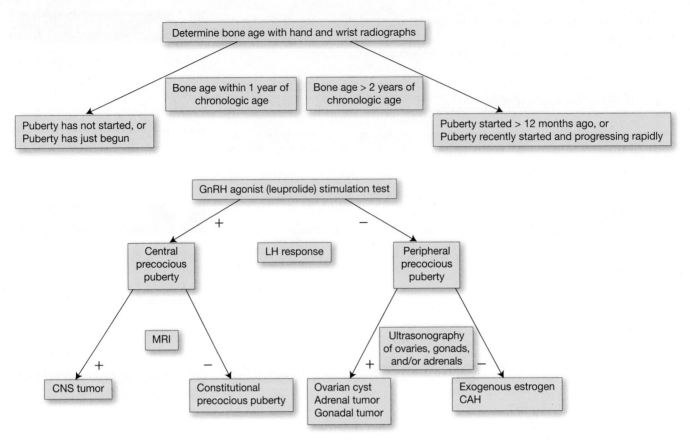

FIGURE 2.12-11. Work-up of precocious puberty.

TREATMENT

- **Central precocious puberty:** Leuprolide is first-line therapy; physical changes regress or cease to progress.
- **Peripheral precocious puberty:** Treat the cause.
  - **Ovarian cysts:** No intervention is necessary, as cysts will usually regress spontaneously.
  - **CAH:** Treat with glucocorticoids. Surgery is not required for the treatment of ambiguous genitalia.
  - **Adrenal or ovarian tumors:** Require surgical resection.
  - **McCune-Albright syndrome:** Antiestrogens (tamoxifen) or estrogen synthesis blockers (ketoconazole or testolactone) may be effective.

Benign Breast Disorders

NONPROLIFERATIVE BREAST LESIONS

Generally, no increased risk for breast cancer. Simple breast cysts are the most common, which involves fluid-filled masses from an exaggerated stromal tissue response to hormones and growth factors.

- Findings include cysts (gross and microscopic), fat necrosis, papillomatosis, adenosis, fibrosis, and ductal epithelial hyperplasia.
  - **Fat necrosis of the breast:** Benign condition that presents radiographically like breast cancer, but biopsy reveals fat globules. No further work-up indicated. Often secondary to trauma to the breast.

- Primarily affects women 30–50 years of age; rarely found in postmeno-pausal women.
- Associated with trauma and caffeine use.

HISTORY/PE

- Cyclic bilateral mastalgia and swelling, most prominent just before menstruation.
- Rapid fluctuation in the size of the masses is common.
  - Fibrocystic change: Multiple, diffuse nodules.
  - Fibroadenoma: Single, well-circumscribed nodule.
- Other symptoms include an irregular, bumpy consistency to the breast tissue.

DIAGNOSIS

- See Figure 2.12-12 for an algorithm of a breast mass work-up.
- First, have patient return after menstruation, because symptoms fluctuate with hormones.
- If unchanged on follow-up, perform ultrasonography to differentiate a mass from fluid-filled vs solid.
- **Best initial test:** Fine-needle aspiration (FNA) of a discrete mass that is suggestive of a cyst is indicated to alleviate pain and to confirm the cystic nature of the mass.
- **Most accurate test:** Excisional biopsy is indicated if no fluid is obtained or if the fluid is bloody on aspiration.
- Mammography is of limited use (especially if < 35 years of age because of density of breast tissue).
- There is no ↑ risk for breast cancer if simple cyst, but ↑ risk if complex cyst (ductal epithelial hyperplasia or cellular atypia), which is rare.

KEY FACT

The differential diagnosis of a breast mass includes fibrocystic disease, fibroadenoma, mastitis/abscess, fat necrosis, and breast cancer.

KEY FACT

Intraductal papilloma and mammary duct ectasia are common causes of bloody nipple discharge.

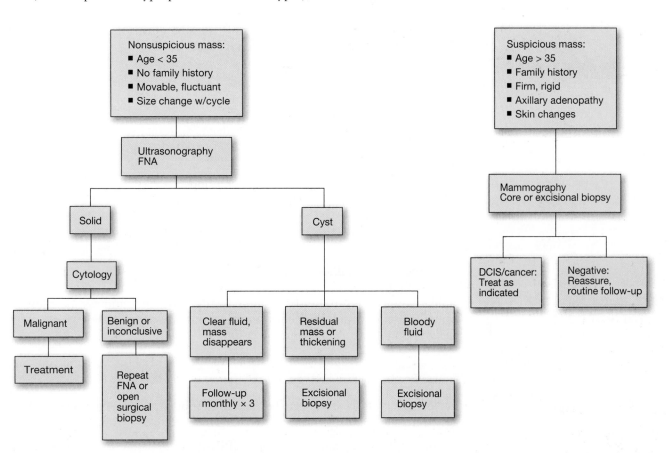

FIGURE 2.12-12.   Work-up of a breast mass.

TREATMENT

- Reassurance.
- If painful: Aspiration, dietary modifications (eg, caffeine restriction), danazol (rarely used because of side effects of acne, hirsutism, edema), and OCPs (↓ hormonal fluctuations).

PROLIFERATIVE BREAST LESIONS WITHOUT ATYPIA

This includes fibroadenomas, intraductal papillomas, sclerosing adenosis, and usual ductal hyperplasia. Associated with a small increased risk for breast cancer. Intraductal papilloma is composed of papillary cells growing from the wall of a cyst into the lumen.

- **Dx:** Diagnosed with core needle biopsy, and surgical excision is required since it can be associated with atypia or DCIS.
- **Tx:** Sclerosing adenosis and usual ductal hyperplasia require no treatment.

FIBROADENOMA

Proliferative breast lesion without atypia. A benign, slow-growing breast tumor with epithelial and stromal components. The most common breast lesion in women < 30 years of age.

HISTORY/PE

- Presents as round, rubbery, discrete, relatively mobile mass 1–3 cm in diameter. Generally nontender, but not always.
- Masses are usually solitary, although up to 20% of patients develop multiple fibroadenomas.
- **Note hormonal relationship:** Can ↑ in size during pregnancy or hormonal therapy and ↓ in size in menopause.

DIAGNOSIS

- Breast ultrasonography to differentiate cystic from solid masses.
- Needle biopsy or FNA.
- Excision with pathologic exam if the diagnosis remains uncertain.

TREATMENT

- Observation and reassurance for most lesions.
- Excision is curative, but recurrence is common.

PHYLLODES TUMOR

Can sometimes be difficult to distinguish from a fibroadenoma. It is generally larger with greater metastatic ability, and the differentiating features are the papillary projections of the stroma, lined with epithelium and associated with hyperplasia and atypia. Phyllodes tumors should be completely excised; axillary lymph node dissection is not necessary (see Figure 2.12-13).

ATYPICAL HYPERPLASIA

Atypical hyperplasia (AH) can be ductal or lobular, filling part but not the entire duct or lobule.

- Similar to a low-grade DCIS or LCIS with a moderate increased risk for breast cancer.

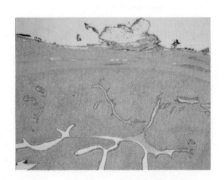

FIGURE 2.12-13. Phyllodes tumor with classic "leaflike" appearance. (Reproduced with permission from Crenshaw SA, et al. Immediate breast reconstruction with a saline implant and AlloDerm, following removal of a Phyllodes tumor. *World J Surg Oncol.* 2011;9:34.)

- A pathologic diagnosis by biopsy often found after mammogram.
- Requires risk reduction, which involves yearly mammograms and tamoxifen or aromatase inhibitor (if postmenopausal).

Breast Cancer

The most common cancer (affects one in eight women) and the second most common cause of cancer death in women (after lung cancer) in the United States. Sixty percent occur in the upper outer quadrant. Half of newly diagnosed patients have risk factors. Risk factors include the following:

- Female gender; older age; white ethnicity.
- A personal history of breast cancer; family history in a first-degree relative; genetic factors (*BRCA1* and *BRCA2* mutations: associated with early onset).
- Alcohol; cigarettes (controversial).
- Exposure to radiation.
- A history of fibrocystic change with cellular atypia.
- ↑ Exposure to estrogen (nulliparity, early menarche, late menopause, first full-term pregnancy after 35 years of age).

HISTORY/PE

Clinical manifestations include the following:

- **Early findings:** Single, nontender, immovable, firm-to-hard mass with ill-defined margins or mammographic abnormalities on routine screening.
- **Later findings/locally advanced:** Axillary lymphadenopathy, breast enlargement, pain, peau d'orange skin findings suggesting inflammation (redness, thickening, dimpling), fixation of the mass to the skin or chest wall.
- **Late findings:**
    - Ulceration; supraclavicular lymphadenopathy; edema of the arm.
    - Prolonged unilateral scaling erosion (with eczematous rash) of the nipple that spreads to the areola with or without discharge (Paget disease of the nipple, specific for ductal carcinoma in situ).
- **Metastatic disease:**
    - Metastases to the bone (pain), lung (dyspnea, cough), and liver (abdominal pain, nausea, jaundice).
    - A firm or hard axillary node > 1 cm.
    - Axillary nodes that are matted or fixed to the skin (stage III); ipsilateral supraclavicular or infraclavicular nodes (stage IV).

DIAGNOSIS

Majority of breast cancers diagnosed from mammography.

- **Screening:**
    - **Postmenopausal women:** Mammography. Look for ↑ density with microcalcifications, irregular borders, and spiculated mass. Mammography can detect lesions roughly 2 years before they become clinically palpable (see Figure 2.12-14A).
    - **Premenopausal women:** Ultrasonography for women < 30 years of age because of density of breast tissue; can distinguish a solid mass from a benign cyst (see Figure 2.12-14C).
    - Women with the following risk factors are recommended by the American Cancer Society to undergo annual MRI screening:
        - Known *BRCA* mutation.
        - First-degree relative who is a *BRCA* carrier.
        - Lifetime risk for breast cancer is 20–25% or greater.

KEY FACT

↑ Exposure to estrogen (early menarche, late menopause, nulliparity) ↑ the risk for breast cancer.

MNEMONIC

Common metastases to bone—

BLT and Kosher Pickle on top

Breast
Lung
Thyroid
Kidney
Prostate

KEY FACT

All hormone-containing contraception is contraindicated in patients with breast cancer. The safest option for contraception is a copper IUD.

Q **1**

A 27-year-old woman palpates a 1 cm × 1 cm new breast mass on self-exam. What is the first step in the work-up of the mass

Q **2**

A 30-year-old woman was in a car accident 1 week ago, and subsequently notices a hardened bump in the left breast. What is this likely to be, and what can be found on biopsy?

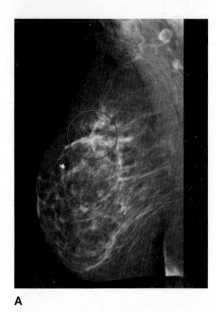
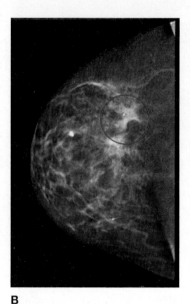
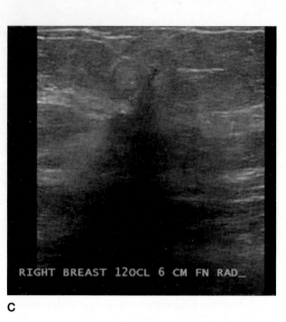

A **B** **C**

FIGURE 2.12-14. **Breast cancer.** Mediolateral oblique (**A**) and craniocaudal (**B**) views from a mammogram demonstrate a spiculated mass with a satellite mass *(circle)* in the central and outer upper right breast. A targeted breast ultrasonogram (**C**) in a different patient demonstrates a hypoechoic mass *(arrow)* that is taller than it is wide and demonstrates dense posterior acoustic shadowing. (Reproduced with permission from USMLE-Rx.com.)

KEY FACT

The first step in the work-up of a suspicious mass in postmenopausal women and in those > 30 years of age is a mammogram. For premenopausal women < 30 years of age, get an ultrasonogram.

1 **A**

Ultrasonography. The patient is < 30 years of age, so ultrasonography is the preferred means of distinguishing a solid mass from a cyst.

2 **A**

This is fat necrosis of the breast. This commonly occurs after trauma that is not always remembered. It is a mimicker of breast cancer in terms of presentation and radiographic findings. Biopsy results differentiate the two and reveal coarse (not micro) calcifications and foamy macrophages.

- **Biopsy of suspicious lesions on mammography:**
  - Perform a mammography-guided FNA or core needle biopsy; full-thickness skin biopsy if signs of inflammation.
  - **FNA:** A good initial biopsy, especially for lesions close to the skin; however, it is a small sample with a high false ⊕ rate. FNA may also be used to follow response to treatment.
  - **Core needle biopsy:** A larger sample that allows testing for receptor status.
  - **Open biopsy:** Less commonly used. Provides tissue for a more accurate diagnosis and allows immediate resection of tumor; however, requires taking the patient to the OR.
- **Receptor status of tumor:** Determine estrogen receptor (ER), progesterone receptor (PR), and human epidermal growth factor 2 (HER2) status.
- **Tumor markers for recurrent breast cancer:** Include CEA and CA 15-3 or CA 27-29.
- **Metastatic disease:**
  - **Labs:** ↑ ESR, ↑ alkaline phosphatase (liver and bone metastases), ↑ calcium.
  - **Imaging:** Chest x-ray (CXR); CT of the chest, abdomen, and pelvis; brain MRI. PET and bone scans can also be useful.

TREATMENT

- **Early-stage:**
  - Breast-conserving surgery + irradiation or mastectomy ± radiation (if cancer in deep margins or axillary lymph nodes).
    - In both cases, must perform sentinel node biopsy for evaluation of axillary lymph nodes.
  - Adjuvant therapy as below.
- **Locally advanced:**
  - Neoadjuvant chemotherapy + trastuzumab (if HER2 ⊕) to reduce size for breast conservation.
  - Breast conservation surgery or mastectomy with sentinel lymph node biopsy.
  - Adjuvant therapy as below.

TABLE 2.12-15. Breast Cancer Stages

PRIMARY TUMOR (T)	REGIONAL LYMPH NODES (N)	METASTASIS (M)
I: Tumor size < 2 cm	I: Movable ipsilateral axillary LN	1: Distant metastasis
II: Tumor size 2–5 cm	II: Fixed ipsilateral axillary LN	
III: Tumor size > 5 cm	III: Ipsilateral infra/supraclavicular LN, or clinically detected LN with axillary LN	
IV: Extension: chest wall, skin		

- **Adjuvant therapy:**
  - All ER/PR ⊕ patients should receive tamoxifen (selective estrogen receptor modulator [SERM] that competitively antagonizes the ER, inhibiting the growth of breast cancer cells) or aromatase inhibitor if postmenopausal (inactivates aromatase that converts peripheral androgens to estrogens).
  - All HER2 ⊕ patients should receive trastuzumab, a monoclonal antibody that binds to HER2 receptors on the cancer cell (watch for cardiotoxicity).
  - ER, PR, and HER2 ⊖ patients should receive chemotherapy if tumor > 0.5 cm. Do not give if patient already received neoadjuvant therapy.
- **Contraindications to breast-conserving therapy (lumpectomy):** Large tumor size, subareolar location, multifocal tumors, fixation to the chest wall, prior radiation to the chest wall, or involvement of the nipple or overlying skin.
- **Stage IV disease:** Treated with radiation therapy and hormonal therapy; mastectomy may be required for local symptom control.

Table 2.12-15 describes the breast cancer stages.

PROGNOSIS

- TNM staging (I–IV) is the most reliable indicator of prognosis.
- ER ⊕ and PR ⊕ status is associated with a favorable prognosis.
- Cancer localized to the breast has a 75–90% cure rate. With spread to the axilla, the 5-year survival rate is 40–50%.
- Aneuploidy is associated with a poor prognosis.

COMPLICATIONS

Pleural effusion occurs in 50% of patients with metastatic breast cancer; edema of the arm is common.

Sexual Assault

The most frequently unreported crime in the United States. Physicians are often required to evaluate sexual assault victims and collect evidence. Most victims are women; however, men can also be victims of sexual assault.

HISTORY/PE

- Take a full history, including contraceptive use, last time of coitus, condom use before the assault, drug or alcohol use, history of STDs, description of the assailant, location and time of the assault, circumstances of the assault (eg, penile penetration, use of condoms, extragenital acts, use or display of weapons), and the patient's actions since the assault (eg, douching, bathing, brushing teeth, urination/defecation, changing clothes).

KEY FACT

In a postmenopausal woman with a new breast lesion, maintain a high degree of clinical suspicion for breast cancer.

KEY FACT

Tamoxifen use is associated with hot flashes, endometrial cancer, and venous thromboembolism because it has mixed antagonist (breast) and agonist (endometrium) activity on estrogen receptors.

KEY FACT

Breast cancer: stage II is associated with tumor size > 2 cm, stage III is associated with nodal involvement, and stage IV is associated with metastases.

KEY FACT

Inflammatory breast carcinoma is rare, but is an aggressive cancer that presents with peau d'orange skin (edematous cutaneous thickening) along with a red and painful breast mass. Axillary lymphadenopathy is typically present.

- Conduct a complete physical exam, making note of any signs of trauma, along with a detailed pelvic exam, including a survey of the external genitals, vagina, cervix, and anus.

DIAGNOSIS

- Gonorrhea and chlamydia smear/culture (including rectal if appropriate); wet mount and culture for trichomonas. On an individual basis, consider serologic testing for HIV, syphilis, HSV, HBV, and CMV.
- Serum pregnancy test.
- Blood alcohol level; urine toxicology screen.

TREATMENT

- Treat traumatic injuries.
- STD treatment/prophylaxis (ceftriaxone plus azithromycin ± metronidazole); Hep B vaccination if patient has not received full series.
- HIV risk assessment and possible postexposure prophylaxis.
- Emergency contraception for pregnancy prevention.
- Refer for psychological counseling.
- Arrange for follow-up with the same physician or with another provider if more appropriate.
- Follow-up should include repeat screening for STDs, repeat screening for pregnancy, and a discussion of coping methods with appropriate referrals for psychiatric care if needed.

Child Development

Pediatric development and growth are very important factors that strongly influence the well-being of the future adult. Although each child is unique and develops differently, there are certain milestone and growth standards tested on the USMLE that are applicable to most children.

DEVELOPMENTAL MILESTONES

Table 2.13-1 highlights major developmental milestones, with commonly tested milestones highlighted in bold. Table 2.13-2 summarizes critical milestones in language development. If language delay is present, audiology exam should be performed.

TABLE 2.13-1. Developmental Milestones

Age[a]	Gross Motor	Fine Motor	Language	Social/Cognitive
2 months	Lifts head/chest when prone	Tracks past midline	Alerts to sound; coos	Recognizes parent; exhibits social smile
4–5 months	Rolls front to back, back to front (4 months)	Grasps rattle	Laughs and squeals; orients to voice; begins to make consonant sounds	Enjoys looking around; laughs
6 months	Sits unassisted	Transfers objects; demonstrates raking grasp	Babbles	Demonstrates stranger anxiety
9–10 months	Crawls; cruises; pulls to stand	Uses three-finger (immature) pincer grasp	Says "mama/dada" (non-specific); says first word at 11 months	Waves bye-bye; plays pat-a-cake
12 months	Walks alone; throws object	Uses two-finger (mature) pincer grasp	Uses 1–3 words	Imitates actions; exhibits separation anxiety Follows one-step commands
2 years	Walks up/down steps; jumps	Builds tower of six cubes	Uses 2-word phrases	Follows two-step commands; removes clothes
3 years	Rides tricycle; climbs stairs with alternating feet (3–4 years)	Copies a circle; uses utensils	Uses 3-word sentences	Brushes teeth with help; washes/dries hands
4 years	Hops	Copies a cross (square at 4.5 years of age)	Knows colors and some numbers	Exhibits cooperative play; plays board games
5 years	Skips; walks backward for long distances	Copies a triangle; ties shoelaces; knows left and right; prints letters	Uses 5-word sentences	Exhibits domestic role playing; plays dress-up

[a]For premature infants < 2 years of age, chronologic age must be adjusted for gestational age. For example, an infant born at 7 months' gestation (2 months early) would be expected to perform at the 4-month level at the chronologic age of 6 months. However, vaccines should be administered based on chronologic age despite prematurity.

Toilet training:

- Most children may start at 2 years of age, with boys usually completing training later than girls.
- Bedwetting (enuresis) is normal until 5 years of age. Positive reinforcement (alarms, rewards) should be provided, along with restricting fluid intake before bed. Desmopressin (ADH analog) and anticholinergic medications may be provided for refractory cases.

GROWTH

At each well-child check, height, weight, and head circumference are plotted on growth charts specific for gender and age:

- **Head circumference:** Measured routinely in the first 2 years. ↑ Head circumference may indicate hydrocephalus or tumor (should be evaluated with brain imaging); ↓ head circumference can point to microcephaly (eg, ToRCHeS infections).
- **Height and weight:** Measured routinely until adulthood. The pattern of growth is more important than the raw numbers. Infants may lose 5–10% of body weight (BW) over the first few days but should return to their BW by 14 days. Infants can be expected to double their BW by 4–5 months, triple by 1 year, and quadruple by 2 years.
- **Failure to thrive (FTT):** Persistent weight less than the fifth percentile for age or "falling off the growth curve" (ie, crossing two major percentile lines on a growth chart). Classified as follows:
  - **Organic:** Caused by an underlying medical condition such as cystic fibrosis, congenital heart disease (CHD), celiac sprue, pyloric stenosis, chronic infection (eg, HIV), or GERD.
  - **Nonorganic:** Primarily caused by psychosocial factors such as poverty, inaccurate mixing of formula (too much water mixed in), maternal depression, neglect, or abuse.
- A careful dietary history and close observation of maternal-infant interactions (especially preparation of formula and feeding) are critical to diagnosis.
- Children should be hospitalized if there is evidence of neglect or severe malnourishment. Calorie counts and supplemental nutrition (if breastfeeding is inadequate) are mainstays of treatment.
- Children 2–12 years of age may have bilateral, intermittent lower extremity cramping and pain that is worse at night, with normal activity levels and normal physical exam. These are growing pains, a benign condition of unknown etiology that requires observation and symptomatic treatment.

SEXUAL DEVELOPMENT

- **Tanner staging:** Performed to assess sexual development in boys and girls. Stage 1 is preadolescent; stage 5 is adult. Increasing stages are assigned for testicular and penile growth in boys and breast growth in girls; pubic hair development is used for both stages.
  - **Girls:** The average age of onset of puberty is 10.5 years. The average age of menarche in US girls is 12.5 years.
  - **Boys:** The average age of onset of puberty is 11.5 years.
- **Variants of normal sexual development** are as follows (see Figure 2.13-1):
  - **Precocious puberty:** Any sign of 2° sexual maturation in girls < 8 years or boys < 9 years of age. Often idiopathic; may be central or peripheral (see the Gynecology chapter).

TABLE 2.13-2. **Major Milestones in Language Development**

AGE	MILESTONE
12 months	1 word, 1-step command
15 months	5 words
18 months	8 words
2 years	2-word phrases, two-step commands Speech 50% (1/2) intelligible
3 years	3-word phrases Speech 75% (3/4) intelligible
4 years	Speech 100% (4/4) intelligible

KEY FACT

Infants with FTT will first fall off the weight curve, then the height curve, and finally the head circumference curve.

KEY FACT

Newborns can lose up to 10% of their birth weight, but will regain the weight by 2 weeks of life.

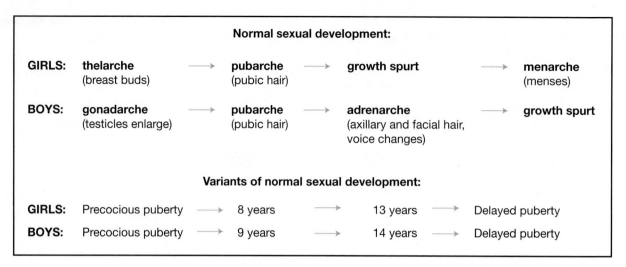

FIGURE 2.13-1. **Patterns of sexual development in girls vs boys.**

TABLE 2.13-3. **Trisomies**

DISEASE	GENETIC ABNORMALITY	PRESENTATION	ASSOCIATED DISEASES	OTHER FACTS
Down syndrome	Trisomy 21 as a result of meiotic nondisjunction (95%), Robertsonian translocation (4%), or mosaicism (1%)	Presents with intellectual disabilities, a flat facial profile, upslanted eyes with epicanthal folds, single palmar crease, general hypotonia, and extra neck folds (nuchal folds are sometimes seen on prenatal ultrasound)	Associated with atlantoaxial instability, duodenal atresia, Hirschsprung disease, and congenital heart disease (CHD); most common cardiac malformation is complete AV canal defect (both systolic ejection murmur and holosystolic murmur present) (60%); atrial septal defects (ASDs), ventricular septal defects (VSDs), patent ductus arteriosus (PDA) (20%), and complex CHD make up the remainder. Also associated with ↑ risk for acute lymphocytic leukemia (ALL), hypothyroidism, and early-onset Alzheimer disease	The most common chromosomal disorder and cause of intellectual disabilities. Associated with advanced maternal age
Edwards syndrome	Trisomy 18	Presents with severe intellectual disabilities, rocker-bottom feet, low-set ears, micrognathia, clenched hands (overlapping of the index finger over the third finger and the pinky over the fourth finger), and a prominent occiput	Associated with CHD (most often VSD). May have horseshoe kidneys	Death usually occurs within 1 year of birth
Patau syndrome	Trisomy 13	Presents with severe intellectual disabilities, microphthalmia, microcephaly, cleft lip/palate, holoprosencephaly, "punched-out" scalp lesions, polydactyly, and omphalocele	Associated with CHD	Death usually occurs within 1 year of birth

- **Delayed puberty:** No testicular enlargement in boys by 14 years, or no breast development or pubic hair in girls by 13 years of age.
- **Constitutional growth delay:** A normal variant, and the most common cause of delayed puberty. The growth curve lags behind others of the same age but remains consistent. There is often a ⊕ family history, and children ultimately achieve target height potential. The key distinguishing feature is delayed bone age.
- **Pathologic puberty delay:** Rarely, caused by systemic disease (eg, inflammatory bowel disease [IBD]), malnutrition (eg, anorexia nervosa), gonadal dysgenesis (eg, Klinefelter syndrome, Turner syndrome), or endocrine abnormalities (eg, hypopituitarism, hypothyroidism, Kallmann syndrome, androgen insensitivity syndrome, Prader-Willi syndrome).

Genetic Disease

Genetic diseases arise from mutations in the DNA and can be inherited or de novo (present for the first time). Tables 2.13-3 to 2.13-6 outline common genetic diseases and their associated abnormalities.

CYSTIC FIBROSIS

An autosomal recessive disorder caused by mutations in the cystic fibrosis transmembrane conductance regulator *(CFTR)* gene (chloride channel) on chromosome 7 and characterized by widespread exocrine gland dysfunction. Cystic fibrosis (CF) is the most common severe genetic disease in the United States and is most frequently found in persons of white ethnicity.

KEY FACT

Androgen insensitivity syndrome (AIS) is a genetic disorder characterized by X-linked mutation of androgen receptor, leading to a phenotypically female appearance in a 46XY individual. AIS-affected individuals will have breast development, no pubic hair, and cryptorchid testes. It is important to perform a gonadectomy after puberty to prevent testicular cancer in these individuals.

A newborn girl presents with lymphedema of the hands and feet, ↓ femoral pulses, a webbed neck, widely spaced nipples, short fourth metacarpals, and nail dysplasia. What form of hormone replacement therapy will the child need in the future?

TABLE 2.13-4. Sex Chromosome Abnormalities

DISEASE	GENETIC ABNORMALITY	PRESENTATION	ASSOCIATED DISEASES	OTHER FACTS
Klinefelter syndrome (male)	47,XXY	Characterized by the presence of an inactivated X chromosome (Barr body) Presents with testicular atrophy, a eunuchoid body shape, tall stature, long extremities, gynecomastia, and female hair distribution	One of the most common causes of hypogonadism in males	Associated with advanced maternal age Treat with testosterone (prevents gynecomastia; improves 2° sexual characteristics)
Turner syndrome (female)	45,XO	Missing one X chromosome; no Barr body Features include short stature, shield chest, widely spaced nipples, a webbed neck, coarctation of the aorta (↓ femoral pulses), and/or bicuspid aortic valve May present with lymphedema of the hands and feet in the neonatal period	The most common cause of 1° amenorrhea; caused by ovarian dysgenesis (treat with estrogen) May have horseshoe kidney	Not associated with advanced maternal age
Double Y males	47,XYY	Often look normal; some patients are very tall with severe acne (seen in 1–2% of XYY male patients)		Observed with ↑ frequency among inmates of penal institutions

A

This newborn has Turner syndrome. Estrogen replacement therapy is required for ovarian dysgenesis. Without exogenous estrogen, this child will be at ↑ risk for delayed puberty and osteoporosis later in life.

History/PE

- Most patients are diagnosed on newborn screening.
- **Presentation:**
    - **Neonates:** Meconium ileus (obstruction of the distal ileum caused by abnormally thick meconium; 15% of presenting cases).
    - **Patients < 1 year of age:** Cough, wheezing, or recurrent respiratory infections. They may also have steatorrhea and/or FTT.
    - **Most patients > 1 year of age:** FTT (caused by pancreatic insufficiency) or chronic sinopulmonary disease/sputum production.
- Affected individuals exhibit recurrent pulmonary infections (especially with *Pseudomonas* as adults and *Staphylococcus aureus* as children) with subsequent cyanosis, digital clubbing, chronic cough (the most common pulmonary symptom), dyspnea, bronchiectasis, hemoptysis, chronic sinusitis, rhonchi, rales, hyperresonance to percussion, and nasal polyposis.

TABLE 2.13-5.   Inherited Metabolic Disorders

Disease	Etiology	Mode of Inheritance/ Notes
Phenylketonuria (PKU)	Caused by ↓ phenylalanine hydroxylase or ↓ tetrahydrobiopterin cofactor Tyrosine becomes essential, and phenylalanine accumulates and is subsequently converted to its ketone metabolites Normal at birth; presents within the first few months of life Presents with intellectual disabilities, fair hair and skin, eczema, blond hair, blue eyes, and a musty urine odor Associated with ↑ risk for heart disease Modify diet by ↓ phenylalanine (artificial sweeteners) and ↑ tyrosine. A mother with PKU who wants to become pregnant must restrict her diet as above before conception	Autosomal recessive PKU is screened for at birth
Fabry disease	Caused by a deficiency of α-galactosidase A that leads to accumulation of ceramide trihexoside in the heart, brain, and kidneys The first sign is severe neuropathic limb pain; also presents with joint swelling Skin involvement takes the form of angiokeratomas and telangiectasias Findings include renal failure and ↑ risk for stroke and MI (thromboembolic events)	X-linked recessive
Krabbe disease	Absence of galactosylceramide and galactoside (caused by galactosylceramidase deficiency), leading to the accumulation of galactocerebroside in the brain Characterized by progressive CNS degeneration, optic atrophy, spasticity, and death within the first 3 years of life	Autosomal recessive
Gaucher disease	Caused by a deficiency of glucocerebrosidase (also known as acid β-glucosidase) that leads to the accumulation of glucocerebroside in the brain, liver, spleen, and bone marrow Gaucher cells have a characteristic "crinkled paper" appearance with enlarged cytoplasm May present with anemia and thrombocytopenia The infantile form results in early, rapid neurologic decline; adult form (more common) is compatible with a normal life span and does not affect the brain	Autosomal recessive
Niemann-Pick disease	A deficiency of sphingomyelinase that leads to the buildup of sphingomyelin cholesterol in reticuloendothelial and parenchymal cells and tissues Death occurs by 3 years of age in patients with type A May present with a cherry-red spot and hepatosplenomegaly	Autosomal recessive No man **PICK**s (Niemann-**PICK**) his nose with his sphinger

(continues)

TABLE 2.13-5.   Inherited Metabolic Disorders *(continued)*

DISEASE	ETIOLOGY	MODE OF INHERITANCE/ NOTES
Tay-Sachs disease	An absence of hexosaminidase A that leads to GM$_2$ ganglioside accumulation Infants may appear normal until 3–6 months of age, when weakness begins and development slows and regresses An exaggerated startle response may be seen Death occurs by 3 years of age Presents with a cherry-red spot but no hepatosplenomegaly The carrier rate is 1 in 30 Jews of European descent (1 in 300 for others)	Autosomal recessive Tay-Sa**X** lacks he**X**osaminidase A
Metachromatic leukodystrophy	A deficiency of arylsulfatase A that leads to the accumulation of sulfatide in the brain, kidney, liver, and peripheral nerves Demyelination leads to progressive ataxia and dementia	Autosomal recessive
Hurler syndrome	A deficiency of α-L-iduronidase Leads to corneal clouding, intellectual disabilities, and gargoylism	Autosomal recessive
Hunter syndrome	A deficiency of iduronate sulfatase A mild form of Hurler syndrome with no corneal clouding and mild intellectual disabilities	**X**-linked recessive Hunters need to see (no corneal clouding) to aim for the **X**
Homocystinemia	A deficiency of cystathionine synthase Causes downward lens subluxation, Marfanoid body habitus, hypercoagulability, and intellectual disability. Treat with anticoagulation	Autosomal recessive

- Patients with pancreatic insufficiency usually have greasy stools and flatulence; other prominent GI symptoms include pancreatitis, rectal prolapse, hypoproteinemia, biliary cirrhosis, jaundice, and esophageal varices.
- Patients who present in late childhood or adulthood are likely to have pancreatic sufficiency; in this case, pulmonary manifestations predominate and the disease tends to have a milder course.

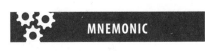
MNEMONIC

Trisomies—

21—Age to **D**rink (**D**own syndrome)
18—Age to vote in **E**lections (**E**dwards syndrome)
13—Age of **P**uberty (**P**atau syndrome)

TABLE 2.13-6.   Other Genetic Diseases

DISEASE	ETIOLOGY	MODE OF INHERITANCE/NOTES
Fragile X syndrome	Caused by a defect affecting the methylation and expression of the *FMR1* gene; a triplet repeat disorder that may show genetic anticipation Presents with large jaw, testes, and ears and with autistic behaviors	X-linked dominant The second most common genetic cause of intellectual disabilities
Friedrich ataxia	Causes gait ataxia, diabetes, and numerous cardiac manifestations (heart failure, myocardial fibrosis)	Autosomal recessive, trinucleotide repeat expansion of GAA causing abnormal frataxin protein
Prader-Willi syndrome	Hypotonia, hyperphagia, obesity, hypogonadism, almond-shaped eyes Deletion of paternal 15q11-q13 Causes sleep apnea, diabetes mellitus [DM] type 2, and obesity-related complications	Deletion of paternal 15q11-q13 (imprinting disorder) Paternal deletion → Prader-Willi

KEY FACT

Almost all cases of meconium ileus are caused by CF.

- **Additional symptoms:** Diabetes mellitus type 2, "salty-tasting" skin, male infertility (agenesis of the vas deferens), and unexplained hyponatremia.
- Patients are at risk for fat-soluble vitamin deficiency (vitamins A, D, E, and K) 2° to malabsorption and may present with manifestations of these deficiencies (ie, night blindness, rickets, neuropathy, coagulopathy).

DIAGNOSIS

- **Best initial test:** Sweat chloride test (pilocarpine electrophoresis).
- Can be confirmed by genetic testing, but diagnosis can be made by positive sweat test and clinical symptoms alone.
- Most states now perform mandatory newborn screening.

TREATMENT

- Pulmonary manifestations are managed with chest physical therapy, bronchodilators, corticosteroids, antibiotics (should cover *Pseudomonas* and *S aureus*; *S aureus* is the main colonizer until 20 years of age), and deoxyribonuclease (DNase).
- Administer pancreatic enzymes and fat-soluble vitamins A, D, E, and K for malabsorption.
- Nutritional counseling and support with a high-calorie and high-protein diet are essential for health maintenance.
- Patients who have severe disease but can tolerate surgery may be candidates for lung or pancreas transplant. Life expectancy was once ~20 years, but with newer treatments it is increasing to past 40 years of age.
- Ivacaftor, a drug that enhances CFTR activity, was recently approved to treat CF.

MNEMONIC

IvAC**a**FT**o**R: A drug used to treat CF by **I**ncreasing **A**ctivity of **CFTR**.

Neonatology

APGAR SCORING

A rapid scoring system that helps evaluate the need for neonatal resuscitation (Table 2.13-7). Each of five parameters is assigned a score of 0–2 at 1 and 5 minutes after birth.

- **Scores of 8–10:** Typically reflect good cardiopulmonary adaptation.
- **Scores of 4–7:** Indicate the possible need for resuscitation. Infants should be observed, stimulated, and possibly given ventilatory support.
- **Scores of 0–3:** Indicate the need for immediate resuscitation.

TABLE 2.13-7. **Apgar Scale (evaluate at 1 and 5 minutes postpartum)**

SIGN	2 POINTS	1 POINT	0 POINTS
Activity (muscle tone)	Active movement	Arms and legs flexed	Absent
Pulse	> 100 bpm	< 100 bpm	Absent
Grimace (reflex irritability)	Active (sneezes, coughs, pulls away)	Some flexion of extremities	Flaccid
Appearance (skin color)	Completely pink	Pink body with blue extremities	Blue/pale all over
Respirations	Vigorous cry	Slow, irregular respirations	Absent

CONGENITAL MALFORMATIONS

Table 2.13-8 describes selected congenital malformations.

NEONATAL JAUNDICE

An elevated serum bilirubin concentration (> 5 mg/dL) caused by ↑ hemolysis or ↓ excretion. Subtypes are as follows:

- **Conjugated (direct) hyperbilirubinemia:** Always pathologic.
- **Unconjugated (indirect) hyperbilirubinemia:** May be physiologic or pathologic. See Table 2.13-9 for differentiating characteristics.
- **Kernicterus:** A complication of unconjugated hyperbilirubinemia that results from irreversible bilirubin deposition in the basal ganglia, pons, and cerebellum. It typically occurs at levels of > 25–30 mg/dL and can be fatal. Risk factors include prematurity, asphyxia, and sepsis.

KEY FACT

Omphalocele is sometimes associated with other congenital anomalies (as in Beckwith-Wiedemann syndrome); gastroschisis is not.

TABLE 2.13-8. Selected Congenital Malformations

MALFORMATION	PRESENTATION	DIAGNOSIS	TREATMENT
Tracheoesophageal fistula	Tract between the trachea and esophagus. Associated with defects such as esophageal atresia and **VACTERL** (**V**ertebral, **A**nal, **C**ardiac, **T**racheal, **E**sophageal, **R**enal, **L**imb) anomalies Polyhydramnios in utero, ↑ oral secretions, inability to feed, gagging, aspiration pneumonia, respiratory distress	Chest x-ray (CXR) showing an NG tube coiled in the esophagus identifies esophageal atresia Presence of air in the GI tract is suggestive; confirm with bronchoscopy	Surgical correction
Congenital diaphragmatic hernia	GI tract segments protrude through the diaphragm into the thorax; 90% are posterior left (Bochdalek) Respiratory distress (from pulmonary hypoplasia and pulmonary hypertension); sunken abdomen; bowel sounds over the left hemithorax	Ultrasound in utero; confirmed by postnatal CXR	High-frequency ventilation or extracorporeal membrane oxygenation to manage pulmonary hypertension; surgical correction
Gastroschisis	Herniation of the intestine only through the abdominal wall next to the umbilicus (usually on the right) with no sac (the GI tract is exposed) Polyhydramnios in utero; often premature; associated with GI stenoses or atresia Presents with erythematous, matted bowel	Diagnosis made clinically	Wrap exposed bowel with saline-soaked gauze, and secure with plastic immediately after birth. Surgical correction is needed in most cases. When primary closure cannot be achieved immediately, a silo bag can be placed to gradually reduce bowel contents into the abdomen until surgery can be performed

(continues)

TABLE 2.13-8. Selected Congenital Malformations (continued)

MALFORMATION	PRESENTATION	DIAGNOSIS	TREATMENT
Omphalocele **A**	Herniation of abdominal viscera through the abdominal wall at the umbilicus into a sac covered by peritoneum and amniotic membrane (see Image A) Polyhydramnios in utero; often premature; associated with other GI and cardiac defects Seen in Beckwith-Wiedemann syndrome and trisomies	Diagnosis made clinically	C-section can prevent sac rupture; if the sac is intact, postpone surgical correction until the patient is fully resuscitated Keep the sac covered/stable with petroleum and gauze. Intermittent NG suction to prevent abdominal distention
Duodenal atresia **B**	Complete or partial failure of the duodenal lumen to recanalize during gestational weeks 8–10 Polyhydramnios in utero; bilious emesis within hours after the first feeding Associated with Down syndrome and other cardiac/GI anomalies (eg, annular pancreas, malrotation, imperforate anus)	X-rays of the abdomens show the "double bubble" sign (air bubbles in the stomach and duodenum [see Image B]) proximal to the site of the atresia	Surgical correction
Jejunal atresia	Vascular accident in utero that prevents canalization of the jejunum Caused by prenatal exposure to cocaine and other vasoconstrictive substances	Triple bubble sign may be seen	Surgical correction

Images reproduced with permission from Brunicardi FC, et al. *Schwartz's Principles of Surgery,* 9th ed. New York, NY: McGraw-Hill; 2010.

TABLE 2.13-9. Physiologic vs Pathologic Jaundice

PHYSIOLOGIC JAUNDICE	PATHOLOGIC JAUNDICE
Not present in the first 24 hours of life	Present in the first 24 hours of life
Bilirubin $\uparrow$ < 5 mg/dL/day	Bilirubin $\uparrow$ > 5 mg/dL/h
Bilirubin peaks at < 14–15 mg/dL	Bilirubin peaks at > 15 mg/dL
Direct bilirubin is < 10% of total	Direct bilirubin is > 10% of total
Resolves by 1 week in term infants and 2 weeks in preterm infants	Persists beyond 1 week in term infants and 2 weeks in preterm infants

HISTORY/PE

See Table 2.13-10.

- History should focus on diet (breast milk or formula), intrauterine drug exposure, and family history (hemoglobinopathies, enzyme deficiencies, RBC defects).
- PE may reveal signs of hepatic or GI dysfunction (abdominal distention, delayed passage of meconium, light-colored stools, dark urine), infection, or birth trauma (cephalohematomas, bruising, pallor, petechiae).
- Kernicterus presents with lethargy, poor feeding, a high-pitched cry, hypertonicity, and seizures; jaundice may follow a cephalopedal progression as bilirubin concentrations ↑.

DIAGNOSIS

- For indirect hyperbilirubinemia, CBC with peripheral blood smear (abnormal RBCs and signs of hemolysis); blood typing of mother and infant (ABO or Rh incompatibility); Coombs test and bilirubin levels.
- For direct hyperbilirubinemia, check LFTs, bile acids, blood cultures, sweat test, and tests for aminoacidopathies and α_1-antitrypsin deficiency. Ultrasound and/or hydroxy iminodiacetic acid (HIDA) scan can confirm suspected cholestatic disease.
- A jaundiced neonate who is febrile, hypotensive, and/or tachypneic needs a full sepsis work-up and ICU monitoring.

MNEMONIC

Crigler-**N**ajjar and **G**ilbert have problems with **CoNjuG**ation of bilirubin while **D**ubin-Johnson and **R**otor have a defective **DooR** for secretion of bilirubin.

KEY FACT

Direct (conjugated) hyperbilirubinemia is always pathologic.

TABLE 2.13-10. Mechanisms of Neonatal Jaundice

MECHANISM	EXAMPLE(S)	PREDOMINANT BILIRUBIN SPECIES
↑ Bilirubin production	Hemolysis (ABO or Rh incompatibility) Erythrocyte enzyme deficiency (G6PD deficiency) Erythrocyte structural defects (sickle cell anemia, hereditary spherocytosis) Ineffective erythropoiesis (thalassemias) Sepsis with DIC	↑ Unconjugated bilirubin
Impaired conjugation of bilirubin	Gilbert syndrome Crigler-Najjar syndrome Newborn physiologic jaundice	↑ Unconjugated bilirubin
Impaired bilirubin uptake and secretion from the liver	Dubin-Johnson syndrome Rotor syndrome	↑ Conjugated bilirubin
↑ Enterohepatic circulation	Poor feeding Breast milk jaundice Pyloric stenosis	↑ Unconjugated bilirubin
Obstruction of biliary tree and ↓ excretion	Biliary/choledochal cyst Biliary atresia Alagille syndrome	↑ Conjugated bilirubin

TREATMENT

■ Treat underlying causes (eg, infection).
■ Treat unconjugated hyperbilirubinemia with phototherapy (for mild elevations) or exchange transfusion (for severe elevations > 20 mg/dL). Start phototherapy earlier (10–15 mg/dL) for preterm infants. Phototherapy is not indicated for conjugated hyperbilirubinemia and can lead to skin bronzing.

RESPIRATORY DISTRESS SYNDROME

KEY FACT

RDS is the most common cause of respiratory failure in preterm infants.

Respiratory distress syndrome (RDS; also known as neonatal respiratory distress syndrome [NRDS]) is the most common cause of respiratory failure in preterm infants (affects > 70% of infants born at 28–30 weeks' gestation); formerly known as hyaline membrane disease. Surfactant deficiency leads to poor lung compliance, alveolar collapse, and atelectasis. Risk factors include maternal DM, male gender, and the second born of twins.

HISTORY/PE

Presents in the first 48–72 hours of life with a respiratory rate > 60/min, progressive hypoxemia, cyanosis, nasal flaring, intercostal retractions, and expiratory grunting.

DIAGNOSIS

■ Check ABGs, CBC, and blood cultures to rule out infection.
■ Diagnosis is clinical and confirmed with characteristic findings on chest x-ray (CXR) (see Table 2.13-11).

TABLE 2.13-11.   Chest X-ray Findings in Neonatal Lung Pathology

DISEASE PROCESS	KEY FINDINGS
NRDS	Ground-glass appearance (see Image A), air bronchograms, and lack of focal opacities
Transient tachypnea of the newborn (retained amniotic fluid in respiratory tract)	Perihilar streaking (see Image B) in interlobular fissures
Meconium aspiration	Coarse, irregular infiltrates (see Image C), lung hyperexpansion, and pneumothorax
Congenital pneumonia	Nonspecific patchy infiltrates

A   B   C

Image A reproduced with permission from Tintinalli JE, et al. *Tintinalli's Emergency Medicine: A Comprehensive Study Guide,* 7th ed. New York, NY: McGraw-Hill; 2010. Image B reproduced with permission from Alorainy IA, Barlas NB, Al-Boukai AA. Pictorial Essay: Infants of diabetic mothers. *Indian J Radiol Imaging.* 2010;20(3):174–181. Image C reproduced with permission from Khan AN, et al. Reading chest radiographs in the critically ill (Part I): Normal chest radiographic appearance, instrumentation and complications from instrumentation. *Ann Thorac Med* 2009;4(2):75–87.

TREATMENT

- Continuous positive airway pressure (CPAP) or intubation and mechanical ventilation.
- Artificial surfactant administration ↓ mortality.
- Pretreat mothers at risk for preterm delivery (24 weeks to 33 6/7 weeks) in the next 7 days with corticosteroids.

COMPLICATIONS

Persistent PDA, bronchopulmonary dysplasia, retinopathy of prematurity, barotrauma from positive pressure ventilation, intraventricular hemorrhage, and NEC are complications of treatment.

Congenital Heart Disease

Intrauterine risk factors for CHD include maternal drug use (alcohol, lithium, thalidomide, phenytoin), maternal infections (rubella), and maternal illness (DM, PKU). CHD can also be caused by fetal genetic anomalies and disorders. See Table 2.13-12 for a list of common disorders and associated causes.

CHD is classified by the presence or absence of cyanosis at birth or shortly after:

- **Acyanotic conditions ("pink babies"):** Have left-to-right shunts in which oxygenated blood from the lungs is shunted back into the pulmonary circulation.
- **Cyanotic conditions ("blue babies"):** Have right-to-left shunts in which deoxygenated blood is shunted into the systemic circulation.

TABLE 2.13-12. Pediatric Heart Conditions and Their Disease Associations

CONDITION	DISORDER
ASD and endocardial cushion defects	Down syndrome
PDA	Congenital rubella
Coarctation of the aorta	Turner syndrome (many also have bicuspid aortic valve)
Coronary artery aneurysms	Kawasaki disease
Congenital heart block	Neonatal lupus
Supravalvular aortic stenosis	Williams syndrome
Conotruncal abnormalities	Tetralogy of Fallot (overriding aorta), truncus arteriosus, DiGeorge syndrome (tetralogy), velocardiofacial syndrome
Ebstein abnormality (apical displacement of the tricuspid valve leading to atrialization of the RV)	Maternal lithium use during pregnancy
Heart failure	Neonatal thyrotoxicosis
Asymmetric septal hypertrophy and transposition of the great vessels	Maternal diabetes

KEY FACT

A venous hum is a benign murmur that can be present in childhood. The murmur is a low-pitched, vibratory murmur that is heard at the upper left sternal border throughout the cardiac cycle. Unlike a PDA, a venous hum murmur is loudest when sitting and disappears with supine position or neck rotation.

MNEMONIC

Noncyanotic heart defects—

The 3 D's

VS**D**
AS**D**
P**D**A

KEY FACT

VSD is the most common type of CHD. They occur most commonly in the membranous septum, and most resolve without intervention.

KEY FACT

The size of the VSD is inversely proportional to the intensity of the murmur. The smaller the VSD, the more intensely the murmur will be heard.

KEY FACT

ASD has a fixed, widely split S2.

KEY FACT

ASDs and VSDs rarely present at birth with findings other than harsh systolic murmur. Remember that ASDs, VSDs, and PDAs are acyanotic conditions unless Eisenmenger syndrome has developed (right-to-left shunt, cyanotic).

KEY FACT

In infants presenting in a shock within the first few weeks of life, look for the following:
- Sepsis
- Inborn errors of metabolism
- Ductal-dependent CHD, usually left-sided lesions (as the ductus is closing)
- Congenital adrenal hyperplasia

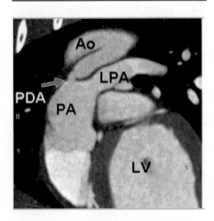

FIGURE 2.13-2.   Patent ductus arteriosus with resultant left-to-right shunting (arrow). (Reproduced with permission from Henjes CR, Nolte I, Wesfaedt P. Multidetector-row computed tomography of thoracic aortic anomalies in dogs and cats: patent ductus arteriosus and vascular rings. *BMC Vet Res.* 2011;7:57. DOI: 10.1186/1746-6148-7-57.)

ACYANOTIC CONDITIONS

Acyanotic congenital heart conditions typically do not present at birth. There is left-to-right shunting, which increases blood flow to the pulmonary system. They typically cause a characteristic murmur and are discovered later in life. Presentation varies with the size of the defect. Increased pulmonary blood flow can eventually lead to Eisenmenger syndrome. In Eisenmenger syndrome, left-to-right shunt leads to pulmonary hypertension and shunt reversal.

SEPTAL DEFECTS

A condition in which an opening in the atrial or ventricular septum allows blood to flow between the atria or ventricles, leading to left-to-right shunting. VSD is the most common type of CHD.

PRESENTATION AND DIAGNOSIS
See Table 2.13-13.

TREATMENT
- Most small ASD/VSDs close spontaneously and do not require treatment. Follow-up echocardiography based on size of ASD/VSD and physical exam.
- Antibiotic prophylaxis is generally not recommended before procedures.
- If CHF develops, best initial treatment involves medical management of CHF using the following:
  - Diuretics.
  - Then positive inotropes and angiotensin-converting enzyme inhibitors.
- Surgical correction is indicated in symptomatic patients who:
  - Fail medical management.
  - < 1 year of age with signs of pulmonary hypertension.
  - Older children with large defects that have not ↓ in size over time.
- Early correction prevents complications such as arrhythmias, right ventricular dysfunction, and Eisenmenger syndrome.

PATENT DUCTUS ARTERIOSUS

Patent ductus arteriosus (Figure 2.13-2) is a failure of the ductus arteriosus to close in the first few days of life, leading to an acyanotic left-to-right shunt from the aorta to the pulmonary artery.

HISTORY/PE
- Typically asymptomatic; patients with large defects may present with FTT, recurrent lower respiratory tract infections, clubbing, and CHF.
- Exam reveals a continuous "machinery murmur" at the second left intercostal space at the sternal border, a loud S2, wide pulse pressure, and bounding peripheral pulses.

DIAGNOSIS
- **Best initial test:** Echocardiogram will demonstrate presence of defect.
- Color flow Doppler will demonstrate blood flow from the aorta into the pulmonary artery.
- With larger PDAs, echocardiography shows left atrial and left ventricular enlargement.
- ECG may show LVH, and CXR may reveal cardiomegaly if lesions are large.

TABLE 2.13-13.   Presentation and Diagnosis of ASD vs VSD

	ASD (See Image A)	VSD (See Image B)
Associated syndromes	Holt-Oram syndrome (absent radii, ASD, first-degree heart block) Fetal alcohol syndrome Trisomy 21	Apert syndrome (cranial deformities, fusion of the fingers and toes) Down syndrome Fetal alcohol syndrome ToRCHeS infections Cri du chat syndrome Trisomies (13, 18, and 21)
Presentation	Small defects: Asymptomatic Large defects: Easy fatigability; frequent respiratory infection; FTT	Small defects: Asymptomatic Large defects: Recurrent respiratory infections; dyspnea; FTT; CHF
Auscultation findings	Wide and fixed split S_2 Systolic ejection murmur at the upper left sternal border ($\uparrow$ flow across pulmonary valve) Mid-diastolic rumble at the left LSB	Harsh holosystolic murmur at lower left sternal border (louder for small defects) Narrow S_2 with $\uparrow P_2$ (large defect) Mid-diastolic apical rumble (caused by increased flow across mitral valve)
CXR findings	Cardiomegaly $\uparrow$ Pulmonary vascular markings	
ECG findings	Right ventricular hypertrophy (RVH) Right atrial enlargement PR prolongation is common	Left ventricular hypertrophy (LVH). RVH may also be found with large defects
Echocardiogram findings	Defect and blood flow across the atrial/ventricular septum	

A

B

Images reproduced with permission from USMLE-Rx.com.

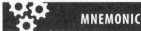

Come **IN** and **CLOSE** the door.
Give **IN**domethacin to **CLOSE** a PDA.

KEY FACT

Coarctation of the aorta and bicuspid aortic valve are associated with Turner syndrome.

TREATMENT

- **Best initial treatment:** Give indomethacin (an NSAID) unless the PDA is needed for survival (eg, transposition of the great vessels, tetralogy of Fallot, hypoplastic left heart), or if indomethacin is contraindicated (eg, intraventricular hemorrhage).
- If indomethacin fails or if the child is > 6–8 months of age, surgical closure is required.

COARCTATION OF THE AORTA

Constriction of a portion of the aorta, leading to ↑ flow proximal to and ↓ flow distal to the coarctation (Figure 2.13-3). Occurs just distal to the left subclavian artery in 98% of patients. The condition is associated with Turner syndrome, berry aneurysms, and male gender. More than two-thirds of patients have a bicuspid aortic valve.

HISTORY/PE

- Often presents in childhood with asymptomatic hypertension (upper extremity hypertension); the classic PE finding is a systolic BP that is higher in the upper extremities; the difference in BP between the left and right arm can indicate the point of coarctation.
- A continuous murmur may be heard diffusely across the torso if well-established collaterals are present.
- Lower-extremity claudication, syncope, epistaxis, and headache may be present.
- Additional findings include weak femoral pulses, radiofemoral delay, a short systolic murmur in the left axilla, and a forceful apical impulse.
- In infancy, critical coarctation requires a PDA for survival. Such infants may present in the first few weeks of life with poor feeding, lethargy, tachypnea, and eventual shocklike state when the PDA closes. Differential cyanosis may be seen with lower O_2 saturation in the left arm and lower extremities (postductal areas) as compared with the right arm (preductal area).

DIAGNOSIS

- Echocardiography with color flow Doppler is the diagnostic test of choice.
- CXR in young children may demonstrate cardiomegaly and pulmonary congestion.

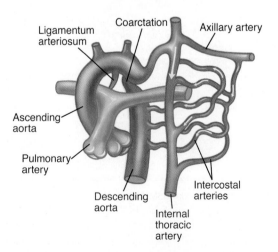

FIGURE 2.13-3. Coarctation of the aorta, causing severe obstruction of flow to the descending thoracic aorta. (Reproduced with permission from USMLE-Rx.com.)

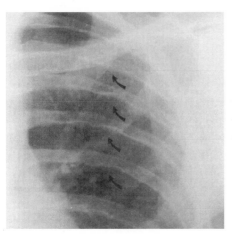
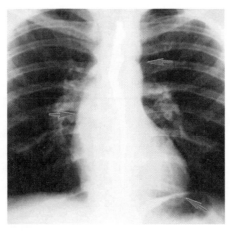

A   **B**

FIGURE 2.13-4.   Coarctation of the aorta. (A) Magnified view of the left upper thorax of a patient with aortic coarctation showing multiple areas of rib notching (*arrows*). (B) Postero-anterior view of another patient with aortic coarctation showing the "3 sign" of the deformed descending aorta and "E sign" on the barium-filled esophagus (*upper arrow*). The lower arrow marks the apex of the enlarged LV. The arrow on the patient's right indicates the dilated ascending aorta. (Reproduced with permission from Fuster V, et al. *Hurst's The Heart*, 13th ed. New York, NY: McGraw-Hill; 2011.)

- In older children, the following compensatory changes may be seen: LVH on ECG; the rib notching of the chest (see Figure 2.13-4A) caused by pre- and postdilatation of the coarctation segment with aortic wall indentation; and the "3" sign on x-ray (see Figure 2.13-4B) caused by collateral circulation through the intercostal arteries.

TREATMENT

- **Best initial treatment:** If severe coarctation presents in infancy, treat with prostaglandin E_1 (PGE_1) to keep the ductus arteriosus open.
- Surgical correction or balloon angioplasty is controversial.
- Monitor for restenosis, aneurysm development, and aortic dissection.

CYANOTIC CONDITIONS

Cyanotic congenital heart conditions typically present with central cyanosis soon after birth.

TRANSPOSITION OF THE GREAT VESSELS

The most common cyanotic congenital heart lesion in the newborn (see Figure 2.13-5). In this condition, the aorta is connected to the right ventricle and the pulmonary artery to the left ventricle, creating parallel pulmonary and systemic circulations. Life is incompatible without a septal defect (ASD or VSD) and/or PDA. A PDA alone is usually not sufficient to allow adequate mixing of blood. Risk factors include diabetic mothers and, rarely, DiGeorge syndrome.

HISTORY/PE

- Critical illness and cyanosis typically present within the first few hours after birth. Reverse differential cyanosis may be seen if left ventricular outflow tract obstruction (eg, coarctation, aortic stenosis) is also present.
- Exam reveals tachypnea, progressive hypoxemia, and extreme cyanosis. Some patients have signs of CHF, and a single loud S_2 is often present.

KEY FACT

Cyanotic CHD does not respond to 100% oxygen challenge (minimal effect on Pao_2), while most lung pathologies will respond to 100% oxygen administration.

KEY FACT

Breath-holding spells are triggered by an emotional trigger and may result in loss of consciousness or cyanosis. Although they may be alarming to the parents, these are benign episodes and not cardiac related. They typically resolve by 5 years of age.

MNEMONIC

Cyanotic heart defects—

The five terrible T's that have right-to-left shunts:

Truncus arteriosus (**1** arterial vessel overriding ventricles)
Transposition of the great vessels (**2** arteries switched)
Tricuspid atresia (**3**)
Tetralogy of Fallot (**4**)
Total anomalous pulmonary venous return (**5** words)
Out of the 5 T's, only transposition presents with severe cyanosis within the first few hours of life.

Q

A 2-year-old boy is brought to the pediatrician because of shortness of breath and easy fatigability during play. Exam is notable for tachypnea and a soft holosystolic murmur over the lower left sternal border. What is the most likely cause of the boy's symptoms?

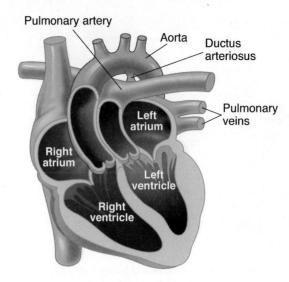

FIGURE 2.13-5. **Complete transposition of the great vessels.** The right ventricle deoxygenated blood is directed to the aorta, and oxygenated blood is directed back to the pulmonary artery. (Reproduced with permission from USMLE-Rx.com.)

A

This boy probably has a large, untreated VSD that has led to Eisenmenger syndrome (and right-to-left shunting). There is less turbulence across a large defect (compared with a small one), leading to a softer murmur.

There may not be a murmur if no VSD is present. If a VSD is present, a systolic murmur may be heard at the left sternal border.

DIAGNOSIS

- **Best initial test:** Echocardiography, which will show abnormal formation of the great arteries.
- CXR may show a narrow heart base, absence of the main pulmonary artery segment, an "egg-shaped silhouette," and ↑ pulmonary vascular markings.

TREATMENT

- **Best initial treatment:** IV PGE to maintain or open the PDA.
- If surgery is not feasible within the first few days of life or if the PDA cannot be maintained with prostaglandin, perform balloon atrial septotomy to create or enlarge an ASD.
- **Most definitive treatment:** Surgical correction (arterial or atrial switch).

TETRALOGY OF FALLOT

Consists of right ventricular outflow tract (RVOT) obstruction, overriding aorta, right ventricular hypertrophy (RVH), and VSD (see Figure 2.13-6). The most common cyanotic CHD in children. Early cyanosis results from right-to-left shunting across the VSD. As right-sided pressures ↓ in the weeks after birth, the shunt direction reverses and cyanosis may ↓. If the degree of pulmonary stenosis is severe, the right-sided pressures may remain high and cyanosis may worsen over time. Risk factors include maternal PKU and DiGeorge syndrome.

HISTORY/PE

- Presents in infancy or early childhood with dyspnea and fatigability. Cyanosis is frequently absent at birth but develops over the first 2 years of life; the degree of cyanosis often reflects the extent of pulmonary stenosis.
- Infants are often asymptomatic until 4–6 months of age, when CHF may develop and manifest as diaphoresis with feeding or tachypnea.

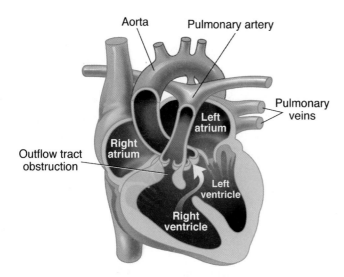

FIGURE 2.13-6. **Tetralogy of Fallot.** Substantial right ventricular outflow tract obstruction resulting in right-to-left shunting through the ventricular septal defect. (Reproduced with permission from USMLE-Rx.com.)

- Children often squat for relief during hypoxemic episodes called "tet spells," which ↑ systemic vascular resistance, thus increasing blood flow to the pulmonary vasculature and improved oxygenation.
- Hypoxemia may lead to FTT or altered mental status.
- Exam reveals a systolic ejection murmur at the upper left sternal border (right ventricular outflow obstruction), a right ventricular heave, and a single S_2.

Diagnosis

- **Best initial test:** Echocardiography and catheterization.
- CXR shows a "boot-shaped" heart with ↓ pulmonary vascular markings. Remember that a VSD may result in ↑ pulmonary vascular markings.
- ECG shows right-axis deviation and RVH.

Treatment

- **Best initial treatment:** If there is severe RVOT obstruction or atresia is immediate, PGE_1 to keep the PDA open along with urgent surgical consultation.
- Treat hypercyanotic "tet spells" with O_2, propranolol, phenylephrine, the knee-chest position, fluids, and morphine.
- Temporary palliation can be achieved through the creation of an artificial shunt (eg, balloon atrial septotomy) before definitive surgical correction (Blalock-Taussig shunt).

Pediatric Gastroenterological Disease

PYLORIC STENOSIS

Hypertrophy of the pyloric sphincter, leading to gastric outlet obstruction. More common in firstborn infant boys; associated with tracheoesophageal fistula, formula feeding, and maternal erythromycin ingestion.

KEY FACT

Both transposition of the great vessels and tetralogy of Fallot are initially treated with PGE_1 but are definitively treated with surgical correction.

Q 1

A 3-day-old boy born at 39 weeks' gestational age via normal spontaneous vaginal delivery has failed to pass meconium and today displays abdominal distention and five episodes of nonbilious vomiting. Rectal exam shows no stool in the rectal vault. Air contrast enema shows an obstruction at the ileum. What is the most likely cause of this patient's symptoms?

Q 2

A 3-week-old ex-term infant boy is brought to the emergency department after experiencing vomiting of increasing frequency and intensity for the past week. His parents state that he now vomits forcefully after every meal and enthusiastically attempts to eat immediately after vomiting. The infant appears lethargic, with sunken fontanelles and decreased skin turgor. The abdomen is soft, nontender, and nondistended; no masses are felt. What is the most likely cause of this infant's symptoms?

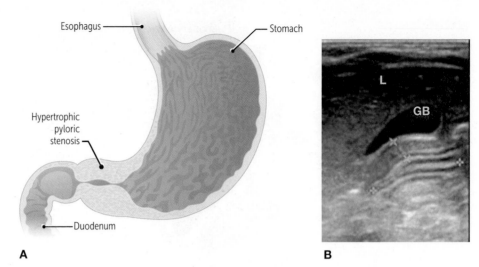

FIGURE 2.13-7. **Hypertrophic pyloric stenosis.** (A) Schematic representation of a hypertrophied pylorus. The arrow denotes protrusion of the pylorus into the duodenum. (B) Longitudinal ultrasound of the pylorus showing a thickened pyloric musculature (*X's*) over a long pyloric channel length (*plus signs*). L, liver; GB, gallbladder. (Reproduced with permission from USMLE-Rx.com.)

HISTORY/PE

- Nonbilious emesis typically begins around 3–5 weeks of age and progresses to projectile emesis after most or all feedings.
- Infants are generally hungry after episodes of vomiting; they initially feed well but eventually suffer from dehydration and malnutrition.
- Exam may reveal a palpable olive-shaped, mobile, nontender epigastric mass and visible gastric peristaltic waves.

DIAGNOSIS

- **Best initial test:** Abdominal ultrasound will reveal a thickened, elongated pylorus (see Figure 2.13-7).
- Laboratory work-up reveals hypochloremic, hypokalemic metabolic alkalosis; emesis results in loss of HCl and renin-angiotensin-aldosterone axis activation.
- Barium studies show a narrow pyloric channel ("string sign") or a pyloric beak.

TREATMENT

- **Best initial treatment:** Keep patient NPO (nothing by mouth), establish IV access, and correct dehydration and acid-base/electrolyte abnormalities.
- **Most definitive treatment:** Surgical correction with pyloromyotomy.

INTUSSUSCEPTION

A condition in which a portion of the bowel invaginates or "telescopes" into an adjacent segment, usually proximal to the ileocecal valve (see Figure 2.13-8A). The most common cause of bowel obstruction in children between 6 months and 3 years of age (boys > girls). Etiology is unclear in most children. Risk factors include conditions with potential lead points, including Meckel diverticulum, intestinal lymphoma (> 6 years of age), submucosal hematoma (as in Henoch-Schönlein purpura), polyps, and CF (lead point is inspissated stool). Antecedent GI or URI is seen in many children, which may cause formation of a lead point through enlargement of Peyer patches.

---

1 **A**

This infant most likely has meconium ileus resulting from CF; however, Hirschsprung disease should remain on the differential diagnosis, as it also can cause delayed meconium passage. Meconium ileus causes obstruction at the level of the ileum, whereas Hirschsprung disease causes rectosigmoid obstruction, and rectal exam may result in the expulsion of stool.

2 **A**

This infant is most likely suffering from pyloric stenosis, an obstruction of the gastric outlet secondary to hypertrophy and hyperplasia of the muscular layers of the pylorus. Note that most (60–80%) but not all infants present with an olive-shaped abdominal mass.

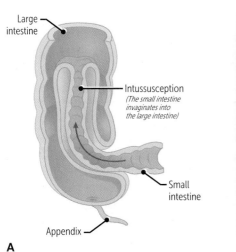
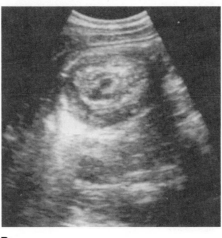

A   **B**

FIGURE 2.13-8.   Intussusception. (A) Ileocolic intussusception, the most common location in children. **(B)** Transabdominal ultrasound shows the classic "target sign" of intussusception in cross-section. (Image A reproduced with permission from USMLE-Rx.com. Image B reproduced with permission from Ma OJ, et al. *Emergency Ultrasound*, 2nd ed. New York, NY: McGraw-Hill; 2008.)

HISTORY/PE

- Presents with abrupt-onset, episodic abdominal pain in apparently healthy children, often accompanied by flexed knees and vomiting. The child may appear well between episodes if intussusception is released.
- The classic triad is severe abdominal pain, vomiting (initially nonbilious, then bilious as obstruction develops), and bloody mucus in stool ("currant jelly stool," a late finding).
- On exam, look for abdominal tenderness, a ⊕ stool guaiac, a palpable "sausage-shaped" RUQ abdominal mass, and "empty" RLQ on palpation (Dance sign).

DIAGNOSIS/TREATMENT

- Ultrasonography is the test of choice and may show a "target sign" (see Figure 2.13-8B); ultrasound must be carried out during a painful episode to diagnose intussusception.
- X-rays of the abdomen are often normal early in the disease, but later they may show small bowel obstruction, perforation, or a soft tissue mass.
- Correct any volume or electrolyte abnormalities, check CBC for leukocytosis, and consider an NG tube for decompression.
- In the setting of high clinical suspicion, perform an air insufflation enema without delay, as it is diagnostic and curative in the vast majority of patients.
- Surgical resection is indicated if the child has peritoneal signs, enema reduction is unsuccessful, or a pathologic lead point is identified.
- Air insufflation enema is preferred over water or barium-contrast enema for diagnosis and management of intussusception, as it is faster and carries a lower risk for complications.

MALROTATION WITH VOLVULUS

Congenital malrotation of the midgut results in abnormal positioning of the small intestine (cecum in the right hypochondrium) and formation of fibrous bands (Ladd bands), which predispose to obstruction and constriction of blood flow.

> **KEY FACT**
>
> The classic triad of abdominal pain, vomiting, and currant jelly stool only occurs in one-third of patients with intussusception.

History/PE

- Often presents in the first month of life with bilious emesis, crampy abdominal pain, distention, and passage of blood or mucus in the stool.
- Postsurgical adhesions can lead to obstruction and volvulus at any point in life.

Diagnosis

- Barium contrast enema may reveal the characteristic "bird-beak" appearance and air-fluid levels but may also appear normal.
- Upper GI series is the study of choice if the patient is stable and shows an abnormal location of the ligament of Treitz. Ultrasound may be used, but its sensitivity is contingent on the experience of the ultrasonographer.

Treatment

- NG tube insertion to decompress the intestine; IV fluid hydration.
- Emergent surgical correction when volvulus is gastric; surgery or endoscopy when volvulus is intestinal.

MECKEL DIVERTICULUM

Caused by failure of the omphalomesenteric (or vitelline) duct to obliterate, resulting in the formation of a true diverticulum (containing all three layers of the small intestine). The heterotopic gastric tissue present in most Meckel diverticula causes intestinal ulceration and painless hematochezia. This is the most common congenital abnormality of the small intestine, affecting up to 2% of children (boys > girls). Most frequently symptomatic in children < 2 years of age.

History/PE

- Typically asymptomatic, and often discovered incidentally.
- Classically presents with painless rectal bleeding.
- Complications include intestinal perforation or obstruction, diverticulitis (which can mimic acute appendicitis), and intussusception.

Diagnosis

- A Meckel scintigraphy scan (technetium-99m pertechnetate; detects ectopic gastric tissue) is diagnostic.
- X-rays have limited value but can be useful in diagnosing obstruction or perforation.

Treatment

- **Most definitive treatment:** Surgical excision of the diverticulum together with the adjacent ileal segment, which may be ulcerated.
- Indications for urgent/emergent surgery include hemorrhage, diverticulitis, intestinal perforation, and obstruction/intussusception.

HIRSCHSPRUNG DISEASE

Characterized by congenital lack of ganglion cells in the distal colon. This leads to decreased motility caused by unopposed smooth muscle tone in the absence of enteric relaxing reflexes and uncoordinated peristalsis (see Figure 2.13-9). Associated with male gender, Down syndrome, Waardenburg syndrome, and multiple endocrine neoplasia type 2.

MNEMONIC

Meckel rule of 2's—

Occurs in **2%** of the population
2% symptomatic by age **2**
2 times more common in boys
Contains **2** types of tissue (gastric and pancreatic)
2 inches long
Found within **2** feet of the ileocecal valve

KEY FACT

Bleeding is the most common complication of Meckel diverticulum; it may be minimal, or severe enough to cause hemorrhagic shock.

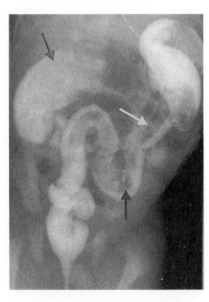

FIGURE 2.13-9. **Hirschsprung disease.** Retrograde barium enema shows small caliber of the left colon (*yellow arrow*) and rectum in comparison to the more dilated transverse colon (*red arrow*). Filling defects in the descending/sigmoid colon represent feces (*blue arrow*). (Reproduced with permission from USMLE-Rx.com.)

HISTORY/PE

- Presentation depends on the extent of the aganglionic segment.
- Neonates present with failure to pass meconium within 48 hours of birth, accompanied by bilious vomiting and FTT; children with less severe lesions may present later in life with chronic constipation.
- PE may reveal abdominal distention and explosive discharge of stool following a rectal exam; lack of stool in the rectum; or abnormal sphincter tone.

DIAGNOSIS

- **Best initial test:** X-rays reveal distended bowel loops with a paucity of air in the rectum.
- Barium enema is the imaging study of choice and reveals a narrowed distal colon with proximal dilation.
- Anorectal manometry detects failure of the internal sphincter to relax after distention of the rectal lumen. It is typically used in atypical presentations or older children.
- **Most accurate test:** Rectal biopsy confirms the diagnosis and reveals absence of the myenteric (Auerbach) plexus and submucosal (Meissner) plexus along with hypertrophied nerve trunks enhanced with acetylcholinesterase stain.

KEY FACT

Definitive diagnosis of Hirschsprung disease requires a rectal biopsy.

TREATMENT

Traditionally a two-stage surgical correction is used involving the creation of a diverting colostomy at the time of diagnosis, followed several weeks later by a definitive "pull-through" procedure connecting the remaining colon to the rectum.

NECROTIZING ENTEROCOLITIS

A condition in which a portion of the bowel (most commonly the terminal ileum/proximal colon) undergoes necrosis. Necrotizing enterocolitis (NEC) is the most common GI emergency in neonates; it is most frequently seen in premature infants but can rarely occur in full-term infants as well. Risk factors include low birth weight, hypotension, and enteral feeding (especially formula).

KEY FACT

Pneumatosis intestinalis on x-rays is pathognomonic for NEC in neonates.

HISTORY/PE

- Symptoms usually present within the first few days or weeks of life and are nonspecific, including feeding intolerance, delayed gastric emptying, abdominal distention, and bloody stools.
- Symptoms can rapidly progress to intestinal perforation, peritonitis, abdominal erythema, and shock. Maintain a high index of suspicion.

DIAGNOSIS

- Lab findings are nonspecific and may show hyponatremia, metabolic acidosis, leukopenia or leukocytosis with left shift, thrombocytopenia, and coagulopathy (DIC with prolonged PT/aPTT and a ⊕ D-dimer).
- X-rays of the abdomen are the imaging modality of choice and may show dilated bowel loops, pneumatosis intestinalis (intramural air bubbles representing gas produced by bacteria within the bowel wall; see Figure 2.13-10), portal venous gas, or abdominal free air (in the case of bowel perforation). Serial x-rays of the abdomen should be taken every 6 hours.
- Ultrasound may also be helpful in discerning free air, areas of loculation, and bowel necrosis.

Q

A 4-day-old boy born at 34 weeks for intrauterine growth restriction has experienced frequent bilious vomiting for the past 24 hours and has passed stool mixed with bright red blood twice today. He initially fed well (consuming formula only) but now refuses the bottle. Exam is notable for lethargy, abdominal distention, and decreased bowel sounds. What is the most likely diagnosis, and what would you expect to see on x-rays of the abdomen?

Posterior urethral valves are the most common congenital urethral obstruction. Classic findings are a male infant with a distended, palpable bladder and low urine output. Can lead to pulmonary hypoplasia and respiratory distress caused by oligohydramnios.

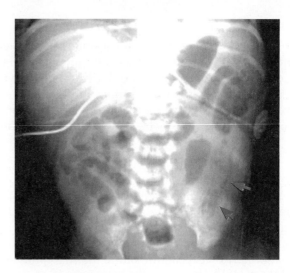

FIGURE 2.13-10. Pneumatosis intestinalis. Short arrows highlight pneumatosis intestinalis on an x-ray of the abdomen for a patient with necrotizing enterocolitis. (Reproduced with permission from Brunicardi FC, et al. *Schwartz's Principles of Surgery*, 9th ed. New York, NY: McGraw-Hill; 2010.)

TREATMENT

- **Best initial treatment:** Initiate supportive measures, including NPO, a nasogastric tube for gastric decompression, correction of dehydration and electrolyte abnormalities, TPN, and IV antibiotics.
- Indications for surgery are perforation (free air under the diaphragm) or worsening radiographic signs on serial abdominal x-rays. An ileostomy with mucous fistula is typically performed, with a reanastomosis later.
- Complications include formation of intestinal strictures and short-bowel syndrome.

Pediatric Urology

VESICOURETERAL REFLUX

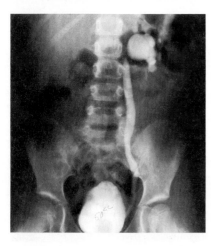

FIGURE 2.13-11. Vesicoureteral reflux. Frontal x-ray from a voiding cystourethrogram shows reflux to the left ureter and intrarenal collecting system with hydronephrosis. Note the absence of reflux on the normal right side. (Reproduced with permission from Doherty GM. *Current Diagnosis & Treatment: Surgery*, 13th ed. New York, NY: McGraw-Hill; 2010.)

Retrograde projection of urine from the bladder to the ureters and kidneys. May be caused by posterior urethral valves, urethral or meatal stenosis, or a neurogenic bladder. Classified as follows:

- **Mild reflux (grades I–II):** No ureteral or renal pelvic dilation. Often resolves spontaneously.
- **Moderate to severe reflux (grade III–V):** Ureteral dilation with associated caliceal blunting in severe cases.

HISTORY/PE

Patients present with recurrent UTIs, typically in childhood. Prenatal ultrasonography may identify hydronephrosis and/or oligohydramnios.

DIAGNOSIS

- Treat UTI first with antibiotics and ultrasound. Follow-up abnormalities with voiding cystourethrogram.
- Obtain a voiding cystourethrogram (VCUG) to detect abnormalities at ureteral insertion sites and to classify the grade of reflux (see Figure 2.13-11) with recurrent UTIs. VCUG should also be performed if there is recurrence of febrile UTI.

A

This infant most likely has necrotizing enterocolitis, given his presentation and risk factors (prematurity, formula feeding). This is a serious diagnosis with up to 40% mortality. X-ray findings can include pneumatosis intestinalis, air in the portal venous system, and free air under the diaphragm (in case of bowel perforation).

TREATMENT

- Treat infections aggressively.
- Surgery (ureteral reimplantation) is generally reserved for children with persistent high-grade (III–V) reflux. Inadequate treatment can lead to progressive renal scarring and end-stage renal disease.
- In children with recurrent UTIs and VUR, daily antibiotic prophylaxis shows limited benefit in reducing the number of febrile UTIs or preventing renal scarring.

CRYPTORCHIDISM

Failure of one or both testes to fully descend into the scrotum. Low birth weight is a risk factor.

HISTORY/PE

Bilateral cryptorchidism is associated with prematurity, oligospermia, congenital malformation syndromes (Prader-Willi, Noonan syndromes), and infertility. Associated with an ↑ risk for testicular malignancy.

DIAGNOSIS

The testes cannot be manipulated into the scrotal sac with gentle pressure (vs retractile testes) and can be palpated anywhere along the inguinal canal or in the abdomen.

TREATMENT

Orchiopexy for prepubertal boys; orchiectomy vs close observation if discovered after puberty to minimize the risk for testicular cancer.

Pediatric Immunology

IMMUNODEFICIENCY DISORDERS

Congenital immunodeficiencies are rare and often present with chronic or recurrent infections (eg, chronic thrush), unusual or opportunistic organisms, incomplete treatment response, or FTT. Categorization is based on the single immune system component that is abnormal (see Table 2.13-14).

- **B-cell deficiencies:** Most common (50%). Typically present after 6 months of age with recurrent sinopulmonary, GI, and urinary tract infections with encapsulated organisms (*Haemophilus influenzae*, *Streptococcus pneumoniae*, *Neisseria meningitidis*). Treat with IVIG (except for IgA deficiencies).
  - Bruton agammaglobulinemia can be confused with transient hypogammaglobulinemia of infancy (THI), as both are characterized by ↑ susceptibility to infections at ~ 6 months of age, when transplacental maternal IgG is no longer active. B cells are ↓ in Bruton, whereas those in THI are normal.
  - Bruton agammaglobulinemia and common variable immunodeficiency (CVID) also have similar symptoms, but the former is found in boys ~ 6 months of age, whereas CVID is seen in older men and women (15–35 years of age), and its symptoms are less severe.
- **T-cell deficiencies:** Tend to present earlier (1–3 months) with opportunistic and low-grade fungal, viral, and intracellular bacterial infections (eg, mycobacteria). 2° B-cell dysfunction can also be seen.

KEY FACT

Children 2–24 months of age with multiple urinary tract infections should first have an ultrasound exam and then have a VCUG only if ultrasonography shows hydronephrosis, scarring, or other findings suspicious for obstruction or high-grade VUR. Evidence is limited for children < 2 months.

KEY FACT

Bringing the testes into the scrotum may lower, but not eliminate, the risk for testicular cancer.

KEY FACT

Flashback to immunology:
- B cells make immunoglobulins and are responsible for immunity against extracellular bacteria.
- T cells are responsible for immunity against intracellular bacteria, viruses, and fungi.

KEY FACT

Untreated Kawasaki disease can lead to coronary aneurysms in up to 25% of patients.

- **Phagocyte deficiencies:** Characterized by mucous membrane infections, abscesses, and poor wound healing. Infections with catalase ⊕ organisms (eg, *S aureus*), fungi, and gram ⊖ enteric organisms are common. See Table 2.13-15.
- **Complement deficiencies:** Present in children with congenital asplenia or splenic dysfunction (sickle cell disease). Characterized by recurrent bacterial infections with encapsulated organisms. See Table 2.13-16.

MNEMONIC

Kawasaki disease symptoms—

CRASH and BURN

Conjunctivitis
Rash
Adenopathy (unilateral)
Strawberry tongue
Hands and feet (red, swollen, flaky skin)
BURN (fever > 40°C [> 104°F] for ≥ 5 days)

KAWASAKI DISEASE

A multisystemic acute vasculitis that primarily affects young children (80% are < 5 years of age), particularly those of Asian ancestry. Divided into acute, subacute, and chronic phases.

HISTORY/PE

- **Acute phase:** 1–2 weeks from onset (see Table 2.13-17 for diagnostic criteria).

TABLE 2.13-14. Pediatric B-Cell and T-Cell Deficiencies

DISORDER	DESCRIPTION	INFECTION RISK/TYPE	DIAGNOSIS/TREATMENT
B-CELL DISORDERS			
Bruton agammaglobulinemia	An X-linked recessive B-cell deficiency found only in boys. Symptoms begin after 6 months of age, when maternal IgG (transferred transplacentally) is no longer active	Life-threatening; characterized by encapsulated *Pseudomonas*, *S pneumoniae*, and *Haemophilus* infections after 6 months of age	Quantitative Ig levels: if low, confirm with B- and T-cell subsets (B cells are absent; T cells are often high). Absent tonsils and other lymphoid tissue may provide a clue. Treat with prophylactic antibiotics and IVIG
Common variable immunodeficiency (CVID)	Usually a combined B- and T-cell defect. All Ig levels are low (in the 20s and 30s). Normal B-cell numbers; ↓ plasma cells. Symptoms usually present later in life (15–35 years of age)	↑ Pyogenic upper and lower respiratory infections. ↑ Risk for lymphoma and auto-immune disease	Quantitative Ig levels; confirm with B- and T-cell subsets. Treat with IVIG
IgA deficiency	Mild; the most common immunodeficiency. ↓ IgA levels only	Usually asymptomatic; patients may develop recurrent respiratory or GI infections (*Giardia*). Anaphylactic transfusion reaction caused by anti-IgA antibodies is a common presentation	Quantitative IgA levels; treat infections. Be careful giving IVIG, as it can lead to the production of anti-IgA antibodies and cause severe allergic reactions; if IVIG is necessary, give IgA-depleted IVI
Hyper-IgM syndrome	Absence of CD40 ligand that allows class-switching from IgM to other Ig classes. ↑ IgM levels, low levels of all other Ig, and normal numbers of lymphocytes	Severe, recurrent sinopulmonary infections caused by impaired Ig	Treat with antibiotic prophylaxis and IVIG

(continues)

TABLE 2.13-14.   Pediatric B-Cell and T-Cell Deficiencies *(continued)*

DISORDER	DESCRIPTION	INFECTION RISK/TYPE	DIAGNOSIS/TREATMENT
T-CELL DISORDERS			
Thymic aplasia (DiGeorge syndrome)	See the mnemonic CATCH 22 Presents with tetany (2° to hypocalcemia) in the first days of life Autosomal dominant	Variable risk for infection ↑↑↑ Infections with viruses, fungi, and pneumocystis pneumonia (PCP) X-ray may show absent thymic shadow	Absolute T-lymphocyte count; mitogen stimulation response; delayed hypersensitivity skin testing Treat with bone marrow transplantation (BMT) and IVIG for antibody deficiency; give PCP prophylaxis Thymus transplantation is an alternative
COMBINED DISORDERS			
Ataxia-telangiectasia	Progressive cerebellar ataxia and oculocutaneous telangiectasias Caused by an autosomal recessive mutation in gene responsible for repair of dsDNA breaks	↑ Incidence of malignancies, including non-Hodgkin lymphoma, leukemia, and gastric carcinoma	No specific treatment; may require IVIG depending on the severity of the Ig deficiency
Severe combined immunodeficiency	Most commonly X-linked recessive Severe lack of B and T cells caused by a defect in stem cell maturation and ↓ adenosine deaminase Referred to as "bubble boy disease," because children are confined to an isolated, sterile environment	Severe, frequent bacterial infections; chronic candidiasis; opportunistic organisms	Treat with bone marrow or stem cell transplantation and IVIG for antibody deficiency Requires PCP prophylaxis
Wiskott-Aldrich syndrome	An X-linked recessive disorder seen only in male patients Symptoms usually present at birth Patients have ↑ IgE/IgA, ↓ IgM, and thrombocytopenia The classic presentation involves bleeding, eczema, and recurrent otitis media Remember the mnemonic **WIPE:** **W**iskott-Aldrich **I**nfections **P**urpura (thrombocytopenic) **E**czema	↑↑ Risk for atopic disorders, lymphoma/leukemia, and infection from *S pneumoniae, S aureus,* and *H influenzae* type b (encapsulated organisms; think back to how IgM functions)	Treatment is supportive (IVIG and antibiotics) Patients are at ↑ risk for developing autoimmune diseases and malignancies Patients rarely survive to adulthood Patients with severe infections may be treated with BMT

- **Subacute phase:** 2–8 weeks from onset. Manifestations are thrombocytosis and ↑ erythrocyte sedimentation rate (ESR). Untreated children may begin to develop coronary artery aneurysms (25%); all patients should be assessed by echocardiography at diagnosis.
- **Chronic phase:** > 8 weeks from onset; begins when all clinical symptoms have disappeared, and lasts until ESR returns to baseline. Untreated children are at risk for aneurysmal expansion and MI.

TABLE 2.13-15. **Pediatric Phagocytic Deficiencies**

DISORDER	DESCRIPTION	INFECTION RISK/TYPE	DIAGNOSIS/TREATMENT
Chronic granulomatous disease (CGD)	An X-linked (2/3) or autosomal-recessive (1/3) disease with deficient superoxide production by polymorphonuclear leukocytes and macrophages. Anemia, lymphadenopathy, and hypergammaglobulinemia may be present	Chronic skin, lymph node, pulmonary, GI, and urinary tract infections; osteomyelitis and hepatitis. Infecting organisms are catalase $\oplus$ (S aureus, Escherichia coli, Candida, Klebsiella, Pseudomonas, Aspergillus). May have granulomas of the skin and GI/GU tracts	Absolute neutrophil count with neutrophil assays. The dihydrorhodamine (DHR) test is diagnostic for CGD; nitroblue tetrazolium test is the previous gold standard and still occasionally used. Treat with daily TMP-SMX; make judicious use of antibiotics during infections. IFN-γ can ↓ the incidence of serious infection. BMT and gene therapy are new therapies
Leukocyte adhesion deficiency	A defect in the chemotaxis of leukocytes. ↓ Phagocytic activity	Recurrent skin, mucosal, and pulmonary infections. May present as omphalitis in the newborn period with delayed separation of the umbilical cord (> 14 days post-birth)	No pus with minimal inflammation in wounds (caused by a chemotaxis defect). High WBCs in blood. BMT is curative
Chédiak-Higashi syndrome	An autosomal recessive disorder that leads to a defect in neutrophil chemotaxis/microtubule polymerization. The syndrome includes partial oculocutaneous albinism, peripheral neuropathy, and neutropenia	↑↑ Incidence of overwhelming pyogenic infections with S pyogenes, S aureus, and Pneumococcus species	Look for giant granules in neutrophils. BMT is the treatment of choice
Job syndrome (Hyperimmunoglobulin E syndrome)	A defect in neutrophil chemotaxis. Remember the mnemonic **FATED:** Coarse **F**acies. **A**bscesses (S aureus). Retained primary **T**eeth. Hyper-Ig**E** (eosinophilia). **D**ermatologic (severe eczema)	Recurrent S aureus infections and abscesses	Treat with penicillinase-resistant antibiotics and IVIG

TABLE 2.13-16. **Pediatric Complement Disorders**

DISORDER	DESCRIPTION	INFECTION RISK/TYPE	DIAGNOSIS/TREATMENT
C1 esterase inhibitor deficiency (hereditary angioedema)	An autosomal dominant disorder with recurrent episodes of angioedema lasting 2–72 hours and provoked by stress or trauma	Can lead to life-threatening airway edema	Total hemolytic complement (CH50) to assess the quantity and function of complement. Purified C1 inhibitor (C1INH) concentrate and FFP can be used before surgery
Terminal complement deficiency (C5–C9)	Inability to form membrane attack complex	Recurrent Neisseria infections, meningococcal or gonococcal. Rarely, lupus or glomerulonephritis	Meningococcal vaccine and appropriate antibiotics

TABLE 2.13-17. **Clinical Manifestations of Kawasaki Disease**

Five days of fever and at least four of the following five criteria:

1. Bilateral, nonexudative, painless conjunctivitis with the limbal sparing
2. Oral mucosal changes (see Image A): erythematous mouth/pharynx, "strawberry tongue", or cracked lips
3. Rash: primarily truncal, polymorphous, erythematous
4. Peripheral extremity changes: induration of hands and feet, erythematous and desquamating palms and soles
5. Cervical lymphadenopathy (> 1.5 cm): generally painful and unilateral

Other manifestations (not required for diagnosis) include sterile pyuria, gallbladder hydrops, hepatitis, and arthritis

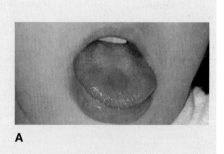

A

Image reproduced with permission from Stagi S, et al. Kawasaki disease in a girl with Turner syndrome: a remarkable association. *Ital J Pediatr.* 2014;40:24.

DIAGNOSIS

- **Laboratory work-up:**
    - **Acute phase:** Normochromic anemia, leukocytosis with left shift, ↑ ESR and CRP.
    - **Subacute phase:** Thrombocytosis. ESR and CRP gradually ↓ during this phase.
- Echocardiogram at time of diagnosis to establish a baseline for longitudinal follow-up of coronary artery morphology. Follow-up for uncomplicated cases usually at 2 weeks and 6–8 weeks after diagnosis.

TREATMENT

- **Best initial treatment:** High-dose aspirin (ASA) (for anti-inflammatory, antipyretic, and antithrombotic effects) and IVIG (to prevent coronary artery aneurysms).
- Low-dose ASA is then continued, usually for 6 weeks. Children who develop coronary aneurysms may require chronic anticoagulation with ASA or other antiplatelet medications. Patients taking ASA are at risk for developing Reye syndrome.
- Corticosteroids may be used in IVIG-refractory cases, but routine use is not recommended.

JUVENILE IDIOPATHIC ARTHRITIS

An autoimmune disorder manifesting as arthritis with "morning stiffness" and gradual loss of motion that is present for at least 6 weeks in a patient < 16 years of age. Formerly known as juvenile rheumatoid arthritis (JRA). Approximately 95% of cases resolve by puberty. More common in girls than in boys. The subtypes of JIA are described in Table 2.13-18.

DIAGNOSIS

See Table 2.13-18.

TREATMENT

- **Best initial treatment:** NSAIDs and strengthening exercises.
- Corticosteroids (for myocarditis) and immunosuppressive medications (methotrexate, anti–tumor necrosis factor agents such as etanercept) are second-line agents.

KEY FACT

Kawasaki disease and scarlet fever may both present with "strawberry tongue," rash, desquamation of the hands and feet, and erythema of the mucous membranes. However, children with scarlet fever have normal lips and no conjunctivitis.

KEY FACT

ASA is only used for Kawasaki disease in the pediatric population in fear of a rare but serious condition called Reye syndrome. Although the exact mechanism is unclear, Reye syndrome results from mitochondrial injury and fatty degenerative liver failure, which leads to hyperammonemia and ultimately encephalopathy.

Q

A 2-year-old boy is brought to the pediatrician for a skin infection that started on his chin and rapidly spread to involve much of his face and neck. This is his third such infection this year, and he is constantly plagued by sinus infections and bouts of pneumonia. There is no family history of recurrent infections. The patient appears uncomfortable, and dermatologic exam is notable for erosions coated in yellow crust that are widespread across the patient's face and neck. He also has patchy white pigmentation of the skin, light blonde hair, and blue eyes. What is the most likely diagnosis?

TABLE 2.13-18. Juvenile Idiopathic Arthritis Subtypes

SUBTYPE	PRESENTATION	RF AND ANA STATUS	NOTES
Pauciarticular (oligoarthritis)	Involves four or fewer joints (usually weight-bearing); no systemic symptoms Uveitis is common; requires slit-lamp exam for diagnosis	ANA ⊕ RF ⊖	Most common presentation of JIA Usually diagnosed in young girls
Polyarthritis	Present in five or more joints; generally symmetric Systemic symptoms rare	RF positivity is rare (indicates severe disease) Young children may be ANA ⊕ with milder disease	Rheumatoid nodules may be seen in children with RF ⊕ disease
Systemic-onset (Still disease)	Recurrent high fever (> 39°C [> 102.2°F]) Hepatosplenomegaly Salmon-colored macular rash	ANA ⊖ RF ⊖	Joint inflammation may not occur for months to years after systemic symptoms appear

Pediatric Infectious Disease

ACUTE OTITIS MEDIA

A suppurative infection of the middle ear cavity that is common in children. Up to 75% of children have at least three episodes by 2 years of age. Common pathogens include *S pneumoniae*, nontypeable *H influenzae*, *Moraxella catarrhalis*, and viruses such as influenza A, respiratory syncytial virus (RSV), and parainfluenza virus.

HISTORY/PE

Symptoms include ear pain, fever, crying, irritability, difficulty feeding or sleeping, vomiting, and diarrhea. Young children may tug on their ears.

DIAGNOSIS

- Diagnosis is made clinically.
- Signs on otoscopic exam reveal an erythematous tympanic membrane (TM), effusion, bulging or retraction of the TM and ↓ TM mobility (test with an insufflator bulb). Viral causes may result in serous otitis media with blue-gray bulging membranes.
- Serous otitis media is the presence of effusion without active infection. Exam shows a dull tympanic membrane.

TREATMENT

- **Best initial treatment:** High-dose amoxicillin (80–90 mg/kg/day) for 10 days for empiric therapy. Resistant cases may require amoxicillin/clavulanic acid.
- Complications include tympanic membrane perforation, mastoiditis, meningitis, cholesteatomas, and chronic otitis media. Recurrent otitis media can cause hearing loss with resultant speech and language delay. Chronic otitis media may require tympanostomy tubes.

BRONCHIOLITIS

An acute inflammatory illness of the small airways of the lower respiratory tract that primarily affects infants and children < 2 years of age, often in the

This child most likely has Chédiak-Higashi syndrome, caused by autosomal recessive defects in the synthesis/maintenance of storage granules in a number of cell types (including leukocytes, platelets, neutrophils, and melanocytes). In addition to partial oculocutaneous albinism, these patients experience hepatosplenomegaly and recurrent, serious infections of the skin and respiratory tract by *S aureus*, *Streptococcus pyogenes,* and *Pneumococcus* species. Chédiak-Higashi syndrome is often fatal in childhood because of overwhelming infection.

fall or winter. RSV is the most common cause; others include parainfluenza, influenza, metapneumovirus, and other viruses. Progression to respiratory failure is a potentially fatal complication. Risk factors for severe RSV infection include < 6 months of age, prematurity, heart or lung disease, neuromuscular disease, and immunodeficiency.

HISTORY/PE

- **Presentation:**
    - **Days 1–3:** Low-grade fever, rhinorrhea, cough. Young infants might have apnea.
    - **Days 4–6:** Respiratory distress, tachypnea, hypoxia.
- **PE:** Tachypnea, hypoxia, intercostal retractions, crackles or coarse breath sounds ("washing machine sounds"), ± wheezing.
- An ↑ respiratory rate is the earliest and most sensitive vital sign change.

DIAGNOSIS

- Predominantly a clinical diagnosis; routine cases do not need any lab or radiologic work-up.
- In severe cases, a CXR can be obtained to rule out pneumonia and may show hyperinflation of the lungs with flattened diaphragms, interstitial infiltrates, and atelectasis.
- Nasopharyngeal aspirate to test for RSV and other viruses is highly sensitive and specific but has little effect on management (infants should be treated for bronchiolitis whether or not a virus is identified).

TREATMENT

- Treatment is primarily supportive with hydration, suctioning, and supplemental O_2.
- For patients with a history or strong family history of asthma, treat with bronchodilators and continue if they improve the patient's symptoms.
- Hospitalize if infant's tachypnea interferes with feeding or signs of severe illness are present.
- Corticosteroids are not indicated.
- Ribavirin is an antiviral drug sometimes used in high-risk infants with underlying heart, lung, or immune disease. The American Academy of Pediatrics recommends against the use of ribavirin in otherwise healthy children.
- RSV prophylaxis with injectable monoclonal antibodies (palivizumab) is recommended in the fall/winter for high-risk patients ≤ 2 years of age (eg, those with a history of prematurity, chronic lung disease, or CHD).

CROUP (LARYNGOTRACHEOBRONCHITIS)

An acute viral inflammatory disease of the larynx, primarily within the sub-glottic space. Pathogens include parainfluenza virus types 1 (most common), 2, and 3, and RSV, influenza, and adenovirus. Bacterial superinfection may progress to tracheitis.

HISTORY/PE

Prodromal URI symptoms are typically followed by low-grade fever, mild dyspnea, inspiratory stridor that worsens with agitation, a hoarse voice, and a characteristic barking cough (that worsens at night).

DIAGNOSIS

- Diagnosed by clinical impression; often based on the degree of stridor and respiratory distress.

KEY FACT

Infants are at risk for foreign body aspiration. Sudden-onset wheezing or respiratory distress are often characteristic. Objects that cause airway compromise or that cause mucosal damage (batteries) should be removed immediately with bronchoscopy, while others can be observed.

KEY FACT

RSV is the most common cause of bronchiolitis. Parainfluenza is the most common cause of croup.

KEY FACT

Young infants are at risk for apnea as a result of RSV bronchiolitis.

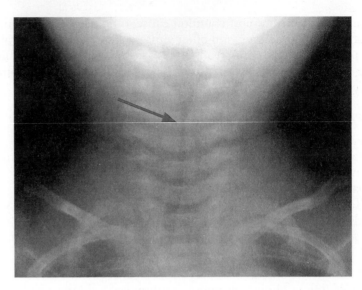

FIGURE 2.13-12. **Croup.** Anteroposterior x-ray of the neck in this 1-year-old child with inspiratory stridor and cough shows the classic "steeple sign" *(arrow)* consistent with the sub-glottic narrowing of laryngotracheobronchitis. (Reproduced with permission from Stone CK, Humphries RL. *Current Diagnosis & Treatment: Emergency Medicine,* 6th ed. New York, NY: McGraw-Hill; 2008.)

- Anteroposterior x-ray of the neck may show the classic "steeple sign" from subglottic narrowing (see Figure 2.13-12), but this finding is neither sensitive nor specific.
- Table 2.13-19 differentiates croup from epiglottitis and tracheitis.

TABLE 2.13-19. **Characteristics of Croup, Epiglottitis, and Tracheitis**

VARIABLE	CROUP	EPIGLOTTITIS	TRACHEITIS
Age group affected	3 months to 3 years	3–7 years	3 months to 2 years
Incidence in children presenting with stridor	88%	8%	2%
Pathogen	Parainfluenza virus	*H influenzae (nontypeable), S pneumoniae*	Often *S aureus;* commonly follows viral URI
Onset	Prodrome (1–7 days)	Rapid (4–12 hours)	Prodrome (3 days) leading to acute decompensation (10 hours)
Fever severity	Low grade	High grade	Intermediate grade
Associated symptoms	Barking cough, inspiratory stridor, hoarseness	Respiratory distress: acute decompensation, toxic appearance, inspiratory stridor, muffled voice, drooling, tripoding	Variable respiratory distress; slower onset than epiglottitis; pseudomembrane
Position preference	None	Seated, neck extended (tripod position)	None
Response to racemic epinephrine	Stridor improves	None	None
Findings on CXR	"Steeple sign" on anteroposterior x-ray	"Thumbprint sign" on lateral film	Subglottic narrowing

TREATMENT

- **Mild cases:** Outpatient management with cool mist therapy and fluids.
- **Moderate cases:** May require supplemental O_2, oral or IM corticosteroids, and nebulized racemic epinephrine.
- **Severe cases** (eg, respiratory distress at rest, inspiratory stridor): Hospitalize and give nebulized racemic epinephrine; consider intubation if there is danger of airway compromise.

EPIGLOTTITIS

A serious and rapidly progressive infection of supraglottic structures (eg, the epiglottis and aryepiglottic folds). Before immunization, *H influenzae* type b was the 1° pathogen. Common causes now include *Streptococcus* species, nontypeable *H influenzae*, and viral agents.

HISTORY/PE

- Presents with acute-onset high fever (39–40°C [102–104°F]), dysphagia, drooling, a muffled voice, inspiratory retractions, cyanosis, and soft stridor.
- Patients sit with the neck hyperextended and the chin protruding ("sniffing dog" position) and lean forward in a "tripod" position to maximize air entry.
- Untreated infection can rapidly lead to life-threatening airway obstruction and respiratory arrest.

DIAGNOSIS

- Diagnosed by clinical impression. The differential diagnosis must include diffuse and localized causes of airway obstruction (see Table 2.13-20).
- The airway must be secured before a definitive diagnosis can be made. In light of potential laryngospasm and airway compromise, do not examine the throat unless an anesthesiologist or otolaryngologist is present.

TABLE 2.13-20.   Retropharyngeal vs Peritonsillar Abscess

VARIABLE	RETROPHARYNGEAL ABSCESS	PERITONSILLAR ABSCESS
Age group affected	From 6 months to 6 years of age	Usually > 10 years of age
History/PE	Acute-onset high fever with sore throat, a muffled "hot potato" voice, trismus, drooling, and cervical lymphadenopathy Usually unilateral; a mass may be seen in the posterior pharyngeal wall on visual inspection	Sore throat, a muffled "hot potato" voice, trismus, drooling, uvula displaced to opposite side
Pathogen	Group A streptococcus (most common), *S aureus, Bacteroides* (often polymicrobial)	Group A streptococcus (most common), *S aureus, S pneumoniae*, anaerobes
Preferred position	Supine with the neck extended (sitting up or flexing the neck worsens symptoms)	None
Diagnosis	On lateral x-ray of the neck, the soft tissue plane should be ≤ 50% of the width of the corresponding vertebral body Contrast CT of the neck helps differentiate abscess from cellulitis	Usually clinical
Treatment	Aspiration or incision and drainage of abscess; antibiotics	Incision and drainage ± tonsillectomy; antibiotics

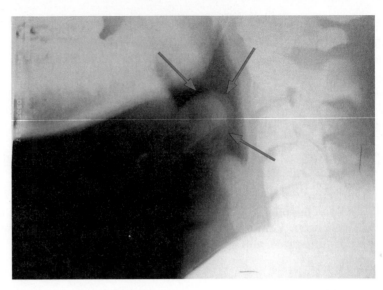

FIGURE 2.13-13. **Epiglottitis.** Lateral x-ray of the neck shows a markedly swollen epiglottis *(arrows)* demonstrating the classic "thumbprint sign," with near-complete airway obstruction. (Reproduced with permission from Stone CK, Humphries RL. *Current Diagnosis & Treatment: Emergency Medicine*, 6th ed. New York, NY: McGraw-Hill; 2008.)

■ Definitive diagnosis is made via direct fiber optic visualization of a cherry-red, swollen epiglottis and arytenoids.
■ Lateral x-ray shows a swollen epiglottis obliterating the valleculae ("thumbprint sign"; see Figure 2.13-13).

TREATMENT

■ This disease is a true emergency, so time should not be wasted on ordering an x-ray.
■ Remember the ABCs; secure the airway first with endotracheal intubation or tracheostomy, and then give IV antibiotics (ceftriaxone or cefuroxime).

KEY FACT

Epiglottitis is a true emergency and can lead to life-threatening airway obstruction.

MENINGITIS

Bacterial meningitis most often occurs in children < 3 years of age; common organisms include *S pneumoniae*, *N meningitidis*, and *E coli*. Enteroviruses are the most common agents of viral meningitis and occur in children of all ages. Risk factors include sinofacial infections, trauma, immunodeficiency, and sepsis.

Most common causes of bacterial meningitis by age are as follows:
■ **Neonates:** Group B streptococci, *E coli*, *Listeria*.
■ **Infants/children:** *S pneumoniae*, *N meningitidis*, *H influenzae*.
■ **Adolescents:** *N meningitidis*, *S pneumoniae*.

HISTORY/PE

■ Bacterial meningitis classically presents with the triad of headache, high fever, and nuchal rigidity.
■ Viral meningitis is typically preceded by a prodromal illness that includes fever, sore throat, and fatigue.
■ Kernig sign (reluctance of knee extension when the hip is flexed) and Brudzinski sign (hips are flexed in response to forced flexion of the neck) are nonspecific signs of meningeal irritation.
■ Additional PE findings may include signs of ↑ intracranial pressure (ICP); (papilledema, cranial nerve palsies) or a petechial rash (*N meningitidis*).

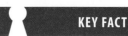

Signs in neonates include lethargy, hyper- or hypothermia, poor tone, a bulging fontanelle, and vomiting.

DIAGNOSIS

- Obtain a head CT to rule out ↑ ICP (risk for brainstem herniation) if the patient is at high risk (ie, exhibits neurologic deficits or has papilledema on funduscopic exam).
- Perform a lumbar puncture (LP); send cell count with differential, glucose and protein levels, Gram stain, and culture.

TREATMENT

- Treat neonates with ampicillin and cefotaxime or gentamicin. Consider acyclovir if there is concern for herpes encephalitis (eg, if the mother had herpes simplex virus [HSV] lesions at the time of the infant's birth or extremely bloody nontraumatic LP).
- Give older children ceftriaxone and vancomycin.

OCULAR INFECTIONS OF THE NEONATE

Infectious conjunctivitis is transmitted as the neonate passes through the birth canal during labor, and the infection often presents during the first weeks of life. The most common causative agents include *Chlamydia trachomatis* and HSV (usually HSV-2). *Neisseria gonorrhoeae* was much more common before the routine use of silver nitrate for prophylaxis; now it only causes < 1% of cases of neonatal conjunctivitis in the United States.

HISTORY/PE

Table 2.13-21 summarizes the clinical presentation of common neonatal ocular infections.

DIAGNOSIS

- Bacterial cultures and Gram stain are the gold standard for suspected gonococcal or chlamydial conjunctivitis.
- HSV polymerase chain reaction is the diagnostic standard for children with corneal ulceration or those with a vesicular eruption anywhere on the body.
- The neonate's mother should undergo cervical Gram stain and culture if a sexually transmitted infection is the suspected cause of conjunctivitis.

TABLE 2.13-21. **Ocular Infections in the Neonatal Period**

CAUSATIVE AGENT	CHARACTERISTICS
Chlamydia trachomatis	Symptoms appear 1–2 weeks after birth Presents with eyelid swelling and relatively scant watery discharge
Neisseria gonorrhoeae	Symptoms appear within 1 week of birth Bilateral purulent conjunctivitis and marked eyelid edema Tends to be more severe than chlamydial conjunctivitis
Herpes simplex virus	Symptoms appear within 2 weeks of birth Presents with conjunctival injection, watery/serosanguineous eye discharge, and vesicular eruptions surrounding the eyes

KEY FACT

Don't be fooled—neonates and young children rarely have meningeal signs on exam!

KEY FACT

Neonates should not be given ceftriaxone in light of the ↑ risk for biliary sludging and kernicterus.

TREATMENT

- Empiric treatment can start before culture results are known.
- For chlamydial conjunctivitis, give topical erythromycin ointment and oral erythromycin; topical antibiotics alone are insufficient, as systemic infection is often present.
- For gonococcal conjunctivitis, give an IV/IM third-generation cephalosporin. Coverage of gonococcus is crucial if the causative agent is unknown, as corneal ulceration (and resultant scarring) can occur within 24–48 hours!
- For HSV conjunctivitis, treat with a 14- to 21-day course of systemic acyclovir, along with a topical agent (such as vidarabine).

PERTUSSIS (WHOOPING COUGH)

A highly infectious form of bronchitis caused by the gram ⊖ bacillus *Bordetella pertussis*. The DTaP vaccine (given in five doses in early childhood) is protective, but immunity wanes by adolescence. Adolescents and young adults serve as the 1° reservoir for pertussis; do not exclude it as a diagnosis in young adults with paroxysms of cough. Transmission is through aerosol droplets and requires airborne precautions with a mask. Pertussis can be life-threatening for young infants but is generally a milder infection in older children and adults.

HISTORY/PE

- Has the following three stages:
  - Catarrhal (mild URI symptoms; lasts 1–2 weeks).
  - Paroxysmal (paroxysms of cough with inspiratory whoop and posttussive emesis; lasts 2–3 months).
  - Convalescent (symptoms wane).
- Patients most often present in the paroxysmal stage but are most contagious in the catarrhal stage.

DIAGNOSIS

- Labs show an elevated WBC count with lymphocytosis (often ≥ 70%).
- **Most accurate test:** Nasopharyngeal culture or PCR.

TREATMENT

- Hospitalize infants < 6 months of age.
- Give azithromycin for 10 days to patients. Exposed newborns are at high risk irrespective of their immunization status because they may not be entirely protected by maternal transplacental immunoglobulins.
- Close contacts (including daycare contacts) should receive prophylactic antibiotics (azithromycin for 5 days).

VIRAL EXANTHEMS

Table 2.13-22 outlines the clinical presentation of common viral exanthems.

TORCHES INFECTIONS

Microbes that can be transmitted vertically (ie, from mother to fetus). Usually transplacental, but can occur perinatally (eg, HSV-2). May cause nonspecific signs such as growth retardation, hepatosplenomegaly, jaundice, and thrombocytopenia.

Table 2.13-23 outlines the common ToRCHeS infections.

KEY FACT

Classic presentation of pertussis is an infant < 6 months of age with paroxysmal coughing, posttussive emesis, and apnea. The typical "whooping" cough is usually absent at this age.

TABLE 2.13-22.   Viral Exanthems

Disease	Cause	Symptoms	Complications
Erythema infectiosum (fifth disease)	Parvovirus B19	Prodrome: None; fever is often absent or low grade Rash: "Slapped-cheek," pruritic, maculopapular, erythematous rash (see Image A) Rash starts on the arms and spreads to the trunk and legs Worsens with fever and sun exposure	Arthropathy in children and adults Congenital infection is associated with fetal hydrops and death Aplastic crisis may be precipitated in children with ↑ RBC turnover (eg, sickle cell anemia, hereditary spherocytosis) or in those with ↓ RBC production (eg, severe iron deficiency anemia)
Measles	Paramyxovirus	Prodrome: Fever (can be as high as 40°C (104°F) with **C**ough, **C**oryza, and **C**onjunctivitis (the **"3 C's"**); Koplik spots (small irregular red spots with central gray specks) appear on the buccal mucosa after 1–2 days Rash: An erythematous maculopapular rash spreads from head to toe (see Image B) Treatment with vitamin A may improve symptoms	Common: Otitis media, pneumonia, laryngotracheitis Rare: Subacute sclerosing panencephalitis Airborne infectious precautions needed because of high level of contagiousness
Rubella ("3-day measles")	Rubella virus	Prodrome: Asymptomatic or tender, generalized lymphadenopathy (clue: posterior auricular lymphadenopathy) Rash: Presents with an erythematous, tender maculopapular rash that also spreads from head to toe (see Image C) In contrast to measles, children with rubella often have only a low-grade fever and do not appear as ill Polyarthritis may be seen in adolescents	Encephalitis, thrombocytopenia (a rare complication of postnatal infection) Congenital infection is associated with congenital anomalies (PDA, deafness, cataracts, intellectual disabilities)
Roseola infantum	HHV-6 and -7	Prodrome: Acute onset of high fever (> 40°C [> 104°F]); no other symptoms for 3–4 days Rash: A maculopapular rash appears as fever breaks (begins on the trunk and quickly spreads to the face and extremities) and often lasts < 24 hours	Febrile seizures may result from rapid fever onset
Varicella (chickenpox)	Varicella-zoster virus (VZV)	Prodrome: Mild fever, anorexia, and malaise precede the rash by 24 hours Rash: Generalized, pruritic, "teardrop" vesicles on red base; lesions are often at different stages of healing (see image D). Rash usually appears on the face and spreads to the rest of the body, sparing the palms and soles Infectious from 24 hours before eruption until lesions crust over	Progressive varicella with meningoencephalitis, pneumonia, and hepatitis in the immunocompromised Skin lesions may develop 2° bacterial infections Reye syndrome (associated with ASA use) Varicella may be prevented with vaccine or with post-exposure prophylaxis for nonimmunized patients > 1 year of age (immunoglobulin for immunocompromised, and vaccine for immunocompetent)

(continues)

TABLE 2.13-22. **Viral Exanthems** *(continued)*

DISEASE	CAUSE	SYMPTOMS	COMPLICATIONS
Varicella zoster	VZV	Prodrome: Reactivation of varicella infection; starts as pain along an affected sensory nerve Rash: Pruritic "teardrop" vesicular rash in a dermatomal distribution Rash uncommon unless the patient is immunocompromised	Encephalopathy, aseptic meningitis, pneumonitis, TTP, Guillain-Barré syndrome, cellulitis, arthritis
Hand-foot-and-mouth disease	Coxsackie A	Prodrome: Fever, anorexia, oral and throat pain Rash: Oral ulcers; maculopapular vesicular rash on the hands and feet and sometimes on the buttocks	Aseptic meningitis, encephalitis, pneumonia, myopericarditis

A   B   C   D

Image A reproduced with permission from Wolff K, Johnson RA. *Fitzpatrick's Color Atlas & Synopsis of Clinical Dermatology,* 6th ed. New York: McGraw-Hill; 2009. Image B reproduced with permission from Wolff K, et al. *Fitzpatrick's Dermatology in General Medicine,* 7th ed. New York: McGraw-Hill; 2008. Image C reproduced courtesy of the US Department of Health and Human Services. Image D modified courtesy of www. badobadop.co.uk.

TABLE 2.13-23. **Common ToRCHeS Infections**

AGENT	MODE OF TRANSMISSION	MATERNAL MANIFESTATIONS	NEONATAL MANIFESTATIONS
Toxoplasma gondii	Cat feces or ingestion of undercooked meat	Usually asymptomatic; lymphadenopathy (rarely)	Classic triad: chorioretinitis, hydrocephalus, and intracranial calcifications, ± "blueberry muffin" rash
Rubella	Respiratory droplets	Rash, lymphadenopathy, arthritis	Classic triad: PDA (or pulmonary artery hypoplasia), cataracts, and deafness, ± "blueberry muffin" rash
CMV	Sexual contact, organ transplants	Usually asymptomatic; mononucleosis-like illness	Hearing loss, seizures, petechial rash, "blueberry muffin" rash, periventricular calcifications
HIV	Sexual contact, needlestick	Variable presentation depending on CD4+ count	Recurrent infections, chronic diarrhea
Herpes simplex virus-2	Skin or mucous membrane contact	Usually asymptomatic; herpetic (vesicular) lesions	Encephalitis, herpetic (vesicular) lesions
Syphilis	Sexual contact	Chancre (1°) and disseminated rash (2°) are the two stages likely to result in fetal infection	Often results in stillbirth, hydrops fetalis; if child survives, presents with cutaneous lesions on the hands/foot, hepatosplenomegaly, jaundice, anemia, and rhinorrhea ("snuffles")

Modified with permission from Le T, et al. *First Aid for the USMLE Step 1 2018.* New York, NY: McGraw-Hill; 2018.

PINWORM INFECTION

Caused by *Enterobius vermicularis*. Pinworm is a parasitic infection that causes perianal pruritus, which is more pronounced at night. Diagnosis is made with the tape test (clear tape is pressed to the anal region in the morning and observed under the microscope for pinworm eggs). Treat patient and all household contacts with albendazole or pyrantel pamoate.

Pediatric Neurologic Disease

CEREBRAL PALSY

A range of nonhereditary, nonprogressive disorders of movement and posture; the most common movement disorder in children. Often results from prenatal neurologic insult, but in most cases the cause is unknown. Risk factors of cerebral palsy (CP) include low birth weight, intrauterine exposure to maternal infection, prematurity, perinatal asphyxia, trauma, brain malformation, and neonatal cerebral hemorrhage. Categories include the following:

- **Pyramidal (spastic):** Spastic paresis of any or all limbs. Accounts for 75% of cases. Intellectual disabilities are also present in up to 90% of cases.
- **Extrapyramidal (dyskinetic):** A result of damage to extrapyramidal tracts. Subtypes are ataxic (difficulty coordinating purposeful movements), choreoathetoid, and dystonic (uncontrollable jerking, writhing, or posturing). Abnormal movements worsen with stress and disappear during sleep.

HISTORY/PE

- May be associated with seizure disorders, behavioral disorders, hearing or vision impairment, learning disabilities, and speech deficits.
- Affected limbs may show hyperreflexia, pathologic reflexes (eg, Babinski), ↑ tone/contractures, weakness, and/or underdevelopment. Definite hand preference before 1 year of age is a red flag.
- Toe walking and scissor gait are common. Hip dislocations and scoliosis may be seen.

DIAGNOSIS

Diagnosed by clinical impression, although imaging can be used to determine the underlying cause of CP in some cases. For instance, ultrasonography may be useful in infants to identify intracranial hemorrhage or structural malformations, and MRI is diagnostic in older children. EEG may be useful in patients with suspected seizures.

TREATMENT

- There is no cure for cerebral palsy. Special education, physical therapy, braces, and surgical release of contractures may help.
- Treat spasticity with diazepam, dantrolene, or baclofen. Baclofen pumps and posterior rhizotomy may alleviate severe contractures.

KEY FACT

The most common presenting symptom of cerebral palsy is delayed motor development.

FEBRILE SEIZURES

Usually occur in children between 6 months and 5 years of age who have no evidence of intracranial infection or other causes. Risk factors include a rapid ↑ in temperature and a history of febrile seizures in a close relative. Febrile seizures recur in approximately one in three patients.

HISTORY/PE

- Seizures usually occur during the onset of fever and may be the first sign of an underlying illness (eg, otitis media, roseola).
- **Classified as simple or complex:**
  - **Simple:** A short-duration (< 15-minute), generalized tonic-clonic seizure with one seizure in a 24-hour period, and returning to neurologic baseline shortly after. A high fever (> 39°C [> 102.2°F]) and fever onset within hours of the seizure are typical.
  - **Complex:** A long-duration (> 15-minute) or focal seizure or multiple seizures in a 24-hour period or not returning to neurologic baseline. A low-grade fever for several days before seizure onset may be present.

DIAGNOSIS

- Focus on finding a source of infection. LP is indicated if there are clinical signs of CNS infection (eg, altered consciousness, meningismus, a tense/bulging anterior fontanelle) after ruling out ↑ ICP.
- No work-up is necessary for first-time simple febrile seizures, and no lab studies are needed if presentation is consistent with febrile seizures in children > 18 months of age. Infants < 6 months of age need a sepsis work-up (CBC; UA; and blood, urine, and cerebrospinal fluid [CSF] culture).
- For atypical presentations, obtain electrolytes, serum glucose, blood cultures, UA, and CBC with differential.

TREATMENT

- Use antipyretic therapy (acetaminophen; avoid ASA in light of the risk for Reye syndrome, acute liver failure, and encephalopathy), and treat any underlying illness. Note that antipyretic therapy does not ↓ the recurrence of febrile seizures.
- For complex seizures, perform a thorough neurologic evaluation, including EEG and MRI. Chronic anticonvulsant therapy (eg, diazepam or phenobarbital) may be necessary.

COMPLICATIONS

- The risk for recurrence is < 30% and is highest within 1 year of the initial episode. For simple febrile seizures, there is no ↑ risk for developmental abnormalities and only slightly higher risk for developing epilepsy.
- Risk factors for the development of epilepsy include complex febrile seizures (~ 10% risk), ⊕ family history of epilepsy, an abnormal neurologic exam, and developmental delay.

KEY FACT

Perform an LP if CNS infection is suspected in a patient with a febrile seizure.

KEY FACT

Simple febrile seizures do not cause brain damage, do not ↑ risk for developmental abnormalities, usually do not recur, and only slightly ↑ the risk for developing epilepsy.

INFANTILE HYPOTONIA

The lack of tone or resistance of muscle movement. It differs from weakness, which is the decrease in active muscle contraction. Common causes of infantile hypotonia are listed in Table 2.13-24.

Pediatric Oncology

LEUKEMIA

A hematopoietic malignancy of lymphocytic or myeloblastic origin. The most common childhood malignancy; 97% of cases are acute leukemias (acute lymphocytic leukemia [ALL] > acute myeloid leukemia [AML]). ALL is most

TABLE 2.13-24.   Common Causes of Infantile Hypotonia

DISORDER	ETIOLOGY	PRESENTATION	TREATMENT
Botulism	Caused by *Clostridium botulinum* toxin Toxin prevents presynaptic release of acetylcholine (ACh) Spores are found in honey or soil	Constipation can be the first presenting sign Symmetric, descending paralysis	Supportive care Botulism immunoglobulin
Spinal muscular atrophy	Mutation in *SMN1* gene Infantile type (type 1; also known as Werdnig-Hoffman disease) Leads to anterior horn cell and motor nuclei degeneration	Progressive muscle weakness and atrophy Presents with tongue fasciculation and symmetric proximal muscle weakness, greater in the lower than upper extremities	Supportive care No cure
Myotonic dystrophy (type 1)	Trinucleotide repeat disorder (CTG) on *DMPK* gene Autosomal dominant disorder that is commonly inherited through the mother	Increasing loss of muscle tone and weakness especially in the facial muscles Can present in infancy as hypotonia Most common onset in the 20s–30s Associated with mental retardation, cataracts, and arrhythmias	Supportive care

common in white boys between 2 and 5 years of age; while AML is seen most frequently in African-American boys throughout childhood. Associated with trisomy 21, Fanconi anemia, prior radiation, severe combined immunodeficiency, and congenital bone marrow failure states.

HISTORY/PE

- Symptoms are abrupt in onset. They are initially nonspecific (anorexia, fatigue) and are followed by bone pain with limp or refusal to bear weight, fever (from neutropenia), anemia, ecchymoses, petechiae, and/or hepatosplenomegaly.
- CNS metastases may be associated with headache, vomiting, and papilledema.
- AML can present with a chloroma, a greenish soft-tissue tumor of leukemic cells on the skin or spinal cord.

DIAGNOSIS

- CBC, coagulation studies, and peripheral blood smear, which shows high numbers of blasts (lymphoblasts are found in 90% of cases). WBC counts can be low, normal, or high.
- A bone marrow aspirate and biopsy for immunophenotyping (TdT assay and a panel of monoclonal antibodies to T- and B-cell antigens) and genetic analysis are necessary to confirm the diagnosis. The diagnosis is made if bone marrow is hypercellular with ↑ lymphoblasts.
- CXR to rule out a mediastinal mass.

TREATMENT

- Chemotherapy based, including induction, consolidation, and maintenance phases.
- Tumor lysis syndrome is common during the initiation of treatment of cancers with high cell turnover (such as leukemias and lymphomas).
  - Caused by the lysis of many neoplastic cells in a short period, resulting in the release of cell contents into the bloodstream.

KEY FACT

ALL is the most common childhood malignancy, followed by CNS tumors and lymphomas.

MNEMONIC

Electrolytes affected by Tumor Lysis Syndrome—

PUKE Calcium

Phosphorus
Uric acid
K (potassium)
Elevated
Calcium (decreased)

- Characterized by hyperkalemia, hyperphosphatemia, hyperuricemia, and hypocalcemia (as calcium is bound by phosphate released from the neoplastic cells). It can result in renal failure, arrhythmias, and death.
- Treat with fluids, diuretics, and allopurinol (which reduces the risk for urate-induced nephropathy). Corticosteroids may precipitate tumor lysis syndrome.

NEUROBLASTOMA

An embryonal tumor of neural crest origin. More than one-half of patients are < 2 years of age, and 70% have distant metastases at presentation. Associated with neurofibromatosis, Hirschsprung disease, and the N-*myc* oncogene.

HISTORY/PE

- Lesion sites are most commonly abdominal, thoracic, and cervical (in descending order).
- Symptoms may vary with location and may include a nontender abdominal mass (may cross the midline), Horner syndrome, hypertension, or cord compression (from a paraspinal tumor).
- Patients may have anemia, FTT, and fever.
- > 50% of patients will have metastases at diagnosis. Signs include bone marrow suppression, proptosis, hepatomegaly, subcutaneous nodules (see Figure 2.13-14), and opsoclonus/myoclonus.

DIAGNOSIS

- Fine-needle aspiration of tumor. Histologically appears as small, round, blue tumor cells with a characteristic rosette pattern.
- Elevated 24-hour urinary catecholamines (vanillylmandelic acid and homovanillic acid).
- CT scan, bone scan, and bone marrow aspirate for staging.

TREATMENT

Local excision plus postsurgical chemotherapy and/or radiation.

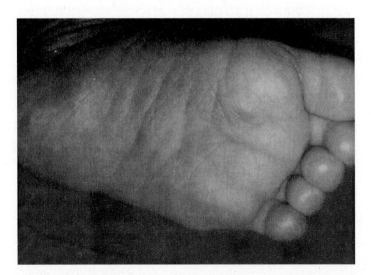

FIGURE 2.13-14. **Neuroblastoma presenting with multiple subcutaneous nodules.**
(Reproduced with permission from the Armed Forces Institute of Pathology, *Atlas of Tumor Pathology*.)

WILMS TUMOR

A renal tumor of embryonal origin that is most commonly seen in children 2–5 years of age. Associated with Beckwith-Wiedemann syndrome (hemihypertrophy, macroglossia, visceromegaly), neurofibromatosis, and **WAGR syndrome** (**W**ilms tumor, **A**niridia, **G**enitourinary abnormalities, mental **R**etardation [now called "intellectual disabilities"]).

HISTORY/PE

- Presents as an asymptomatic, nontender, smooth abdominal mass that does not usually cross the midline.
- Abdominal pain, fever, hypertension, and microscopic or gross hematuria may be seen.

DIAGNOSIS

- **Most accurate test:** Biopsy or fine-needle aspiration is required for definitive diagnosis.
- Abdominal ultrasonography.
- CT scans of the chest and abdomen are used to detect metastases.

TREATMENT

Local resection and nephrectomy with postsurgical chemotherapy and radiation depending on stage and histology.

CHILDHOOD BONE TUMORS

It is critical to distinguish between Ewing sarcoma and osteosarcoma (see Table 2.13-25).

Langerhans histiocytosis is a rare pediatric malignancy presenting with solitary, painful lytic bone lesions surrounded by edema with hypercalcemia. "Tennis racket" granules may be seen on pathology.

Pediatric Musculoskeletal Disorders

COMMON PEDIATRIC ORTHOPEDIC INJURIES

Table 2.13-26 outlines the presentation and treatment of common pediatric orthopedic injuries.

DUCHENNE MUSCULAR DYSTROPHY

An X-linked recessive disorder resulting from a deficiency of dystrophin, a cytoskeletal protein. Onset is usually at 3–5 years of age. Female carriers can be symptomatic depending on severity of disease.

HISTORY/PE

- Affects axial and proximal muscles more than distal muscles.
- May present with progressive clumsiness, fatigability, difficulty standing or walking, difficulty walking on toes (gastrocnemius shortening), Gowers maneuver (using the hands to push off the thighs when rising from the floor), and waddling gait.

Q

A 2-year-old girl is brought to the pediatrician by her mother for increasing irritability and a 4-pound weight loss in the last month. PE is notable for an ill-appearing child with a well-defined, nodular mass in the left flank that crosses the midline. What is the most likely diagnosis?

TABLE 2.13-25. Ewing Sarcoma vs Osteosarcoma

VARIABLE	OSTEOSARCOMA	EWING SARCOMA	
Origin	Osteoblasts (mesenchyme)	Sarcoma (neuroecto-derm); associated with chromosome 11:22 translocation	
Epidemiology	Commonly seen in male adolescents	Commonly seen in white male adolescents	
History/PE	Local pain and swelling Systemic symptoms are rare	Local pain and swelling Systemic symptoms (fever, anorexia, fatigue) are common	**A**
Location	Metaphyses of long bones (distal femur, proximal tibia, prox-imal humerus) Metastases to lungs in 20%	Midshaft of long bones (femur, pelvis, fibula, humerus)	
Diagnosis	↑ Alkaline phosphatase "Sunburst" lytic bone lesions (see Image A) CT of the chest to rule out pulmonary metastases	Leukocytosis, ↑ ESR Lytic bone lesion with "onion skin" peri-osteal reaction on x-ray (see Image B)	
Treatment	Local excision, chemotherapy	Local excision, che-motherapy, and radiation	**B**

Images reproduced with permission from Kantarjian HM, et al. *MD Anderson Manual of Medical Oncology.* New York, NY: McGraw-Hill; 2006.

- Pseudohypertrophy of the gastrocnemius muscles is also seen.
- Intellectual disabilities are common.

Table 2.13-27 outlines the differential diagnosis of DMD and Becker muscular dystrophy.

DIAGNOSIS

- Elevated CK levels suggests DMD.
- Confirmation is made with genetic testing.
- Optional muscle biopsy shows necrotic muscle fibers with absence of dystrophin protein.
- ⊖ Dystrophin immunostain; ↑ CK.
- EMG shows polyphasic potentials and ↑ recruitment.

A

This patient most likely has neuroblastoma arising from the left adrenal gland. It is the most common solid tumor of childhood and is derived from neural crest cells. Unlike Wilms tumor (nephroblastoma), neuroblastoma is accompanied by systemic symptoms and often crosses the midline. The majority of children have metastases at the time of diagnosis.

TABLE 2.13-26. Orthopedic Injuries in Children

INJURY	MECHANICS	TREATMENT
Clavicular fracture	The most commonly fractured long bone in children. May be birth related (especially in large infants); can be associated with brachial plexus palsies and subclavian artery injury (angiography should be done to rule out injury) Usually involves the middle third of the clavicle, with the proximal fracture end displaced superiorly as a result of the pull of the sternocleidomastoid	Sling
Greenstick fracture	Incomplete fracture involving the cortex of only one side (tension/trauma side) of the bone	Reduction with casting Order x-rays at 10–14 days
Nursemaid's elbow	Radial head subluxation secondary to being pulled or lifted by the hand Pain, pronation, and refusal to bend the elbow	Manual reduction by gentle forearm hyperpronation. Alternatively, supination of the forearm at 90 degrees of flexion No immobilization
Torus fracture	Buckling of the compression side of the cortex 2° to trauma Usually occurs in the distal radius or ulna from a fall	Cast immobilization for 3–5 weeks
Supracondylar humerus fracture	The most common pediatric elbow fracture Tends to occur at 5–8 years of age Proximity to the brachial artery ↑ the risk for Volkmann contracture (results from compartment syndrome of the forearm) Beware of brachial artery entrapment (check radial pulse) 	Cast immobilization; closed reduction with percutaneous pinning if significantly displaced
Osgood-Schlatter disease	Overuse apophysitis of the tibial tubercle. Causes localized pain, especially with quadriceps contraction, in active young boys	↓ Activity for 2–3 months or until asymptomatic Neoprene brace for symptomatic relief
Salter-Harris fracture	Fractures of the growth plate in children. Classified by fracture pattern: I: Physis (growth plate) II: Metaphysis and physis III: Epiphysis and physis IV: Epiphysis, metaphysis, and physis V: Crush injury of the physis	Closed vs open reduction to obtain appropriate alignment, followed by immobilization

Image reproduced with permission from USMLE-Rx.com.

TABLE 2.13-27. DMD vs Becker Muscular Dystrophy

CHARACTERISTIC	DMD	BECKER MUSCULAR DYSTROPHY
Onset	3–5 years	5–15 years and beyond
Life expectancy	Teens	30s–40s
Intellectual disabilities	Common	Uncommon
Western blot	Dystrophin is markedly ↓ or absent	Dystrophin levels are normal, but protein is abnormal

TREATMENT

Physical therapy is necessary to maintain ambulation and to prevent contractures. Liberal use of tendon release surgery may prolong ambulation.

COMPLICATIONS

Mortality is caused by high-output cardiac failure (stemming from cardiac fibrosis).

MYOTONIC MUSCULAR DYSTROPHY

Autosomal dominant disorder causing impaired muscle relaxation (look for "abnormally-long handshake" on USMLE). Other symptoms include dysphagia, balding, testicular atrophy, and cardiac conduction abnormalities. Type 1 is caused by trinucleotide repeat disorder (CTG) on the *DMPK* gene.

SPONDYLOLISTHESIS

Developmental disorder caused by forward slipping of vertebrae (L5 over S1) that causes bowel and bladder symptoms, lower back pain, and a palpable "step-off" on PE.

METATARSUS ADDUCTUS

Congenital deformity of the lower extremity, where the forefoot is turned inward. If the foot is flexible, no treatment is indicated and the condition may be observed for spontaneous resolution.

CLUBFOOT (TALIPES EQUINOVARUS)

Congenital deformity of the lower extremity presenting with forefoot adduction and varus of calcaneum, talus, and midfoot. In contrast to metatarsus adductus, the foot is not flexible and requires immediate treatment with serial casting. Surgery is performed within 3–6 months if it does not resolve.

DEVELOPMENTAL DYSPLASIA OF THE HIP

Also called congenital hip dislocation. Excessive hip flexion in utero (eg, breach presentation) leads to excessive stretching of the posterior hip capsule causing lax musculature and contractures. Can result in subluxation or dislocation of femoral heads, leading to early degenerative joint disease.

HISTORY/PE

- Most commonly found in firstborn girls born in the breech position. ↑ Risk with family history.
- **Barlow maneuver:** Posterior pressure is placed on inner aspect of the abducted thigh, and then the hip is adducted, leading to an audible "clunk" as the femoral head dislocates posteriorly.
- **Ortolani maneuver:** Thighs are gently abducted from the midline with anterior pressure on the greater trochanter. A soft click signifies a reduction of the femoral head into the acetabulum.
- **Allis (Galeazzi) sign:** The knees are at unequal heights when the hips and knees are flexed (the dislocated side is lower).
- Asymmetric inguinal skin folds that extend beyond the anus and limited abduction of the affected hip are also seen.

DIAGNOSIS

- Early detection with PE is critical to allow for proper hip development.
- Perform ultrasonography before 6 months of age given lack of ossification of the femoral head.
- X-rays are appropriate at > 4–6 months of age.

TREATMENT

- Begin treatment early. May self-resolve before 2 weeks of age.
- **< 6 months:** Splint with a Pavlik harness (maintains the hip flexed and abducted). To prevent avascular necrosis (AVN), do not flex the hips > 60 degrees.
- **6–15 months:** Spica cast.
- **15–24 months:** Open reduction followed by spica cast.

COMPLICATIONS

- Joint contractures and AVN of the femoral head.
- Without treatment, a significant defect is likely in patients < 2 years of age.

LEGG-CALVÉ-PERTHES DISEASE

Idiopathic AVN and osteonecrosis of the femoral head (see Figure 2.13-15). Most common in boys 4–10 years of age. Can be a self-limited disease in younger patients, with symptoms lasting < 18 months.

HISTORY/PE

- Generally asymptomatic at first, but patients can develop a painless limp, antalgic gait, and thigh muscle atrophy.
- If pain is present, it can be in the groin or anterior thigh, or it may be referred to the knee.
- Limited abduction and internal rotation; atrophy of the affected leg.
- Usually unilateral (85–90%).

DIAGNOSIS

Initial x-rays can be normal but later can show a flattened and fragmented femoral head.

TREATMENT

- Observation is sufficient if limited femoral head involvement or if full ROM is present.

KEY FACT

Legg-Calvé-Perthes disease typically presents as painLESS, while SCFE can be painFULL.

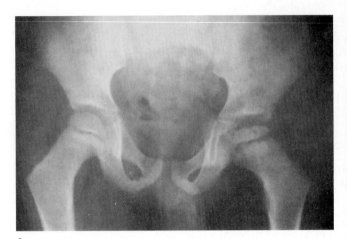
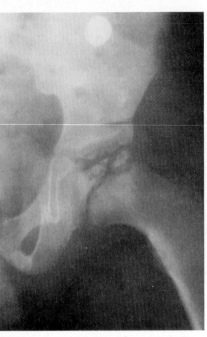

A   **B**

FIGURE 2.13-15. **Legg-Calvé-Perthes disease.** Avascular necrosis of the femoral head. (Reproduced with permission from Skinner HB. *Current Diagnosis & Treatment in Orthopedics,* 2nd ed. Stamford, CT: Appleton & Lange; 2000.)

MNEMONIC

Differential diagnosis of pediatric limp—

STARTSS HOTT

Septic joint
Tumor
Avascular necrosis (Legg-Calvé-Perthes)
Rheumatoid arthritis/JIA
Tuberculosis
Sickle cell disease
SCFE
Henoch-Schönlein purpura
Osteomyelitis
Trauma
Toxic synovitis

- If extensive or ↓ ROM, consider bracing, hip abduction with a Petrie cast, or an osteotomy.
- The prognosis is favorable if the patient is < 6 years of age and has full ROM, ↓ femoral head involvement, and a stable joint.

SLIPPED CAPITAL FEMORAL EPIPHYSIS

Displacement of the femoral epiphysis from the femoral neck, through the growth plate. The name slipped capital femoral epiphysis (SCFE) is misleading because the epiphysis remains within the acetabulum while the metaphysis moves anteriorly and superiorly. Presents in obese children 10–16 years of age. Associated with hypothyroidism and other endocrinopathies.

HISTORY/PE

- Insidious onset of dull hip pain, or referred knee pain, and a painful limp.
- Restricted ROM and inability to bear weight (differentiates unstable from stable SCFE).
- Bilateral in 40–50% of cases.
- Limited internal rotation and abduction of the hip. Patients hold hip in passive external rotation.

DIAGNOSIS

- X-rays of both hips in anteroposterior and frog-leg lateral views reveal posterior and inferior displacement of the femoral head (see Figure 2.13-16).
- In patients under the 10th percentile of height, rule out hypothyroidism with TSH.

TREATMENT

- The disease is progressive, so treatment should begin promptly.
- Immediate surgical screw fixation to reduce risk for AVN.
- No weight bearing should be allowed until the defect is surgically stabilized.

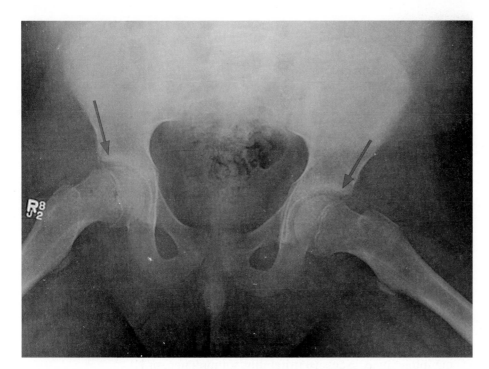

FIGURE 2.13-16. **Slipped capital femoral epiphysis.** Frog-leg anteroposterior x-ray demonstrates medial and inferior displacement of the right femoral epiphysis *(red arrow)* relative to the femoral neck. In comparison, the left side *(blue arrow)* is normal. (Reproduced with permission from USMLE-Rx.com.)

COMPLICATIONS

Chondrolysis, AVN of the femoral head, and premature hip osteoarthritis requiring arthroplasty.

SCOLIOSIS

A lateral curvature of the spine > 10 degrees. It is sometimes associated with kyphosis or lordosis. Most commonly idiopathic, developing in early adolescence. Other etiologies are congenital or associated with neuromuscular, vertebral, or spinal cord disease. The male-to-female ratio is 1:7 for curves that progress and require treatment.

HISTORY/PE

- Idiopathic disease is usually identified during school physical screening.
- Vertebral and rib rotation deformities are accentuated by the Adams forward bending test.

DIAGNOSIS

X-rays of the spine (posterior, anterior, and full-length views).

TREATMENT

- Close observation for < 20 degrees of curvature.
- Spinal bracing for 20–49 degrees of curvature in patients with remaining growth. Curvature may progress even with bracing.
- Surgical correction for > 50 degrees of curvature.

COMPLICATIONS

Severe scoliosis can create restrictive lung disease.

KEY FACT

Suspect sexual abuse if there is genital trauma, bleeding, or discharge. In girls, consider vaginal foreign body as an alternative diagnosis, especially in the setting of a foul-smelling vaginal discharge, bleeding, and pain. Also consider if children have an excessive preoccupation/knowledge of adult sexual behaviors.

KEY FACT

Osteogenesis imperfecta (OI) is a great mimicker of child abuse and is often tested on the USMLE. It is a genetic disease that affects type I collagen. Those with OI can present with a broad spectrum of clinical features. The most classically described form of OI presents with blue sclera, easy bruising, opalescent teeth, conductive hearing loss, skeletal anomalies, and easily fractured bones.

Child Abuse

Also known as non-accidental trauma (NAT); includes neglect and physical, sexual, and psychological maltreatment of children. Suspect abuse if the history is discordant with physical findings or if there is a delay in obtaining appropriate medical care. Certain injuries in children, such as retinal hemorrhages and specific fracture types, are highly suspicious for abuse.

HISTORY/PE

- Suspect abuse if the story is not consistent with the injury pattern or with the child's developmental age. For example, take note if the parents claim that their 2-month-old child "rolled off the couch" (2-month-olds cannot roll yet). Also suspect abuse if the story continually changes or is very vague.
- Look for bruising on fleshy areas, patterns of bruises (indicative of the object used), bruises of different ages and color, and burns that are well circumscribed.
- **Risk factors:** Look for parents with a history of alcoholism or drug use, children with complex medical problems, infants with colic (excessive crying for > 3 hours per day for > 3 days per week), and repeated hospitalizations.
- **Infants:** Abuse or neglect in infants may present as apnea, seizures, feeding intolerance, excessive irritability, somnolence, or FTT.
- **Older children:** Neglect in older children may present as poor hygiene or behavioral abnormalities.

See Table 2.13-28 for exam findings.

DIAGNOSIS

- An x-ray skeletal survey and bone scan can show fractures in various stages of healing. X-rays may not show fractures until 1–2 weeks after injury

TABLE 2.13-28.   **Common Presentations and Mimics of Child Abuse**

TYPE OF ABUSE	PRESENTATION/IMAGING FINDINGS	MIMICS	
Bruises	Most common physical finding Often located on head and torso May be in pattern reflecting implement (hand, belt)	Mongolian spots (see Image A) Coining/cupping (alternative treatments in certain cultures) Bleeding diathesis	
Burns	Contact burns: cigarette/curling iron Immersion burns: hot water, appear on buttocks, sparing of flexor surfaces, or stocking-glove distribution	Scalded skin syndrome, severe contact dermatitis	
Fractures	Spiral fractures: humerus/femur. Epiphyseal-metaphyseal "bucket" fractures Posterior rib fractures: indicate squeezing	Osteogenesis imperfecta (blue sclerae, hearing loss, opalescent teeth)	
Abusive head trauma	Lethargy, feeding difficulty, apnea, seizures, retinal hemorrhage, subdural/epidural hematoma	Accidental head trauma	A

Image reproduced with permission from Wolff K, et al. *Fitzpatrick's Dermatology in General Medicine,* 7th ed. New York, NY: McGraw-Hill; 2008.

(although they may show evidence of prior trauma in children < 3 years of age); by contrast, bone scans may show fractures within 48 hours.

- If sexual abuse is suspected, test for gonorrhea, syphilis, chlamydia, HIV, and sperm (within 72 hours of assault).
- Rule out abusive head trauma (formerly referred to as shaken baby syndrome) by performing an ophthalmologic exam for retinal hemorrhage and a noncontrast CT for subdural hematoma. Infants with abusive head trauma often do not exhibit external signs of abuse.
- Consider an MRI to visualize white-matter changes associated with violent shaking and the extent of intra- and extracranial bleeds.

TREATMENT

- Document injuries, including location, size, shape, color, and the nature of all lesions, bruises, or burns.
- Notify Child Protective Services for possible removal of the child from the home.
- Hospitalize if necessary to stabilize injuries or to protect the child.
- Antibiotics and high-dose oral contraceptives for those with sexual abuse.

Well-Child Care

ANTICIPATORY GUIDANCE

An important aspect of every well-child visit. Commonly tested advice includes the following:

- Keep the water heater at < 48.8°C (< 120°F).
- Babies should sleep on their backs without any stuffed animals or other toys in the crib (to ↓ the risk for SIDS).
- Car safety seats should be rear facing and should be placed in the back of the car (seats can face forward if the child is > 2 years of age and weighs > 40 pounds).
- No solid foods should be given before 6 months of age; they should then be introduced gradually and one at a time. Do not give cow's milk before 12 months of age.
- Syrup of ipecac (an emetic) is no longer routinely recommended for accidental poisoning. Poison control should be contacted immediately for assistance.

HEARING AND VISION SCREENING

- Objective hearing screening (otoacoustic emissions and/or auditory brainstem response) for newborns before discharge is standard of care.
- Objective hearing screening is indicated for children with a history of meningitis, ToRCHeS infections, measles and mumps, and recurrent otitis media. The most common cause of childhood conductive hearing loss is repeated ear infections.
- The red reflex should be checked at birth. Leukocoria is the lack of a red reflex and can indicate the presence of retinoblastoma. Can also be an incidental finding in a baby's first photos.
- Strabismus (ocular misalignment) is normal until 3 months of age; beyond 3 months of age, children should be evaluated by a pediatric ophthalmologist and may require corrective lenses, occlusion, and/or surgery to prevent amblyopia (suppression of retinal images in a misaligned eye, leading to permanent vision loss). Treatment of strabismus includes occluding the normal eye with an eye patch.

CHILDHOOD VACCINATIONS

The Epidemiology chapter summarizes CDC-recommended vaccinations for the pediatric population. Contraindications and precautions in this population are as follows:

- **Contraindications:**
    - Severe allergy to a vaccine component or a prior dose of vaccine. Patients who have life-threatening allergies to eggs may receive MMR and influenza vaccinations under observation. Exercise caution in administering yellow fever vaccinations to those with egg allergies.
    - Encephalopathy within 7 days of prior pertussis vaccination.
    - Personal history of intussusception is a contraindication for the rotavirus vaccine.
    - Avoid live vaccines (rotavirus, oral polio vaccine, varicella, MMR, intranasal influenza, yellow fever) in immunocompromised and pregnant patients (exception: HIV patients may receive MMR and varicella).
    - Weight < 2 kg for hepatitis B vaccine in newborns.
- **Precautions:**
    - Current moderate to severe illness (with or without fever).
    - Prior reactions to pertussis vaccine (fever > 40.5°C [> 104.9°F]), a shocklike state, persistent crying for > 3 hours within 48 hours of vaccination, or seizure within 3 days of vaccination.
    - History of receiving IVIG in the past year.
- **The following are not contraindications to vaccination:**
    - Mild illness and/or low-grade fever.
    - Current antibiotic therapy.
    - Prematurity. All vaccines should be given based on the child's chronologic age, even if the child is premature.

A

The most likely cause of this infant's apnea is abusive head trauma, which is most common in 3- to 4-month-old infants and presents early with nonspecific symptoms (lethargy, irritability, poor feeding, vomiting) and later with seizures or apnea. There is generally no reported history of head trauma. Subdural hematoma and edema account for most neurologic findings. In babies with abusive head trauma, there is a 50–70% chance of prior abuse.

LEAD POISONING

Most exposure in children is caused by lead-contaminated household dust from lead paint. Screening should be routinely performed at 12 and 24 months for patients living in high-risk areas (pre-1950s homes or zip codes with high percentages of elevated blood lead levels); universal screening is not recommended.

HISTORY/PE

- Children are usually asymptomatic.
- With high levels, they present with irritability, headache, hyperactivity or apathy, anorexia, intermittent abdominal pain, constipation, intermittent vomiting, and peripheral neuropathy (wrist or foot drop).
- Acute encephalopathy (usually with levels > 70 µg/dL) is characterized by ↑ ICP, vomiting, confusion, seizures, and coma.

DIAGNOSIS

- Do a fingerstick test as an initial screen at 1 or 2 years of age; If elevated, then obtain a serum lead level.
- CBC and peripheral blood smear show microcytic, hypochromic anemia and basophilic stippling (see Figure 2.13-17). Sideroblastic anemia may also be present.

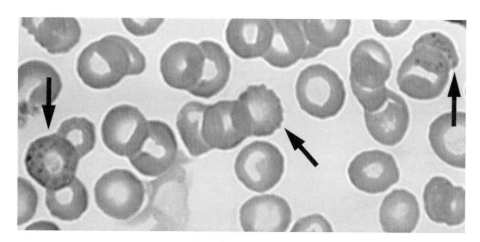

FIGURE 2.13-17. Basophilic stippling *(arrows)* in lead poisoning. (Reproduced courtesy of van Dijk HA, Fred HL. Images of memorable cases: case 81. Connexions Web site. December 3, 2008. Available at https://cnx.org/contents/MZa_Ph4e@4/Images-of-Memorable-Cases-Case.)

TREATMENT

- **Blood lead levels:**
  - **< 5 µg/dL:** Family education and annual test of blood lead levels.
  - **5–14 µg/dL:** Retest at 1–3 months, remove sources of lead exposure.
  - **15–44 µg/dL:** Retest within 1–4 weeks, remove sources of lead exposure.
  - **45–69 µg/dL:** Retest within 48 hours along with further workup (x-ray of the abdomen, electrolytes, etc), begin chelation therapy (oral succimer is recommended).
  - **> 70 µg/dL:** Retest within 24 hours, urgent evaluations, hospitalization, and chelation therapy (succimer + $CaNa_2EDTA$).

NOTES

PSYCHIATRY

Childhood and Adolescent Disorders

ATTENTION-DEFICIT HYPERACTIVITY DISORDER

A persistent pattern of excessive inattention and/or hyperactivity/impulsivity. Typically presents between 3 and 13 years of age; more common in men; often shows a familial relationship.

HISTORY/PE

- Presents with core symptoms that can be divided into the following two categories:
  - **Inattention**: Exhibits a poor/short attention span in schoolwork/play; displays poor attention to detail or careless mistakes; has difficulty following instructions or finishing tasks; is forgetful and easily distracted.
  - **Hyperactivity/impulsivity**: Fidgets; leaves seat in classroom; runs around inappropriately; cannot play quietly; talks excessively; does not wait for his or her turn; interrupts others.

DIAGNOSIS

- Symptoms must be present for ≥ 6 months in at least two independent settings (eg, home and school).
- **Age < 17 years**: Diagnosis requires ≥ 6 symptoms from either category of core symptoms.
- **Age ≥ 17 years**: Diagnosis requires ≥ 5 symptoms from either category of core symptoms.
  - **Inattention**: See above.
  - **Hyperactivity/impulsivity**: See above.
- Symptoms must be present before 12 years of age.
- Symptoms must cause functional impairment (social, academic, or occupational).
- Alternative causes of inattention and/or hyperactivity must be ruled out (such as substance abuse, organic [eg, lead toxicity], hearing/visual impairment, thyroid disorders, sleep disorders, absence seizures).

TREATMENT

- **4–5 years of age**:
  - **Best initial treatment**: Behavior therapy. Add medication if behaviors do not improve.
- **≥ 6 years of age**:
  - **Best initial treatment**: Pharmacologic therapy + behavior therapy.
    - **First line**: CNS stimulants (eg, methylphenidate, dextroamphetamine, amphetamine salts [dextroamphetamine and amphetamine combo]).
      - Adverse effects: Weight loss (↓ appetite), insomnia, anxiety, irritability, headache, tic exacerbation, and ↓ growth velocity (normalizes when medication is stopped).
  - **Alternatives**: Nonstimulants.
    - Atomoxetine (norepinephrine reuptake inhibitor): Can be tried first because of the negative side-effect profile of CNS stimulants.
    - Clonidine/guanfacine (α_2-agonist), bupropion, and tricyclic antidepressants (TCAs).
- **All ages**: Continue regular diet. Sugar and food additives are not considered etiologic factors.

KEY FACT

Children must exhibit ADHD symptoms in two or more settings (eg, home and school).

AUTISM SPECTRUM DISORDER

Developmental disorder characterized by impairments in two major domains: 1) social interaction and communication and 2) repetitive/restricted behavior, interests, or activities. More common in men. Severity is based on the level of support required for each domain. The *DSM-5* does not distinguish among the pervasive developmental disorders.

HISTORY/PE

- **Deficits in social interaction and communication:** Reduced interest in socialization, reduced empathy, inability to form relationships, impaired language development, inability to understand social cues, poor eye contact.
  - Prognosis is best determined by language development.
- **Restricted/repetitive patterns of behavior, interests, or activities:** Highly fixated or restricted interests, inflexibility to change, hand flapping, increased/decreased response to sensory input (eg, indifference to temperature, excessive touching/smelling, adverse response to sounds).
- Symptoms must impair function (eg, academic, social).
- Symptoms must be present in the early developmental period (typically < 3 years of age).
- Conditions that produce symptoms suggestive of autism spectrum disorder (ASD) must be excluded:
  - **Intellectual disability** or global developmental delay.
  - **Hearing impairment:** Rule out with audiometry before making diagnosis.
  - **Selective mutism:** Refusal to speak only in social situations.
  - **Rett syndrome:** Similar to ASD. X-linked disorder characterized by marked physical and psychomotor regression at approximately 6 months of age after normal development.
    - Predominantly seen in girls. Patients have stereotyped hand-wringing movements.

TREATMENT

- Intensive special education, behavioral management, and symptom-targeted medications (eg, neuroleptics for aggression; SSRIs for stereotyped behavior).
- Family support and counseling are crucial.

KEY FACT

If you see ASD, think about associated congenital conditions such as Rett syndrome, tuberous sclerosis, and fragile X syndrome.

DISRUPTIVE BEHAVIORAL DISORDERS

Includes conduct disorder, oppositional defiant disorder, and disruptive mood dysregulation disorder. More common in men and in patients with a history of abuse. Psychiatric comorbidities are common (eg, posttraumatic stress disorder [PTSD], depression, substance abuse, somatoform conditions, personality disorders).

HISTORY/PE

- **Oppositional defiant disorder (ODD):** A pattern of negative, defiant, disobedient, and hostile behavior toward authority figures (eg, losing temper, arguing) for ≥ 6 months. May progress to conduct disorder.
- **Conduct disorder:** A repetitive, persistent pattern of violating the basic rights of others or age-appropriate societal norms/rules for ≥ 1 year in

children < 18 years of age. Behaviors can be aggressive (eg, rape, robbery, animal cruelty) or nonaggressive (eg, destruction of property, stealing, lying, deliberately annoying others).
  - After 18 years of age, conduct disorder is considered antisocial personality disorder.
- **Disruptive mood dysregulation disorder (DMDD):** A pattern of severe, recurrent verbal (eg, screaming) or behavioral (eg, physical aggression) outbursts that are out of proportion to the situation and a persistently irritable or angry mood between outbursts; symptoms must occur for ≥ 1 year; may progress to depression in adulthood. DMDD should not be diagnosed before 6 years of age or after 18 years of age.

TREATMENT

Psychotherapy is the first-line treatment for all disruptive behavioral disorders.

INTELLECTUAL DEVELOPMENTAL DISORDER

Disorder of cognitive, social, and practical functioning. Associated with male gender, chromosomal abnormalities, congenital infections, teratogens (including alcohol/illicit substances), and inborn errors of metabolism.

- Down syndrome (Trisomy 21) is the most common chromosomal cause of intellectual disability.
- Fetal alcohol syndrome (FAS) is the most common preventable cause of intellectual disability.
- Fragile X syndrome is the most common inherited form of intellectual disability.
- No identifiable cause is found in most patients with intellectual disability.

HISTORY/PE

- Patients have deficiencies in multiple domains as follows:
  - **Intellectual deficits:** Poor performance on standardized testing.
  - **Adaptive functioning deficits:** Poor hygiene, social functioning, activities of daily living (ADLs).
- **Onset:** During developmental period (< 18 years of age).
- **Severity of intellectual disability:** Determined by level of support required to address impaired adaptive functioning (IQ is no longer used with the *DSM-5*).
  - Mild (independent in ADLs); moderate (some teaching and support for ADLs); severe (significant support for ADLs); profound (dependent on support for all ADLs).
- **Differential diagnosis:** Specific learning disorder (reading, math, or writing skills that are significantly lower than expected for age and intelligence).
  - Reading disorder is the most common.

TREATMENT

- **Primary prevention:** Educating the public about possible causes of intellectual disability and providing optimal prenatal screening and care to mothers.
- **Treatment measures:** Family counseling and support; speech and language therapy; occupational/physical therapy; behavioral intervention; educational assistance; and social skills training.
  - **Learning disorder:** Remedial therapy directed toward patient's deficiency.

TOURETTE SYNDROME

Disorder characterized by both motor and vocal tics. More common in men; shows a genetic predisposition. Associated with ADHD, learning disorders, and obsessive-compulsive disorder (OCD).

HISTORY/PE

Symptoms begin < 18 years of age and cause social or occupational impairment.

DIAGNOSIS

Diagnosis requires the following:

- Multiple motor tics (eg, blinking, grimacing).
- One or more vocal tics (eg, grunting, coprolalia, echolalia, throat clearing, coughing).
- Tics present for > 1 year.
- Tics must be recurrent (occur many times per day and/or nearly every day).

TREATMENT

- **Best initial treatment:** Behavior therapy (habit reversal therapy is most effective).
- If behavior therapy fails or tics are severe/disabling, the next step is pharmacologic management.
  - **Antidopaminergic agents:**
    - **Dopamine-depleting agents** (eg, tetrabenazine [VMAT-2 inhibitor; results in ↓ uptake of monoamines]): Preferred over dopamine-blocking agents; does not cause tardive dyskinesia (TD).
    - **Dopamine-blocking agents:** Antipsychotics (eg, fluphenazine, risperidone, haloperidol, pimozide).
      - Severe, refractory tics: Treat with haloperidol or pimozide (typical antipsychotics).
  - **α_2-agonists** (eg, clonidine, guanfacine): Less effective at tic reduction; more favorable side-effect profile.

KEY FACT

Coprolalia = repetition of obscene words
Echolalia = repetition of words spoken by others

Psychotic Disorders

SCHIZOPHRENIA

Disorder of thought process. Characterized by psychotic symptoms, which are further divided into positive symptoms (hallucinations, delusions, disorganized thought/behavior) and negative symptoms (flat affect, social withdrawal, apathy).

- **Epidemiology:** Prevalence is approximately 1% (M=F). Peak onset is earlier in men (18–25 years of age) than in women (25–35 years of age). Schizophrenia in first-degree relatives also ↑ risk. Up to 50% of patients attempt suicide, and 10% of those affected complete suicide.
- **Etiology:** Unknown; theories focus on neurotransmitter abnormalities such as dopamine dysregulation (frontal hypoactivity and limbic hyperactivity) and brain abnormalities on CT and MRI (enlarged ventricles and ↓ cortical volume).

KEY FACT

Psychosis (hallucinations and/or delusions without insight) ≠ schizophrenia. Differential diagnosis must also include medical diseases, other psychiatric illnesses, and substance-induced psychosis.

HISTORY/PE

- Presents with chronic or recurrent psychosis, disorganization, and/or negative symptoms.

Terms used to describe components of psychosis are as follows:

- Delusion: A fixed false idiosyncratic belief.
- Hallucination: Perception without an existing external stimulus.
- Illusion: Misperception of an actual external stimulus.

MNEMONIC

Evolution of EPS—

4 and A

4 hours: **A**cute dystonia
4 days: **A**kinesia
4 weeks: **A**kathisia
4 months: Tardive dyskinesia (often permanent)

- Cognitive impairment in multiple areas (eg, processing speed, working memory, attention, social cognition) may be present.
- Mood and anxiety symptoms are common.

DIAGNOSIS

Requires two or more of the following symptoms for ≥ 6 months with social or occupational dysfunction:

- Hallucinations (most often auditory).
- Delusions.
- Disorganized speech.
- Disorganized or catatonic behavior.
- **Negative symptoms:** Flattened affect, social withdrawal, anhedonia, apathy, ↓ emotion. May mimic depression.
  - **5A's:** Affect (flat), avolition, asociality, anhedonia, apathy.

See Table 2.14-1 for the differential diagnosis of psychosis.

TREATMENT

- Antipsychotics (see Table 2.14-2); long-term follow-up.
- Supportive psychotherapy, training in social skills, vocational rehabilitation, and illness education may help.
- Negative symptoms may be more difficult to treat than positive symptoms; atypical antipsychotics are the drug of choice.

TABLE 2.14-1. **Differential Diagnosis of Psychosis**

DISORDER	DURATION/CHARACTERISTICS
Psychotic disorders	Brief psychotic disorder: 1 day – 1 month
	Schizophreniform disorder: 1–6 months
	Note: Both have the same presentation as schizophrenia, but are usually preceded by stressors, have no prior episodes, are less likely to have negative symptoms, and have better lifetime prognosis
	Schizophrenia: > 6 months
	Schizoaffective disorder: Psychosis + mood disorder (mania or depression)
	Requires history/presence of both:
	Psychosis plus mood episode AND
	Psychosis for ≥ 2 weeks without mood episode
Personality disorders	Schizotypal: "Magical thinking"
	Schizoid: "Loners"
Delusional disorder	Persistent delusions (often nonbizarre) without disorganized thought process, hallucinations, or negative symptoms of schizophrenia; subtypes are jealous, paranoid, somatic, erotomanic, or grandiose
	Symptoms must be present ≥ 1 month
	Day-to-day functioning mostly unaffected
	Folie à deux: A shared delusion (commonly between parent and child)
	The best course of action is to separate the patient pair and treat individually

TABLE 2.14-2. Antipsychotic Medications

Drug Class	Mechanism	Examples	Indications	Side Effects
Typical antipsychotics	D_2 antagonist (High potency)	Haloperidol[a], fluphenazine[a]	Psychotic disorders, acute agitation, acute mania, Tourette syndrome Thought to be more effective for positive symptoms of schizophrenia If compliance is a major issue, consider antipsychotics available in long-acting depot form[a]	Extrapyramidal symptoms (EPS) > anticholinergic symptoms (dry mouth, urinary retention, constipation) QTc prolongation and torsades, especially IV haloperidol Neuroleptic malignant syndrome (see Table 2.14-3)
	D_2 antagonist (Low potency)	Thioridazine, chlorpromazine	Same as high potency	Anticholinergic > EPS More sedating Greater risk for orthostatic hypotension Thioridazine causes dose-dependent QTc prolongation and irreversible retinal pigmentation
Atypical antipsychotics	D_2 antagonist, 5-HT_{2A} antagonist	Risperidone[a], quetiapine, olanzapine[a], paliperidone[a], ziprasidone, clozapine	First-line treatment for schizophrenia given fewer EPS and anticholinergic effects Clozapine is reserved for severe treatment resistance and severe tardive dyskinesia	↓ EPS (d/t 5-HT_{2A} antagonism) Weight gain, dyslipidemia, type 2 diabetes mellitus, somnolence, sedation, and QTc prolongation (ziprasidone), hyperprolactinemia (risperidone) Clozapine can cause agranulocytosis; requires weekly CBC monitoring during first 6 months
	D_2 partial agonist, 5-HT_{1A} partial agonist, 5-HT_{2A} antagonist	Aripiprazole[a]	Same as other atypicals	Same as other atypicals

[a] Also available as a long-acting depot injection.

- Catatonia (awkward posturing, mutism, and immobility) may be seen in severe disease; treated with benzodiazepine challenge and electroconvulsive therapy (ECT).

Dissociative Disorders

Includes dissociative identity disorder, depersonalization/derealization disorder, and dissociative amnesia. See Table 2.14-4 for an overview of the dissociative disorders.

TREATMENT

- **Best initial treatment:** Psychotherapy.
- Appropriate pharmacologic treatment can be added to address comorbidities (eg, depression, anxiety, substance abuse, PTSD).

Q

A 24-year-old woman has been "hearing voices" and has isolated herself from her friends and family. She first noticed the voices about 2 months ago when she was feeling sad and reported sleeping poorly. She reports that her mood has since improved and denies any current sleep disturbances. What is her most likely diagnosis?

TABLE 2.14-3. **EPS and Treatment**

Subtype	Description	Time of Onset	Treatment
Acute dystonia	Prolonged, painful tonic muscle contraction or spasm (eg, torticollis, oculogyric crisis)	Hours	Anticholinergics (benztropine or diphenhydramine) for acute therapy; patients who are prone to dystonic reactions may need regular prophylactic dosing (eg, benztropine)
Akathisia	Subjective/objective restlessness that is perceived as being distressing	Days	↓ Neuroleptic; β-blockers (propranolol) Benzodiazepines or anticholinergics may help
Dyskinesia	Pseudoparkinsonism (eg, shuffling gait, cogwheel rigidity)	Weeks	Anticholinergics (benztropine) or dopamine agonist (amantadine) ↓ The dose of neuroleptic or discontinue (if tolerated)
Tardive dyskinesia	Stereotypic, involuntary, painless oral-facial movements Probably from dopamine receptor sensitization from chronic dopamine blockade Often irreversible (50%)	Months	Discontinue or ↓ the dose of neuroleptic; consider changing neuroleptic (eg, to clozapine or risperidone) Giving anticholinergics or ↓ neuroleptic dose may initially worsen tardive dyskinesia
Neuroleptic malignant syndrome	Fever, muscle rigidity, autonomic instability, elevated creatine kinase and white blood cells, delirium	Anytime	Stop medication; provide supportive care in the ICU; administer dantrolene or bromocriptine

A

This patient most likely has schizoaffective disorder, which is characterized by psychosis and intermittent mood symptoms. The diagnosis requires: 1) psychotic symptoms AND mood symptoms, and 2) at least 2 weeks when psychotic symptoms are present WITHOUT mood symptoms. Patients often have chronic psychotic symptoms, even after mood symptoms have resolved.

TABLE 2.14-4. **Overview of Dissociate Disorders**

Disorder	Characteristics
Dissociative identity disorder (multiple personality disorder)	Disruption in identity characterized by ≥ 2 distinct personalities Associated with history of trauma and child abuse
Depersonalization/ derealization disorder (DDD)	Recurrent or persistent[a] experiences of ≥ 1 of the following: Depersonalization: Feeling of detachment from one's self; may feel like an outside observer Derealization: Experiencing one's surroundings as unreal
Dissociative amnesia	Inability to recall memories or important personal information, usually after a traumatic or stressful event Not better explained by substances or another medical condition Dissociative fugue: Subtype of dissociative amnesia Characterized by sudden, unexpected travel in a dissociated state and subsequent amnesia of the travel

[a]Transient depersonalization/derealization may occur during times of severe stress; does not meet diagnostic criteria for DDD.

Anxiety Disorders

GENERALIZED ANXIETY DISORDER

Uncontrollable, excessive anxiety or worry about multiple activities or events that leads to significant impairment or distress.

HISTORY/PE

Clinical onset is usually in the early 20s; it is more common in women. The male-to-female ratio is 1:2.

DIAGNOSIS

- Excessive anxiety or worry about multiple activities, occurring on most days for ≥ 6 months.
- Symptoms of anxiety/worry are associated with at ≥ 3 somatic symptoms: restlessness, easy fatigue, difficulty concentrating, irritability, muscle tension, sleep disturbances.
- Symptoms cause a clinically significant impairment (eg, social, occupational).
- Disturbances are not caused by substances (eg, drug of abuse [cocaine], medication [amphetamines]).
- Disturbance is not better explained by another psychiatric disorder (eg, excessive worry about panic attacks).

TREATMENT

- **Best initial treatment:** Selective serotonin reuptake inhibitors (SSRIs; eg, fluoxetine, sertraline, escitalopram). See Table 2.14-5.

TABLE 2.14-5. Anxiolytic Medications

DRUG CLASS	INDICATIONS	SIDE EFFECTS
SSRIs (eg, fluoxetine, sertraline, paroxetine, citalopram, escitalopram)	First-line treatment for GAD, OCD, panic disorder	Nausea, GI upset, somnolence, sexual dysfunction, agitation
5-HT partial agonist (eg, buspirone)	Not first-line treatment for GAD, social phobia	Headaches, dizziness, nausea. No tolerance, dependence, or withdrawal
β-blocker (propranolol)	Performance only social anxiety disorder	Bradycardia, hypotension
Benzodiazepines (eg, clonazepam, alprazolam)	Anxiety (short-term), insomnia, alcohol withdrawal, muscle spasm, night terrors, sleepwalking	↓ Sleep duration; risk for abuse, tolerance, and dependence; disinhibition in young or old patients; confusion. Abruptly stopping a short-acting benzodiazepine (eg, alprazolam) can result in seizures

- **Alternative treatment:** Serotonin norepinephrine reuptake inhibitors (SNRIs; eg, venlafaxine, duloxetine), buspirone, tricyclic antidepressants (TCAs), benzodiazepines (short-term treatment).
- **Nonpharmacologic interventions:** Psychotherapy, lifestyle changes.

PANIC DISORDER

Characterized by recurrent, unexpected periods of intense fear that last for several minutes and causes excessive worry about having another panic attack.

HISTORY/PE

- Recurrent episodes of intense fear and discomfort; symptoms usually last ≤ 30 minutes.
- May lead to agoraphobia in 30–50% of cases (fear/anxiety of developing paniclike symptoms in situations where it may be difficult to escape or get help, resulting in avoidance of those situations).
  - The modifiers "with agoraphobia" or "without agoraphobia" are no longer included in *DSM-5*. Panic disorder and agoraphobia are now separate diagnoses.
- More common in women; average age of onset is 25 years, but may occur at any age.

DIAGNOSIS

- **Panic attacks:** Discrete periods of intense fear or discomfort in which ≥ 4 of the following symptoms develop abruptly and peak within 10 minutes:
  - Tachycardia or palpitations, diaphoresis, chest pain, shortness of breath, nausea, trembling, dizziness, fear of dying or "going crazy," depersonalization, hot flashes, chills or heat sensation, paresthesia.
- **Panic disorder:**
  - Recurrent, unexpected panic attacks.
  - Attacks followed by ≥ 1 month of least one of the following:
    - Persistent worry/concern of having additional attacks.
    - Maladaptive change in behavior (avoidance of unfamiliar situations).
  - Not explained by substances, medications, or another medical condition.

TREATMENT

- See Table 2.14-5 for medications.
- **Best initial treatment:** Benzodiazepines (eg, clonazepam). Avoid long-term use due to concerns of potential dependence and abuse. Taper benzodiazepines as soon as long-term treatment is initiated.
- **Long-term treatment:** SSRIs (eg, sertraline).
  - **Psychotherapy:** Cognitive behavioral therapy (CBT); higher rates of response and sustained effects compared with placebo and pharmacotherapy alone.

PHOBIAS (SOCIAL AND SPECIFIC)

Disorders characterized by excessive fear that is unreasonable and stimulated by the presence or anticipation of a specific object or situation. Patients recognize the fear is excessive.

HISTORY/PE

- **Social phobia (social anxiety disorder):** Presents with excessive fear of criticism, humiliation, and embarrassment in multiple situations requiring social interaction.

- **Social anxiety disorder, performance only:** Symptoms provoked only by performance situations (eg, public speaking, test taking, sexual intercourse).
    - Symptoms are persistent, usually lasting ≥ 6 months.
- **Specific phobia:** Excessive anxiety and fear provoked by exposure to a feared object or situation (eg, animals, heights, airplanes). Most cases begin in childhood.

TREATMENT

- **Social phobia (social anxiety disorder):** First-line treatment is CBT, involving desensitization through incremental exposure to the feared object or situation along with relaxation techniques.
    - **Best initial treatment:** SSRIs. Alternatives include benzodiazepines with exposure techniques.
- **Social anxiety disorder, performance only:** First-line treatment with β–blockers (eg, propranolol). Alternatives include CBT, benzodiazepines, and/or SSRIs.
- **Specific phobias:** First-line treatment is CBT. Alternatives include SSRIs, benzodiazepines.

Obsessive-Compulsive Disorder and Related Disorders

OBSESSIVE-COMPULSIVE DISORDER

Characterized by obsessions and/or compulsions that lead to significant distress and dysfunction in social or personal areas. Typically presents in late adolescence or early adulthood; prevalence is equal in male and female patients. Often chronic and difficult to treat.

HISTORY/PE

- **Obsessions:** Persistent, unwanted, and intrusive ideas, thoughts, impulses, or images that lead to marked anxiety or distress (eg, fear of contamination, fear of harming oneself or loved ones).
- **Compulsions (or rituals):** Repeated mental acts or behaviors that neutralize anxiety from obsessions (eg, handwashing, elaborate rituals for ordinary tasks, counting, excessive checking).
- Patients recognize their behaviors as excessive and irrational (vs obsessive-compulsive personality disorder, or OCPD; see Table 2.14-6).
- Patients wish they could get rid of the obsessions and/or compulsions.

KEY FACT

Many patients with OCD initially present to a nonpsychiatrist—eg, they may consult a dermatologist with a skin complaint 2° to overwashing hands.

TABLE 2.14-6.   OCD vs OCPD

OCD	OCPD
Characterized by obsessions and/or compulsions	Patients are excessively conscientious and inflexible
Patients recognize the obsessions/compulsions and want to be rid of them (ego dystonic)	Patients do not recognize their behavior as problematic (ego syntonic)

TREATMENT

- **Best initial treatment:** SSRIs (high-dose).
  - **Alternative:** Clomipramine (TCA).
- CBT using exposure and desensitization relaxation techniques.
- Patient education is imperative.

OBSESSIVE-COMPULSIVE–RELATED DISORDERS

See Table 2.14-7 for a listing of OCD-related disorders and their characteristics. All OCD-related disorders can be treated with CBT and SSRIs.

Trauma and Stressor-Related Disorders

POSTTRAUMATIC STRESS DISORDER

Disorder characterized by clinically significant distress or impairment in daily functioning caused by exposure to an extreme, life-threatening traumatic event (eg, war, assault, injury, rape, accident, violent crime). Event can be directly experienced or witnessed.

HISTORY/PE

- Patients experience severe psychological distress when exposed to stimuli that remind them of the event, resulting in avoidance of situations where exposure to triggers is possible.
- High incidence of substance abuse, anxiety, and/or depression.

KEY FACT

Top causes of PTSD in male patients are (1) sexual assault and (2) war.
Top causes of PTSD in female patients are (1) childhood abuse and (2) sexual assault.

TABLE 2.14-7. Obsessive-Compulsive–Related Disorders

DISORDER	CHARACTERISTICS
Body dysmorphic disorder	Preoccupation with imagined or slight defects in physical appearance that are usually imperceptible to others, leading to significant distress/impairment Suspect in patients with extensive history of cosmetic procedures
Hoarding disorder	Difficulty discarding possessions, regardless of value. Attempts at discarding objects causes significant distress. Results in accumulation of objects and can lead to an unsafe living environment
Excoriation (skin picking) disorder	Recurrent skin picking resulting in skin lesions that causes clinically significant distress or impairment in social functioning. Patient may report repeated attempts to stop or decrease Differential diagnosis: Pruritus caused by a medical condition (eg, primary biliary cholangitis [PBC])
Trichotillomania (hair pulling disorder)	Recurrent hair pulling leading to hair loss that causes clinically significant distress or impairment in social functioning. Patients may report repeated attempts to stop or decrease Differential diagnosis: Tinea capitis, alopecia

DIAGNOSIS

- Exposure to a traumatic event and the presence of the following:
    - **Intrusive symptoms:** Re-experiencing the event through nightmares, flashbacks, intrusive memories.
    - Avoidance of stimuli associated with the trauma.
    - Negative alterations in mood and cognition: Numbed responsiveness (eg, detachment, anhedonia), guilt, self-blame.
    - Changes in arousal and reactivity: ↑ Arousal (eg, hypervigilance, exaggerated startle response), sleep disturbances, aggression/irritability, and poor concentration.
- Symptoms lead to significant distress or impairment in functioning.
- Symptoms must persist for > 1 month.
    - Acute stress disorder is diagnosed if symptoms are present for ≤ 1 month.
        - Clinical presentation is the same as PTSD.
        - Symptoms last ≥ 3 days, but < 1 month.
        - Symptoms present within 1 month of experiencing the traumatic event.

TREATMENT

- **Best initial treatment:** Trauma-focused CBT, with or without pharmacotherapy.
    - **Pharmacotherapy:** SSRIs, SNRIs.
        - Prazosin (α_1-blocker) is used to treat PTSD-related nightmares.

Neurocognitive Disorders

Disorders that affect memory, orientation, judgment, and attention.

DEMENTIA (MAJOR NEUROCOGNITIVE DISORDER)

A decline in cognitive functioning with global deficits. Level of consciousness is stable (vs delirium). Prevalence is highest among those > 85 years of age. The course is persistent and progressive. The most common causes are Alzheimer disease (65%) and vascular dementia (20%). Other causes are outlined in the mnemonic **DEMENTIASS**.

HISTORY/PE

- Patients with dementia are usually not concerned about their cognitive decline and are often accompanied to the doctor visit by a family member or friend (versus major depressive disorder [MDD]/pseudodementia).
- Characterized by progressive memory impairment that can be classified into the following four stages:
    - **Preclinical:** Slight forgetfulness, fully oriented, and capable of self-care.
    - **Mild:** Moderate memory loss, impaired executive function, impaired function at home, but can maintain most chores. Personal hygiene may need prompting.
    - **Moderate:** Severe memory loss, inability to recognize friends (agnosia), impaired social judgement, requires assistance with dressing and personal hygiene.
    - **Severe:** Severe memory loss, oriented only to person, completely dependent on others for ADLs, and may develop aphasia and become incommunicable.
- Personality, mood, and behavior changes are common (eg, wandering and aggression).

KEY FACT

In patients with a history of substance abuse, benzodiazepines should be avoided in view of their high addictive potential.

MNEMONIC

Causes of dementia—

DEMENTIASS

Degenerative diseases (Parkinson, Huntington, dementia with Lewy bodies [DLB])

Endocrine (thyroid, parathyroid, pituitary, adrenal)

Metabolic (alcohol, electrolytes, vitamin B_{12} deficiency, glucose, hepatic, renal, Wilson disease)

Exogenous (heavy metals, carbon monoxide, drugs)

Neoplasia

Trauma (subdural hematoma)

Infection (meningitis, encephalitis, endocarditis, syphilis, HIV, prion diseases, Lyme disease)

Affective disorders (pseudodementia)

Stroke/**S**tructure (vascular dementia, ischemia, vasculitis, normal-pressure hydrocephalus)

DIAGNOSIS

- Diagnosis is clinical.
  - History, PE, and Mini-Mental State Exam (MMSE) or Montreal Cognitive Assessment (MoCA).
  - **Rule out treatable causes of dementia/delirium:** Obtain UA, CBC, ESR, B$_{12}$, folate, CMP, TFTs, HIV, RPR, and a head CT/MRI.
- Definitive diagnosis requires autopsy and histopathologic exam (rarely performed).
- Table 2.14-8 outlines key characteristics distinguishing dementia from delirium.

TREATMENT

- **Pharmacotherapy:**
  - **Best initial treatment:** Cholinesterase inhibitors (donepezil, rivastigmine, galantamine).
  - **Moderate/severe Alzheimer dementia (AD):** Add memantine (N-methyl-D-aspartate [NMDA] antagonist).
  - **Aggression/psychosis:** Low-dose antipsychotics (use with caution in elderly; black box warning for increased mortality).
  - Avoid benzodiazepines, which may exacerbate disinhibition and confusion.
- Provide environmental cues and a rigid structure for the patient's daily life.
- Family, caregiver, and patient education and support are imperative.

TABLE 2.14-8. Delirium vs Dementia

CHARACTERISTIC	DELIRIUM	DEMENTIA
Level of attention	Impaired (fluctuating)	Usually alert
Onset	Acute	Gradual
Course	Fluctuating from hour to hour, "sundowning"	Progressive deterioration
Consciousness	Clouded	Intact
Hallucinations	Present (often visual or tactile)	Occur in approximately 30% of patients in highly advanced disease
Prognosis	Reversible	Largely irreversible, but up to 15% of cases are a result of treatable causes and are reversible
Treatment	Treat underlying causes Environmental changes (eg, ↓ stimuli, frequent orientation to day/time, shades up during daytime to reestablish circadian rhythm) Low-dose antipsychotics for disruptive behaviors (agitation, combativeness)	Cholinesterase inhibitors; low-dose antipsychotics (primarily for behavior disturbances) Environmental changes

DELIRIUM

An acute disturbance of consciousness with altered cognition that develops over a short period (usually hours to days). Children, the elderly, and hospitalized patients (eg, ICU psychosis) are particularly susceptible. Major causes are outlined in the mnemonic **I WATCH DEATH**. Symptoms are potentially reversible if the underlying cause can be treated.

HISTORY/PE

- Presents with acute onset of waxing and waning consciousness with lucid intervals and perceptual disturbances (hallucinations, illusions, delusions).
- Patients may be combative, anxious, paranoid, or stuporous.
- Patients have ↓ attention span and short-term memory, a reversed sleep-wake cycle, and ↑ symptoms at night (sundowning).

DIAGNOSIS

- **Best initial test:** Investigate common causes of delirium.
  - Perform history, physical, and neurologic exam.
  - Check vital signs, pulse oximetry, electrolytes, glucose, CBC, and UA.
    - UTI is a common cause of delirium in the elderly.
  - Note recent medication additions/changes (eg, narcotics, anticholinergics, steroids, benzodiazepines).
  - Evaluate for substance abuse and medical problems (eg, renal failure, liver failure).

TREATMENT

- Treat underlying causes (delirium is often reversible).
- Normalize fluids and electrolytes.
- Optimize the sensory environment, and provide necessary visual and hearing aids.
- Use low-dose antipsychotics (eg, haloperidol) for agitation and psychotic symptoms.
- Conservative use of physical restraints may be necessary to prevent harm to the patient or others.

Mood Disorders

Also known as affective disorders.

MAJOR DEPRESSIVE DISORDER

A mood disorder characterized by one or more major depressive episodes (MDEs). The male-to-female ratio is 1:2; lifetime prevalence ranges from 15% to 25%. Onset is usually in the mid-20s; in the elderly, prevalence ↑ with age. Chronic illness and stress ↑ risk. Approximately 2–9% of patients die by suicide.

HISTORY/PE

Diagnosis requires depressed mood or anhedonia (loss of interest/pleasure) and ≥ 5 signs/symptoms from the SIG E CAPS mnemonic for ≥ 2 weeks. Table 2.14-9 outlines the differential diagnosis of conditions that can be mistaken for depression. Select depression subtypes include the following:

- **Psychotic features:** Generally mood-congruent delusions/hallucinations. Psychosis only occurs during the MDD episode (distinguished from schizoaffective disorder).

MNEMONIC

Major causes of delirium—

I WATCH DEATH
Infection
Withdrawal
Acute metabolic/substance **A**buse
Trauma
CNS pathology
Hypoxia
Deficiencies
Endocrine
Acute vascular/MI
Toxins/drugs
Heavy metals

KEY FACT

It is common for delirium to be superimposed on dementia.

MNEMONIC

Symptoms of a depressive episode—

SIG E CAPS

Sleep (hypersomnia or insomnia)
Interest (loss of interest or pleasure in activities)
Guilt (feelings of worthlessness or inappropriate guilt)
Energy (↓) or fatigue
Concentration (↓)
Appetite (↑ or ↓) or weight (↑ or ↓)
Psychomotor agitation or retardation
Suicidal ideation

KEY FACT

Major depressive episodes can be present in major depressive disorder or in bipolar disorder types I and II.

TABLE 2.14-9. Differential Diagnosis of Major Depression

Disorder	Description and Examples
Mood disorder caused by a medical condition	Hypothyroidism, Parkinson disease, CNS neoplasm, other neoplasms (eg, pancreatic cancer), stroke (especially anterior cerebral artery stroke), dementias, parathyroid disorders
Substance-induced mood disorder	Illicit drugs, alcohol, antihypertensives, corticosteroids, OCPs
Adjustment disorder with depressed mood	A constellation of symptoms that resemble an MDE but does not meet the criteria for MDE Occurs within 3 months of an identifiable stressor
Normal bereavement	Occurs after the loss of a loved one. Involves no severe impairment/suicidality. "Waves" of grief at reminders of loved one Usually lasts < 6 months; should resolve within 1 year May lead to MDD that requires treatment Illusions/hallucinations of the deceased can be normal as long as the person recognizes them as such
Dysthymia	Milder, chronic depression with depressed mood (≥ 2 depressive symptoms) present most of the time for ≥ 2 years; often resistant to treatment

KEY FACT

SIG E CAPS = Major depressive disorder
DIG FAST = Mania/bipolar disorder

MNEMONIC

TCA toxicity—

Tri-C's

Convulsions
Coma
Cardiac arrhythmias

- **Postpartum:** Occurs within 1 month postpartum; has a 10% incidence and a high risk for recurrence. Psychotic symptoms are common (see Table 2.14-10).
- **Atypical:** Characterized by weight gain, hypersomnia, and rejection sensitivity.
- **Seasonal:** Depressive episodes occur during a specific season (most commonly winter). Responds well to light therapy with or without antidepressants.

TREATMENT

- **Pharmacotherapy: Best initial treatment** is with an SSRI (eg, fluoxetine, sertraline, paroxetine, citalopram, escitalopram).
  - Allow 2–6 weeks to take effect; adjust dose as needed.
  - Continue for at least 6 months (at the same effective dose) beyond the time of achieving full remission.
  - If a patient fails to respond to the initial antidepressant, switch to another first-line agent (SSRI).
    - See Table 2.14-11 for alternatives.
- **Most accurate treatment:** Psychotherapy + antidepressants is more effective than either treatment alone.

TABLE 2.14-10. Differential Diagnosis of Postpartum Disorders

Subtype	Time of Onset	Symptoms
Postpartum "blues"	Within 2 weeks of delivery	Sadness, moodiness, emotional lability No thoughts about hurting self or baby
Postpartum depression	1–3 months postdelivery	Same as above plus sleep disturbances and anxiety May have thoughts about hurting self and/or baby
Postpartum psychosis	2–3 weeks postdelivery	Delusions, disorganized behavior May have thoughts about hurting baby

TABLE 2.14-11. Indications and Side Effects of Common Antidepressants

Drug Class	Examples	Indications	Side Effects
SSRIs	Fluoxetine, sertraline, paroxetine, citalopram, escitalopram, fluvoxamine	Depression, anxiety	Sexual side effects, GI distress, agitation, insomnia, tremor, diarrhea Serotonin syndrome (fever, myoclonus, hyperreflexia, altered mental status, cardiovascular collapse) can occur if SSRIs are used with MAOIs, illicit drugs, or herbal medications Paroxetine should be avoided during pregnancy; can cause cardiac defects (first trimester) and pulmonary hypertension (third trimester) in the fetus Discontinuation syndrome (flulike symptoms, nausea, insomnia, sensory disturbances) occurs with abrupt cessation of shorter-acting agents
Atypical antidepressants	Bupropion, mirtazapine, trazodone	Depression, anxiety Smoking cessation (bupropion)	Bupropion: ↓ Seizure threshold; minimal sexual side effects Contraindicated in patients with eating disorders and seizure disorders Mirtazapine: Weight gain, sedation, minimal sexual side effects Trazodone: Highly sedating; priapism
SNRIs	Venlafaxine, duloxetine	Depression, anxiety, neuropathic pain	Noradrenergic side effects at higher doses Venlafaxine: Diastolic hypertension
TCAs	Nortriptyline, desipramine, amitriptyline, imipramine, clomipramine	Depression, anxiety, neuropathic pain, migraine headaches, enuresis (imipramine), OCD (clomipramine)	Antihistaminic effects: Sedation, weight gain Anticholinergic effects: Dry mouth, tachycardia, urinary retention Antiadrenergic effects: Orthostatic hypotension TCA overdose can be lethal and cause convulsions (seizures), coma, cardiotoxicity (prolonged conduction through AV node, prolonged QRS), hyperpyrexia, and respiratory depression Treatment: sodium bicarbonate if prolonged QRS (> 100 msec), hypotensive, or ventricular arrhythmia Alleviates depressant effect of TCA on cardiac fast sodium channels
MAOIs	Phenelzine, tranylcypromine, selegiline (also available in patch form)	Depression, especially atypical	Hypertensive crisis if taken with high-tyramine foods (aged cheese, red wine) Sexual side effects, orthostatic hypotension, weight gain

- **ECT:** Small electrical current is used to produce a generalized seizure under anesthesia. Safe and highly effective treatment option for severe depression. Usually requires 2–3 treatments per week for a total of 6–12 treatments.
  - **Indications are as follows:**
    - Refractory or treatment-resistant depression.
    - Major depression with psychotic features.
    - Need for rapid improvement: Actively suicidal, refusal to eat/drink, catatonia, pregnancy.
    - Bipolar depression or mania.
  - No absolute contraindications. Relative contraindications include recent MI/stroke, intracranial mass, and high anesthetic risk.
  - **Adverse effects:** Anterograde amnesia, postictal confusion, arrhythmias, and headache.
- **Phototherapy:** Effective for depression with seasonal pattern.

KEY FACT

Discontinue SSRIs at least 2 weeks before starting an MAOI. Wait 5 weeks if the patient was on fluoxetine.

PERSISTENT DEPRESSIVE DISORDER (DYSTHYMIA)

HISTORY/PE

- Chronic depressed mood that is present on most days for > 2 years.
- Patients often feel depressed for as long as they can remember.
- **Double depression:** Diagnosed if patient meets criteria for MDD during dysthymic periods.

TREATMENT

- Psychotherapy is the most effective treatment.
- Often resistant to treatment. Consider antidepressants (eg, SSRIs) and ECT.

ADJUSTMENT DISORDER

Clinically significant distress following a profound life change (eg, divorce, unemployment, financial issues, romantic breakup); it is not severe enough to meet criteria for another mental disorder.

HISTORY/PE

- Patients develop anxiety or depressive symptoms (eg, anhedonia, depressed mood, weight loss) following a stressful life event (eg, divorce, death of family member, change in school/work).
  - Event is not life threatening.
  - Symptoms present within 3 months after onset of the stressor. Resolves within 6 months after event is over.
  - Causes social or occupational dysfunction, as opposed to normal stress reaction.

TREATMENT

- **Best initial treatment:** Psychotherapy focusing on coping skills and supportive counseling.
- No pharmacologic treatment.

BIPOLAR AND RELATED DISORDERS

Psychiatric illnesses characterized by episodes of mania or hypomania ± MDE. A family history significantly ↑ risk. The average age of onset is 20 years, and the frequency of mood episodes tends to ↑ with age. Up to 10–15% of those affected complete suicide. Classified into the following subtypes: bipolar I, bipolar II, or cyclothymic disorder.

HISTORY/PE

- The mnemonic **DIG FAST** outlines the clinical presentation of mania. See Table 2.14-12 to differentiate mania from hypomania.
  - May report excessive engagement in pleasurable activities (eg, excessive spending or sexual activity), reckless behaviors, and/or psychotic features.
- Patients may or may not have history of a major depressive episode (**SIG E CAPS** mnemonic).
- Antidepressants may trigger manic episodes (without a mood stabilizer).

DIAGNOSIS

- Symptoms must not be caused by substance abuse or a medical condition.
- **Bipolar I:**
  - Manic episode.
  - Major depressive episode not required for diagnosis.

MNEMONIC

Symptoms of mania—

DIG FAST

Distractibility
Insomnia (↓ need for sleep)
Grandiosity (↑ self-esteem)/more **G**oal directed
Flight of ideas (or racing thoughts)
Activities/psychomotor **A**gitation
Sexual indiscretions/other pleasurable activities
Talkativeness/pressured speech

TABLE 2.14-12. Mania vs Hypomania

MANIA	HYPOMANIA
More severe symptoms	Less severe symptoms
Symptoms present for ≥ 1 week, or hospitalization is necessary	Symptoms present for ≥ 4 days. No hospitalization is required
Significant impairment in social/occupational functioning	No significant impairment in social/occupational functioning
May develop psychotic features	No psychotic features

- Bipolar II:
  - Hypomanic episode.
  - ≥ 1 major depressive episode.
- Cyclothymic disorder:
  - Alternating periods of the following symptoms for at least 2 years:
    - Hypomanic symptoms that do not meet criteria for hypomania.
    - Depressive symptoms that do not meet criteria for major depressive episode.

TREATMENT

- Bipolar I and Bipolar II:
  - **Maintenance therapy:** Mood stabilizers (see Table 2.14-13). Most patients require lifelong mood stabilizer treatment.
    - **Best initial treatment:** Lithium.
  - **Acute mania:** Considered a psychiatric emergency because of impaired judgment and risk for harm to self or others.
    - Mild to moderate mania: Atypical antipsychotics (olanzapine, quetiapine).

> **Q**
>
> A 23-year-old woman complains of difficulty falling asleep and worsening anxiety that began 2 months earlier after she was involved in a minor biking accident (bike vs car) in which she did not suffer any injuries. Since the accident, she has refused to participate in any outdoor activities. What is her most likely diagnosis?

TABLE 2.14-13. Mood Stabilizers

DRUG CLASS	INDICATIONS	SIDE EFFECTS
Lithium	First-line mood stabilizer Used for acute mania (in combination with antipsychotics), for prophylaxis in bipolar disorder, and for augmentation in depression treatment Also ↓ suicide risk	Thirst, polyuria, diabetes insipidus, tremor, weight gain, hypothyroidism, nausea, diarrhea, seizures, teratogenicity (if used in the first trimester, 0.1% risk for Ebstein anomaly), acne, vomiting Narrow therapeutic window (0.8–1.2 mEq/L) Lithium toxicity (blood level > 1.5 mEq/L): Presents with ataxia, dysarthria, delirium, and acute renal failure Contraindicated in patients with ↓ renal function,
Lamotrigine	Second-line mood stabilizer; anticonvulsant	Blurred vision, GI distress, Stevens-Johnson syndrome. ↑ Dose slowly to monitor for rashes
Carbamazepine	Alternative mood stabilizer; anticonvulsant; trigeminal neuralgia	Nausea, skin rash, leukopenia, AV block. Teratogenicity (0.5–1% neural tube defect) Rarely, aplastic anemia (monitor CBC biweekly). Stevens-Johnson syndrome
Valproic acid	Bipolar disorder; anticonvulsant	GI side effects (nausea, vomiting), tremor, sedation, alopecia, weight gain, teratogenicity (3–5% risk for neural tube defect) Rarely, pancreatitis, thrombocytopenia, fatal hepatotoxicity, and agranulocytosis Contraindicated in patients with hepatic disease

- Severe mania: Mood stabilizer (lithium/valproate) + antipsychotic.
- Refractory mania: ECT.
- Mania/hypomania in pregnancy: Antipsychotics; typical antipsychotics (eg, haloperidol) are generally first line and have fewer risks to the developing fetus than mood stabilizers.
  - ECT can be used for severe or refractory mania in pregnancy.
- **Bipolar depression:** Mood stabilizers with or without antidepressants. Start mood stabilizer first to avoid inducing mania. May also try combination of mood stabilizer and antipsychotic if monotherapy fails.

Adjustment disorder, which consists of emotional and behavioral symptoms that develop in response to an identifiable stressor, lasts > 1 month and < 6 months, and does not have five or more symptoms of major depressive disorder.

Personality Disorders

Personality can be defined as an individual's set of emotional and behavioral traits, which are generally stable and predictable. Personality disorders are defined when one's traits become chronically rigid and maladaptive, leading to social or occupational dysfunction. Disorders are outlined in Table 2.14-14.

TABLE 2.14-14.   Signs and Symptoms of Personality Disorders

DISORDER	CHARACTERISTICS	CLINICAL PRESENTATION
CLUSTER A: "WEIRD"		
Paranoid	Distrustful, suspicious; interpret others' motives as malevolent Note: These patients will use projection as a defense mechanism	59-year-old man who lives alone constantly feels that his neighbor's children are spying on him and plotting to break into his home. He has installed security cameras all around his property to obtain proof. He feels he cannot trust the police to do a good job because they will probably take the side of his neighbors
Schizoid	Isolated, detached "loners" who prefer to be alone Restricted emotional expression	66-year-old man who moves to Thailand alone after retirement, has no desire to remain in contact with his family, and is very distant in his interactions. He stays in his remote accommodations without unnecessary travel and does not crave interaction with the locals
Schizotypal	Odd behavior, perceptions, and appearance Magical thinking; ideas of reference Note: Remember, in contrast to OCD, these patients do not feel their behavior is problematic (ego syntonic). They also do not have true obsessions and compulsions.	35-year-old man with very strange ideas regarding the importance of crystals and their effect on health. He meticulously mines and collects crystals, feeling that they will one day prevent him from acquiring cancer
CLUSTER B: "WILD"		
Borderline	Unstable mood, relationships, and self-image; feelings of emptiness Impulsive History of suicidal ideation or self-harm Note: These patients often employ splitting as a defense mechanism	28-year-old woman presents to clinic after having praised her new clinician as better than all the others. She reveals that she fired her last therapist, as he was not really helping. You notice she has fresh cuts in a row on her forearm

(continues)

TABLE 2.14-14.   Signs and Symptoms of Personality Disorders *(continued)*

Disorder	Characteristics	Clinical Presentation
Cluster B: "Wild"		
Histrionic	Excessively emotional and attention seeking Sexually provocative; theatrical	35-year-old woman presents to clinic wearing a very low-cut blouse, adjusting her position to draw attention to herself. When she does not get attention, she breaks into tears, saying that no one notices her, not even her friends
Narcissistic	Grandiose; need admiration; have sense of entitlement Lack empathy	45-year-old man sits impatiently tapping his foot in the waiting room of your office. He approaches the receptionist, demands to know where the doctor is, and tells her that he will have her fired and the doctor reported if he is not seen shortly. You are all wasting his time
Antisocial	Violate rights of others, social norms, and laws; impulsive; lack remorse Must be > 18 years of age Evidence of conduct disorder before 15 years of age	22-year-old man who was in juvenile detention for theft as a teenager and presents to your office now via court order after a brutal assault. He says that he does not need to be seen by a shrink and that the victim offended him and deserved the assault
Cluster C: "Worried and Wimpy"		
Obsessive-compulsive	Preoccupied with perfectionism, order, and control at the expense of efficiency Inflexible morals and values Note: Remember, in contrast to OCD, these patients do not feel their behavior is problematic (ego-syntonic). They also do not have true obsessions and compulsions	35-year-old woman presents to your office at the request of her boss, who feels she is too focused on minute details on team projects and does not allow others to participate for fear of unwanted errors. She does not see anything wrong with this style of work, as she believes her coworkers cannot be trusted to pay adequate attention to detail
Avoidant	Socially inhibited; rejection sensitive Fear of being disliked or ridiculed, yet desires to have friends and social interactions	33-year-old man stays at home to avoid an office party, as he fears having to make small talk. He wants to go, though he is more afraid that he will be inadequate or rejected by others
Dependent	Submissive, clingy; feel a need to be taken care of Have difficulty making decisions Feel helpless	30-year-old woman presents to your office in crisis, saying that her parents just kicked her out of their house and she is struggling to survive on her own. She says she cannot make her own choices at the grocery store, as her mother would always care for her, and now these decisions are overwhelming. She has been sitting outside of their house daily, hoping they will let her live there again

Defense mechanisms are methods of dealing with anxiety or conflicts of the ego (eg, anger, guilt, inadequacy, grief). These can be immature (more primitive) or mature (more sophisticated). Immature defense mechanisms are **common in personality disorders.** Important defense mechanisms are outlined in Table 2.14-15.

DIAGNOSIS

Diagnosis is clinical, and detailed history taking is imperative. Collateral information may be helpful. Patients typically deny or do not realize they have a problem (ego syntonic).

Q

A 22-year-old man frequently washes his hands, refuses to sit on chairs in public places, and will not use public transportation for fear of contracting diseases. He does not think his behaviors are abnormal, nor does he think his behaviors interfere with his daily activities. What is the diagnosis?

TABLE 2.14-15. Defense Mechanisms

IMMATURE	
Acting out	Expressing unacceptable feelings and thoughts through actions
Denial	Acting as if an aspect of reality does not exist; refusal to accept the situation
Displacement	Transferring feelings or impulses to a more neutral object
Intellectualization	Using facts and logic to avoid stressful thoughts or emotions
Passive aggression	Demonstrating hostile feelings in a nonconfrontational manner
Projection	Attributing an unacceptable internal impulse to others (vs displacement) Associated with paranoid personality disorder
Rationalization	Explaining unacceptable behaviors in a rational or logical manner
Reaction formation	Behaving in a manner opposite to one's true feelings and thoughts
Regression	Involuntarily reverting to an earlier developmental stage Associated with dependent personality disorder
Splitting	Believing that people are either all bad or all good Associated with borderline personality disorder

MATURE	
Sublimation	Channeling an unacceptable thought/wish with socially acceptable behaviors
Altruism	Coping with difficult stressors by meeting the needs of others
Suppression	Intentionally avoiding unwanted thoughts or feelings to deal with reality
Humor	Joking about an uncomfortable or anxiety-provoking situation

MNEMONIC

Characteristics of personality disorders—

MEDIC

Maladaptive
Enduring
Deviate from cultural norms
Inflexible
Cause impairment in social or occupational functioning

A

This person suffers from obsessive-compulsive personality disorder (OCPD). These patients are perfectionists, are preoccupied with rules and order, and are often inflexible. Unlike patients with obsessive-compulsive disorder, those with OCPD typically are not disturbed by their disease.

TREATMENT

- **Best initial treatment:** Psychotherapy.
- Pharmacotherapy is reserved for cases with comorbid mood, anxiety, or psychotic signs/symptoms.

Substance Use Disorders

Substance use disorder is a maladaptive pattern of substance use that leads to clinically significant impairment. It can be applied to most substances of abuse. The patient must meet ≥ 2 of the 11 criteria within a 1-year period for diagnosis. The criteria can be grouped into four categories of symptoms and are as follows:

- **Impaired control:**
  - Consumption of greater amounts of the substance than intended.
  - Failed attempts to cut down use or abstain from the substance.

- Increased amount of time spent acquiring, using, or recovering from effects.
  - Craving.
- **Social impairment:**
  - Failure to fulfill responsibilities at work, school, or home.
  - Continued substance use despite recurrent social or interpersonal problems 2° to the effects of such use (eg, frequent arguments with spouse over the substance use).
  - Isolation from life activities.
- **Risky use:**
  - Use of substances in physically hazardous situations (eg, driving while intoxicated).
  - Continued substance abuse despite recurrent physical or psychological problems 2° to the effect of the substance use.
- **Pharmacologic:**
  - Tolerance and use of progressively larger amounts to obtain the same desired effect.
- Withdrawal symptoms when not taking the substance.

Tolerance and withdrawal are not needed to make the diagnosis.

DIAGNOSIS/TREATMENT

- Diagnosis is typically clinical, and detailed history taking is imperative.
- **Lab tests:** Urine and blood toxicology screens, LFTs, and serum EtOH.
- Severity is determined by number of symptoms present.
  - **Mild:** 2–3, moderate 4–5, severe: ≥ 6.
- Management of intoxication for selected drugs is described in Table 2.14-16.

KEY FACT

Pinpoint pupils are not always a reliable sign of opioid ingestion, because co-ingestions can lead to normal or enlarged pupils. Also look for a ↓ respiratory rate, track marks, and ↓ breath sounds.

TABLE 2.14-16. **Signs and Symptoms of Substance Abuse**

DRUG	INTOXICATION	WITHDRAWAL
Alcohol	Disinhibition, emotional lability, slurred speech, ataxia, aggression, blackouts, hallucinations, memory impairment, impaired judgment, coma	Tremor, tachycardia, hypertension, malaise, nausea, seizures, delirium tremens (DTs), agitation
Opioids	Euphoria leading to apathy, CNS depression, constipation, pupillary constriction, and respiratory depression (life-threatening in overdose) Naloxone and naltrexone are opioid receptor antagonists and reverse the effects of opioids; may require redosing because of short half-life	Dysphoria, insomnia, anorexia, myalgias, fever, lacrimation, diaphoresis, dilated pupils, rhinorrhea, piloerection, nausea, vomiting, stomach cramps, diarrhea, yawning Opioid withdrawal is not life-threatening, "hurts all over," and does not cause seizures
Amphetamines	Psychomotor agitation, impaired judgment, hypertension, pupillary dilation, tachycardia, fever, diaphoresis, anxiety, angina, euphoria, prolonged wakefulness/attention, arrhythmias, delusions, seizures, hallucinations MDMA ("ecstasy") is an amphetamine with hallucinogenic properties; popular at dance parties or "raves." Intoxication: As above, plus hyperthermia, heat exhaustion, hyponatremia, may also precipitate serotonin syndrome Haloperidol can be given for severe agitation and symptom-targeted medications (eg, antiemetics, NSAIDs)	Post-use "crash" with anxiety, lethargy, headache, stomach cramps, hunger, fatigue, depression/dysphoria, sleep disturbance, nightmares

(continues)

TABLE 2.14-16.   Signs and Symptoms of Substance Abuse *(continued)*

DRUG	INTOXICATION	WITHDRAWAL
Cocaine	Psychomotor agitation, euphoria, impaired judgment, tachycardia, pupillary dilation, hypertension, paranoia, hallucinations, "cocaine bugs" (the feeling of bugs crawling under one's skin), sudden death Chronic use causes weight loss, erythema of the nasal turbinates and septum, and behavioral changes ECG changes from ischemia are often seen ("cocaine chest pain") Treat with haloperidol for severe agitation along with symptom-specific medications (eg, to control hypertension)	Post-use "crash" with hypersomnolence, depression, malaise, severe craving, angina, suicidality, ↑ appetite, nightmares
Phencyclidine hydrochloride (PCP)	Assaultive/combative, belligerence, psychosis, violence, impulsiveness, psychomotor agitation, fever, tachycardia, vertical/horizontal nystagmus, hypertension, impaired judgment, ataxia, seizures, delirium Give benzodiazepines or haloperidol for severe symptoms; otherwise reassure Gastric lavage can help eliminate the drug	Recurrence of intoxication symptoms caused by reabsorption in the GI tract; sudden onset of severe, random violence
LSD	Marked anxiety or depression, delusions, visual hallucinations, flashbacks, pupillary dilation, impaired judgment, diaphoresis, tachycardia, hypertension, heightened senses (eg, colors become more intense) Supportive counseling; traditional antipsychotics for psychotic symptoms; benzodiazepines for anxiety	None
Marijuana (cannabis)	Euphoria, laughter, slowed sense of time, impaired judgment, social withdrawal, ↑ appetite, dry mouth, conjunctival injection, hallucinations, anxiety, paranoia, ↓ motivation	None
Barbiturates	Low safety margin; respiratory depression	Anxiety, seizures, delirium, life-threatening cardiovascular collapse
Benzodiazepines	Interactions with alcohol, amnesia, ataxia, somnolence, mild respiratory depression Avoid using for insomnia in the elderly; can cause paradoxical agitation even in relatively low doses	Rebound anxiety, seizures, tremor, insomnia, hypertension, tachycardia, death
Caffeine	Restlessness, insomnia, diuresis, muscle twitching, arrhythmias, tachycardia, flushed face, psychomotor agitation	Headache, lethargy, depression, weight gain, irritability, craving
Nicotine	Restlessness, insomnia, anxiety, arrhythmias	Irritability, headache, anxiety, weight gain, craving, bradycardia, difficulty concentrating, insomnia
Synthetic opioids	Contains MPTP (synthetic heroin) leading to Parkinson-like disorder and loss of pigmented neurons in the substantia nigra	None
Bath salts (synthetic cathinones)	Stimulant drug that causes agitation, combativeness, delirium, and psychosis that may last for weeks	None

ALCOHOL USE DISORDER

Occurs more often in men (4:1) and in those 21–34 years of age, although the incidence in women is rising. Associated with a positive family history.

HISTORY/PE

See Table 2.14-16 for the symptoms of intoxication and withdrawal. Look for palmar erythema or telangiectasias and for other signs and symptoms of end-organ complications. Patients often present with sleep disturbances or anxiety symptoms caused by mild withdrawal.

DIAGNOSIS

- Screen with the CAGE questionnaire. Monitor vital signs for evidence of withdrawal.
- Labs may reveal ↑ LFTs (classically AST:ALT ratio > 2:1), ↑ LDH, ↑ carbohydrate-deficient transferrin, and ↑ mean corpuscular volume.

TREATMENT

- **Abstinence:**
  - **Best initial treatment:** Naltrexone (μ-opioid receptor blocker).
    - ↓ Cravings. Can start while patient is still drinking.
  - Long-term rehabilitation (eg, Alcoholics Anonymous).
- **Aversion:**
  - Disulfiram (acetaldehyde dehydrogenase inhibitor): Produces an unpleasant response (eg, flushing, nausea, vertigo, palpitations) when EtOH is consumed.
- **Withdrawal:**
  - Stabilize vital signs; correct electrolyte abnormalities.
  - Thiamine (administer before glucose to prevent Wernicke encephalopathy), glucose, and folic acid.
  - Start medium-length benzodiazepine taper (eg, lorazepam, diazepam, chlordiazepoxide).
  - Add haloperidol for hallucinations and psychotic symptoms.

COMPLICATIONS

- Gastritis (GI bleeds, ulcers), varices, or Mallory-Weiss tears.
- Pancreatitis, liver disease, DTs, alcoholic hallucinosis (see Table 2.14-17), peripheral neuropathy, Wernicke encephalopathy, Korsakoff psychosis, fetal alcohol syndrome, cardiomyopathy, anemia, aspiration pneumonia, ↑ risk for sustaining trauma (eg, subdural hematoma).

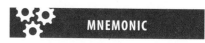

MNEMONIC

CAGE questionnaire:

1. Have you ever felt the need to **C**ut down on your drinking?
2. Have you ever felt **A**nnoyed by criticism of your drinking?
3. Have you ever felt **G**uilty about drinking?
4. Have you ever had to take a morning **E**ye opener?

More than one "yes" answer makes alcoholism likely.

KEY FACT

Naltrexone is a first-line pharmacotherapy to reduce the craving for alcohol. It works by blocking the μ-opioid receptor and can be given to patients who are still drinking.

TABLE 2.14-17. Alcoholic Hallucinosis vs Delirium Tremens

ALCOHOLIC HALLUCINOSIS	DELIRIUM TREMENS
12–24 hours since last drink	48–96 hours since last drink
Visual, auditory, and tactile hallucinations	Autonomic instability (hyperadrenergic state; ↑ BP, ↑ HR)
	Disorientation, agitation
	Hallucinations

Eating Disorders

ANOREXIA NERVOSA

Risk factors include female gender, low self-esteem, and high socioeconomic status. Associated with OCD, MDD, anxiety, and careers/hobbies such as modeling, gymnastics, ballet, and running.

HISTORY/PE

- Patients are often perfectionists and high-achieving. They have a distorted body image and fear of gaining weight. Divided into two subtypes:
    - **Restrictive:** Severe restriction of food intake is primary method of weight loss.
    - **Binge eating/purging:** Food intake is compensated by purging (eg, excessive exercise, vomiting, laxative/diuretic abuse).
- **Signs and symptoms:** Cachexia, body mass index (BMI) < 18.5 kg/m², lanugo, dry skin, bradycardia, lethargy, hypotension, cold intolerance, and hypothermia (as low as 35°C [95°F]).
- See Table 2.14-18 to differentiate anorexia nervosa from bulimia nervosa.

DIAGNOSIS

- Measure height and weight; check BMI; check CBC, electrolytes, endocrine levels, and ECG.
- Perform a psychiatric evaluation to screen patients for comorbid conditions.

TREATMENT

See Table 2.14-18.

COMPLICATIONS

See Table 2.14-19. Mortality from suicide or medical complications is > 10%.

> **KEY FACT**
>
> Bupropion should be avoided in the treatment of patients with eating disorders, as it is associated with a ↓ seizure threshold.

TABLE 2.14-18.   Anorexia Nervosa vs Bulimia Nervosa

CHARACTERISTIC	ANOREXIA NERVOSA	BULIMIA NERVOSA
Presentation	Persistent restriction of caloric intake resulting in low body weight, an intense fear of gaining weight, and a distorted body image (patients perceive themselves as fat)	Episodes of binge eating followed by compensatory behaviors (eg, purging, fasting, excessive exercise) Episodes occur at least once a week for ≥ 3 months
Weight	Patients are underweight (BMI < 18.5 kg/m²)	Patients are of normal weight or are overweight (BMI > 18.5 kg/m²)
Attitude toward illness	Patients are typically not distressed by their illness and may thus be resistant to treatment	Patients are typically distressed about their symptoms and are thus easier to treat
Treatment	Monitor calorie intake and weight gain; hospitalize if necessary Watch for refeeding syndrome (electrolyte abnormalities [↓ phosphate], arrhythmias, respiratory failure, and seizures after sudden ↑ in caloric intake) Psychotherapy: Address maladaptive family dynamics Antidepressants (SSRIs) are not effective Treat comorbidities. Avoid bupropion because of risk for seizure	Psychotherapy ± antidepressants (SSRIs) Treat comorbidities. Avoid bupropion because of risk for seizure

TABLE 2.14-19.   Medical Complications of Eating Disorders

Constitutional	Cardiac	GI	GU	Other
Cachexia	Arrhythmias	Dental erosions and decay	Amenorrhea	Dermatologic: lanugo
Hypothermia	Sudden death		Nephrolithiasis	Hematologic: leukopenia
Fatigue	Hypotension	Abdominal pain		Neurologic: seizures
Electrolyte abnormalities (hypokalemia, pH abnormalities)	Bradycardia	Delayed gastric emptying		Musculoskeletal: osteoporosis, stress fractures
	Prolonged QT interval			

BULIMIA NERVOSA

Eating disorder characterized by recurrent episodes of binge eating and compensatory purging behavior (eg, vomiting, laxative/diuretic abuse, excessive exercise). More common in women; associated with low self-esteem, mood disorders, and OCD.

HISTORY/PE

- Patients often have a long history of other comorbid psychiatric conditions (eg, anxiety, depression) and are concerned about their behaviors.
- **Signs:** Dental enamel erosion, enlarged parotid glands, scars on the dorsal hand surfaces (if there is a history of repeated induced vomiting), and BMI > 18.5 kg/m^2.
- See Table 2.14-18 to differentiate anorexia nervosa from bulimia nervosa.

TREATMENT

See Table 2.14-18.

COMPLICATIONS

See Table 2.14-19.

KEY FACT

Patients with bulimia tend to be more disturbed by their behavior than patients with anorexia and are more easily engaged in therapy. Patients with anorexia often deny health risks associated with their behavior, making them resistant to treatment.

Miscellaneous Disorders

SEXUAL DISORDERS

Sexual Changes with Aging

- Interest in sexual activity usually does not $\downarrow$ with aging.
- Men usually require $\uparrow$ stimulation of the genitalia for longer periods of time to reach orgasm; intensity of orgasm $\downarrow$, and the length of the refractory period before the next orgasm $\uparrow$.
- In women, estrogen levels $\downarrow$ after menopause, leading to vaginal dryness and thinning, which may result in discomfort during coitus. May be treated with hormone replacement therapy, estrogen vaginal suppositories, or other vaginal creams.

Paraphilic Disorders

- Preoccupation with or engagement in unusual sexual fantasies, urges, or behaviors for > 6 months with clinically significant impairment in one's life. There are eight classified disorders, characterized by disordered courtship (voyeurism, exhibitionism, and frotteurism), disordered preferences (pedophilia, transvestic fetishism, fetishism), and pleasure in inflicting/receiving pain (sadism, masochism). See Table 2.14-20.

TABLE 2.14-20. **Features of Common Paraphilic Disorders**

DISORDER	CLINICAL MANIFESTATIONS
Exhibitionistic	Sexual arousal from exposing one's genitals to a stranger
Pedophilic	Urges or behaviors involving sexual activities with children
Voyeuristic	Observing unsuspecting persons unclothed or involved in sex
Fetishistic	Use of nonliving objects (often clothing) for sexual arousal
Transvestic	Cross-dressing for sexual arousal
Frotteuristic	Touching or rubbing one's genitalia against a nonconsenting person (common in crowded places)
Sexual sadism	Sexual arousal from inflicting suffering on sexual partner
Sexual masochism	Sexual arousal from being hurt, humiliated, bound, or threatened

- **Tx:** includes insight-oriented psychotherapy and behavioral therapy. Antiandrogens (eg, medroxyprogesterone injection) have been used for hypersexual paraphilic activity.

Gender Dysphoria

- Strong, persistent cross-gender identification and discomfort with one's assigned sex or gender role of the assigned sex in the absence of intersexual disorders. Patients may have a history of dressing like the opposite sex, taking sex hormones, or pursuing surgeries to reassign their sex.
- More common in men than in women. Associated with depression, anxiety, substance abuse, and personality disorders.
- **Tx:** Educate the patient about culturally acceptable behavior patterns. Address comorbidities, psychotherapy, sex-reassignment surgery, or hormonal treatment (eg, estrogen for men, testosterone for women).
  - In teens, hormone-suppression therapy can be offered to delay puberty, but this decision should be made with support from family, if possible.

Sexual Dysfunction

- Problems in sexual arousal, desire, or orgasm, or pain with sexual intercourse.
- Prevalence is 30%; one-third of cases are attributable to biologic factors and another third to psychological factors.
- **Tx:** Depends on the condition. Pharmacologic strategies include PDE5 inhibitors (eg, sildenafil, tadalafil). If dysfunction is caused by antidepressants (SSRI), switch to bupropion. Psychotherapeutic strategies include sensate focusing.

SLEEP DISORDERS

Up to one-third of all American adults suffer from some type of sleep disorder during their lives. Dyssomnia describes any condition that leads to a disturbance in the normal rhythm or pattern of sleep. Insomnia is the most common example. Risk factors include female gender, the presence of mental and medical disorders, substance abuse, and advanced age.

Normal age-related sleep changes include more frequent awakenings, decreased total time asleep, and increased napping.

1° Insomnia

Affects up to 30% of the general population; causes sleep disturbance that is not attributable to physical or mental conditions. Often exacerbated by anxiety, and patients may become preoccupied with getting enough sleep.

DIAGNOSIS

Patients present with a history of nonrestorative sleep or difficulty initiating or maintaining sleep that is present at least three times per week for 1 month.

TREATMENT

- **Best initial treatment:** Initiate good sleep hygiene measures.
- **Next best treatment:** Pharmacotherapy; should be initiated with care for short periods of time (< 2 weeks). Pharmacologic agents include diphenhydramine, zolpidem, zaleplon, and trazodone.

1° Hypersomnia

DIAGNOSIS

Diagnosed when a patient complains of excessive daytime sleepiness or nighttime sleep that occurs for > 1 month. The excessive somnolence cannot be attributable to medical or mental illness, medications, poor sleep hygiene, insufficient sleep, or narcolepsy.

TREATMENT

- **Best initial treatment:** CNS stimulants (eg, amphetamines).
- Antidepressants such as SSRIs may be useful in some patients.

Narcolepsy

Onset typically occurs by young adulthood, generally before 30 years of age. Some forms of narcolepsy may have a genetic component.

DIAGNOSIS

- Manifestations include excessive daytime somnolence and ↓ REM sleep latency daily for at least 3 months. Sleep attacks are the classic symptom; patients cannot avoid falling asleep.
- Characteristic excessive sleepiness may be associated with the following:
  - **Cataplexy:** Sudden loss of muscle tone that leads to collapse.
  - **Hypnagogic hallucinations:** Occur as the patient is falling asleep.
  - **Hypnopompic hallucinations:** Occur as the patient awakens.
  - **Sleep paralysis:** Brief paralysis upon awakening.

TREATMENT

Treat with a regimen of scheduled daily naps plus stimulant drugs such as amphetamines or modafinil; give SSRIs for cataplexy.

Sleep Apnea

- Occurs 2° to disturbances in breathing during sleep that lead to excessive daytime somnolence and sleep disruption. Etiologies can be either central or peripheral.
  - **Central sleep apnea (CSA):** A condition in which both airflow and respiratory effort cease. CSA is linked to morning headaches, mood changes, and repeated awakenings during the night.
  - **Obstructive sleep apnea (OSA):** A condition in which airflow ceases as a result of obstruction along the respiratory passages. OSA is strongly associated with snoring.
    - Risk factors: Male gender, obesity, prior upper airway surgeries, a deviated nasal septum, a large uvula or tongue, and retrognathia (recession of the mandible).

KEY FACT

Recommended sleep hygiene measures: Stimulus control therapy to reestablish a circadian (24-hour) sleep/wake cycle.

- Establishment of a regular sleep schedule.
- Limiting of caffeine intake.
- Avoidance of daytime naps.
- Warm baths in the evening.
- Use of the bedroom for sleep and sexual activity only.
- Exercising early in the day.
- Relaxation techniques.
- Avoidance of large meals near bedtime.

- In both forms, arousal results in cessation of the apneic event.
- Associated with sudden death in infants and the elderly, headaches, depression, ↑ systolic BP, and pulmonary hypertension.

DIAGNOSIS

Sleep study (polysomnography) to document the number of arousals, obstructions, and episodes of ↓ O_2 saturation; distinguish OSA from CSA; and identify possible movement disorders, seizures, or other sleep disorders.

TREATMENT

- **OSA:** Nasal continuous positive airway pressure (CPAP). Weight loss if obese. In children, most cases are caused by tonsillar/adenoidal hypertrophy, which is corrected surgically.
- **CSA:** Mechanical ventilation (eg, BiPAP) with a backup rate for severe cases.

Circadian Rhythm Sleep Disorder

A spectrum of disorders characterized by a misalignment between desired and actual sleep periods. Subtypes include jet-lag type, shift-work type, delayed sleep-phase type ("night owls"), and unspecified.

TREATMENT

- Jet-lag type usually resolves within 2–7 days without specific treatment.
- Shift-work type and delayed sleep-phase type may respond to light therapy. Modafinil is approved for shift-work type sleep disorder.
- Oral melatonin may be useful if given 30 minutes before the desired bedtime.

SOMATIC SYMPTOM AND RELATED DISORDERS

Somatic Symptom Disorder

Patients often present with excessive thoughts, anxiety, and behaviors driven by the presence of somatic symptoms that is distressing and negatively affects daily life. This may occur with or without any medical illness present. High health care utilization is often present.

TREATMENT

- Regularly scheduled appointments with one clinician as 1° caregiver.
- Avoid unnecessary diagnostics, but legitimize symptoms.
- Psychotherapy focusing on reducing psychosocial stressors.

Conversion Disorder

Characterized by symptoms or deficits of voluntary motor or sensory function (eg, blindness, seizurelike movements, paralysis) incompatible with medical processes. Close temporal relationship to stress or intense emotion.

DIAGNOSIS

- Symptoms unexplained by other medical or neurologic causes.
- Physical exam signs suggesting nonorganic cause of symptoms:
  - Presence of Hoover sign (extension of affected leg when asked to raise the unaffected contralateral leg) when attempting to rule out leg paralysis.

KEY FACT

Factitious disorders and malingering are distinct from somatoform disorders in that they involve conscious and intentional processes.

- Eyes closed and resistant to opening during seizure; negative simultaneous EEG.
- Tremor disappears with distraction.
- **La belle indifference:** Patients are strangely indifferent to their symptoms.

TREATMENT

- Psychotherapy, PT/OT, treating comorbid psychiatric issues (anxiety, depression, trauma).
- Goal is to improve function.

FACTITIOUS DISORDERS AND MALINGERING

DIAGNOSIS

- **Factitious disorder:** Characterized by the fabrication of symptoms or self-injury to assume the sick role (primary gain).
  - Factitious disorder imposed on another (formerly Munchausen by proxy): Caregiver exaggerates or falsifies medical/psychiatric symptoms or intentionally induces illness in someone else to receive benefit by taking on the role of concerned caregiver.
- **Malingering:** Patients intentionally cause or feign symptoms for secondary gain (eg, financial, housing, legal).

TREATMENT

- Psychotherapy.
- Minimal diagnostics and treatment to avoid reinforcement of behaviors.
- Contact appropriate legal authorities (factitious disorder imposed on another).

KEY FACT

In malingering, patients intentionally simulate illness for personal gain.

SEXUAL AND PHYSICAL ABUSE

- Most frequently affects women < 35 years of age who:
  - Are experiencing marital discord and have a personal history of, or partner with, substance abuse.
  - Are pregnant, have low socioeconomic status, or have obtained a restraining order.
- Victims of childhood abuse are more likely to become adult victims of abuse.

HISTORY/PE

- Patients typically have multiple somatic complaints, frequent emergency department visits, and unexplained injuries with delayed medical treatment. They may also avoid eye contact or act afraid or hostile.
- Children may exhibit precocious sexual behavior, genital or anal trauma, STDs, UTIs, and psychiatric/behavioral problems.
- Other clues include a partner who answers questions for the patient or refuses to leave the exam room.

TREATMENT

- Perform a screening assessment of the patient's safety domestically and in her or his close personal relationships.
- Provide medical care, emotional support, and counseling.
- Educate the patient about support services, and refer appropriately.
- Documentation is crucial. Know local laws for reporting suspected child/elder abuse.

KEY FACT

Sexual abusers are usually male and are often known to the victim (and are often family members).

Q

A 57-year-old morbidly obese man presents to his physician with concerns about ↑ daytime sleepiness and ↓ work productivity. He recently received multiple divorce threats from his wife for excessive snoring that sounds like "the snort of a steam engine." What long-term complications are of concern for this patient?

SUICIDALITY

Accounts for 45,000 deaths per year in the United States; the 10th overall cause of death in the United States. Approximately one suicide occurs every 11 minutes.

- **Risk factors:** Male gender, > 45 years of age, psychiatric disorders (major depression, presence of psychotic symptoms), history of psychiatric hospitalization, previous suicide attempt (primary risk factor), history of violent behavior, ethanol or substance abuse, recent severe stressors, poor social support, and a family suicide history (see the mnemonic **SAD PERSONS**).
- Women are more likely to attempt suicide. Men use more lethal methods (eg, firearms) and are more likely to complete suicide.

DIAGNOSIS

- Perform a comprehensive psychiatric evaluation.
- Ask about family history, previous attempts, ambivalence toward death, and hopelessness.
- Ask directly about suicidal ideation, intent, and plan, and look for available means.

TREATMENT

- A patient who endorses suicidality requires emergent inpatient hospitalization even against his or her will.
- Suicide risk may ↑ after antidepressant therapy is initiated because a patient's energy to act on suicidal thoughts can return before the depressed mood lifts.

PULMONARY

KEY FACT

Beware—all that wheezes is not asthma! Other conditions that can cause wheezes are foreign body inhalation and COPD (ie, anything causing airway constriction).

 KEY FACT

Asthma should be suspected in children with multiple episodes of croup and URIs associated with dyspnea. Childhood eczema is also associated with asthma.

 KEY FACT

Asthma triggers include allergens, URIs, cold air, exercise, drugs, and stress.

Obstructive Lung Disease

Characterized by airway narrowing or collapse that causes impaired expiration; results in air trapping. Figure 2.15-1 illustrates the role of lung volume measurements in the diagnosis of lung disease; Table 2.15-1 and Figure 2.15-2 contrast obstructive with restrictive lung diseases.

ASTHMA

Reversible airway obstruction 2° to bronchial hyperreactivity, airway inflammation, mucous plugging, and smooth muscle hypertrophy. Most often diagnosed in childhood or early adulthood but can present later.

HISTORY/PE

- Usually presents with dry cough, episodic wheezing, dyspnea, and/or chest tightness, often worsening at night or in early morning.
- **PE:** Wheezing, prolonged expiration ($\downarrow$ I/E ratio), increased accessory muscle use, tachypnea, tachycardia, hyperresonance, and possible pulsus paradoxus (severe).
- **Late signs:** $\downarrow$ Breath sounds, cyanosis, and $\downarrow$ O_2 saturation, hypercapnia ($\uparrow$ $Paco_2$).
- **Aspirin-exacerbated respiratory disease:** Samter's triad of asthma and chronic rhinosinusitis with nasal polyps that is exacerbated with aspirin or NSAID use.
  - Pseudoallergic reaction (not IgE mediated).

DIAGNOSIS

- **Best initial test:** Spirometry/PFTs; obstructive pattern that is reversible with short-acting β-agonists (SABA).
  - $FEV_1/FVC < 70\%$, $\downarrow$ FEV_1, normal/$\downarrow$ FVC, $\uparrow$ RV and TLC, normal/$\uparrow$ DLCO (diffusing capacity of the lung for carbon monoxide). Increase in $FEV_1 \geq 12\%$ with SABA (albuterol). PFTs are often normal between exacerbations.
- **Methacholine challenge:** Tests for bronchial hyperresponsiveness; useful when PFTs are normal but asthma is still suspected. Considered positive with $\geq 20\%$ decrease in FEV_1.

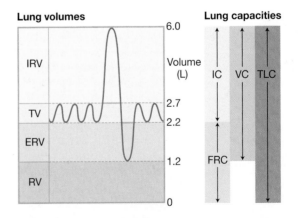

FIGURE 2.15-1. **Lung volumes in the interpretation of PFTs.** (Reproduced with permission from USMLE-Rx.com.)

TABLE 2.15-1.   Obstructive vs Restrictive Lung Disease

Test	Normal	Obstructive	Restrictive
FEV_1/FVC (FEV_1 %)	> 0.70	↓	Normal/↑
FEV_1 (% of predicted)	80–120%	↓	↓
FVC (% of predicted)	80–120%	Normal/↓	↓
FRC (% of predicted)	80–120%	↑	↓
TLC (% of predicted)	80–120%	↑	↓

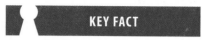

KEY FACT

FEV_1/FVC ratio < 70% suggests obstructive ventilatory defect. FEV_1/FVC ratio ≥ 70% suggests restrictive ventilatory defect.

KEY FACT

Summary of asthma medications:
- PRN medications—short-acting bronchodilators (eg, albuterol).
- Long-term medications—inhaled corticosteroids, long-acting β_2-agonists (eg, salmeterol), long-acting muscarinic antagonists (LAMAs), and PO corticosteroids.

- **Arterial blood gas (ABG):**
  - Early exacerbation: Respiratory alkalosis caused by hyperventilation (↓ $Paco_2$, ↑ pH, mild hypoxemia).
  - Late/severe exacerbation (impending respiratory failure): Respiratory muscle fatigue results in respiratory acidosis caused by inability to ventilate (normalizing $Paco_2$, normalizing pH, ↓ Pao_2).
- **Chest x-ray (CXR):** Normal appearance to hyperinflation with flattening of the diaphragm.

TREATMENT

In general, avoidance of allergens or any potential triggers. See Tables 2.15-2 and 2.15-3 for asthma medications and management guidelines.

- **Acute exacerbation:**
  - O_2, SABA (albuterol is first-line), systemic glucocorticoids. SABA/ipratropium and magnesium can be used in severe exacerbations.
    - Never use ipratropium alone in asthma treatment.
  - Consider intubation in severe cases (cyanosis, inability to maintain respiratory effort, altered mental status) or acutely in patients with a $Paco_2 > 50$ mmHg or a $Pao_2 < 50$ mmHg.

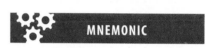

MNEMONIC

Meds for asthma exacerbations—

ASTHMA

Albuterol
Steroids
Theophylline (rare)
Humidified O_2
Magnesium (severe exacerbations)
Anticholinergics

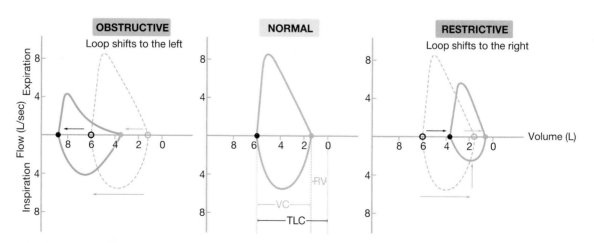

FIGURE 2.15-2.   Obstructive vs restrictive lung disease. Shown are typical alterations in lung volumes and capacities in restrictive and obstructive diseases. (Reproduced with permission from USMLE-Rx.com.)

TABLE 2.15-2. Common Asthma Medications and Their Mechanisms

DRUG	MECHANISM OF ACTION
β_2-agonists	Albuterol: Short acting (SABA). Relaxes bronchial smooth muscle (β_2-adrenoceptors) Salmeterol: Long-acting (LABA) agent for maintenance therapy
Corticosteroids	Inhaled corticosteroids are first-line treatment for long-term control of asthma Beclomethasone, prednisone: Inhibit the synthesis of cytokines
Muscarinic antagonists	Ipratropium: Short acting (SAMA). Competitively blocks muscarinic receptors, preventing bronchoconstriction Tiotropium: Long-acting (LAMA)
Methylxanthines	Theophylline: Causes bronchodilation by inhibiting phosphodiesterase, thereby $\downarrow$ cAMP hydrolysis and $\uparrow$ cAMP levels Usage is limited because of its narrow therapeutic-toxic index (cardiotoxicity, neurotoxicity)
Cromolyn	Prevents the release of vasoactive mediators from mast cells Useful for exercise-induced bronchospasm Effective only for the maintenance of asthma; not effective during an acute attack. Toxicity is rare
Antileukotrienes	Zileuton: A 5-lipoxygenase pathway inhibitor; blocks conversion of arachidonic acid to leukotrienes Montelukast, zafirlukast: Block leukotriene receptors
Anti-IgE	Omalizumab: Monoclonal antibody against IgE; inhibits IgE binding to IgE receptor (FcεRI) on mast cells. Used in patients with allergic asthma
Anti-IL-5	Mepolizumab: Monoclonal antibody against IL-5 (potent chemoattractant for eosinophils)

TABLE 2.15-3. Medications for the Chronic Treatment of Asthma

TYPE	SYMPTOMS (DAY/NIGHT)	FEV$_1$	MEDICATIONS
Mild intermittent	$\leq$ 2 days/week $\leq$ 2 nights/month	$\geq$ 80%	Step 1: ▪ No daily medications ▪ SABA (albuterol) PRN
Mild persistent	> 2 times/week but < 1 time/day > 2 nights/month	$\geq$ 80%	Step 2: ▪ Daily low-dose ICS ▪ SABA (albuterol) PRN
Moderate persistent	Daily > 1 night/week	60–80%	Step 3: ▪ Low-dose ICS + LABA or ▪ Medium-dose ICS ▪ SABA (albuterol) PRN
Severe persistent	Continual, frequent	$\leq$ 60%	Step 4: Medium-dose ICS + LABA Step 5 (if unable to control symptoms): High-dose ICS + LABA Step 6 (if still unable to control symptoms): High-dose ICS + LABA + PO SABA (albuterol) PRN for all steps

- **Maintenance therapy:** Determined by the classification of asthma severity. See Table 2.15-3.
  - **Step 1:** Inhaled SABA (albuterol) as needed for symptom control is first-line.
  - **Step 2:** Add daily medication for long-term control. Low-dose inhaled corticosteroids (ICS) are preferred. Alternatives include cromolyn, leukotriene receptor antagonist (LTRA), or theophylline. Continue albuterol PRN.
  - **Step 3:** Add long-acting β-agonist (LABA) such as salmeterol to low-dose ICS or ↑ dose of ICS to medium-dose. Continue albuterol PRN.
  - **Step 4:** Medium-dose ICS + LABA. Continue albuterol PRN.
  - **Step 5:** High-dose ICS + LABA. Consider omalizumab (anti-IgE) or mepolizumab (anti-IL-5) for patients with allergies (↑ IgE). Continue albuterol PRN.
  - **Step 6:** High-dose ICS + LABA + oral corticosteroid. Continue albuterol PRN.

BRONCHIECTASIS

A disease caused by recurrent cycles of infection and inflammation in the bronchi/bronchioles that leads to fibrosis, remodeling, and permanent dilation of bronchi (see Figure 2.15-3).

HISTORY/PE

- Presents with chronic productive cough accompanied by frequent bouts of yellow or green sputum production, dyspnea, and possible hemoptysis and halitosis.
- Associated with a history of cystic fibrosis (CF), pulmonary infections, hypersensitivity, immunodeficiency, localized airway obstruction, aspiration, autoimmune disease, or IBD, but seen more closely in allergic bronchopulmonary aspergillosis, tuberculosis, and nontuberculous mycobacterium such as *Mycobacterium avium complex* (MAC).
- Exam reveals rales, wheezes, rhonchi, purulent mucus, and occasional hemoptysis.

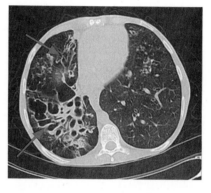

FIGURE 2.15-3. Bronchiectasis. Chest CT demonstrates markedly dilated and thick-walled airways (*arrows*) consistent with bronchiectasis in this CF patient. (Reproduced with permission from USMLE-Rx.com.)

DIAGNOSIS

- **CXR:** Shows ↑ bronchovascular markings and tram lines (parallel lines outlining dilated bronchi as a result of peribronchial inflammation and fibrosis).
- **Most accurate test:** High-resolution CT; dilated airways (ie, larger than pulmonary arteries) and ballooned cysts are seen at the end of the bronchus (mostly lower lobes).
- **Spirometry/PFTs:** Obstructive pattern with ↓ FEV_1/FVC ratio.

TREATMENT

- **Medications:** Antibiotics (↓ bacterial load and airway/systematic inflammatory mediators).
  - **Empiric therapy:** Respiratory fluoroquinolone (levofloxacin, moxifloxacin).
  - Tailor treatment to sputum culture results, if available.
  - **Allergic bronchopulmonary aspergillosis (ABPA):** Systemic glucocorticoids and antifungals (voriconazole, itraconazole).
- **Lifestyle:** Bronchopulmonary hygiene (cough promotion, postural drainage, chest physiotherapy).
- **Surgery:** Consider lobectomy for localized disease or lung transplantation for severe disease.

KEY FACT

In patients with COPD and chronic hypercapnia, excess supplemental oxygen can decrease ventilatory drive, resulting in worsening hypercapnia and respiratory acidosis.

KEY FACT

Consider α_1-antitrypsin deficiency in a patient who is < 60 years of age, has minimal or no smoking history, or has basilar-predominant COPD.

KEY FACT

Supplemental O_2 and smoking cessation are the only interventions proven to improve survival in patients with COPD.

CHRONIC OBSTRUCTIVE PULMONARY DISEASE

A disease with ↓ lung function associated with airflow obstruction. Can be divided into two major subtypes:

- **Chronic bronchitis:** Productive cough for > 3 months per year for 2 consecutive years (clinical diagnosis).
- **Emphysema:** Destruction and dilation of structures distal to the terminal bronchioles (pathologic diagnosis) that may be 2° to smoking (centrilobular) or to α_1-antitrypsin deficiency (panlobular).

HISTORY/PE

- Symptoms are minimal or nonspecific until the disease is advanced.
- The clinical spectrum is shown in Table 2.15-4 (most patients are a combination of the two phenotypes).
- Look for the classic barrel chest, use of accessory chest muscles, jugular vein distention (JVD), end-expiratory wheezing, dyspnea on exertion, and muffled breath sounds.

DIAGNOSIS

- **Best initial test:** Spirometry (PFTs); obstructive pattern that is nonreversible with SABA.
  - FEV_1/FVC <70%, ↓ FEV_1, normal/↓ FVC, ↑ RV and TLC. Minimal (< 12%) to no change in FEV_1 with SABA (albuterol).
    - ↓ DLCO (emphysema or late-stage COPD). Normal DLCO (chronic bronchitis).
- **CXR:** Hyperinflated lungs, ↓ lung markings with flat diaphragms, and a thin-appearing heart and mediastinum are sometimes seen. Parenchymal bullae or subpleural blebs (pathognomonic of emphysema) are also seen (see Figure 2.15-4).
- **ABGs:** Hypoxemia with acute or chronic respiratory acidosis (↑ Pco_2).
- **Gram stain and sputum culture:** Consider if bacterial infection is suspected (eg, fever, productive cough, new infiltrate on CXR).

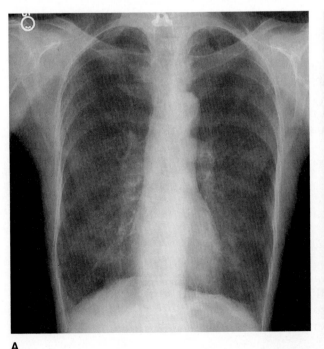

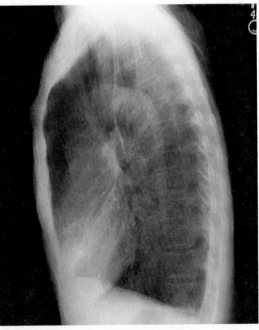

A   **B**

FIGURE 2.15-4. **COPD.** (A) PA and (B) lateral radiographs of a patient with emphysema show hyperinflation with large lung volumes, flattening of the diaphragm, and minimal peripheral vascular markings. (Reproduced with permission from USMLE-Rx.com.)

TABLE 2.15-4. **COPD Subtypes**

COPD Type	Nickname	Definition	Appearance	Acid-Base Status
Emphysema	"Pink puffer"	Terminal airway destruction and dilation	Thin, wasted appearance with pursed lips, minimal cough	Late hypercarbia/ hypoxia (hence pink)
Chronic bronchitis	"Blue bloater"	Productive cough > 3 months for 2 years	Overweight, edematous	Early hypercarbia/ hypoxia (hence blue)

TREATMENT

See Table 2.15-5.

TABLE 2.15-5. **COPD Treatment**

	TREATMENT

Acute exacerbation	■ Supplemental O_2 (titrate Spo_2 to 88–92%)
	■ Inhaled bronchodilators
	  ■ SABA (albuterol) and anticholinergics (ipratropium)
	■ Systemic corticosteroids (prednisone)
	■ Add antibiotics if ≥ 2 cardinal symptoms:
	  ■ ↑ Dyspnea
	  ■ ↑ Cough
	  ■ Sputum production (change from baseline)
	■ Severe exacerbations (respiratory failure, severe hypoxemia or respiratory acidosis, altered mental status):
	  ■ Noninvasive positive-pressure ventilation (NPPV) with BiPAP (bilevel positive airway pressure) first
	  ■ If NPPV fails, the next step is tracheal intubation

Chronic COPD	■ Lifestyle modifications: Smoking cessation, pneumococcal vaccine, influenza vaccine (PPSV23 = polysaccharide; PCV13 = conjugate)
	  ■ < 65 years of age: PPSV 23 alone
	  ■ ≥ 65 years of age: PCV 13 + PPSV 23
	  ■ All ages: influenza annually
	■ Inhaled bronchodilators
	  ■ SABA (albuterol), LABA (salmeterol), anticholinergics (ipratropium, tiotropium)
	■ If ≥ 2 exacerbations per year, consider adding ICS
	■ Long-term oxygen therapy (LTOT)
	  ■ Indications:
	    ■ Spo_2 ≤ 88% or Pao_2 ≤ 55 mmHg
	    ■ Spo_2 ≤ 89% or Pao_2 ≤ 59 mmHg if evidence of cor pulmonale, right heart failure, or polycythemia (Hct > 55%) is present
	  ■ Supplemental O_2 can worsen hypercapnia. The goal oxygen saturation is 90–93%

KEY FACT

Treatments for acute asthma and COPD exacerbations both involve β_2-agonists and corticosteroids. During an acute COPD exacerbation, antibiotics may also be given. During an acute asthma exacerbation, magnesium can be given.

MNEMONIC

Treatment for COPD—

COPD

Corticosteroids
Oxygen (if resting Spo_2 < 88% or < 89% with cor pulmonale)
Prevention (smoking cessation, pneumococcal and influenza vaccines)
Dilators (β_2-agonists, anticholinergics)

MNEMONIC

Etiology of restrictive lung disease—

If the lungs AIN'T compliant

Alveolar (edema, hemorrhage, pus)

Interstitial lung disease (ILD) (idiopathic interstitial pneumonias), **I**nflammatory (sarcoid, cryptogenic organizing pneumonia), **I**diopathic pulmonary fibrosis (IPF)

Neuromuscular (myasthenia, phrenic nerve palsy, myopathy)

Thoracic wall (kyphoscoliosis, obesity, ascites, pregnancy, ankylosing spondylitis)

KEY FACT

Medications and interventions that can cause or contribute to ILD include amiodarone, busulfan, nitrofurantoin, bleomycin, methotrexate, radiation, and long-term high O_2 concentration (eg, Pao_2 ventilators).

Restrictive Lung Disease

Characterized by a loss of lung compliance, restrictive lung diseases result in ↑ lung stiffness and ↓ lung expansion. Table 2.15-1 and Figure 2.15-2 contrast obstructive with restrictive lung disease. The etiologies of restrictive lung disease are shown in the mnemonic **AIN'T.**

INTERSTITIAL LUNG DISEASE

A heterogeneous group of disorders characterized by inflammation and/or fibrosis of the interstitium. In advanced disease, cystic spaces can develop in the lung periphery, which gives the characteristic "honeycomb" pattern seen on CT (see Figure 2.15-5A). Also called diffuse parenchymal lung disease (DPLD).

Subgroups:

- **Exposure related:** Asbestosis, silicosis, berylliosis, coal worker's pneumoconiosis, medications (eg, amiodarone, bleomycin), hypersensitivity pneumonitis, radiation-induced injury.
- **ILD associated with systemic disease or connective tissue diseases:** Polymyositis/dermatomyositis, sarcoidosis, amyloidosis, vasculitis, CREST syndrome.
- **Idiopathic:** Idiopathic pulmonary fibrosis, cryptogenic organizing pneumonia, acute interstitial pneumonia.

HISTORY/PE

- Presents with shallow, rapid breathing; progressive dyspnea with exertion; and a chronic nonproductive cough.
- Patients may have cyanosis, inspiratory squeaks, fine or "velcro-like" crackles, clubbing, or right heart failure.

DIAGNOSIS

- **Best initial test:** CXR; reticular, nodular, or ground-glass pattern.
  - **Next best step:** If CXR is suspicious of ILD, then high-resolution CT. CT shows "honeycomb" pattern (severe disease).

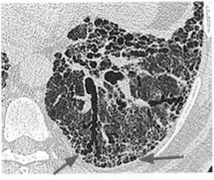
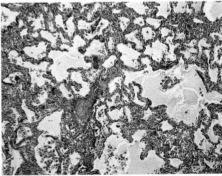

A **B**

FIGURE 2.15-5. Idiopathic pulmonary fibrosis. (A) Chest CT showing the characteristic "honeycomb" lung that is seen in advanced disease. **(B)** Lung biopsy specimen demonstrating increased interstitial fibrosis and nonspecific inflammation with alveolar thickening. (Reproduced with permission from USMLE-Rx.com.) (Image A reproduced with permission from Walsh SLF, Wells AU, Sverzellati N, et al. Relationship between fibroblastic foci profusion and high-resolution CT morphology in fibrotic lung disease. *BMC Med.* 2015;13:241. Image B reproduced with permission from USMLE-Rx.com).

- **PFTs**: Restrictive pattern.
  - Normal/↑ FEV₁/FVC, ↓ FVC, ↓ FEV₁, ↓ TLC, ↓ FVC, ↓ DLCO.
- If systemic disease is suspected as the cause, consider serologic testing (eg, ANA, anti-CCP, CK, aldolase, anti-Jo1, ANCA, anti-topoisomerase, anti-dsDNA).
- **Most accurate test:** Surgical biopsy; often to confirm a diagnosis of IPF (see Figure 2.15-5B).
  - Only performed when diagnosis is uncertain (eg, atypical CT findings, equivocal PFTs).

TREATMENT

- **Supportive:** Avoid exposure to causative agents.
- **Medications:** Anti-inflammatory/immunosuppressive agents for some disease (eg, corticosteroids), antifibrotic agents (pirfenidone, nintedanib) for IPF.
- **Surgery:** Lung transplantation may be indicated at late stages of IPF.

SYSTEMIC SARCOIDOSIS

A multisystem disease of unknown etiology characterized by infiltration of non-caseating granulomas. Most commonly found in African-American women and Northern European whites; most often arises in the third or fourth decade of life.

HISTORY/PE

- Can present with fever, cough, dyspnea, malaise, weight loss, and arthritis.
  - **Lofgren syndrome:** Erythema nodosum, hilar adenopathy, migratory polyarthralgias, and fever.
- Extrapulmonary manifestations can involve the following organs: Liver, eyes (uveitis), skin (erythema nodosum, violaceous skin plaques), nervous system, heart (third-degree heart block, arrhythmias), and kidneys.

DIAGNOSIS

- **Best initial test:** CXR shows bilateral hilar adenopathy and reticular opacities (upper lobe predominant). High-resolution CT is usually done following suspicious CXR.
  - **Next best step:** If CXR/CT is suspicious, then lymph node biopsy. Noncaseating granulomas is diagnostic in presence of correct clinical picture with exclusion of other diseases.
- **PFTs:** Restrictive pattern and ↓ DLCO.
- **Other findings:** ↑ Serum ACE levels (neither sensitive nor specific), hypercalcemia, hypercalciuria, ↑ alkaline phosphatase (with liver involvement), lymphopenia, cranial nerve defects, arrhythmias.

TREATMENT

- **Asymptomatic:** Observation.
- **Symptomatic:** Systemic corticosteroids are indicated for deteriorating respiratory function, constitutional symptoms, hypercalcemia, or extrathoracic organ involvement.
- **Refractory disease:** Immunosuppressants (eg, methotrexate, azathioprine, TNFα inhibitors).
- **Lofgren Syndrome:** NSAIDs and supportive therapy.

MNEMONIC

Learning the features of sarcoid can be GRUELING—

Granulomas
a**R**thritis
Uveitis
Erythema nodosum
Lymphadenopathy (particularly hilar, seen on CXR)
Interstitial fibrosis
Negative TB test
Gammaglobulinemia

KEY FACT

Lofgren syndrome is a type of sarcoidosis with the following triad: arthritis, erythema nodosum, and bilateral hilar adenopathy.

A 10-year-old child with a history of asthma on daily fluticasone has been using an albuterol inhaler once a day for several weeks. What changes should be made to the current regimen?

HYPERSENSITIVITY PNEUMONITIS

Alveolar thickening and noncaseating granulomas 2° to environmental exposure (eg, mold, hot tubs, birds, down feather antigens).

HISTORY/PE

- **Acute:** Dyspnea, fever, malaise, shivering, and cough starting 4–6 hours after exposure. Gather a job/travel history to determine exposure.
- **Chronic:** Patients present with progressive dyspnea; exam reveals fine bilateral rales.

DIAGNOSIS

Appearance on CXR/CT is variable, but upper lobe fibrosis is a common feature of chronic disease.

TREATMENT

Avoid ongoing exposure to inciting agents; give corticosteroids to ↓ chronic inflammation.

PNEUMOCONIOSIS

Risk factors include prolonged occupational exposure and inhalation of small inorganic dust particles.

HISTORY/PE/DIAGNOSIS

Table 2.15-6 outlines the findings and diagnostic criteria associated with common pneumoconioses.

TREATMENT

Avoid triggers; supportive therapy and supplemental O_2.

EOSINOPHILIC PULMONARY SYNDROMES

A diverse group of disorders characterized by eosinophilic pulmonary infiltrates and abnormal peripheral blood eosinophilia. Includes ABPA, Löffler syndrome, acute eosinophilic pneumonia, and drug-induced (eg, NSAIDs, nitrofurantoin, sulfonamides).

HISTORY/PE

Presents with dyspnea, cough, potentially blood-tinged sputum, and/or fever.

DIAGNOSIS

- **CBC:** May reveal peripheral eosinophilia.
- **CXR:** Shows pulmonary infiltrates.
- **Bronchoalveolar lavage:** ↑ Eosinophils (> 25%).

TREATMENT

Removal of the extrinsic cause or treatment of underlying infection (eg, helminths) if identified. Corticosteroid treatment may be used.

This child has moderate persistent asthma with daily symptoms. The patient will benefit from an inhaled corticosteroid and a long activating β₂-agonist, such as salmeterol, for prevention of symptoms.

TABLE 2.15-6.   Diagnosis of Pneumoconioses

DISORDER	HISTORY	IMAGING FINDINGS[a]	COMPLICATIONS
Asbestosis	Work involving the manufacture of tile or brake linings, insulation, construction, demolition, or shipbuilding Presents 15–20 years after initial exposure	Linear opacities at lung bases and interstitial fibrosis; calcified pleural plaques (see Images A and B) are indicative of benign pleural disease. Image C shows ferruginous bodies in alveolar septum	↑ Risk for mesothelioma (rare) and lung cancer; the risk for lung cancer is higher in smokers. The most common malignancy associated with asbestos exposure is bronchogenic carcinoma
Coal worker's disease	Work in underground coal mines	Small nodular opacities (< 1 cm) in upper lung zones	Progressive massive fibrosis
Silicosis	Work in mines or quarries or with glass, pottery, or silica	Small (< 1-cm) nodular opacities in upper lung zones; eggshell calcifications	↑ Risk for TB; need annual TB skin test Progressive massive fibrosis
Berylliosis	Work in high-technology fields such as aerospace, nuclear, and electronics plants; ceramics industries; foundries; plating facilities; dental material sites; and dye manufacturing	Diffuse infiltrates; hilar adenopathy	Requires chronic corticosteroid treatment

A   B   C

Image A reproduced with permission from Dr. Yale Rosen. Image B reproduced with permission from Miles SE, Sandrini A, Johnson AR, et al. Clinical consequences of asbestos-related diffuse pleural thickening: a review. *J Occup Med Toxicol* 2008;3:20. Image C reproduced with permission from Nephron.

[a]Spirometry, consistent with restrictive disease.

Acute Respiratory Failure

HYPOXEMIA

↓ PaO_2; causes include ventilation-perfusion (V/Q) mismatch, right-to-left shunt, hypoventilation, low inspired O_2 content (high altitudes), and diffusion impairment.

History/PE

Findings depend on the etiology. ↓ SpO_2, cyanosis, tachypnea, shortness of breath, pleuritic chest pain (caused by wheezing, coughing), and altered mental status may be seen.

Q

A 25-year-old African-American woman presents with painful bumps on her shins, weight loss, and cough. Exam reveals a prominent 1-cm right axillary lymph node. What is the next best step for diagnosis?

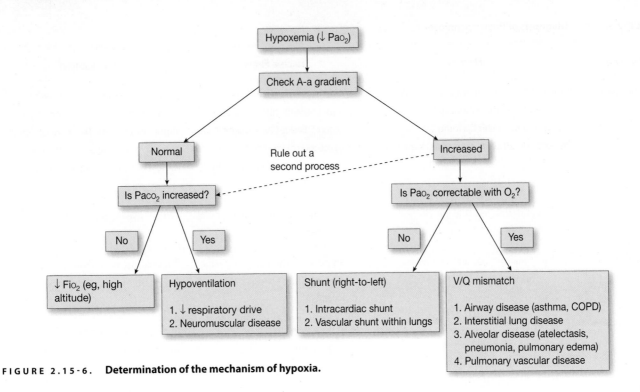

FIGURE 2.15-6. **Determination of the mechanism of hypoxia.**

TABLE 2.15-7. **Mechanical Ventilator Parameters Affecting Oxygenation and Ventilation**

↑ OXYGENATION	↑ VENTILATION
↑ FiO_2	↑ Respiratory rate
↑ PEEP	↑ Tidal volume

DIAGNOSIS

- **Best initial test:** ABGs; show ↓ PaO_2. Calculate the alveolar-arterial (A-a) oxygen gradient: $([P_{atm} - 47] \times FiO_2 - [PaCO_2/0.8]) - PaO_2$.
- **CXR:** To evaluate for an infiltrative process (eg, pneumonia), atelectasis, a large pleural effusion, or pneumothorax and to assess for acute respiratory distress syndrome (ARDS). An ↑ A-a gradient suggests shunt, V/Q mismatch, or diffusion impairment. Figure 2.15-6 summarizes the approach toward hypoxemic patients.

TREATMENT

- Address the underlying etiology.
- Administer O_2 before initiating evaluation.
- ↑ Oxygenation parameters if the patient is on mechanical ventilation (see Table 2.15-7).
- In hypercapnic patients, ↑ ventilation (↑ RR or ↑ TV) to ↑ CO_2 exchange.

ACUTE RESPIRATORY DISTRESS SYNDROME

Respiratory failure with refractory hypoxemia, ↓ lung compliance, and non-cardiogenic pulmonary edema with a $PaO_2/FiO_2 \leq 300$. Pathogenesis is thought to be dependent on endothelial injury.

Common triggers are as follows:

- Sepsis (most common), pneumonia, aspiration, multiple blood transfusions (> 15 units), inhaled/ingested toxins, drowning, and trauma. Overall mortality is 30–40%.

HISTORY/PE

- Presents with acute-onset (12–48 hours) tachypnea, dyspnea, and tachycardia ± fever, cyanosis, labored breathing, diffuse high-pitched rales, and hypoxemia in the setting of one of the systemic inflammatory causes or exposure.

This is presumed sarcoidosis. Biopsy of the right axillary lymph node is the next best step for diagnosis and is less invasive than transbronchial lung biopsy.

- Additional findings are as follows:
  - **Phase 1 (acute injury):** Normal physical exam; possible respiratory alkalosis.
  - **Phase 2 (6–48 hours):** Hyperventilation, hypocapnia, widening A-a gradient.
  - **Phase 3:** Acute respiratory failure, tachypnea, dyspnea, ↓ lung compliance, scattered rales, diffuse chest opacity on CXR (see Figure 2.15-7).
  - **Phase 4:** Severe hypoxemia unresponsive to therapy; ↑ intrapulmonary shunting; metabolic and respiratory acidosis.

DIAGNOSIS

The criteria for ARDS diagnosis (according to the Berlin definition) are as follows:

- Acute onset (< 1 week) of respiratory distress.
- **Ground-glass appearance on CXR:** Bilateral alveolar infiltrate consistent with pulmonary edema.
  - Pulmonary edema on CXR < 24 hours after insult suggests pulmonary contusion instead of ARDS.
- A PaO_2/FiO_2 ratio ≤ 300 with positive end-expiratory pressure (PEEP)/CPAP ≥ 5 cm H_2O.
- Respiratory failure not completely explained by heart failure.

TREATMENT

- Treat the underlying disease, and maintain adequate perfusion to prevent end-organ damage.
- Mechanical ventilation with low tidal volumes (4–6 cc/kg of ideal body weight) to minimize ventilator-induced lung injury by overdistention of alveoli.
- Use PEEP to recruit collapsed alveoli, and titrate PEEP and FiO_2 to achieve adequate oxygenation.
  - To ↑ PaO_2, ↑ PEEP.
  - Keep FiO_2 ≤ 60% (0.6), if possible to prevent oxygen toxicity.
- Goal oxygenation is PaO_2 > 55 mmHg or SpO_2 > 88%.
- Extubation may be attempted if:
  - The cause of respiratory failure has been improved.
  - Ventilator support required is minimal (low PEEP, low pressure support).
  - Oxygen supplementation is easily accomplished without the support of PEEP or other adjuvant treatments.
  - Patient passes a spontaneous breathing trial.

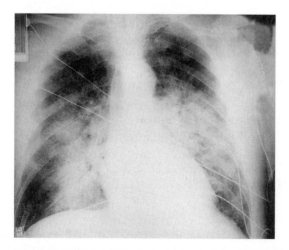

FIGURE 2.15-7.   Anteroposterior CXR showing a diffuse alveolar filling pattern 2° to ARDS. (Reproduced with permission from Kasper DL, et al. *Harrison's Principles of Internal Medicine,* 16th ed. New York, NY: McGraw-Hill; 2005.)

Q

A 25-year-old man in the ICU is intubated following an acute asthma exacerbation. A repeat ABG is sent after intubation and shows a pH of 7.5, a $PaCO_2$ of 33 mm Hg, and an HCO_3^- of 26 mEq/L. What adjustments, if any, would you make to the ventilator settings?

Pulmonary Vascular Disease

PULMONARY HYPERTENSION/COR PULMONALE

- **Pulmonary hypertension (PH):** Elevated pulmonary arterial pressure (> 25 mmHg) at rest.
    - Classified into the following groups by etiology:
        - Group 1: Pulmonary arterial hypertension (PAH).
        - Group 2: ↑ Pulmonary venous pressure from left-sided heart disease.
        - Group 3: Hypoxic vasoconstriction 2° to chronic lung disease.
        - Group 4: Chronic thromboembolic disease.
        - Group 5: Pulmonary hypertension with an unclear, multifactorial etiology.
- **Cor pulmonale:** Alteration in structure and function of the right ventricle (RV) of the heart caused by a primary disorder of the respiratory system, most commonly PH.
    - Right-sided heart failure can occur in severe cases.

HISTORY/PE

- Presents with dyspnea and syncope on exertion, and fatigue, lethargy, chest pain, and symptoms of right-sided CHF (edema, abdominal distention, JVD).
- **Hx:** COPD, interstitial lung disease, heart disease, sickle cell anemia, emphysema, and pulmonary emboli.
- **PE:** Loud, palpable S2 (often split), a flow murmur, an S4, or a parasternal heave. Patient may also be hypoxemic, especially on exertion.

DIAGNOSIS

- **Best initial test:** Echocardiogram estimates pulmonary artery (PA) pressure and assesses RV function.
- **CXR:** Shows enlargement of central pulmonary arteries with rapid tapering of the distal vessels (pruning).
- **ECG:** Demonstrates right ventricular hypertrophy (RVH).
- **Most accurate test:** Right heart catheterization; mean pulmonary artery pressure > 25 mmHg (normal: 8–20 mmHg).

TREATMENT

- Treat underlying disease. Supplemental O_2, diuretics, anticoagulation, digoxin, and exercise should be considered in all groups.
    - **Group 1 (Primary PAH):** IV Prostanoids; endothelin receptor antagonists (bosentan), and phosphodiesterase (PDE) inhibitors can be added for further symptom relief.
        - Some patients have vasoreactivity and respond well to calcium channel blockers.
    - **Group 4 (thromboembolic disease):** Surgical thrombectomy; anticoagulation and thrombolytics are alternatives for individuals who cannot undergo surgery.

PULMONARY THROMBOEMBOLISM

An occlusion of the pulmonary vasculature by a blood clot. Ninety-five percent of emboli originate from deep venous thrombosis (DVT) in the deep leg veins (eg, femoral vein). May lead to pulmonary infarction, right heart failure, and hypoxemia.

KEY FACT

Causes of PH include left heart failure, mitral valve disease, and ↑ resistance in the pulmonary veins, including hypoxic vasoconstriction.

KEY FACT

Other etiologies of embolic disease include postpartum status (amniotic fluid emboli), fracture (fat emboli), cardiac surgery (air emboli), and endovascular procedure (cholesterol emboli).

MNEMONIC

VIRchow triad—

Vascular trauma
Increased coagulability
Reduced blood flow (stasis)

This patient has an uncompensated respiratory alkalosis caused by ↑ ventilation. To ↓ ventilation, tidal volume can be ↓ or respiratory rate can be slowed, however reducing tidal volume can trigger an ↑ in ventilatory rate, exacerbating the situation.

TABLE 2.15-8. Virchow Triad for Venous Thrombosis

Venous Stasis	Endothelial Injury	Hypercoagulability
Immobility	Trauma	Pregnancy, postpartum
CHF	Surgery	Cigarette use
Obesity	Recent fracture	OCP use
↑ Central venous pressure	Previous DVT	Coagulation disorders (eg, protein C/protein S deficiency, factor V Leiden)
		Malignancy
		Severe burns

TABLE 2.15-9. Modified Wells Criteria for Pulmonary Embolism

Criteria	Points
Signs/symptoms of DVT	3
PE is most likely clinical diagnosis	3
Tachycardia (HR > 100/ min)	1.5
Immobilization (≥ 3 days) or surgery in last month	1.5
Previous PE/DVT	1.5
Hemoptysis	1
Malignancy	1

Traditional Clinical Probability Assessment	
High	> 6
Moderate	2 to 6
Low	< 2

Simplified Clinical Probability Assessment	
PE likely	> 4
PE unlikely	≤ 4

History/PE

- Factors predisposing to thromboembolism are summarized by the Virchow triad (see Table 2.15-8).
- Presents with sudden onset or subacute dyspnea, pleuritic chest pain, low-grade fever, cough, tachypnea, tachycardia, and rarely, hemoptysis (indicates pulmonary infarction).
- May have history of immobility (eg, long plane ride, bed-bound).
- Exam may reveal a loud P_2 and prominent jugular A waves with right heart failure.
- Patients with acute massive pulmonary embolism (PE) will present with hypotension, JVD, and new-onset right bundle branch block.

Diagnosis

- Best initial step: Calculate modified Wells score (Table 2.15-9).
  - PE unlikely (modified Wells score ≤ 4):
    - Best initial test: D-dimer used to rule out PE. High negative predictive value and sensitivity; not specific.
      - If ↑ D-dimer (≥ 500 ng/mL) → CT chest with contrast (or V/Q).
      - If normal D-dimer → PE excluded.
  - PE likely (modified Wells score > 4):
    - Best initial test: CT chest with contrast has high sensitivity and specificity (see Figure 2.15-8).

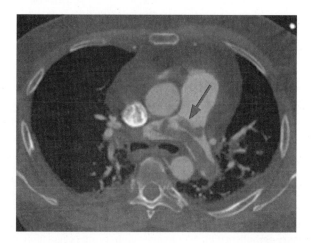

FIGURE 2.15-8. **Pulmonary embolus.** Axial slice from a CT pulmonary angiogram shows a pulmonary embolus extending from the main pulmonary artery into the right and left pulmonary arteries, consistent with a saddle embolus. (Reproduced with permission from Chen MY, et al. *Basic Radiology*, 2nd ed. New York, NY: McGraw-Hill; 2011.)

Dyspnea, tachycardia, and a normal CXR in a hospitalized and/or bedridden patient should raise suspicion of PE.

MNEMONIC

Wells criteria—

SHIT PMH

Symptoms of DVT: 3 points
History of DVT or PE: 1.5 points
Immobilization (≥ 3 days): 1.5 points
Tachycardia (HR > 100/min): 1.5 points
Post-op (surgery within previous 4 weeks): 1.5 points
Malignancy: 1 point
Hemoptysis: 1 point
Total point value = 11

- **V/Q scan:** Used when CT scan is contraindicated (↑ Cr [contraindication to contrast], pregnancy [contraindication to radiation]). May reveal areas of V/Q mismatch to predict low, indeterminate, or high probability of PE. Sensitive for PE, but not specific, especially if there is underlying lung disease.
- **ABGs:** Respiratory alkalosis caused by hyperventilation (↓ Pao_2 [< 80 mm Hg], ↓ $Paco_2$).
- **CXR:** Most often normal. May show atelectasis, pleural effusion, Hampton hump (a wedge-shaped infarct), Westermark sign (oligemia/collapse of vessels seen distal to PE).
- **ECG:** Most commonly reveals sinus tachycardia. The classic triad of S1Q3T3 is rare (acute right heart strain with an S wave in lead I, a Q wave in lead III, and an inverted T wave in lead III).
- **Lower extremity venous ultrasound:** Specific and sensitive for DVT that may be the cause of the PE. Not used in the diagnosis of PE.

TREATMENT

- **Anticoagulation:** See Figure 2.15-9.
    - **Acute:** Unfractionated heparin, subcutaneous low-molecular weight heparin (LMWH), subcutaneous fondaparinux, or direct oral anticoagulants (rivaroxaban, apixaban). In patients with high probability of PE, anticoagulation should be given before confirmatory testing.
        - Use unfractionated heparin in patients with renal failure.
    - **Chronic:** LMWH, direct oral anticoagulants, or warfarin (goal INR = 2–3).
        - Use LMWH in pregnancy (warfarin is contraindicated).

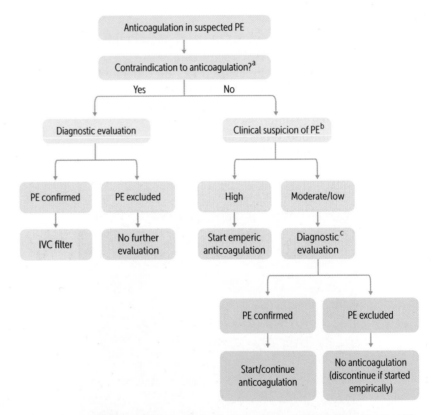

FIGURE 2.15-9. Guide to anticoagulation in hemodynamically stable patients with a suspected pulmonary embolism (PE). [a]Contraindications to anticoagulation include recent surgery, hemorrhagic stroke, active bleeding (eg, GI bleed) and aortic dissection. [b]Clinical suspicion of PE is determined using the modified Wells criteria: high > 6, moderate 2–6, low < 2. [c]If diagnostic evaluation cannot be completed within 4 hours, start empiric anticoagulation. (Reproduced with permission from USMLE-Rx.com.)

- **IVC filter:** Indicated in patients with a documented lower extremity DVT/PE if anticoagulation is contraindicated or if patients experience recurrent emboli while anticoagulated.
- **Thrombolysis:** Indicated in cases of massive PE causing right heart failure and hemodynamic instability (saddle PE).
- **DVT prophylaxis:** Treat all immobile patients; give subcutaneous heparin or low-dose LMWH, intermittent compression of the lower extremities (less effective), and early ambulation (most effective).

Neoplasms of the Lungs

SOLITARY PULMONARY NODULES

Commonly found on CXR. History, physical exam, and imaging features help guide treatment (see Table 2.15-10).

History/PE

- Often asymptomatic; may present with chronic cough, dyspnea, and shortness of breath.
- Always inquire about smoking and exposure history, which are associated with ↑ cancer risk.

Diagnosis & Treatment

- **Best initial test:** Chest CT. Obtain noncontrast chest CT if nodule was discovered on another modality.
  - If nodule has fat or calcifications characteristic of a benign lesion (eg, hamartoma, granuloma), then no further evaluation.
  - If nodule does not have characteristics of a benign lesion, then next step is to review medical record for a previous CT (if available).
    - If nodule is old and size is stable (> 2 years), then no further evaluation.
    - If nodule is new, increasing in size, or no prior CT scans are available, then determine risk for malignancy (see Table 2.15-11).
      - Low risk: Serial CT scans.
      - Intermediate risk: Further investigation required with biopsy or PET.
      - High risk: Surgical resection.

KEY FACT

Lung nodule clues based on the history:
- Recent immigrant—think TB.
- From the southwestern United States—think coccidioidomycosis.
- From the Ohio River Valley—think histoplasmosis or blastomycosis.

TABLE 2.15-10.   Characteristics of Benign and Malignant Lung Nodules

Benign	Malignant
Age < 35 years	> 45–50 years of age
Nonsmoker	Smoker
No change from old films	New or enlarging lesions
Central, uniform, or popcorn calcification	Absent or irregular calcification
Smooth margins	Irregular margins (scalloped, spiculated)
Size < 2 cm	Size > 2 cm

Q

A 25-year-old woman presents with dyspnea, chest pain, and leg pain. She takes birth control pills regularly. She returned from Asia 3 days ago. What is the next step?

TABLE 2.15-11. Risk for Malignancy in Patients with Solitary Pulmonary Nodules

Variable	Low	Intermediate	High
Diameter of nodule (cm)	< 0.8	0.8–2	≥ 2
Age (years)	< 45	45–60	> 60
Smoker?	Never	Yes	Yes
Years since smoking cessation	> 15	5–15	< 5
Nodule characteristics	Smooth	Scalloped	Corona radiata or spiculated

LUNG CANCER

The leading cause of cancer death in the United States. Risk factors include tobacco smoke (except for bronchioalveolar carcinoma) and radon or asbestos exposure. Types are as follows (see also Table 2.15-12):

- **Small cell lung cancer (SCLC):**
  - Highly correlated with cigarette exposure. Central location (see Figure 2.15-10), neuroendocrine origin; associated with paraneoplastic syndromes (see Table 2.15-13).
  - Metastases are often found on presentation in intrathoracic and extrathoracic sites such as brain, liver, and bone.
- **Non–small cell lung cancer (NSCLC):** Group of cancers, with the most common types being adenocarcinoma, squamous cell carcinoma (SCC), and large cell carcinoma. These cancers are less likely than SCLC to metastasize at an early stage.
  - **Adenocarcinoma:** Most common lung cancer; peripheral location.
    - Bronchioalveolar carcinoma (BAC): Subtype of adenocarcinoma; has unique pathologic and clinical features. Associated with multiple nodules, interstitial infiltration, and prolific sputum production (often confused with pneumonia). Good prognosis, ↓ association with smoking.
  - **SCC:** Has a central location; strongly associated with smokers.

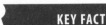

KEY FACT

Squamous and **S**mall cell cancers are **S**entral lesions.

The next step is to treat with a heparin bolus. When there is high clinical suspicion (birth control, history of long flight, multiple symptoms) for a DVT, one should treat first and follow with imaging (CT angiogram). With patients who have lower clinical suspicion, imaging is warranted first before treatment.

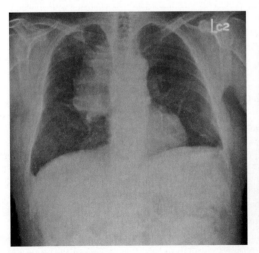

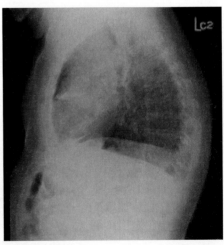

A

B

FIGURE 2.15-10. **Small cell lung cancer.** Note the central location of the tumor in the posteroanterior (**A**) and lateral (**B**) x-rays of the chest. (Reproduced with permission from Kantarjian HM, et al. *MD Anderson Manual of Medical Oncology.* New York, NY: McGraw-Hill; 2006.)

TABLE 2.15-12.   **Small Cell and Non–Small Cell Lung Cancers**

Type	Location	Characteristics	Histology
Small Cell			
Small cell (oat cell) carcinoma	Central	Undifferentiated → very aggressive May produce **A**CTH (Cushing syndrome), SI**A**DH, or **A**ntibodies against presynaptic Ca^{2+} channels (Lambert-Eaton myasthenic syndrome) or neurons (paraneoplastic myelitis/encephalitis) Amplification of *myc* oncogenes common Inoperable; treat with chemotherapy	Neoplasm of neuroendocrine Kulchitsky cells → small dark blue cells (see Image A) Chromogranin A ⊕
Non–Small Cell			
Adenocarcinoma	Peripheral	Most common lung cancer in nonsmokers and overall (except for metastases). Activating mutations include *KRAS, EGFR*, and *ALK* Associated with hypertrophic osteoarthropathy (clubbing) Bronchioloalveolar subtype (adenocarcinoma in situ): CXR often shows hazy infiltrates similar to pneumonia; favorable prognosis	Glandular pattern on histology, often stains mucin ⊕ (see Image B) Bronchioloalveolar subtype: grows along alveolar septa → apparent "thickening" of alveolar walls
Squamous cell carcinoma	Central	Hilar mass arising from bronchus (see Image C); cavitation; cigarettes; hypercalcemia (produces PTHrP)	Keratin pearls (see Image D) and intercellular bridges
Large cell carcinoma	Peripheral	Highly anaplastic undifferentiated tumor; poor prognosis. Less responsive to chemotherapy; removed surgically	Pleomorphic giant cells Can secrete β-hCG
Bronchial carcinoid tumor	—	Favorable prognosis; metastasis rare Symptoms usually caused by mass effect; occasionally carcinoid syndrome (5-HT secretion → flushing, diarrhea, wheezing)	Nests of neuroendocrine cells; chromogranin A ⊕

A   B   C   D

Reproduced with permission from Le T, et al. *First Aid for the USMLE Step 1 2015.* New York, NY: McGraw-Hill; 2015. Images A and D reproduced with permission from USMLE-Rx.com. Image B reproduced with permission from the US Department of Health and Human Services and Armed Forces Institute of Pathology. Image C reproduced with permission from Dr. James Heilman.

- **Large cell carcinoma:** Highly anaplastic undifferentiated tumor with poor prognosis.
- **Bronchial carcinoid tumor:** Neuroendocrine tumor with favorable prognosis.

History/PE

- **Presentation:** Cough, hemoptysis, dyspnea, wheezing, pneumonia, chest pain, weight loss, and possible abnormalities on respiratory exam (crackles, atelectasis).

MNEMONIC

Lung cancer mets are often found in LABBs—

Liver
Adrenals
Brain
Bone

TABLE 2.15-13. Paraneoplastic Syndromes of Lung Cancer

CLASSIFICATION	SYNDROME	HISTOLOGIC TYPE
Endocrine/metabolic	Cushing syndrome (ACTH)	Small cell
	SIADH leading to hyponatremia	Small cell
	Hypercalcemia (PTHrP)	Squamous cell
	Gynecomastia	Large cell
Skeletal	Hypertrophic pulmonary osteoarthropathy (including digital clubbing)	Non–small cell
Neuromuscular	Peripheral neuropathy	Small cell
	Subacute cerebellar degeneration	Small cell
	Myasthenia (Lambert-Eaton syndrome)	Small cell
	Dermatomyositis	All
Cardiovascular	Migratory thrombophlebitis	Adenocarcinoma
	Nonbacterial verrucous endocarditis	Adenocarcinoma
Hematologic	Anemia	All
	DIC	All
	Eosinophilia	All
	Thrombocytosis	All
	Hypercoagulability	Adenocarcinoma
Cutaneous	Acanthosis nigricans	All

- **Superior sulcus tumors (Pancoast tumors):** Tumor at the apex of the lung, adjacent to the subclavian vessels. Presentation is dependent on which of the following structures are compressed:
  - **Brachial plexus:** Shoulder pain (most common initial symptom) and arm pain (C8–T2 radicular pain).
  - **Paravertebral sympathetic chain and inferior cervical (stellate) ganglion:** Horner syndrome (miosis, ptosis, anhidrosis).
- **SVC syndrome:** Obstruction of the SVC with supraclavicular venous engorgement and facial swelling (see Figure 2.15-11).
- **Hoarseness:** 2° to recurrent laryngeal nerve involvement.
- Many paraneoplastic syndromes (see Table 2.15-13).

DIAGNOSIS

- **Best initial test:** CXR or chest CT.
- If initial test is suspicious of malignancy, obtain tissue sample next.
- **Most accurate tests:** Fine-needle aspiration (CT guided) for peripheral lesions and bronchoscopy (biopsy or brushing) for central lesions.

TREATMENT

- **SCLC:** Unresectable. Often responds to radiation and chemotherapy initially but usually recurs; has a low median survival rate.
- **NSCLC:** Surgical resection in early stages. Supplement surgery with radiation or chemotherapy (depending on the stage). Palliative radiation and/or chemotherapy is appropriate for symptomatic but unresectable disease.

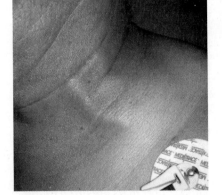

FIGURE 2.15-11. SVC syndrome. Prominent JVD is seen in SVC syndrome 2° to obstruction of the SVC by a central malignant lesion. (Reproduced with permission from Tintinalli JE, et al. *Tintinalli's Emergency Medicine: A Comprehensive Study Guide,* 7th ed. New York, NY: McGraw-Hill; 2011.)

TABLE 2.15-14. **Causes of Pleural Effusions**

TRANSUDATES	EXUDATES
CHF	Pneumonia (parapneumonic effusion)
Cirrhosis (hepatic hydrothorax)	TB
Nephrotic syndrome	Malignancy
	PE
	Collagen vascular disease (rheumatoid arthritis, SLE)
	Pancreatitis
	Trauma
	Chylothorax (↑ triglycerides)

Pleural Disease

PLEURAL EFFUSION

An abnormal accumulation of fluid in the pleural space.

Classified as follows:

- **Transudate:** 2° to ↑ pulmonary capillary wedge pressure (PCWP) or ↓ oncotic pressure.
- **Exudate:** 2° to ↑ pleural vascular permeability.

Table 2.15-14 lists the possible causes of both transudates and exudates.

HISTORY/PE

Presents with dyspnea, pleuritic chest pain, and/or cough. Exam reveals dullness to percussion and ↓ breath sounds over the effusion (see Table 2.15-15). A pleural friction rub may be present.

DIAGNOSIS

- **Best initial test:** CXR; blunting of the costophrenic angle. Lateral decubitus view is most sensitive; also used to assess for loculation.
- **Next step:** Thoracentesis indicated for new effusions > 1 cm in decubitus view, except with bilateral effusions and other clinical evidence of CHF.

TABLE 2.15-15. **Pulmonary Physical Exam Findings**

	LUNG CONSOLIDATION (EG, LOBAR PNEUMONIA)	PLEURAL EFFUSION	PNEUMOTHORAX
Percussion	Dull	Dull	Hyperresonant
Tactile fremitus	↑	↓	↓
Breath sounds	Bronchial	↓	↓/Absent
Voice transmission	Bronchophony Egophony	↓	↓
Crackles	Present (often)	Absent	Absent

A 65-year-old patient with a 30-pack-year history presents with a 2-week history of facial swelling. Biopsy reveals a hilar SCLC. What is the next step in treatment?

TABLE 2.15-16. Light's Criteria for Pleural Effusions[a]

Measure	Value
Pleural protein/serum protein	> 0.5
Pleural LDH/serum LDH	> 0.6
Pleural fluid LDH	> ⅔ the upper limit of normal serum LDH > 60 U/L[b]

[a]An effusion is an exudate if any of the above criteria are met.
[b]Using normal serum LDH: 45–90 U/L

- Use Light's criteria to determine if the effusion is transudative or exudative (see Table 2.15-16).
  - Transudative effusions: Typically have a pH of 7.4–7.55.
  - Exudative effusions: Typically have a pH of 7.30–7.45.
- Effusion is an exudate if it meets any of Light's criteria (see Table 2.15-16).
  - Exudative effusions: Require further workup (eg, pleural fluid glucose, amylase, cytology, cell count, culture, Gram stain, AFB, TB antigen, RF, CCP, ANA).
- **Complications:**
  - Parapneumonic effusion and empyema: Pleural effusions that arise as result of pneumonia, lung abscess, or bronchiectasis. See Table 2.15-17.
  - Recurrent effusion.

TREATMENT

- Treat the underlying cause of the effusion.
- See Table 2.15-17 for treatment of parapneumonic effusions and empyemas.
- **Recurrent effusions:** May require pleurodesis (procedure to obliterate pleural space).

KEY FACT

Complicated parapneumonic effusions necessitate chest tube drainage.

TABLE 2.15-17. Parapneumonic Effusions and Empyemas

	Uncomplicated Parapneumonic Effusion	Complicated Para-pneumonic Effusion	Empyema
Etiology	Fluid movement into pleural space (caused by inflammation associated with pneumonia)	Persistent bacterial invasion into pleural space	Bacterial colonization of pleural space
Appearance	Clear/cloudy	Cloudy	Purulent
Pleural fluid Analysis	pH > 7.2 Glucose: Normal/↓ LDH Ratio > 0.6	pH < 7.2 Glucose: ↓ LDH Ratio > 0.6	pH < 7.2 Glucose: ↓ LDH Ratio > 0.6
Pleural fluid Gram stain and culture	Negative	Negative	Positive
Treatment	Antibiotics	Antibiotics Chest tube	Antibiotics Chest tube

The mainstay of therapy for SCLC is chemotherapy, which yields high rates of response.

PNEUMOTHORAX

Collection of air in the pleural space that can lead to pulmonary collapse. Etiologies are the following:

- **1° Spontaneous pneumothorax:** 2° to rupture of subpleural apical blebs (usually found in tall, thin young men).
- **2° Pneumothorax:** 2° to COPD, trauma, infections (TB, *Pneumocystis jirovecii*), and iatrogenic factors (thoracentesis, subclavian line placement, positive-pressure mechanical ventilation, bronchoscopy).
- **Tension pneumothorax:** A pulmonary or chest wall defect acts as a one-way valve causing air trapping in the pleural space. Buildup of air pushes the mediastinum to the opposite side of the chest, which can obstruct venous return to the heart, leading to cardiac arrest and hemodynamic instability. Shock and death occur unless immediately treated.

HISTORY/PE

- Presents with acute onset of unilateral pleuritic chest pain and dyspnea.
- Exam reveals tachypnea, diminished or absent breath sounds, hyperresonance, ↓ tactile fremitus, and JVD 2° to compression of the SVC. See Table 2.15-15.
- **Tension pneumothorax:** Presents with respiratory distress, hypoxia, tracheal deviation, and hemodynamic instability.

DIAGNOSIS

- The diagnosis of a tension pneumothorax should be made clinically and should be followed by immediate decompression for treatment.
- CXR shows the presence of a visceral pleural line and/or lung retraction from the chest wall (best seen in end-expiratory films; see Figure 2.15-12). In an ED or ICU setting, bedside ultrasound can be used and has a high sensitivity and specificity.

TREATMENT

- **Tension pneumothorax:** Requires immediate needle decompression (second intercostal space at the midclavicular line) followed by chest tube placement.
- **Small pneumothorax (≤ 2 cm):** Observation ± supplemental O_2. It may resorb spontaneously.

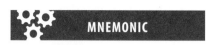

MNEMONIC

Presentation of pneumothorax—

P-THORAX

Pleuritic pain
Tracheal deviation
Hyperresonance
Onset sudden
Reduced breath sounds (and dyspnea)
Absent fremitus (asymmetric chest wall)
X-ray shows collapse.

KEY FACT

Treatment of a tension pneumothorax requires needle decompression first, then chest tube placement.

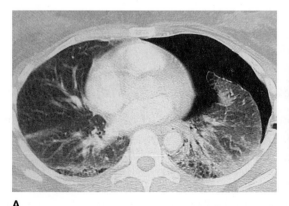
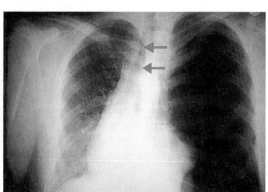

A   **B**

FIGURE 2.15-12. **Pneumothorax. (A)** Pneumothorax. CT shows collapsed left lung. **(B)** Tension pneumothorax. Note the hyperlucent left lung field with low left hemidiaphragm *(below the field of view)* and rightward mediastinal/tracheal shift *(arrows).* (Reproduced with permission from Le T, et al. *First Aid for the USMLE Step 1 2015.* New York, NY: McGraw-Hill; 2015.)

- **Large (> 3 cm), symptomatic pneumothorax:** Needle aspiration.
- **Unstable patients or recurrent pneumothorax:** Chest tube placement.

Pulmonary Sleep Disorders

OBSTRUCTIVE SLEEP APNEA

OSA is a sleep disorder characterized by transient obstruction of the upper airway that causes hypoxemia. Etiology may be central (eg, stroke), secondary (eg, obesity), or mixed. Risk factors include male gender, older age, obesity, craniofacial abnormalities, upper airway abnormalities (adenotonsillar hypertrophy [children]), sedative use (eg, alcohol, benzodiazepines), smoking, and many others.

HISTORY/PE

- **Cardinal features:**
    - **Irregular respiratory pattern during sleep:** Obstructive apneas, hypopneas, or respiratory effort–related arousals (RERAs).
    - **Daytime symptoms related to poor sleep:** Somnolence, fatigue, poor concentration, morning headaches.
    - **Signs of disturbed sleep:** Snoring, gasping, choking, restlessness.
- **Complications:**
    - ↑ Cardiovascular morbidity (systemic hypertension, PAH, coronary artery disease, arrhythmias, heart failure, polycythemia, and stroke).
    - ↑ Risk for insulin resistance and type 2 diabetes mellitus.
    - ↑ Risk for motor vehicle collisions caused by impaired alertness.

DIAGNOSIS

- **Best initial test:** Polysomnography (sleep study); based on apnea-hypopnea index (AHI = apneas + hypopneas/total hours of sleep) and presence or absence of related symptoms.
- **Diagnosis is confirmed with the following:**
    - AHI ≥ 5 PLUS symptoms.
    - AHI ≥ 15 regardless of symptoms.

TREATMENT

- **Best initial therapy:** Weight loss (if applicable) and continuous positive airway pressure (CPAP).
- **Alternatives:** Uvulopalatopharyngoplasty (surgical removal of excess oropharyngeal tissue), oral appliances, and hypoglossal nerve stimulation.
- **Last resort:** Tracheostomy.

OBESITY HYPOVENTILATION SYNDROME

OHS is a sleep disorder defined as awake alveolar hypoventilation in an obese individual that cannot be attributed to other conditions associated with alveolar hypoventilation.

HISTORY/PE

- Presents with hypersomnolence and obesity. Further characterized by coexisting sleep disturbances:
    - **OHS with OSA (90% of patients):** Presents with symptoms of OSA (see above).

- **OHS with sleep-related hypoventilation (10%):** Presents the same as OHS + OSA but witnessed apneas during sleep are uncommon.

DIAGNOSIS

- Diagnosis of exclusion; patient must meet all of the following criteria:
  - Obesity (BMI > 30 kg/m^2).
  - Awake alveolar hypoventilation (Paco$_2$ > 45 mmHg).
  - Exclusion of alternative causes of hypercapnia and hypoventilation.

TREATMENT

- **Best initial treatment:** Weight loss and noninvasive positive airway pressure (PAP).
  - **OHS + OSA:** CPAP.
    - Initiate bilevel positive airway pressure (BiPAP) if initial management with CPAP fails.
  - **OHS + hypoventilation:** BiPAP.
- **Next best treatment:**
  - Bariatric surgery.
  - Tracheostomy (last resort).

NOTES

Electrolyte Disorders

HYPERNATREMIA

Serum sodium > 145 mEq/L. Usually caused by free water loss rather than sodium gain. Refer to the Endocrinology chapter for a review of diabetes insipidus, an important cause of hypernatremia.

HISTORY/PE

Presents with thirst (caused by hypertonicity), neurologic symptoms including altered mental status, weakness, focal neurologic deficits, and seizures.

DIAGNOSIS

See Figure 2.16-1 for the hypernatremia diagnostic algorithm. Diagnosis is based on urine osmolality and urine sodium.

TREATMENT

- Determine volume status. If hypovolemic with unstable vital signs, use isotonic 0.9% NaCl before correcting free water deficits. If normal volume status and asymptomatic, can treat with D_5W, 0.45% NaCl or enteral fluids.
- Use isotonic 0.9% NaCl until the patient is euvolemic, even with stable vital signs.
- Determine free water deficit. Water deficit = Total body water × ([serum Na/140] − 1).
    - Total body water (TBW) is ± 60% of lean body weight.
    - Replace with D_5W, 0.45% NaCl, or enteral water.
- Determine rate of replacement. Correction of chronic hypernatremia (> 48 hours) should be accomplished gradually over 48–72 hours (≤ 0.5 mEq/L/h) to prevent neurologic damage secondary to cerebral edema.
- Euvolemic and hypervolemic hypernatremia are rare and treated with a combination of diuretics and D_5W to remove excess Na.

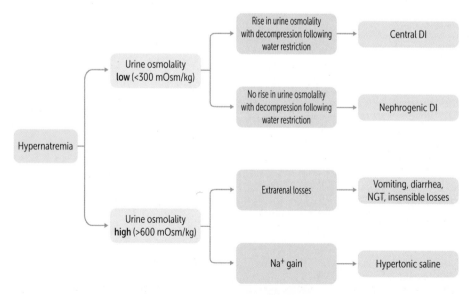

FIGURE 2.16-1. **Diagnostic algorithm for hypernatremia.** Diagnosis of central DI and nephrogenic DI also established by use of the DDAVP replacement test (see Endocrinology chapter). Intermediate values (300–600 mOsm/kg) often caused by osmotic diuresis, though can occasionally be seen in DI. Urine sodium measurement can also be helpful to distinguish extrarenal losses (urine sodium < 25 mEq/L) from sodium gain (> 100 mEq/L). DI, diabetes insipidus; NGT, nasogastric tube. (Reproduced with permission from USMLE-Rx.com)

HYPONATREMIA

Serum sodium < 135 mEq/L. Hyponatremia is most commonly caused by ↑ ADH; however, there are some ADH-independent etiologies, like primary polydipsia, starvation (solute deficiency), and the presence of a non-sodium effective osmole in the extracellular fluid.

HISTORY/PE

- May be asymptomatic or may present with confusion, lethargy, muscle cramps, and nausea.
- Can progress to seizures, coma, or brainstem herniation.

DIAGNOSIS

- **Best initial test:** Measure serum osmolality (S_{osm}) as the first step in evaluation. If the measured serum osmolality is higher than the calculated $S_{osm} = (2 \times \text{serum Na}) + (\text{BUN}/2.8) + (\text{glucose}/18)$ by more than 10–15 mOsm, then this indicates an exogenous osmole (a nonsodium osmole) diluting the serum sodium.
- Correct sodium in hyperglycemia. Sodium decreases by 1.6 mEq/L for every 100 mg/dL elevation in glucose.
- Hypotonic hyponatremia is the most common and is further categorized by volume status. See Figure 2.16-2 for the full diagnostic algorithm.

KEY FACT

Consider using hypertonic saline only if a patient has seizures caused by hyponatremia, and when serum Na^+ is < 120 mEq/L. In most cases, NS is the best replacement fluid.

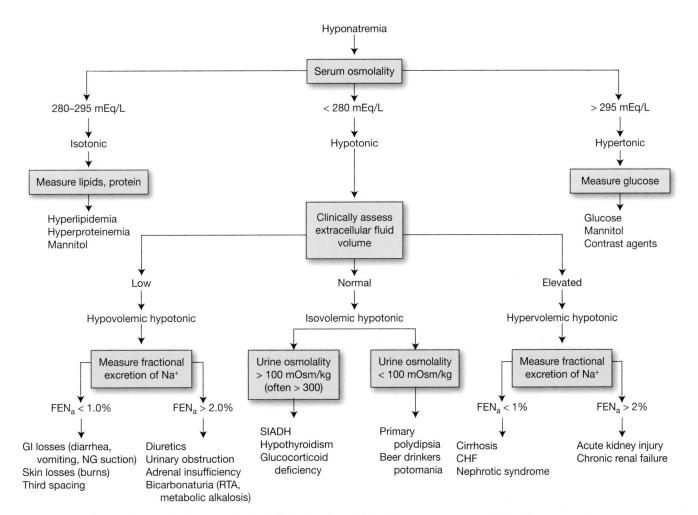

FIGURE 2.16-2.   Diagnostic algorithm for hyponatremia. Boxes highlighted in yellow represent key lab tests to perform.

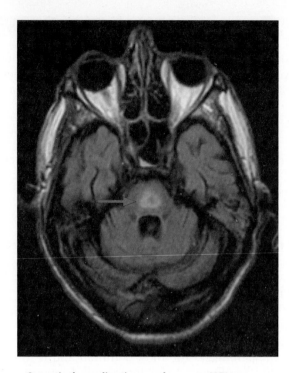

FIGURE 2.16-3. **Osmotic demyelination syndrome on MRI.** (Reproduced with permission from Dr. Frank Gaillard.)

TREATMENT

■ Treat underlying disorder. Treat hyponatremia from hypervolemic and euvolemic etiologies with water restriction ± diuretics. If hypovolemic, replete volume with NS. If severe hyponatremia (Na < 120 mEq/L), consider 3% hypertonic saline, particularly if symptomatic.
■ Correct chronic hyponatremia (> 72 hours' duration) slowly (< 8−10 mEq/L/day) to prevent osmotic demyelination syndrome (symptoms include paraparesis/quadriparesis, dysarthria, and coma). See Figure 2.16-3.

HYPERKALEMIA

Serum potassium (K^+) > 5 mEq/L. Etiologies are as follows:

■ **Spurious:** Hemolysis of blood samples, fist clenching during blood draws, delays in sample analysis, extreme leukocytosis or thrombocytosis.
■ **↓ Excretion:** Renal insufficiency, drugs (eg, spironolactone, triamterene, amiloride, ACE inhibitors (ACEIs), trimethoprim, NSAIDs, β-blockers), hypoaldosteronism, type IV renal tubular acidosis (RTA), calcineurin inhibitors.
■ **Cellular shifts:** Cell lysis, tissue injury (rhabdomyolysis), tumor lysis syndrome, insulin deficiency, acidosis, drugs (eg, succinylcholine, digitalis, arginine, β-blockers), hyperosmolality, exercise, resorption of blood (hematomas, GI bleeding).
■ **↑ Intake:** Food (most fruits, potatoes), iatrogenic.

HISTORY/PE

May be asymptomatic or may present with nausea, vomiting, intestinal colic, areflexia, weakness, flaccid paralysis, arrhythmias, and paresthesia.

DIAGNOSIS

- Confirm hyperkalemia with a repeat blood draw for suspected spurious results. In the setting of extreme leukocytosis or thrombocytosis, check plasma K^+.
- **Other work-up:** ECG to evaluate for cardiac complications. ECG findings include tall, peaked T waves; a wide QRS; PR prolongation; and loss of P waves (see Figure 2.16-4). Can progress to sine waves, ventricular dysrhythmias, and cardiac arrest.

TREATMENT

- Treatment is listed in the mnemonic C BIG K and is summarized as follows:
  - **Best initial treatment:** always give calcium gluconate for cardiac cell membrane stabilization if $K^+ > 6.5$ mEq/L or ECG changes.
  - Give insulin (with glucose to avoid hypoglycemia), β-agonists (eg, albuterol), and/or alkali (eg, bicarbonate) to temporarily shift K^+ into cells. Most rapid way to shift K^+ into cells.
  - Eliminate K^+ from diet, medications (eg, penicillin has K^+), and IV fluids.
  - Remove K^+ from the body. Historically, kayexalate (sodium polystyrene sulfonate) has been used to remove K^+ from the body.
    - Contraindications: Ileus, bowel obstruction, ischemic gut, or pancreatic transplants (can cause bowel necrosis).
  - Because of serious adverse effects, kayexalate is falling out of favor. IV saline (in hypovolemic settings) and loop diuretics (in normo- or hypervolemic settings) can enhance urinary excretion of K^+.
- Dialysis is needed for patients with renal failure and hyperkalemia refractory to the above medical management.

HYPOKALEMIA

Serum $K^+ < 3.6$ mEq/L. Etiologies are as follows:

- **Transcellular shifts:** Insulin, β$_2$-agonists, and alkalosis all cause K^+ to shift intracellularly (see Figure 2.16-5).
- **GI losses:** Diarrhea, chronic laxative abuse, vomiting, nasogastric tube suction.

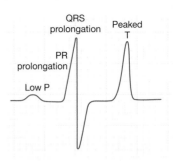

FIGURE 2.16-4. Hyperkalemia on ECG. Electrocardiographic manifestations include peaked T waves, PR prolongation, and a widened QRS complex. (Reproduced with permission from USMLE-Rx.com.)

KEY FACT

Hypokalemia is usually caused by renal +/− GI losses.

Q **1**

A 26-year-old woman with a history of depression presents to the emergency department with altered mental status, tinnitus, nausea, and vomiting. An ABG shows a pH of 7.4, Paco$_2$ of 22, and a HCO$_3$− of 13. What is the most likely diagnosis, and what is her acid-base disorder?

Q **2**

A 37-year-old homeless man was found unconscious on a park bench. Upon waking, he complains of severe muscle soreness and red urine. His urine dipstick is ⊕ for blood. What is the likely cause of this finding, and what is the best next step?

Q **3**

A 29-year-old woman with a history of bipolar disorder presents to the emergency department with altered mental status. On exam, she has dry mucous membranes and ↓ skin turgor with a BP of 92/40 mm Hg and HR of 106 bpm. Her serum sodium level is 154 mEq/L. What is the next best step in management?

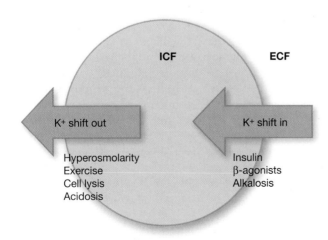

FIGURE 2.16-5. Causes of transcellular K^+ shifts.

If a patient is on digitalis, K⁺ levels must be carefully monitored. Hypokalemia sensitizes the heart to digitalis toxicity, because K⁺ and digitalis compete for the same sites on the Na⁺/K⁺ pump.

If hypokalemia is not responding to K⁺ repletion, check magnesium levels.

1 **A**

Aspirin overdose. Though her pH is normal, she has a mixed metabolic acidosis and respiratory alkalosis. Her bicarbonate is low, indicating a metabolic acidosis. Winter's formula predicts that her $Paco_2$ under normal compensation should be 29 ($Paco_2 = 1.5 (HCO_3-) + 8$). Her $Paco_2$ is lower than this at 22, which indicates a concurrent respiratory alkalosis.

2 **A**

This patient probably has rhabdomyolysis, and the urine dipstick is detecting myoglobin. He should be managed with saline hydration, mannitol, bicarbonate, and an ECG to rule out life-threatening hyperkalemia.

3 **A**

This patient probably has nephrogenic diabetes insipidus from presumed lithium use. She is hypovolemic with unstable vital signs; therefore, she should be treated initially with NS and switched to D_5W once her volume status improves.

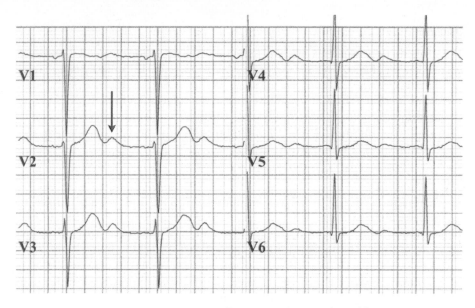

FIGURE 2.16-6. **Hypokalemia on ECG.** Prominent U wave indicated by *arrow*. (Reproduced with permission from Van Beers EJ, Stam J, van den Bergh WM. Licorice consumption as a cause of posterior reversible encephalopathy syndrome: a case report. Crit Care. 2011;15(1):R64.)

- **Renal losses:** Diuretics (eg, loop or thiazide), 1° mineralocorticoid excess or 2° hyperaldosteronism, ↓ circulating volume (stimulates RAAS- and mineralocorticoid-associated K⁺ secretion), Bartter and Gitelman syndromes, drugs (eg, gentamicin, amphotericin), diabetic ketoacidosis, hypomagnesemia, type I and type II RTA.

HISTORY/PE

Presents with fatigue, muscle weakness or cramps, ileus, hyporeflexia, paresthesias, rhabdomyolysis, and ascending paralysis.

DIAGNOSIS

Other work-up: ECG may show T-wave flattening, U waves (an additional wave after the T wave), and ST-segment depression, leading to AV block and subsequent cardiac arrest. See Figure 2.16-6.

TREATMENT

- Treat the underlying disorder.
- Oral and/or IV K⁺ repletion. Oral is the preferred route for safety purposes. If IV is necessary, a continuous rate of K⁺ as an additive is preferred over an IV K⁺ bolus. Reserve IV boluses for symptomatic hypokalemia or ECG changes. Do not exceed 20 mEq/L/h.
- Replace magnesium, as this deficiency makes K⁺ repletion more difficult.

HYPERCALCEMIA

Serum calcium > 10.2 mg/dL (corrected for serum albumin). The most common causes are the following:

- Hyperparathyroidism.
- Malignancy (eg, breast cancer, squamous cell carcinoma, multiple myeloma).
- Other causes are summarized in the mnemonic **CHIMPANZEES.**

History/PE

Usually asymptomatic but can present with bones (osteopenia, fractures), stones (kidney stones), abdominal groans (anorexia, constipation), and psychiatric overtones (weakness, fatigue, irritability, altered mental status).

Diagnosis

- **Best initial test:** total/ionized calcium, albumin, phosphate, PTH. Also electrolytes, BUN, creatinine, magnesium, and alkaline phosphatase levels.
- **Also consider:** Parathyroid hormone–related peptide (PTHrP) if malignancy suspected, serum protein electrophoresis for multiple myeloma, vitamin D (total 25 Vit D and 1,25 vitamin D levels) if granulomatous disease (eg, sarcoidosis), iatrogenic vitamin D intake, or TB suspected.
- **Other work-up:** ECG may show prolonged QT interval.

Treatment

- If serum calcium > 14 mg/dL, treat urgently with isotonic IV fluids ($+/-$ furosemide) and calcitonin; bisphosphonates (eg, zoledronic acid, pamidronate) should be considered as well. High sodium intake (in isotonic fluids) facilitates renal calcium excretion and prevents renal complications (stones).
- Treat the underlying disorder including steroids for some of the granulomatous diseases.

HYPOCALCEMIA

Serum calcium < 8.5 mg/dL. Etiologies include the following:

- **Parathyroid-related:** Hypoparathyroidism (postsurgical, idiopathic), 2° hyperparathyroidism (chronic kidney disease [CKD]), and pseudohypoparathyroidism. In infants, consider DiGeorge syndrome.
- Malnutrition, vitamin D deficiency.
- **Other:** hypomagnesemia, acute pancreatitis, and chelation from citrate found in blood products.

History/PE

- Presents with abdominal muscle cramps, dyspnea, tetany, perioral and acral paresthesias, and convulsions.
- Facial spasm elicited from tapping of the facial nerve (Chvostek sign) and carpal spasm after arterial occlusion by a BP cuff (Trousseau sign) are classic findings that are most commonly seen in severe hypocalcemia.

Diagnosis

- **Most accurate test:** Ionized Ca^{2+} and PTH. See Endocrinology chapter for interpretation of PTH levels.
- If the patient has had a thyroidectomy, review the operative note to determine if there was any potential damage to the parathyroid glands.
- **Labs:** Mg^{2+} (low levels can induce PTH resistance), albumin, 25-OH vitamin D, 1,25-OH vitamin D levels, and electrolytes. BUN, creatinine, and alkaline phosphatase may also be helpful to test, depending on clinical situation.
- **Other work-up:** ECG may show prolonged QT interval.

Treatment

- Treat the underlying disorder.
- In most cases, will need to administer oral calcium supplements; give oral and IV calcium for severe symptoms or signs.
- Ensure magnesium repletion.

MNEMONIC

Causes of hypercalcemia—

CHIMPANZEES

Calcium supplementation
Hyperparathyroidism/**H**ypothyroidism
Iatrogenic (eg, thiazides, parenteral nutrition)/**I**mmobility (especially in the ICU setting)
Milk-alkali syndrome
Paget disease
Adrenal insufficiency/**A**cromegaly
Neoplasm
Zollinger-Ellison syndrome (eg, MEN type 1)
Excess vitamin A
Excess vitamin D
Sarcoidosis and other granulomatous disease

KEY FACT

Loop diuretics (furosemide) **L**ose calcium. **T**hiazide diuretics ↑ **T**ubular reabsorption of calcium.

KEY FACT

A classic case of hypocalcemia is a patient who develops cramps and tetany following thyroidectomy because of parathyroidectomy as a complication.

KEY FACT

Serum calcium levels may be falsely low in hypoalbuminemia; check ionized calcium. Corrected Ca^{2+} = Total serum Ca^{2+} + 0.8 (4 − serum albumin).

KEY FACT

Alcoholics are the most common patient population with hypomagnesemia.

KEY FACT

ASA (salicylate) overdose can cause both metabolic acidosis and respiratory alkalosis.

MNEMONIC

Specific treatments for anion-gap causes of metabolic acidosis—

MUDPILES

Methanol: FOMEPIZOLE
Uremia: Dialysis
Diabetic ketoacidosis: Insulin, isotonic IV fluids, K+ repletion
Paraldehyde, **P**henformin
Iron, **INH**: GI lavage, charcoal (INH)
Lactic acidosis: Correct underlying cause; if from ischemia, then responds to repletion of circulating volume
Ethylene glycol: Fomepizole
Salicylates: Isotonic IV fluids with added sodium bicarbonate to alkalinize urine

KEY FACT

Ethylene glycol presentation = Urine calcium oxalate (envelope-shaped) crystals
Methanol presentation = Vision loss, optic disc hyperemia
Both present with ↑ osmolal gap (Measured osmolality-calculated osmolality > 10 mOsmol/L)

KEY FACT

A history of AKI and nephrotoxin exposure should make you suspect a diagnosis of ATN.

MNEMONIC

Indications for urgent dialysis—

AEIOU

Acidosis
Electrolyte abnormalities (hyperkalemia)
Ingestions (salicylates, theophylline, methanol, barbiturates, lithium, ethylene glycol)
Overload (fluid)
Uremic symptoms (pericarditis, encephalopathy, bleeding, nausea, pruritus, myoclonus)

HYPOMAGNESEMIA

Serum magnesium < 1.5 mEq/L. Etiologies are as follows:

- ↓ **Intake:** Malnutrition, malabsorption, short bowel syndrome, TPN, PPIs.
- ↑ **Loss:** Diuretics, diarrhea, vomiting, hypercalcemia, alcoholism.
- **Miscellaneous:** Diabetic ketoacidosis, pancreatitis, extracellular fluid volume expansion.

HISTORY/PE

In severe cases, symptoms may include hyperactive reflexes, tetany, paresthesias, irritability, confusion, lethargy, seizures, and arrhythmias.

EVALUATION

- Lab results may show concurrent hypocalcemia and hypokalemia.
- ECG may reveal prolonged PR and QT intervals.

TREATMENT

- Generally most causes respond to IV and/or oral supplements, depending on severity.
- Hypokalemia and hypocalcemia will not correct without magnesium correction.

Acid-Base Disorders

See Figure 2.16-7 for a diagnostic algorithm of acid-base disorders.

Renal Tubular Acidosis

A net ↓ in either tubular H+ secretion or HCO_3^- reabsorption that leads to a non–anion-gap metabolic acidosis. There are three main types of RTA; type IV (aldosterone deficient/resistant) is the most common form (see Table 2.16-1).

Acute Kidney Injury

Formerly known as acute renal failure, acute kidney injury (AKI) is defined as a ↓ in renal function compared with a previous baseline within a period of < 3 months, leading to the retention of creatinine. ↓ Urine output (oliguria, defined as <0.5 mL/kg/h) is not required for AKI, but if present can be part of the diagnostic criteria. Complications include metabolic acidosis, electrolyte abnormalities, uremia, and volume overload (see **AEIOU** mnemonic). Many cases of AKI will recover with treatment and/or supportive care, but each episode of AKI can lead to chronic impacts and scarring and progressively develop into chronic kidney disease (especially with very severe or recurrent AKI). See Table 2.16-2 for the work-up of AKI.

Chronic Kidney Disease

CKD is defined as > 3 months of GFR < 60 mL/min or signs of chronic kidney damage (structural/functional abnormalities), even with normal GFR (> 90 mL/min). In adults, most commonly caused by diabetes mellitus (DM), hypertension, analgesia abuse (ASA, naproxen), and glomerulonephritis.

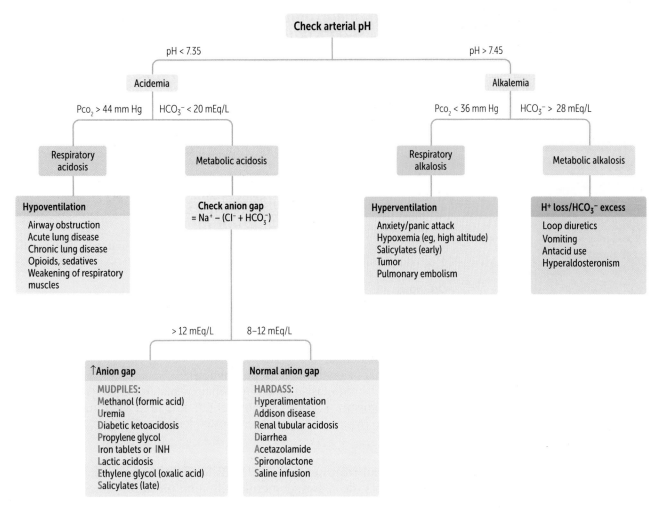

FIGURE 2.16-7. **Diagnostic algorithm for acid-base disorders.** (Reproduced with permission from USMLE-Rx.com.)

TABLE 2.16-1. **Types of RTA**

VARIABLE	TYPE I (DISTAL)	TYPE II (PROXIMAL)	TYPE IV (IMPAIRED MINERALOCORTICOID EFFECT)
Defect	H⁺ secretion	HCO₃⁻ reabsorption	Aldosterone deficiency or resistance
Serum K⁺	Low	Low	High
Urinary pH	> 5.5	5.5 or high at onset, but can be < 5.5 once serum is in its acidotic state	Variable (not typically used to differentiate)
Etiologies (most common)	Autoimmune disorders, hypercalciuria, amphotericin B, ifosfamide, genetic disorders	Multiple myeloma, amyloidosis, all other causes of Fanconi syndrome (eg genetic and acquired), aminoglycosides, ifosfamide, cisplatin, acetazolamide	Hypoaldosteronism, angiotensin II inhibition (ACEIs/ARBs), urinary tract obstruction, heparin
Treatment	K⁺ bicarbonate supplementation	Treat underlying cause, often needs sodium and K⁺ bicarbonate supplementation	Depending on etiology, may need mineralocorticoid replacement, sodium bicarbonate supplementation, or K⁺ wasting diuretics
Complications	Nephrolithiasis	Rickets, osteomalacia	

KEY FACT

Do not give metformin to septic patients or those with renal or hepatic failure, because it can worsen the metabolic acidosis.

KEY FACT

Cardiovascular disease is the most common cause of death in dialysis and renal transplant patients (> 50%). Infectious complications is the second most common cause (and most common cause of death in pediatric dialysis and transplant patients).

Polycystic kidney disease (PKD) is a significant cause and the most common hereditary cause of CKD. In children, the most common cause is congenital anomalies of the kidney and urinary tract (CAKUT).

HISTORY/PE

- Generally asymptomatic until GFR is < 30 mL/min, but patients gradually experience the signs and symptoms of electrolyte disorders such as hyperkalemia and metabolic acidosis, secondary hyperparathyroidism, anemia of CKD, and uremia (anorexia, nausea, vomiting, uremic pericarditis, "uremic frost," delirium, seizures, coma), the latter at a very late stage (GFR <10).
- Depending on the etiology, signs of fluid retention (hypertension, edema) often develop, especially with primary glomerular etiologies like diabetic nephropathy.
- With congenital anomalies, obstructions, and PKD, patients may continue to have polyuria even at very low GFRs.

DIAGNOSIS

- Common metabolic derangements include the following:
  - Azotemia (↑ BUN).
  - Metabolic acidosis.
  - Hyperkalemia.
  - Anemia (↓ erythropoietin production).
- Abnormal hemostasis caused by impaired platelet aggregation. 2° Hyperparathyroidism (↓ phosphate excretion; impaired vitamin D production leading to hypocalcemia and renal osteodystrophy).

TREATMENT

- **Best initial treatment:** ACEIs/ARBs for tight control of hypertension and proteinuria (decreases glomerular filtration pressures) have been shown to ↓ the progression of CKD.
- Erythropoietin analogues for anemia of chronic disease. Supportive dietary management of fluids, sodium, K^+, and phosphate (as applicable for patients; some require restrictions, but those with PKD or polyuria may actually need fluid supplementation).
- Oral phosphate binders (calcium acetate, calcium carbonate, sevelamer, lanthanum) and calcitriol (1,25-OH vitamin D) for renal osteodystrophy.

TABLE 2.16-2. Acute Kidney Injury

	PRERENAL	INTRINSIC	POSTRENAL
Pathophysiology	↓ Renal perfusion	Injury within the nephron	Urinary outflow obstruction
Common etiologies	Hypovolemia, shock/sepsis, decreased intravascular volume (cirrhosis, nephrotic syndrome), renal artery stenosis, hepatorenal syndrome, drugs (NSAIDs, ACEIs), CHF (especially with diuretic treatment)	Acute tubular necrosis (ATN) from ischemia or nephrotoxins, AIN, glomerulonephritis, embolic disease, rhabdomyolysis Interstitial nephritis (drugs: penicillins, cephalosporins, NSAIDs, sulfa drugs, PPIs, allopurinol)	Prostatic disease, pelvic tumors, intratubular obstruction from crystalluria (acyclovir), bilateral stones, congenital obstructions
History/PE	Symptoms of hypovolemia (tachycardia, hypotension) or other underlying disease process (liver failure, nephrotic syndrome)	History of drug exposure (aminoglycosides, NSAIDs, penicillins), contrast media.	Suprapubic and/or flank pain, distended bladder, bladder scan shows post-void residual > 50 mL

(continues)

TABLE 2.16-2.   Acute Kidney Injury (continued)

	PRERENAL	INTRINSIC	POSTRENAL
LAB VALUES			
BUN/Creatinine ratio	> 20:1	< 15:1	Varies
Fractional excretion of sodium (Fe_{Na})	< 1%	> 2%	Varies
Urine sodium	< 20 mEq/L	> 40 mEq/L	Varies
Urine Osms	> 500 mOsm/kg	< 350 mOsm/kg (isosthenuria, damaged tubules cannot reabsorb water or concentrate urine)	Varies
Urine sediment	Hyaline casts (see Image A) (normal finding, but ↑ in volume depletion)	RBC casts/dysmorphic RBCs (see Image B) (glomerulonephritis), WBCs/eosinophils, WBC casts (see Image C) (AIN), "muddy-brown or granular casts" (see Image D) (ATN), WBC casts (pyelonephritis), fatty casts (nephrotic syndrome)	
Treatment	For all etiologies, dialyze if meet **AEIOU** criteria and refractory to medical management (see mnemonic)		
	Fluids to replete circulating volume if hypovolemic. Avoid nephrotoxic drugs (metformin, NSAIDs). IV fluids will not help hepatorenal syndrome, nephrotic syndrome, or CHF, or other causes of increased total body volume	Prevent contrast nephropathy with IV fluids or nonionic contrast agents. Discontinue offending medications	Urgent bladder scan and catheterization or relief of obstruction, as applicable

A   B   C   D

Image A reproduced with permission from USMLE-Rx.com. Images B and D reproduced with permission from Dr. Adam Weinstein. Image C reproduced with permission from Perazella MA. Diagnosing drug-induced AIN in the hospitalized patient: a challenge for the clinician. *Clin Nephrol.* 2014;81(6):381–388. DOI: 10.5414/CN108301.

- Use desmopressin in cases of abnormal bleeding (complication of uremia).
- Renal replacement therapy options include hemodialysis, peritoneal dialysis, and renal transplantation.

COMPLICATIONS

Cardiovascular complications (MI, CHF, sudden cardiac death) are the most common cause of death, followed by infectious complications. Acquired renal cystic disease can occur in patients undergoing long-term dialysis.

Post-infectious glomerulonephritis will present 2–6 weeks after an infection and has a low C3; IgA nephropathy will present concurrent with an infection and has a normal C3.

KEY FACT

Granulomatosis with polyangiitis = kidney + lung + sinus
Microscopic polyangiitis = kidney + lung
Churg-Strauss syndrome = kidney + asthma

MNEMONIC

Nephritic syndrome findings—

PHAROH

Proteinuria
Hematuria
Azotemia
RBC casts
Oliguria
Hypertension

Diuretics

Table 2.16-3 summarizes the mechanisms of action and side effects of commonly used diuretics. Figure 2.16-8 provides a review of nephron physiology with diuretic sites of action.

Glomerular Disease

NEPHRITIC SYNDROME

A disorder of glomerular inflammation, also called glomerulonephritis. Proteinuria may be present but is variable. If severe glomerular inflammation, it can exceed 2.0 g/day and lead to a concurrent nephrotic syndrome. Most cases of glomerulonephritis are usually associated with less proteinuria, often < 1.5 g/day. Causes are summarized in Table 2.16-4.

HISTORY/PE

The classic findings are macroscopic/microscopic hematuria (tea- or cola-colored urine), hypertension, and edema (can also present with pulmonary edema).

DIAGNOSIS

- Urinalysis (UA) shows hematuria and variable degrees of proteinuria.
- In most severe cases, patients may have a ↓ GFR with elevated BUN and creatinine. See Table 2.16-4 for pertinent labs.
- Renal biopsy may be needed for histologic evaluation and treatment and prognosis considerations.
- Findings are shown in Figure 2.16-9.

TABLE 2.16-3. Mechanism of Action and Side Effects of Diuretics

TYPE	DRUGS	SITE OF ACTION	MECHANISM OF ACTION	SIDE EFFECTS
Carbonic anhydrase inhibitors	Acetazolamide	Proximal convoluted tubule	Inhibit carbonic anhydrase, ↑ H+ reabsorption, block Na+/H+ exchange	Proximal (Type II) RTA, sulfa allergy
Osmotic agents	Mannitol, urea	Entire tubule	↑ Tubular fluid osmolarity	↓ Na+
Loop agents	Furosemide, ethacrynic acid, bumetanide, torsemide	Ascending loop of Henle	Inhibit Na+/ K+/2Cl− transporter	Water loss, metabolic alkalosis, ↓ K+, ↓ Ca2+, ↓ Mg+, ototoxicity, sulfa allergy (except ethacrynic acid), hyperuricemia
Thiazide agents	Hydrochlorothiazide, chlorothiazide, chlorthalidone	Distal convoluted tubule	Inhibit Na+/Cl− transporter	Water loss, metabolic alkalosis, ↓ Na+, ↓ K+, ↑ glucose, ↑ Ca2+, ↑ uric acid, ↑ LDL cholesterol, sulfa allergy, pancreatitis
K+-sparing agents	Spironolactone, triamterene, amiloride	Cortical collecting tubule	Aldosterone receptor antagonist (spironolactone); block sodium channel (triamterene, amiloride)	Metabolic acidosis; ↑ K+; antiandrogenic effects, including gynecomastia (spironolactone)

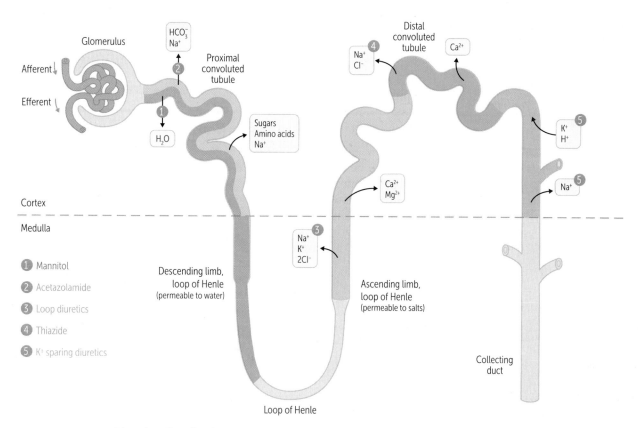

FIGURE 2.16-8. **Diuretics: Site of action.** (Reproduced with permission from USMLE-Rx.com.)

TREATMENT

- If present, treat hypertension, fluid overload, with salt restriction, RAAS blockade, +/− diuretics.
- In some cases, depending on the etiology, corticosteroids +/− other immunosuppressant agents are a necessary treatment to reduce glomerular inflammation.

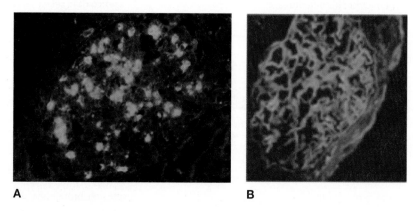

FIGURE 2.16-9. **Findings in nephritic syndromes. (A)** "Lumpy-bumpy" immunofluorescence found in postinfectious glomerulonephritis. **(B)** Linear immunofluorescence seen in Goodpasture syndrome. (Image A reproduced with permission from Oda T, Yoshizawa N, Yamakami K, et al. The role of nephritis-associated plasmin receptor (NAPLR) in glomerulonephritis associated with streptococcal infection, Biomed Biotechnol. 2012;2012:417675. Image B reproduced with permission from Kasper D, et al. *Harrison's Principles of Internal Medicine,* 19th ed. New York, NY: McGraw-Hill; 2015.)

Q

A 17-year-old boy with a history of asthma presented to the emergency department with severe shortness of breath. His arterial pH has gone from 7.49 to 7.38 and Pco₂ from 30 to 50 mmHg since the time of admission. What is the next best step in management?

This is a sign of respiratory muscle fatigue and may require urgent intubation.

NEPHROTIC SYNDROME

Nephrotic syndrome is defined as follows:

- Hyperproteinuria ($\geq$ 3.5 g/day).
- Hypoproteinemia/Hypoalbuminemia—albumin levels fall caused by protein loss.
- Hyperlipidemia (accelerated atherosclerosis).
- Edema (morning periorbital edema).

Thrombosis can be seen too, but is not part of the definition. Occurs because of loss of antithrombin III, protein C, and protein S in urine.

Approximately one-third of all cases result from systemic diseases such as DM, SLE, or amyloidosis. In children, the most common cause is minimal change disease, a primary disease of the kidney and not a systemic disease. Causes and findings are summarized in Table 2.16-5.

TABLE 2.16-4. **Causes of Nephritic Syndrome**

DISORDER	DESCRIPTION	HISTORY/PE	LABS/HISTOLOGY	TREATMENT/ PROGNOSIS
IMMUNE COMPLEX				
Postinfectious glomerulonephritis	Classically associated with recent group A β-hemolytic streptococcal infection, but can be seen with many other infections (usually 2–4 weeks after the infectious trigger). Most common cause in children	Tea- or cola-colored urine, hypertension, edema, and occasional oliguria	Low serum C3 that normalizes 6–8 weeks after presentation; ↑ ASO and/or anti-DNase titers (if strep associated); lumpy-bumpy immunofluorescence	Supportive with diuretics to treat fluid overload and/or hypertension. Most patients have a complete recovery
IgA nephropathy (Berger disease)	Most common cause of glomerulonephritis in adults; typically occurs concurrent with an upper respiratory or GI infection (IgA producing mucosa). Henoch-Schönlein purpura is a vasculitis whose renal manifestation is pathologically the same as IgA nephropathy	Episodic gross hematuria with respiratory and/or GI infections. Often with persistent microscopic hematuria between infections. May also have chronic hypertension and low to moderate levels of proteinuria	Normal C3. IgA deposits on immunofluorescence	ACEIs in patients with persistent hypertension and/or proteinuria. Glucocorticoids in select severe inflammatory presentations. Nonresponsive patients have slow progression to ESRD
Henoch-Schönlein purpura	Small vessel vasculitis, often seen in childhood	Triad: Palpable purpura, arthralgias, abdominal pain + IgA nephropathy (the renal manifestation)	Identical to IgA nephropathy	Supportive therapy ± ACE-I (for persistent hypertension, proteinuria) ± glucocorticoids and immunosuppressants for severe inflammatory presentations

(continues)

T A B L E 2 . 1 6 - 4 . **Causes of Nephritic Syndrome** *(continued)*

Disorder	Description	History/PE	Labs/Histology	Treatment/ Prognosis
Pauci-Immune (No Ig deposits on immunofluorescence)				
Granulomatosis with polyangiitis ([GPA] formerly Wegener granulomatosis)	Granulomatous inflammation of the respiratory tract (with nasopharyngeal involvement) and kidney with necrotizing vasculitis of glomerular capillaries	Respiratory and sinus symptoms. Cavitary pulmonary lesions bleed and lead to hemoptysis. Renal manifestation often acute kidney injury, hypertension, sometimes gross hematuria, oliguria	Presence of PR3-ANCA/ c-ANCA (anti-proteinase 3). Segmental necrotizing glomerulonephritis with crescents on light microscopy	High-dose corticosteroids, cytotoxic agents, or rituximab. Patients tend to have frequent relapses. Life-threatening cases are treated with plasmapheresis
Microscopic polyangiitis	Small vessel vasculitis similar to GPA. No granulomas	Similar to GPA but no nasopharyngeal involvement. Renal manifestation often acute kidney injury, hypertension, sometimes gross hematuria, oliguria	MPO-ANCA/p-ANCA (antimyeloperoxidase). Necrotizing glomerulonephritis with crescents on light microscopy	Glucocorticoids, cyclophosphamide, or rituximab. Life-threatening cases are treated with plasmapheresis
Eosinophilic granulomatosis with polyangiitis (Churg-Strauss syndrome)	Small vessel vasculitis similar to GPA (no granulomas)	Asthma, sinusitis, skin nodules/purpura, peripheral neuropathy. Renal manifestation often acute kidney injury, hypertension, sometimes gross hematuria, oliguria	MPO-ANCA, ↑ eosinophils, ↑ IgE. Necrotizing glomerulonephritis with crescents on light microscopy	Glucocorticoids. cyclophosphamide, or rituximab. Life-threatening cases are treated with plasmapheresis
Anti-GBM Disease				
Goodpasture syndrome	Rapidly progressing glomerulonephritis with pulmonary hemorrhage; peak incidence is in men in their mid-20s	Hemoptysis, dyspnea, possible respiratory failure. No upper respiratory tract involvement. Renal manifestation often acute kidney injury, hypertension, sometimes gross hematuria, oliguria	Linear anti-GBM deposits on immunofluorescence; iron deficiency anemia; hemosiderin-filled macrophages in sputum; pulmonary infiltrates on chest x-ray (CXR). Necrotizing glomerulonephritis with crescents on light microscopy	Plasma exchange therapy; pulsed steroids and cyclophosphamide. Very severe, life- threatening, and may not be responsive to treatment and progress to ESRD
Alport syndrome	Hereditary glomerulonephritis; 80% of cases X-linked and thus more often presents in boys; typically diagnosed between 5 and 20 years of age	Asymptomatic persistent microscopy hematuria, gross hematuria in setting of intercurrent illness or systemic stressors, progressive proteinuria as condition progresses, associated with acquired sensorineural deafness and eye disorders (related to the same loss of function of type IV collagen)	GBM splitting on electron microscopy	Progresses to renal failure but ACE-I can slow progression by controlling proteinuria and hypertension. After kidney transplant, since these patients do not have normal GBMs, with a normal renal allograft (and normal GBMs). Anti-GBM nephritis may develop

TABLE 2.16-5. **Causes of Nephrotic Syndrome**

DISORDER	DESCRIPTION	HISTORY/PE	LABS/HISTOLOGY	TREATMENT/PROGNOSIS
Minimal-change disease	The most common cause of nephrotic syndrome in children Idiopathic etiology; 2° causes include NSAIDs and hematologic malignancies (eg, Hodgkin disease)	Sudden onset of edema	Light microscopy appears normal; electron microscopy shows effacement of epithelial foot processes (*arrows* in Image A; for reference, Image B shows a normal glomerulus)	Steroids; favorable prognosis
Focal segmental glomerulosclerosis	Idiopathic, but also can be secondary to IV drug use (heroin), HIV, sickle cell disease, and obesity. The most common cause of nephrotic syndromes in adults, but especially in African-American individuals	Presents with hypertension and often with edema	Biopsy shows focal glomerular sclerosis in capillary tufts (*arrows* in Image C)	Prednisone, immunosuppressant therapy, ACEIs/ARBs to ↓ proteinuria and treat hypertension
Membranous nephropathy	Accounts for ± 30% of nephrotic syndromes in adults. Most common cause of nephrotic syndrome in white adults	May be secondary to solid-tumor malignancies, infections (HBV, malaria), autoimmune diseases (SLE), drugs (NSAIDs, gold) Presents with severe anasarca and, of all causes of nephrotic syndrome, has the highest rate of thrombosis, likely related to severity of protein losses	"Spike-and-dome" appearance caused by granular deposits of IgG and C3 at the subepithelial side of the basement membrane. On light microscopy, GBM thickening are seen. (*arrows* in Image D). Anti-phospholipase A_2 receptor (PLA2R) antibodies are associated with primary membranous nephropathy	RAAS inhibition is first line. Prednisone and immunosuppressive therapy for severe disease refractory to RAAS inhibition alone
Diabetic nephropathy	Has two characteristic forms: diffuse hyalinization and nodular glomerulosclerosis (Kimmelstiel-Wilson lesions)	Patients generally have long-standing, poorly controlled DM with evidence of other organ system complications, such as retinopathy and/or neuropathy	Thickened GBM; ↑ mesangial matrix. Kimmelstiel-Wilson lesions are seen (*arrows* in Image E)	Tight control of blood sugar; ACEIs or ARBs Screen for diabetic nephropathy with random urine microalbumin/creatinine ratio
Lupus nephritis	Classified as WHO types I–VI. The severity of renal disease often determines overall prognosis	Hematuria and/or proteinuria may be found during evaluation of SLE patients, or SLE patients may present with gross hematuria, hypertension, and/or edema. Lupus nephritis is often associated with severe, nephrotic levels of proteinuria, so it is a nephritis that often presents with a nephrotic syndrome	Mesangial proliferation; subendothelial and/or subepithelial immune complex deposition Low serum C3 and C4	Prednisone and cytotoxic or immunosuppressant therapy are the mainstays of treatment. RAAS inhibition is also often given

(continues)

TABLE 2.16-5.   Causes of Nephrotic Syndrome *(continued)*

DISORDER	DESCRIPTION	HISTORY/PE	LABS/HISTOLOGY	TREATMENT/PROGNOSIS
Renal amyloidosis	1° (plasma cell dyscrasia) and 2° (infectious or inflammatory) are the most common	Patients may have multiple myeloma or a chronic inflammatory disease (eg, rheumatoid arthritis, TB)	Nodular glomerulosclerosis; EM reveals amyloid fibrils; apple-green birefringence with Congo red stain	Prednisone and melphalan. Bone marrow transplantation may be used for multiple myeloma
MEMBRANOPROLIFERATIVE NEPHROPATHY				
Type I/III (nomenclature is changing, but these are the classic terms)	May be primary MPGN (especially in children) or secondary to HBV, HCV, cryoglobulinemia	May present with gross hematuria, hypertension, and/or edema. Lupus nephritis is often associated with severe, nephrotic levels of proteinuria, so it is a nephritis that often presents with a nephrotic syndrome	"Tram-track," double-layered basement membrane (*arrow* in Image F). Subendothelial and mesangial deposits. Low serum C3	Prednisone +/− immunosuppressant therapy are the mainstays of treatment; RAAS inhibition is often given
Type II (nomenclature is changing, but this is the classic term)	May be primary MPGN (especially in children) or secondary to HBV, HCV, cryoglobulinemia	May present with gross hematuria, hypertension, and/or edema. Lupus nephritis is often associated with severe, nephrotic levels of proteinuria, so it is a nephritis that often presents with a nephrotic syndrome	Intramembranous dense deposits. "Tram-track," double-layered basement membrane may also be present (*arrows* in Image F). Occurs by way of C3 nephritic factor	Prednisone +/− immunosuppressant therapy are the mainstays of treatment; RAAS inhibition is often given

(Images A and B reproduced with permission from Le T, et al. *First Aid for the USMLE Step 1 2018.* New York, NY: McGraw-Hill Education; 2018. Image C courtesy of Dr. Michael Bonert. Images D and F reproduced with permission from USMLE-Rx.com. Image E reproduced with permission from Doc Mari.)

HISTORY/PE

- Presents with generalized edema. Sometimes patients will notice they have foamy urine. In severe cases, dyspnea and ascites and other complications from anasarca may develop.
- Patients have ↑ susceptibility to infection and hypercoagulable states with an ↑ risk for venous thrombosis and pulmonary embolism (caused by loss of antithrombin 3, increased platelet aggregation, and changes in protein C and S levels). Commonly manifests as renal vein thrombosis.

DIAGNOSIS

- UA shows proteinuria (≥ 3.5 g/day) and lipiduria (Maltese crosses signifying lipids on microscopic urine exam). It is now more common for clinicians to use a spot protein-to-creatinine ratio rather than 24-hour urine. Cutoff for nephrotic syndrome is 2.0 mg/mg on this ratio.
- Blood chemistry shows ↓ albumin (< 3 g/dL) and hyperlipidemia.
- Evaluation should include work-up for 2° causes.
- Renal biopsy may also be needed to definitively diagnose the underlying etiology.

TREATMENT

- Treat with salt restriction and judicious diuretic therapy.
- If hypertensive, can use RAAS blockade and/or diuretic therapy.
- If nephrotic syndrome is chronic, may need to treat with statins.
- Steroids and/or other immunosuppressant medications may be useful for certain etiologies.
- ACEIs ↓ proteinuria and diminish the progression of renal disease in patients with renal scarring (especially in patients with diabetes).
- Vaccinate with 23-polyvalent pneumococcus vaccine (PPV23), as patients are at ↑ risk for *Streptococcus pneumoniae* infection based on hypogammaglobulinemia from immunoglobulin losses in urine and edema (pulmonary edema, ascites).

Nephrolithiasis

Renal calculi. Stones are most commonly calcium oxalate, but many other types exist (see Table 2.16-6.). Risk factors include a ⊕ family history, low fluid intake, gout, medications (allopurinol, chemotherapy, loop diuretics), postcolectomy/postileostomy, specific enzyme deficiencies, type I RTA (caused by alkaline urinary pH and associated hypocitruria), and hyperparathyroidism. Most common in older men.

HISTORY/PE

- Presents with acute onset of severe, colicky flank pain that may radiate to the groin and is associated with nausea and vomiting.
- Patients are unable to get comfortable and shift position frequently (as opposed to those with peritonitis, who lie still).

DIAGNOSIS

- UA may show gross or microscopic hematuria (85%).
- Noncontrast abdominal CT scan is the **gold standard** for the diagnosis of kidney stones (see Figure 2.16-10). However, plain x-rays of the abdomen are still useful for following the progression/treatment of larger stones. Contrast should be avoided.

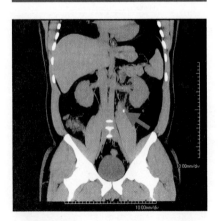

FIGURE 2.16-10.   Nephrolithiasis. CT scan shows a dense 1-cm calcification *(arrow)* in the left ureter, consistent with nephrolithiasis. (Reproduced with permission from Tintinalli JE, et al. Tintinalli's *Emergency Medicine: A Comprehensive Study Guide,* 7th ed. New York, NY: McGraw-Hill; 2011.)

TABLE 2.16-6. **Types of Nephrolithiasis**

Type	Frequency	Etiology and Characteristics	Urinary pH	Treatment
Calcium oxalate/calcium phosphate	83%	Most common causes are idiopathic hypercalciuria and 1° Hyperparathyroidism. Can also see in fat malabsorption (↑ oxalate absorption, eg, Crohn disease). Alkaline urine. Radiopaque	↑ pH (calcium phosphate precipitates) ↓ pH (calcium oxalate precipitates with hypoci-trituria, the latter of which is often associated with low urine pH)	Hydration, dietary sodium restriction, thiazide diuretics. Do not ↓ calcium intake (can lead to hyperoxaluria and ↑ risk for osteoporosis). For calcium oxalate stones, may also treat with citrate supplements, but be careful not to raise urine pH too high
Struvite (Mg-NH$_4$-PO$_4$) or "triple phosphate"	9%	Associated with urease-producing organisms (eg, *Proteus*). Form staghorn calculi. Alkaline urine. Radiopaque	↑ pH	Hydration; treat UTI if present; surgical removal of staghorn stone
Uric acid	7%	Associated with gout, xanthine oxidase deficiency, and high purine turnover states (eg, chemotherapy). Acidic urine (pH < 5.5). Radiolucent on plain film, but can be detectable with CT (still not as bright as calcium stones on CT)	↓ pH	Hydration; alkalinize urine with citrate, which is converted to HCO$_3^-$ in the liver; dietary purine restriction and allopurinol
Cystine	1%	Caused by a defect in renal transport of certain amino acids (**COLA: C**ystine, **O**rnithine, **L**ysine, and **A**rginine). Hexagonal crystals. ⊕ Urinary cyanide nitroprusside test. Partially radiopaque (may need a CT to see; not always seen on x-ray)	↓ pH	Hydration, dietary sodium restriction, alkalinization of urine, penicillamine or tiopronin

(Images reproduced with permission from Le T, et al. *First Aid for the USMLE Step 1 2018.* New York, NY: McGraw-Hill Education; 2018.)

- Ultrasonography is preferred for pregnant patients and children, in whom radiation from CT should be avoided.
- KUB (kidney/ureter/bladder) radiography identifies radiopaque stones but will often miss stones that are smaller or radiolucent.
- Intravenous pyelogram (IVP) is rarely used.

TREATMENT

- **Best initial treatment:** Hydration and analgesia.
- α_1-receptor blockers (eg, tamsulosin) and calcium channel blockers (eg, nifedipine) reduce ureteral spasm and facilitate stone passage of ureteral stone < 10 mm, reducing the need for analgesics.
- Treatment varies according to the size and diameter of the stone:
  - < 5 mm: May pass spontaneously.
  - < 10 mm: Higher rate of spontaneous passage with α-blocker or calcium channel blocker therapy.
  - 5–20 mm: May be treated with shock wave lithotripsy or ureteroscopy.
  - > 20 mm: percutaneous nephrolithotomy.
- Dietary changes to prevent calcium stones include ↑ fluid intake (most important), normal calcium intake (RDA recommended intake), and ↓ sodium intake. If caused by hyperoxaluria, then ↓ oxalate intake.

Polycystic Kidney Disease

Characterized by the presence of progressive cystic dilation of the renal tubules:

- **Autosomal dominant polycystic kidney disease (ADPKD):**
  - Most common.
  - Usually asymptomatic until patients are > 30 years of age, though about 10% of these patients present in childhood.
  - Most common presenting symptoms are hypertension or gross hematuria.
  - Cysts may form in other organs, especially the liver and pancreas.
  - One-half of ADPKD patients will have ESRD requiring dialysis by 60 years of age, but other patients may simply have mildly reduced renal function and only require supportive care and BP control.
  - Associated with ↑ risk for cerebral aneurysm, especially in patients with a ⊕ family history.
- **Autosomal recessive polycystic kidney disease (ARPKD):**
  - Less common but more severe.
  - Presents in infants and young children with renal failure, liver fibrosis, and portal hypertension; can lead to death in the first few days of life if associated with in utero oliguria (oligohydramnios) leading to Potter's sequence.

HISTORY/PE

- **ADPKD:**
  - Hypertension, flank pain, and gross hematuria are the most common presenting symptoms. Sharp, localized pain may result from cyst rupture, infection, or passage of renal calculi.
  - Additional findings include hepatic cysts, cerebral berry aneurysms, diverticulosis, and mitral valve prolapse.
- **ARPKD:** Hypertension, abdominal distension, and flank masses are the most common presenting findings. It is most commonly identified prenatally.

ADPKD and ARPKD:

- Patients may have large, palpable kidneys on abdominal exam.
- A single, simple renal cyst does not suggest ADPKD and does not require further evaluation.

DIAGNOSIS

Based on ultrasonography (most common) or CT scan (see Figure 2.16-11). Multiple bilateral cysts will be present throughout the renal parenchyma, and renal enlargement will be visualized. Genetic testing for ADPKD (*PKD1* and *PKD2* genes) and ARPKD (*PKHD* gene) is available but often not necessary.

TREATMENT

- Prevent complications and ↓ the rate of progression to ESRD. Early management of urinary tract infection (UTI) is critical to prevent renal cyst infection. BP control (ACEIs, ARBs) is necessary to ↓ hypertension-induced renal damage and control proteinuria.
- Dialysis and renal transplantation are used to manage patients with ESRD.
- High fluid intake is helpful to prevent development of kidney stones and may be helpful at slowing cyst progression too (ADH may stimulate cyst growth).

Hydronephrosis

Dilation of the urinary tract. Usually occurs secondary to obstruction of the urinary tract. In pediatric patients, the obstruction is often at the ureteropelvic junction but may also be at ureterovesicular junction (at the insertion into the bladder) or at the bladder outlet (eg from "posterior urethral valves"). In adults, it may be caused by benign prostatic hyperplasia (BPH), neurogenic bladder (spinal cord injuries), tumors, aortic aneurysms, or renal calculi. Apart from obstruction, hydronephrosis can also be caused by excessively high-output urinary flow and vesicoureteral reflux.

HISTORY/PE

May be asymptomatic, or may present with flank/back pain, abdominal pain, and UTIs.

DIAGNOSIS

Ultrasonography or CT scan to detect dilation of the renal pelvis and calyces (see Figure 2.16-12A), and/or ureter.

TREATMENT

- Some pediatric causes will spontaneously resolve. Otherwise the only treatment is to surgically correct any anatomic obstruction or reflux; or if neurogenic bladder, starting a clean intermittent catheterization regimen for bladder emptying.
- Ureteral stent placement across the obstructed area of the urinary tract and/or percutaneous nephrostomy tube placement to relieve pressure may be appropriate if the urinary outflow tract is not sufficiently cleared of obstruction. Foley or suprapubic catheters may be required for lower urinary tract obstruction (eg, BPH).

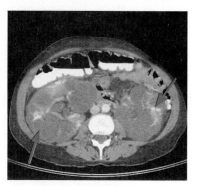

A

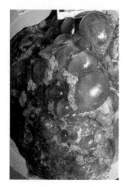

B

FIGURE 2.16-11. Autosomal dominant polycystic kidney disease. (**A**) Contrast-enhanced CT scan demonstrates bilaterally enlarged kidneys that have been almost entirely replaced by cysts (*arrows*). (**B**) Gross specimen of a right kidney from a patient with ADPKD who underwent renal transplantation. (Image A reproduced with permission from Fauci AS, et al. Harrison's Principles of Internal Medicine, 17th ed. New York, NY: McGraw-Hill; 2008. Image B reproduced with permission from USMLE-Rx.com.)

 KEY FACT

Left untreated, hydronephrosis resulting from urinary obstruction leads to hypertension, acute or chronic renal failure, or sepsis, and has a very poor prognosis.

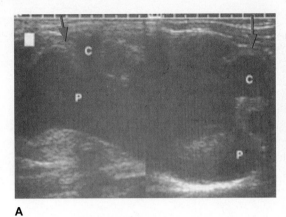
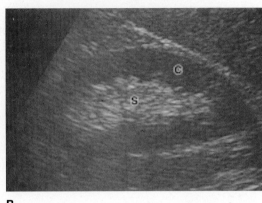

FIGURE 2.16-12. **Hydronephrosis.** **(A)** Ultrasound of a renal transplant shows severe hydronephrosis, with dilation of the renal pelvis (P) and the renal calyces (C). The overlying renal cortex is severely thinned *(arrows)*. **(B)** Normal renal ultrasound for comparison. C, cortex; S, sinus fat. (Reproduced with permission from Tanagho EA, McAninch JW. Smith's General Urology, 17th ed. New York, NY: McGraw-Hill; 2008.)

Scrotal Swelling

- Painless etiologies → hydrocele (remnant of processus vaginalis), varicocele (dilatation of pampiniform plexus, ↑ with standing/Valsalva).
- Painful etiologies → epididymitis (STDs, prostatitis), testicular torsion (twisting of the spermatic cord).

HISTORY/PE

Physical exam reveals "bag of worms" in varicocele, more often in left testicle than right. ⊕ Prehn sign (↓ pain with scrotal elevation) in epididymitis, ⊖ Prehn sign in torsion.

DIAGNOSIS

- Hydrocele will transilluminate on flashlight test; varicocele will not.
- Doppler ultrasonography shows normal to ↑ blood flow to testes in epididymitis, ↓ blood flow in torsion (see Figure 2.16-13).
- UA and culture may show *Neisseria gonorrhoeae, Escherichia coli,* or *Chlamydia* in epididymitis. Culture required to direct therapy in acute prostatitis. Chronic prostatitis/chronic pelvic pain syndrome will present with culture ⊖ irritation on voiding.

TREATMENT

- **Hydrocele:** Typically resolve within 12 months. Hydroceles that do not resolve should be removed surgically because of risk for inguinal hernia.
- **Varicocele:** May need surgery if large or symptomatic.
- **Epididymitis and acute prostatitis:** Antibiotics (ceftriaxone, doxycycline, fluoroquinolones); NSAIDs; scrotal support for pain.
- **Testicular torsion:** Immediate surgery (< 6 hours) to salvage testis. Attempt manual detorsion only if surgery is unavailable or if it will not delay surgery. Orchiopexy of both testes to prevent future torsion.
- **Chronic prostatitis/chronic pelvic pain syndrome:** α-Blockers, 5-α-reductase inhibitors.

KEY FACT

A tender, boggy prostate on rectal exam in the setting of fever is diagnostic for prostatitis.

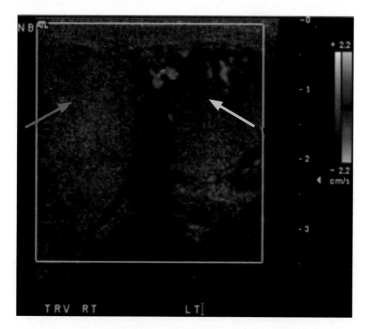

FIGURE 2.16-13. **Testicular torsion.** Transverse Doppler image through the scrotum demonstrates asymmetric swelling and decreased blood flow to the right testis *(red arrow)* compared with the left testis *(yellow arrow)* in this patient with acute right testicular pain. (Reproduced with permission from USMLE-Rx.com.)

Urinary Incontinence

See Table 2.16-7.

Interstitial Cystitis

Chronic, painful bladder condition that is associated with psychiatric disorders and other pain syndromes (eg, fibromyalgia). The onset is gradual.

TABLE 2.16-7. **Types of Urinary Incontinence and Associated Treatment**

TYPE	RISK FACTORS	SYMPTOMS	TREATMENT
Stress	Trauma during vaginal delivery	↑ Intraabdominal pressure (eg, laughing, sneezing, Valsalva) causing leakage	Lifestyle modifications and pelvic floor exercises (for all types of incontinence) Topical estrogen Pessary Surgery (eg, midurethral sling)
Urge	Older age, detrusor hyperactivity (eg, spinal cord injury)	Sudden need to urinate followed closely by leakage	Topical estrogen Antimuscarinics or mirabegron
Overflow	Detrusor underactivity (eg, diabetic neuropathy), bladder outlet obstruction	Constant leakage	Depending on underlying etiology: cholinergic agents, intermittent catheterization, sacral nerve stimulation

Bladder pain exacerbated by exercise, sexual intercourse, and alcohol consumption. Pain is relieved with voiding.

HISTORY/PE
- UA normal.
- Symptoms for >6 weeks.

DIAGNOSIS
Primary clinical.

TREATMENT
- Avoiding triggers (behavioral modification).
- Amitriptyline for refractory symptoms.

Erectile Dysfunction

Found in 10–25% of middle-aged and elderly men. Classified as failure to initiate (eg, psychological, endocrinologic, neurologic), failure to fill (eg, arteriogenic), or failure to store (eg, veno-occlusive dysfunction). Risk factors include DM, atherosclerosis, medications (eg, β-blockers, SSRIs, TCAs, diuretics), hypertension, heart disease, surgery or radiation for prostate cancer, and spinal cord injury.

HISTORY/PE
- Ask about risk factors (diabetes, peripheral vascular disease), medication use, recent life changes, and psychological stressors.
- The distinction between psychological and organic erectile dysfunction (ED) is based on the presence of nocturnal or early-morning erections (if present, it is nonorganic) and on situation dependence (ie, occurring with only one partner).
- Evaluate for neurologic dysfunction (eg, anal tone, lower extremity sensation) and for hypogonadism (eg, small testes, loss of 2° sexual characteristics).

DIAGNOSIS
- Clinical diagnosis.
- **Other work-up:** Testosterone and gonadotropin levels may be abnormal. Elevated prolactin can result in ↓ androgen activity.

TREATMENT
- **Best initial treatment:** Patients with psychological ED may benefit from psychotherapy involving discussion and exercises with the partner.
- Oral sildenafil, vardenafil, and tadalafil are phosphodiesterase-5 (PDE-5) inhibitors that result in prolonged action of cGMP-mediated smooth muscle relaxation and ↑ blood flow in the corpora cavernosa.
    - While sildenafil is useful for patients with ED 2° to cardiovascular disease, use with nitrates is contraindicated.
- Testosterone is a useful therapy for patients with hypogonadism of testicular or pituitary origin; it is discouraged for patients with normal testosterone levels.
- Vacuum pumps, intracavernosal prostaglandin injections, and surgical implantation of semirigid or inflatable penile prostheses are alternatives for patients for whom PDE5 therapy fails.

KEY FACT

"**P**oint and **S**hoot": The **P**arasympathetic nervous system mediates erection; the **S**ympathetic nervous system mediates ejaculation.

KEY FACT

Nitrates and phosphodiesterase 5 inhibitors are a dangerous combination → significant ↓ BP can lead to myocardial ischemia.

Benign Prostatic Hyperplasia

Enlargement of the prostate that is a normal part of the aging process and is seen in > 80% of men by 80 years of age. Most commonly presents in men > 50 years of age. BPH can coexist with prostate cancer, but BPH does not cause prostate cancer.

HISTORY/PE

- **Obstructive symptoms:** Hesitancy, weak stream, intermittent stream, incomplete emptying, urinary retention, bladder fullness, acute urinary retention following surgery.
- **Irritative symptoms:** Nocturia, daytime frequency, urge incontinence, opening hematuria.
- On digital rectal exam (DRE), the prostate is uniformly enlarged with a rubbery texture. Suspect cancer if the prostate is hard or has irregular lesions.

DIAGNOSIS

- Obtain a UA and urine culture to rule out infection and hematuria.
- Initial prostate-specific antigen (PSA) testing is controversial, though often ↑ in BPH. Further work-up needed if ↑ PSA correlates with other findings suspicious for prostate cancer.
- Consider creatinine levels to rule out obstructive uropathy and renal insufficiency. Similarly, consider testing electrolytes for any signs of renal tubular dysfunction from an obstruction.

TREATMENT

- Medical therapy:
  - **Best initial treatment:** α-blockers (eg, tamsulosin, terazosin), which relax smooth muscle in the prostate and bladder neck.
  - **Next best treatment:** 5α-reductase inhibitors (eg, finasteride), which inhibit the production of dihydrotestosterone.
- Transurethral resection of the prostate (TURP) or open prostatectomy is appropriate for patients with moderate to severe symptoms/complications (including renal insufficiency, recurrent UTIs, bladder stones).

Urologic Cancer

PROSTATE CANCER

The most common cancer in men and the second leading cause of cancer death in men (after lung cancer). Risk factors include advanced age and a ⊕ family history.

HISTORY/PE

- Usually asymptomatic, but may present with obstructive urinary symptoms and with lymphedema caused by obstructing metastases, constitutional symptoms, and back pain caused by bone metastases.
- DRE may reveal a palpable nodule or an area of induration (see Figure 2.16-14). Early carcinoma is usually not detectable on exam.

KEY FACT

BPH most commonly occurs in the central (periurethral) zone of the prostate and may not be detected on DRE.

KEY FACT

Leading causes of cancer death in men:
1. Lung cancer
2. Prostate cancer
3. Colorectal cancer
4. Pancreatic cancer

 Q **1**

A 68-year-old woman with a history of hepatitis and CKD presents with RUQ abdominal pain. A CT scan identifies liver cirrhosis. Two days later, her creatinine levels have doubled. What is the likely cause, and what could have prevented this outcome?

 Q **2**

A 19-year-old man with a history of recurrent kidney stones presents with acute left flank pain. His father also has a history of kidney stones. A urinary cyanide nitroprusside test is ⊕. A CT scan confirms nephrolithiasis. What is the most likely diagnosis?

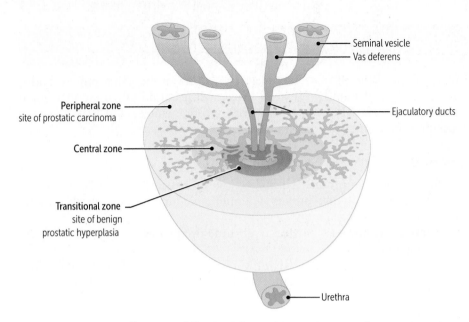

FIGURE 2.16-14. **Structure of the prostate.** (Reproduced with permission from USMLE-Rx.com.)

DIAGNOSIS

- Suggested by clinical findings and/or a markedly ↑ PSA (> 4 ng/mL).
- **Most accurate test:** Ultrasound-guided transrectal biopsy.
- Tumors are graded by the Gleason histologic system, which sums the scores (from 1 to 5) of the two most dysplastic samples (10 is the highest grade).
- Look for metastases with CT of the abdomen/pelvis and bone scan (metastatic lesions show an osteoblastic or ↑ bone density).

TREATMENT

- Watchful waiting may be the best approach for elderly patients with low-grade tumors, as many cases of prostate cancer are slow to progress.
- Radical prostatectomy is associated with ↑ risk for incontinence and/or ED.
- Radiation therapy (eg, brachytherapy or external beam) is associated with ↑ risk for radiation proctitis and GI symptoms.
- PSA, while controversial as a screening test, is used to follow a patient's posttreatment to evaluate for disease recurrence.
- Treat metastatic disease with androgen ablation (eg, gonadotropin-releasing hormone agonists, orchiectomy, flutamide) and chemotherapy.
- Radiation therapy is useful to manage bone pain from metastases after androgen ablation.

PREVENTION

Screening guidelines remain controversial. Men should discuss the pros and cons of annual DRE and/or PSA testing starting at 50 years of age. Screening should begin earlier in African-American men and in those with a first-degree relative with prostate cancer.

BLADDER CANCER

The second most common urologic cancer and the most frequent malignant tumor of the urinary tract; usually a transitional cell carcinoma (see Figure 2.16-15). Most prevalent in men during the sixth and seventh decades. Risk factors include smoking, diets rich in meat and fat, schistosomiasis, past treatment with cyclophosphamide, and occupational exposure to aniline dye.

KEY FACT

An ↑ PSA can be caused by BPH, prostatitis, prostatic trauma, or carcinoma.

1 | **A**

The patient probably has contrast-induced nephropathy and would have benefited from isotonic saline hydration before and during the CT scan.

2 | **A**

Cystinuria. Decreased cystine reabsorption caused by a defect in proximal tubular amino acid transport. You would also probably see hexagonal crystals on UA.

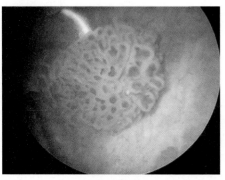
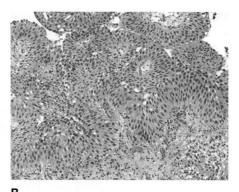

A   **B**

FIGURE 2.16-15.   Transitional cell carcinoma of the bladder. (**A**) Cystoscopic image of bladder wall mass. (**B**) Papillary growth lined by transitional epithelium with mild nuclear atypia and pleomorphism. (Part A modified with permission from Geavlete B, Stanescu F, Moldoveanu C, et al. NBI cystoscopy and bipolar electrosurgery in NMIBC management—an overview of daily practice. J Med Life. 2013;6(2):140–145. Part B reproduced with permission from Le T, et al. First Aid for the USMLE Step 1 2015. New York, NY: McGraw-Hill; 2015.)

HISTORY/PE

- Gross, painless hematuria is the most common presenting symptom. Terminal hematuria (end of voiding) suggests bleeding from bladder.
- Other urinary symptoms, such as frequency, urgency, and dysuria, can also be seen, but most patients are asymptomatic in the early stages of disease.

DIAGNOSIS

- Screening is not recommended.
- Cystoscopy with biopsy is diagnostic and is recommended in the evaluation of older adults to rule out malignancy.
- UA often shows hematuria (macro- or microscopic).
- Cytology may show dysplastic cells.
- MRI, CT, and bone scan are important tools with which to define invasion and metastases.

TREATMENT

Treatment depends on the extent of spread beyond the bladder mucosa.

- **Carcinoma in situ:** Intravesicular chemotherapy.
- **Superficial cancers:** Complete transurethral resection or intravesicular chemotherapy with mitomycin-C or BCG (the TB vaccine).
- **Large, high-grade recurrent lesions:** Intravesicular chemotherapy.
- **Invasive cancers without metastases:** Radical cystectomy or radiation therapy for patients who are deemed poor candidates for radical cystectomy and for those with unresectable local disease.
- **Invasive cancers with distant metastases:** Chemotherapy alone.

RENAL CELL CARCINOMA

An adenocarcinoma from tubular epithelial cells (~ 80–90% of all malignant tumors of the kidney). Tumors can spread along the renal vein to the IVC and can metastasize to lung and bone. Risk factors include male gender, smoking, obesity, acquired cystic kidney disease in ESRD, and certain genetic conditions, such as von Hippel–Lindau disease.

HISTORY/PE

- Presenting signs include gross hematuria, flank pain, and a palpable flank mass. Metastatic disease can present with weight loss and malaise.

MNEMONIC

Differential for hematuria—

I PEE RBCS

Infection (UTI)
Polycystic kidney disease
Exercise
External trauma
Renal glomerular disease
Benign prostatic hyperplasia
Cancer, **C**ongenital anomalies/obstruction, **C**ysts, Hyper**C**alciuria, **C**rystals
Stones, **S**ickle cell

KEY FACT

The next best step for diagnosis in an adult patient with unexplained hematuria is cystoscopy to evaluate for bladder cancer.

KEY FACT

The classic triad of renal cell carcinoma is hematuria, flank pain, and a palpable flank mass, but only 5–10% present with all three components of the triad.

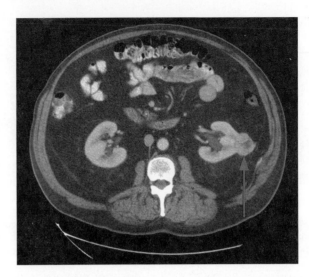

FIGURE 2.16-16. **Renal cell carcinoma.** A contrast-enhanced CT through the abdomen demonstrates an enhancing exophytic mass *(arrow)* in the left kidney that proved on pathology to be renal cell carcinoma. (Reproduced with permission from Doherty GM. Current Diagnosis & Treatment: Surgery, 13th ed. New York, NY: McGraw-Hill; 2010.)

KEY FACT

In a middle-aged smoker with a left-sided varicocele, think renal cell carcinoma!

- Many patients have fever or other constitutional symptoms. Left-sided varicocele can be seen in men (caused by tumor blockage of the left gonadal vein, which empties into the left renal vein; the right gonadal vein empties directly into the IVC).
- Anemia is common at presentation, but polycythemia caused by ↑ erythropoietin production can be seen in 5–10% of patients.

DIAGNOSIS

Best initial test: Diagnosed via CT (see Figure 2.16-16) to characterize the renal mass and stage for lymph nodes/metastases. Ultrasonography rarely used. Diagnosis is then confirmed by histology on nephrectomy specimen.

TREATMENT

- Surgical resection may be curative in localized disease. Metastasectomy may improve survival in metastatic disease.
- Response rates from radiation or chemotherapy are only 15–30%. Newer tyrosine kinase inhibitors (sorafenib, sunitinib), which ↓ tumor angiogenesis and cell proliferation, have shown promising results.

TESTICULAR CANCER

A heterogeneous group of neoplasms. Some 95% of testicular tumors derive from germ cells, and virtually all are malignant. Cryptorchidism is associated with an ↑ risk for neoplasia in both testes. Klinefelter syndrome is also a risk factor. Testicular cancer is the most common malignancy in men 15–34 years of age.

HISTORY/PE

- Patients most often present with painless enlargement of the testes.
- Most testicular cancers occur between 15 and 30 years of age, but seminomas have a peak incidence between 40 and 50 years of age.

TABLE 2.16-8.   Tumor Markers in Testicular Cancer

TYPE	TUMOR MARKER
GERM CELL TUMORS (95% OF ALL TESTICULAR TUMORS)	
Seminoma (most common testicular tumor)	Usually ⊖, ↑ β-hCG in some cases
Yolk sac (endodermal sinus tumor)	↑ AFP
Choriocarcinoma	↑ β-hCG
Teratoma	AFP and/or β-hCG
NON–GERM CELL TUMORS (5% OF ALL TESTICULAR TUMORS)	
Leydig cell	↑ Testosterone and estrogen (causing ↓ LH and FSH)
Sertoli cell	None
Testicular lymphoma	None. Arises from metastasis to testes

DIAGNOSIS

- Testicular ultrasonography.
- Chest x-ray (CXR) and CT of the abdomen/pelvis to evaluate for metastasis.
- Tumor markers are useful for diagnosis and in monitoring treatment response (see Table 2.16-8).

TREATMENT

- Radical orchiectomy and classify into seminoma or nonseminomatous germ cell tumor (NSGCT).
  - Seminoma: Radiation therapy for low-stage disease.
  - NSGCT: Retroperitoneal lymph node dissection for low-stage disease.
- Platinum-based chemotherapy is used for advanced disease of either type.

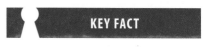

KEY FACT

β-hCG in men = choriocarcinoma

NOTES

SURGERY AND EMERGENCY MEDICINE

Trauma Management

The Advanced Trauma Life Support (ATLS) algorithm divides management into two phases: the primary survey focuses on resuscitation and gross identification of injuries, while the secondary survey serves as a more detailed, head-to-toe assessment of the patient. Many USMLE questions on trauma depend on knowing the order of the primary and secondary surveys. Remember, establishing and maintaining airway patency takes precedence over all other treatment.

PRIMARY SURVEY

Airway

- **Assessment:** If the patient can speak clearly, the airway is intact. If not, consider these indications for emergency airway management:
    - **Structural airway damage:** Subcutaneous emphysema in neck, gurgling noises during breathing, or major facial trauma with blood in airway.
    - **Airway compression:** Expanding neck hematoma.
    - **Somnolence:** Glasgow Coma Scale (GCS) 8 or less (see Table 2.17-1).
    - **Thermal or inhalation injury:** Suspect in patients with singed facial hairs, facial burns, or soot in the posterior oropharynx or sputum.
- **Management:** Emergency airway:
    - **Endotracheal intubation:** Preferred method, even in setting of cervical spinal trauma.
    - **Nasotracheal intubation w/fiberoptic bronchoscope:** Preferred if tracheobronchial tree is ruptured. Contraindicated if basilar skull fracture (risk for intracranial penetration).
    - **Emergency cricothyroidotomy:** Attempt only if other methods are ineffective.
    - **Emergency tracheostomy:** In general, never do this. Choose cricothyroidotomy instead.

Breathing

- **Assessment:** Breath sounds, chest rise, oxygen saturation.
- **Management:**
    - If patient has unilateral breath sounds, think pneumothorax or hemothorax. Differentiate using percussion (dullness = hemothorax; resonance

TABLE 2.17-1. Glasgow Coma Scale Scoring

SCORE	EYE OPENING RESPONSE (4 POINTS, [FOUR-EYES])	VERBAL RESPONSE (5 POINTS, [JACKSON-5])	MOTOR RESPONSE (6 POINTS [V6 ENGINE])
6			Follows commands
5		Oriented	Localizes pain
4	Spontaneous	Confused speech	Withdraws to pain
3	Opens to command	Inappropriate words	Flexion
2	Opens to pain	Incomprehensible	Extension
1	None	None	None

= pneumothorax). Can verify with chest x-ray (CXR) only if patient is hemodynamically stable. Insert chest tube to expand lung.

- If patient has unilateral breath sounds on the right after intubation, consider right main stem bronchus cannulation. CXR may show endotracheal tube below carina. Withdraw tube above carina to oxygenate both lungs.
- If patient has bilateral breath sounds and good chest rise but cannot oxygenate, intubate and mechanically ventilate.

Circulation

- **Assessment:** Assess for shock (systolic blood pressure [SBP] < 90 mmHg, fast and weak pulse, pallor, diaphoresis).
- **Management:** Three causes of shock in trauma are as follows:
  - **Hemorrhage** (most common): There are only 5 places you can bleed enough to cause shock: the chest, abdomen, pelvis, extremities, and the floor (external hemorrhage). Intracranial hemorrhage (ICH) will never cause hypovolemic shock. Place two large-bore IVs (16 gauge or larger) and bolus 2 L isotonic crystalloid. If still unstable, transfuse PRBCs and look for source of bleeding. Transfuse FFP if > 6 units PRBCs given.
  - **Tension pneumothorax:** Diagnose clinically if hypotension, tracheal deviation, ↓ O₂ saturation, unilateral decreased breath sounds/hyperresonance. Needle decompress with IV catheter, and then place chest tube. **Do not wait for CXR to intervene** (see Figure 2.17-2).
  - **Cardiac tamponade:** Suspect if hypotension, muffled heart sounds, and jugular venous distension. Confirm with ultrasound (see Figure 2.17-1). Surgical intervention via pericardial window, pericardiocentesis, or thoracotomy.

Deformities

Assessment: Assess for traumatic brain injury using GCS and pupillary exam. Assess for spinal cord injury by examining movement and gross sensation in extremities.

Exposure

- **Assessment:** Assess visible injuries, take body temperature, logroll the patient, and perform rectal exam.
- **Management:** Remove clothing, and cover with warm blankets.

KEY FACT

Hemodynamic instability in the trauma setting is defined as systolic blood pressure < 90 mmHg.

KEY FACT

When IV access is necessary but cannot be obtained after multiple attempts, place an interosseous line.

KEY FACT

A fourth rare cause of shock in trauma is neurogenic shock from high spinal cord injury. Disrupted sympathetic outflow ↓ total peripheral resistance (TPR). Suspect after ruling out three main causes of shock in a patient with motor deficits. Treat with vasopressors to ↑ TPR.

KEY FACT

A rough estimate of SBP can be made based on palpated pulses. Palpable carotid = 60 mmHg, femoral = 70 mmHg, and radial = 80 mmHg.

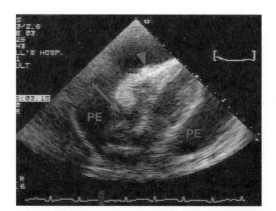

FIGURE 2.17-1. Cardiac tamponade. Echocardiogram in a patient with cardiac tamponade shows a large pericardial effusion (PE) with right atrial (*arrow*) and right ventricular (*arrowhead*) collapse. (Reproduced with permission from Hall JB, et al. *Principles of Critical Care*, 3rd ed. New York, NY: McGraw-Hill; 2005.)

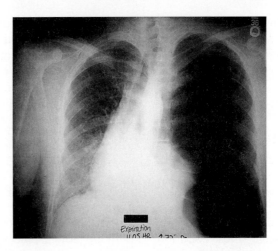

FIGURE 2.17-2. **Tension pneumothorax.** Note the hyperlucent left hemithorax, flattening and inferior displacement of the left diaphragm, and rightward shift of the mediastinal structures. These are typical radiographic findings in patients with tension pneumothorax.

SECONDARY SURVEY

- After the patient's ABCDEs are managed, conduct a full head-to-toe exam.
- **Adjuncts to survey:**
  - CXR, x-ray of the pelvis, and focused abdominal sonography for trauma (FAST) to identify source in a bleeding patient.
  - Pertinent labs should address mechanism of injury, intoxication or overdose, and medical history (type and cross-match all patients of concern or with hemorrhage).
  - Place Foley catheter to monitor urine output in hemodynamically unstable patients to guide resuscitation and those undergoing surgery.
  - Place orogastric tube for patients requiring mechanical ventilation.
- **Order radiologic studies based on the assessment of hemodynamically stable patients:**
  - Head CT for any patient with head trauma, loss of consciousness, drowsiness/altered mental status, structural skull damage, or neurologic deficits.
  - C-spine CT is needed for all patients with neck pain or tenderness, or anyone getting a head CT.

Penetrating Trauma

This section describes management of specific trauma injuries after initial evaluation using primary and secondary surveys. These considerations generally assume ABCDEs are previously secured.

NECK

- In patients with signs of arterial injury (eg, active bleed, expanding hematoma, neurologic deficit, or hematemesis) or hemodynamic instability, immediately secure airway and take to the operating room (OR) for exploration.
- Stable patients should receive CT angiography (CTA) of the neck. Identified vascular injuries are treated with surgery or embolization.

KEY FACT

Always rule out urethral injury before placing a Foley catheter. Blood at the meatus, high-riding prostate, and scrotal hematoma are signs of urethral injury. Perform retrograde urethrogram to identify injury.

KEY FACT

Only wounds that violate the platysma are considered true penetrating neck trauma. Other superficial wounds are treated with conservative wound care.

▪ Patients with suspected injury to the trachea or esophagus (eg, gurgling breath sounds, bubbling wound, pneumomediastinum) should be evaluated via direct visualization using bronchoscopy or esophagoscopy. Alternatively, barium swallow esophagography can evaluate the esophagus.

CHEST

Penetrating chest injuries are often treated during the primary survey since they often can compromise breathing or cause hemodynamic instability. The treatment of tension pneumothorax and cardiac tamponade are therefore discussed previously.

HISTORY/PE

▪ If a previously stable chest trauma patient becomes rapidly unstable, suspect air embolism.
▪ A new diastolic murmur after chest trauma suggests aortic dissection.
▪ Massive air leak into tube thoracostomy suggests tracheobronchial injury.

DIAGNOSIS

▪ Perform CXR in any patient with penetrating chest trauma to evaluate for pneumothorax or hemothorax not found in primary survey. Aortic disruption, diaphragmatic tear, or esophageal injury may also be evident on CXR.
▪ Chest injuries between the nipples require evaluation of mediastinal structures. Order echocardiography for the heart, CTA for the aorta and its branches, bronchoscopy for the upper airway, and esophagograph/esophagogram for the esophagus.

TREATMENT

▪ Insert tube thoracostomy for pneumothorax or hemothorax.
▪ 1500 mL output initially or 300 mL/h for 3 consecutive hours from tube thoracostomy warrants thoracotomy.
▪ Aortic, diaphragmatic, esophageal, or tracheobronchial injury also warrant surgical correction.
▪ Immediate thoracotomy without transport to OR may be indicated for patients with penetrating chest trauma and cardiac arrest.

ABDOMEN

Penetrating trauma to the abdomen is defined as any object (typically gunshot or knife) that violates the peritoneum. An important step in management is determining whether peritoneal signs (guarding, rigidity, rebound tenderness) are present. These injuries are managed according to the mechanism.

▪ Gunshot wounds below the nipple (fourth intercostal space) require immediate exploratory laparotomy.
▪ Abdominal stab wounds warrant immediate exploratory laparotomy if the patient exhibits hemodynamic instability, peritoneal signs, or extruded bowel or omentum.
  ▪ If the patient does not have these indications, explore the wound to identify violation of peritoneum. If a defect is found, laparotomy is generally indicated.
  ▪ If peritoneum is not violated, observe the patient for 24 h. Perform laparotomy if the patient develops hemodynamic instability, peritoneal signs, drop in Hb > 3mg/dL, or leukocytosis.

KEY FACT

Leave impaled objects in place until the patient is taken to the OR, as such objects may tamponade further blood loss.

Q   1

A 25-year-old man walks into the ED holding a blood-soaked towel against his neck after being shot. The patient is anxious, appears pale, and states he heard multiple gunshots. Vital signs after 2 L of crystalloid are BP 86/55 mm Hg, HR 122 bpm, RR 16/min, and Spo$_2$ 99%. Physical exam reveals that the neck wound does not extend through the platysma muscle. What is the next step in management?

Q   2

A 22-year-old woman is brought to the ED after a motor vehicle collision in which she was the restrained driver. She receives 2 L of crystalloid en route and has a BP of 65/40 mm Hg and a HR of 135 bpm on arrival. She has ↓ breath sounds on the right, flat neck veins, and dullness to percussion on the right side. What is the most likely diagnosis?

EXTREMITIES

- Neurovascular assessment is critical; check pulses using palpation and Doppler, motor function, and sensory function.
  - For hard signs of vascular injury (eg, expanding hematoma, pulsatile bleeding, absent pulse), immediately explore and repair in OR.
  - For soft signs of vascular injury (neurologic deficit, significant bleeding, weak pulse), perform CTA.
- Extremities with multiples injuries are generally treated in the following order:
  - Fixation of broken bones.
  - Revascularization of arterial injuries.
  - Reapproximation of injured nerves.
- If an injury separates an appendage from the body, parts should be placed in gauze moistened with saline, sealed inside a plastic bag, and placed on ice to maximize tissue viability.
- Contaminated wounds require early wound irrigation and tissue débridement. Also, administer antibiotics and tetanus prophylaxis.
- Long-term complications include high-output heart failure caused by formation of an arteriovenous fistula (AVF). Despite ↑↑ cardiac output, patients present with signs and signs and symptoms of CHF.

Blunt and Deceleration Trauma

HEAD

- All patients with loss of consciousness need CT head without contrast.
- Look for signs of ↑ ICP (eg, bradycardia, hypertension, respiratory depression, fixed and dilated pupil[s], vomiting, and/or papilledema). Treat ↑ ICP with head elevation, hyperventilation, and IV mannitol.
- **Linear skull fractures:** Treat nonoperatively with wound care and closure if open. Surgery is reserved for displaced or comminuted fractures.
- **Epidural hematomas:** Lenticular or biconvex shape on head CT (see Figure 2.17-3A). Blood from the middle meningeal artery fills the potential space between the dura and skull. These hemorrhages cannot cross suture lines (dura is anchored to sutures) but can expand rapidly causing uncal herniation and death. Patients classically lose consciousness immediately after the injury and undergo a "lucid interval" after which they become

1 **A**

Administer blood products, and search for source of bleeding other than the neck. The management of this patient begins with the primary survey. The patient can speak, so airway is intact. RR and Spo₂ are within normal limits, so breathing is assumed to be stable. The patient remains hemodynamically unstable despite 2 L of crystalloid, so blood products are administered, and a source of bleeding is sought. The platysma is not violated, so the neck wound is not the cause of significant bleeding despite the blood-soaked towel. There is likely an additional gunshot wound that needs to be identified.

2 **A**

Hemothorax. Hemodynamic instability with ↓ breath sounds are concerning for hemothorax and tension pneumothorax. Flat neck veins are more consistent with hemothorax since tension pneumothorax causes ↑ intrathoracic pressure → ↓ ventricular filling → ↑ CVP and distended neck veins. Dullness to percussion also shifts the diagnosis toward hemothorax. Each hemothorax can hold 40% of a patient's circulating blood volume, and patients may therefore present in hypovolemic shock.

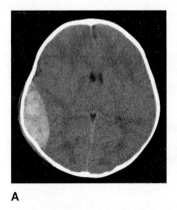
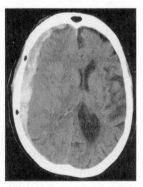

A   **B**

FIGURE 2.17-3. **Acute epidural and acute subdural hematoma.** (**A**) Noncontrast CT showing a right temporal acute epidural hematoma. Note the characteristic biconvex shape. (**B**) Noncontrast CT demonstrating a right acute hemispheric subdural hematoma. Note the characteristic crescentic shape. (Image A reproduced with permission from Doherty GM. *Current Diagnosis & Treatment: Surgery*, 13th ed. New York, NY: McGraw-Hill; 2010. Image B reproduced with permission from Chen MY, et al. *Basic Radiology*, 1st ed. New York, NY: McGraw-Hill; 2004.)

comatose. Exam may show ipsilateral blown pupil and ipsilateral hemiparesis. Perform emergent craniotomy.

- **Subdural hematomas:** Crescent-shaped bleed on head CT (see Figure 2.17-3B). Blood from the dural bridging veins fills potential space between the dura and arachnoid mater. These hemorrhages cross suture lines. They may present acute (immediate), subacute (days), or chronic (weeks). Perform craniotomy if CT shows midline shift. Otherwise, manage ICP and use fluids judiciously to limit cerebral edema.
- **Diffuse axonal injury:** Often occurs with severe rapid-deceleration head injuries. CT characteristically shows blurring and punctate hemorrhaging along the gray–white matter junction. Prognosis is hard to predict. Reduce 2° injury by limiting cerebral edema and increases in ICP.

CHEST

Tracheobronchial Disruption

- Most often caused by deceleration shearing forces.
- Physical findings include respiratory distress, hemoptysis, sternal tenderness, and subcutaneous emphysema.
- Radiographs may show a large pneumothorax or pneumomediastinum (see Figure 2.17-4).
- Air may persistently pour into chest tube when hooked to wall suction.

Blunt Cardiac Injury

- Also known as myocardial contusion, may present as a new bundle branch block, ectopy or dysrhythmia, or hypotension.
- Severe contusion can present with LV dysfunction and cardiogenic shock. Serum cardiac biomarkers are often elevated.
- Treatment is largely supportive, sometimes requiring inotropes.

Pulmonary Contusion

- May lead to hypoxia from damage to capillaries causing interstitial fluid accumulation. Hypoxia, therefore, tends to worsen with fluid hydration.
- Look for patchy alveolar opacities on CXR.
- Intubate if necessary, and be judicious about IV fluids.
- More common in children because of a less rigid, protective chest wall.

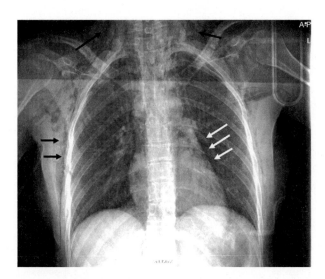

FIGURE 2.17-4. CXR reveals pneumomediastinum *(white arrows)* and subcutaneous emphysema *(black arrows)*. (Reproduced with permission from Van Heijl M, et al. Unique case of esophageal rupture after a fall from height. *BMC Emerg Med.* 2009;9:24.)

Q   **1**

A 36-year-old man is brought to the ED following a motor vehicle collision in which he was an unrestrained passenger. X-rays show multiple fractures. Several hours later he develops fever, respiratory distress, and a rash consisting of small red and purple 1- to 2-mm macules covering his arms and shoulders. What is the most likely diagnosis?

Q   **2**

A 10-year-old boy is brought to the ED 5 hours after he hit his head on a concrete sidewalk while skateboarding. He briefly lost consciousness at the scene, but his neurologic exam and head CT are normal. What is the next step in ED management?

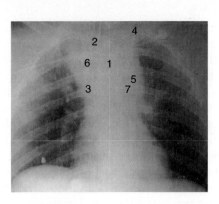

FIGURE 2.17-5. **Aortic disruption.** CXR of hypotensive man injured in a high-speed motor vehicle collision. Findings: (1) widened mediastinum; (2) deviation of the trachea to the right; (3) widening of the right paratracheal stripe; (4) left apical cap; (5) blurring of the aortic knob; (6) deviation of the NG tube to the right; (7) obliteration of the aortopulmonary window. (Reproduced with permission from Stone CK, Humphries RL. *Current Diagnosis & Treatment: Emergency Medicine,* 7th ed. New York, NY: McGraw Hill; 2011.)

KEY FACT

Since complete aortic rupture is rapidly fatal (85% die at the scene), patients with aortic disruption seen in the ED usually have a contained hematoma within the adventitia.

KEY FACT

Hoarseness of the voice can be caused by aortic disruption as expansion of the hematoma impinges on the left recurrent laryngeal nerve.

KEY FACT

Marfan syndrome, syphilis, and Ehlers-Danlos syndrome weaken the aortic wall and predispose to aortic injury.

Aortic Disruption

- Classically caused by rapid deceleration injury (eg, high-speed motor vehicle accidents, ejection from vehicles, fall from heights).
- Injury is most common in the proximal thoracic aorta near the ligamentum arteriosum, which anchors the aorta in place. The adjacent aorta displaces forward, creating shear force.
- CXR reveals a widened mediastinum (> 8 cm), loss of aortic knob, pleural cap, deviation of the trachea and esophagus, and depression of the left main stem bronchus (see Figure 2.17-5).
- Ultrasonography can diagnose concurrent pericardial tamponade.
- Confirm with CTA in stable patients. Unstable patients may undergo transesophageal echocardiogram or intraoperative evaluation.
- Emergency surgery is required for any defect.

Flail Chest

- Three or more adjacent ribs are fractured at two points causing paradoxical movement of the segment. The segment moves **in**ward with **in**spiration and outward during exhalation (see Figure 2.17-6).

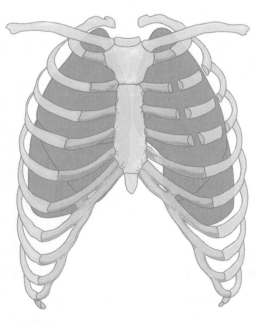

FIGURE 2.17-6. **Flail chest.** (Reproduced with permission from USMLE-Rx.com.)

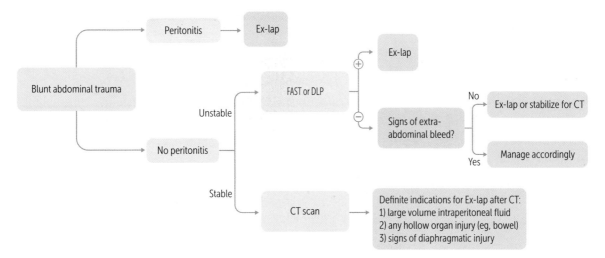

FIGURE 2.17-7.   Blunt abdominal trauma algorithm. (Reproduced with permission from USMLE-Rx.com.)

- Respiratory compromise in flail chest occurs because of underlying pulmonary contusion rather than the flail chest itself.
- Pain control and positive pressure ventilation compose the mainstay of treatment for flail chest. Ribs can be fixed surgically, especially in severe cases.

ABDOMEN

Figure 2.17-7 describes the diagnostic work-up for blunt abdominal trauma (BAT). The FAST exam is preferred over diagnostic peritoneal lavage (DPL) in unstable patients, but DPL is used for unequivocal FAST or if FAST is unavailable. Assess hemodynamically stable patients with CT scan. Patients with minor BAT (no seatbelt sign [see Figure 2.17-8], mild tenderness) may be observed with serial abdominal scans. While management of specific organ damage is beyond the scope of Step 2 CK, some common associations come in handy (see Table 2.17-2).

- Anticoagulation and cardiac catheterization place patients at risk for retroperitoneal hematoma. Look for back pain and hemodynamic instability.
- In patients with spinal cord injuries, catheterization placement is diagnostic and therapeutic for acute urinary retention.

PELVIS

Pelvic Fractures

Most commonly occur after high-speed traumas such as motor vehicle accidents or falls from heights. Can cause significant hemorrhage leading to hypotension and shock.

DIAGNOSIS

- Apply pressure to the anterior superior iliac spine bilaterally to test for unstable or open book fracture.
- X-ray of the pelvis may confirm the fracture. In a stable patient, CT scan of the pelvis will better define the extent of injury.
- Always rule out injuries to other pelvic structures. Perform rectal exam and/or proctoscopy for the rectum, retrograde cystogram for the bladder, pelvic exam for the vagina in women, and retrograde urethrogram for urethra in men.

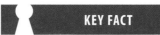

KEY FACT

First rib, scapula, and sternum are thick, strong bones and difficult to break. Blunt trauma causing these injuries is associated with aortic disruption.

KEY FACT

Diaphragmatic irritation can cause referred pain to the shoulder since the phrenic nerve shares origins with the brachial plexus. Irritation is caused by blood, air, or rupture.

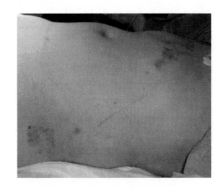

FIGURE 2.17-8.   Seat belt sign. Adult restrained driver with abdominal seat belt sign. (Reproduced with permission from Abbas AK, Hefny AF, Abu-Zidan FM. Seatbelts and road traffic collision injuries. *World J Emerg Surg* 2011;6:18.)

TABLE 2.17-2. **Commonly Injured Abdominal Organs**

ORGAN	NOTES
Spleen	Most commonly injured organ in BAT Often associated with fractured left ribs 9–11 Give vaccines 2 weeks later if spleen is removed (pneumococcal [PCV and PPSV], HiB, and meningococcal)
Liver	Second most commonly injured organ in BAT Often associated with right lower rib fractures
Kidney	Kidneys do not grow back, so try not to remove them
Duodenum	Susceptible to compression injury caused by position adjacent to spinal column. Look for retroperitoneal air on x-ray Suspect duodenal hematoma in a child who wrecks his or her bike and falls on handlebars. Patient presents with epigastric pain + bilious vomiting
Pancreas	Also common in children with handlebar injuries
Diaphragm	Diaphragm most commonly ruptures on the left since liver protects the right side Look for abdominal viscera in thorax on CXR

TREATMENT

- Transfuse as necessary. More than 40% of patients with pelvic fractures require transfusion.
- Management of unstable patients is controversial, but external pelvic binder (provides stability and tamponade effect) and angiographic embolization is probably the safest answer.
- External and internal pelvic fixation are also options, but surgery on a bleeding pelvis is risky. This may be the answer in a stable patient or if pelvic binder is not an option.

COMPLICATIONS

- **Bladder injuries:** Classified based on whether the injury communicates with the peritoneal cavity (intraperitoneal) or stays confined to the pelvis (extraperitoneal).
  - **Extraperitoneal bladder injury:** Rupture of bladder neck/trigone. Pain is localized in the lower abdomen and pelvis. Causes gross hematuria. Treat nonoperatively with Foley catheter.
  - **Intraperitoneal bladder injury:** Rupture of the dome of the bladder. Abdominal pain is diffuse +/− guarding and rigidity. Urine output is low or absent despite aggressive rehydration. Treat with surgical correction.
- **Rectal and vaginal:** Usually managed nonoperatively unless reconstruction is necessary.

KEY FACT

Because of the ringlike structure of the pelvic anatomy, pelvic fractures tend to occur in multiples rather than singular fractures.

Acute Abdomen

Defined as any patient that presents with new-onset, severe abdominal pain and tenderness. These patients usually require surgery, but many nonsurgical mimics exist. Do not be fooled by alternate diagnoses (see Table 2.17-3) that

TABLE 2.17-3. Nonsurgical Causes of Acute Abdomen

Etiology	Cause
Extra-abdominal	MI, PE, pneumonia (all cause right or left upper quadrant pain)
Hematologic	Sickle cell crisis, leukemia
Metabolic	Diabetic ketoacidosis, uremia
Genetic/familial	Familial Mediterranean fever, acute intermittent porphyria
Toxic	Lead and heavy metal poisoning, black widow spider bite

present with acute abdominal pain and additional bizarre features. Always consider the gynecologic etiology in women.

History/PE

- In general, four pathologies contribute to acute abdomen and present with characteristic symptoms. Considering these mechanisms along with location (see Figure 2.17-9) and associated history/physical exam findings may help delineate the diagnosis.
- Rectal exam for everyone and pelvic exam for women are always indicated.
- **Perforation or rupture**: Sudden onset of diffuse, excruciating pain. Patients will lie still to minimize pain. Peritoneal signs are prominent.
  - **Esophageal perforation (Boerhaave syndrome)**: Associated with recurrent vomiting/hematemesis. Commonly presents with retrosternal and epigastric pain.

KEY FACT

There are only two indications to defer a rectal exam: (1) patient does not have a rectum, and (2) you do not have a finger.

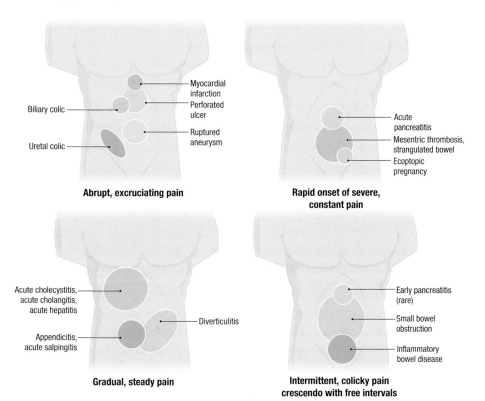

Abrupt, excruciating pain
- Biliary colic
- Ureteral colic
- Myocardial infarction
- Perforated ulcer
- Ruptured aneurysm

Rapid onset of severe, constant pain
- Acute pancreatitis
- Mesentric thrombosis, strangulated bowel
- Ecoptopic pregnancy

Gradual, steady pain
- Acute cholecystitis, acute cholangitis, acute hepatitis
- Appendicitis, acute salpingitis
- Diverticulitis

Intermittent, colicky pain crescendo with free intervals
- Early pancreatitis (rare)
- Small bowel obstruction
- Inflammatory bowel disease

FIGURE 2.17-9. Acute abdomen. The location and character of pain can be helpful in the differential diagnosis of the acute abdomen. (Reproduced with permission from USMLE-Rx.com.)

Q

A 65-year-old male smoker is brought to the ED for sudden-onset abdominal and back pain. The anxious patient complains of "ripping pain." Physical exam reveals a large, pulsatile mass behind the umbilicus. The patient's BP is 80/50 mm Hg and heart rate 125 bpm. You begin crystalloid and blood infusions. What is the most appropriate next step in management?

- **Other GI perforation:** Associated with peptic ulcer disease (PUD), cancer, diverticulitis, and inflammatory bowel disease (IBD).
- **Ruptured AAA:** Most common in male smokers > 55 years of age. Patient may describe periumbilical pain that radiates to the back. Abdominal exam may reveal pulsatile mass.
- **Ruptured ectopic pregnancy/ovarian cyst:** Common in women of childbearing age.
- **Obstruction:** Sudden onset of severe, colicky, intermittent pain. Patients cannot sit still. Peritoneal signs are usually absent.
  - **Small bowel obstruction:** Most commonly from adhesions after surgery, incarcerated hernias, or in patients with IBD or cancer. Patient may complain of obstipation (failure to pass stool or gas).
  - **Volvulus:** Patient may complain of obstipation.
  - **Ureteric/biliary obstruction:** Nephrolithiasis causes colicky pain, but it usually radiates to the groin and may cause hematuria/pyuria. May also cause costovertebral angle tenderness (CVAT). Biliary colic is most common in multiparous, overweight women (female, forty, fertile, and fat). Fatty meals exacerbate pain. No signs of peritoneal irritation.
- **Inflammation:** Gradual onset (over 10–12 h) of constant, poorly localized pain that later localizes to problem area. Patients lie still to minimize pain. Peritoneal signs are prominent.
  - **Appendicitis:** Detailed later.
  - **Cholecystitis:** Same demographics as biliary colic. Pain is constant. Peritoneal irritation is evident. Murphy sign causes pain on inspiration.
  - **Diverticulitis:** Prominent LLQ pain, change in bowel habits, and +/– nausea/vomiting. Palpation or rectal exam may reveal mass (abscess).
  - **Pelvic inflammatory disease (PID):** Associated with history of GC/Chlamydia or in young women with unsafe sexual practices. Pelvic exam elicits cervical motion tenderness and adnexal tenderness.
- **Ischemia:** Variable presentation, dependent on specific etiology.
  - **Acute mesenteric ischemia:** Sudden onset of pain and hematochezia in a patient with history of atrial fibrillation.
  - **Ischemic colitis:** Postprandial abdominal pain +/– hematochezia/melena in a patient with significant atherosclerotic disease (prior MI/stroke, peripheral artery disease).
  - **Strangulated hernia:** Irreducible bulge in abdominal wall.
  - **Ovarian torsion:** Sudden onset of adnexal pain +/– nausea/vomiting. Character of pain is variable. Palpation usually reveals a mass. Have a high index of suspicion in women since clinical presentation is variable.

DIAGNOSIS

- **Rule out OB/GYN causes in women:** Urine β-hCG for ectopic pregnancy; pelvic ultrasound for ovarian torsion, ruptured cyst, or fibroids; pelvic exam +/– swab for PID.
- **Rule out extra-abdominal mimics in patients with upper abdominal pain:** Troponins and ECG for MI, D-dimer/CT angiogram for pulmonary embolism, CXR for pneumonia.
- **Rule out nonsurgical abdominal causes, if appropriate:** Amylase/lipase in patient consistent with pancreatitis (nausea/vomiting, epigastric pain, hunched over), CT abdomen without contrast in patient consistent with kidney stones/pyelonephritis (hematuria, flank pain, radiation to groin), paracentesis for patient consistent with SBP (ascites, fever).
- **Additional diagnostic tests to rule in surgical diagnoses:**
  - **X-ray of the abdomen:** Perforation (see Figure 2.17-10), small bowel obstruction, volvulus.

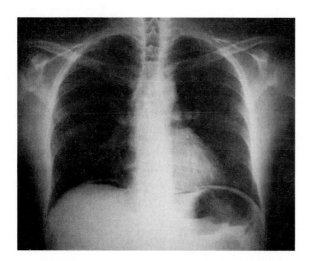

FIGURE 2.17-10. **Pneumoperitoneum.** CXR showing multiple small bowel perforations from CMV ileitis in a young man infected with HIV. (Reproduced with permission from Michalopoulos N, et al. Small bowel perforation caused by CMV enteritis infection in an HIV-positive patient. *BMC Res Notes* 2013;6:45.)

- **CT w/contrast:** Appendicitis, diverticulitis, IBD, abscess, cancer, AAA, and so on.
- **RUQ ultrasound:** Cholecystitis, biliary colic, choledocholithiasis.

MANAGEMENT

A detailed approach to management is beyond the scope of this section, but general concepts are as follows:

- In the presence of peritoneal signs or shock, generally perform exploratory laparotomy.
- Type and cross-match all unstable patients and those in whom you suspect potential hemorrhage.
- Give broad-spectrum antibiotics to patients with perforation or signs of sepsis. They are also indicated for patients with infectious processes (eg, cholecystitis, diverticulitis, pyelonephritis).
- In stable patients, expectant management may include NPO status, nasogastric (NG) tube placement (for decompression of bowel in the setting of obstruction or acute pancreatitis), IV fluids, placement of a Foley catheter (to monitor urine output and fluid status), and vital sign monitoring with serial abdominal exams and serial labs.

Acute Appendicitis

The inciting event is obstruction of the appendiceal lumen with subsequent inflammation and infection. Rising intraluminal pressure leads to vascular compromise of the appendix, ischemia, necrosis, and possible perforation. Etiologies include hypertrophied lymphoid tissue (55–65%), fecalith (35%), foreign body, tumor (eg, carcinoid tumor), and parasites. Incidence peaks in the early teens (most patients 10–30 years of age), and the male-to-female ratio is 2:1.

HISTORY/PE

- Classically presents with dull periumbilical pain lasting 1–12 hours that leads to sharp RLQ pain at McBurney point.

KEY FACT

The McBurney point is located one-third of the distance from the anterior superior iliac spine to the umbilicus.

- Can present with nausea, vomiting, anorexia, and low-grade fever.
- Psoas, obturator, and Rovsing signs are not sensitive tests, but their presence ↑ the likelihood of appendicitis. Remember that Psoas abscess can present very similarly to appendicitis but with a more insidious onset over days. CT can distinguish the two.
- In perforated appendicitis, partial pain relief is possible, but peritoneal signs (eg, rebound, guarding, hypotension, ↑ WBC count, fever) will ultimately develop.
- Children, the elderly, pregnant women, and those with retrocecal appendices may have atypical presentations that may result in misdiagnosis and ↑ mortality.

DIAGNOSIS

- Appendicitis is a clinical diagnosis in patients with classic history (described earlier), fever, and leukocytosis. No imaging is necessary.
- If the clinical picture is uncertain, investigate with CT with PO and IV contrast (see Figure 2.17-11) or RLQ ultrasound (preferred in children and pregnant women).

TREATMENT

- Immediately start IV antibiotics with anaerobic and gram ⊖ coverage (eg, cefoxitin or cefazolin plus metronidazole). The patient should be NPO and receive IV hydration, analgesia, and antiemetics.
- **Uncomplicated appendicitis:** Perform immediate open or laparoscopic appendectomy. If appendicitis is not found, complete exploration of the abdomen is performed. There is no need to administer antibiotics postoperatively.
- **Perforation:** Perform immediate open or laparoscopic appendectomy. Administer antibiotics postoperatively until the patient is afebrile with a normalized WBC count. If open approach is used, the incision should be closed by delayed 1° closure.
- **Abscess:** Treat with broad-spectrum antibiotics and CT-guided drainage; interval appendectomy should be performed 6–8 weeks after resolution of abscess.

KEY FACT

Surgical incisions can be closed by the following:

- Primary closure (primary intent): Surgical approximation using sutures or staples.
- Secondary closure (secondary intent): No approximation, typically packed with gauze, filled in with granulation tissue.
- Delayed primary closure (tertiary intent): Observation for several days to ensure no infection and surgical approximation later.

MNEMONIC

Initial treatment for appendicitis—

PAIN

Pain management
Antibiotics
IVF
NPO

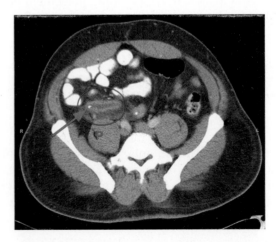

FIGURE 2.17-11. Acute appendicitis. Contrast-enhanced CT image through the lower abdomen in a 30-year-old woman with RLQ pain demonstrates an enlarged, hyperenhancing appendix (circle) with peri-appendiceal fat stranding located just anterior to the right psoas muscle (*P*). An appendicolith (*arrow*) is noted near the base of the appendix. (Reproduced with permission from USMLE-Rx.com.)

TABLE 2.17-4.   Special Considerations in Chemical and Electric Burns

TYPE OF BURN	COMPLICATIONS	MANAGEMENT
Chemical	pH abnormalities	Copiously irrigate for 20–30 minutes before transferring to hospital
Electrical	Deep muscle injury → rhabdomyolysis, compartment syndrome	Early prophylactic fasciotomies and débridement can prevent compartment syndrome and rhabdomyolysis
	Thrombosis of blood vessels → limb ischemia	Closely observe pulses and kidney function
	Electrolyte abnormalities, arrhythmias	Amputation may be necessary
		Monitor electrolytes (especially potassium); obtain ECG

Burns

A leading cause of death in children. Patients with serious burns should be treated in an ICU setting. Burns can be chemical, electrical, or thermal. Chemical and electric burns require special considerations found in Table 2.17-4. Burns of all types are categorized by depth of tissue destruction (see Figure 2.17-12):

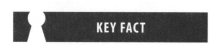

KEY FACT

Superinfection in burns is commonly caused by *Pseudomonas* or gram ⊕ cocci.

- **First degree (eg, sunburn):** Only the epidermis is involved. The area is painful and erythematous without blisters. Capillary refill is intact.

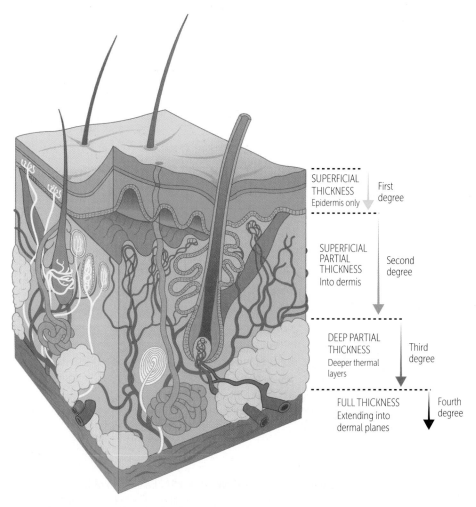

SUPERFICIAL THICKNESS
Epidermis only — First degree

SUPERFICIAL PARTIAL THICKNESS
Into dermis — Second degree

DEEP PARTIAL THICKNESS
Deeper thermal layers — Third degree

FULL THICKNESS
Extending into dermal planes — Fourth degree

FIGURE 2.17-12.   Depth of burn wounds. (Reproduced with permission from USMLE-Rx.com.)

- **Second degree (eg, boiling water):** The epidermis and partial thickness of the dermis are involved. The area is painful and blistered.
- **Third degree (eg, fire):** The epidermis, the full thickness of the dermis, and potentially deeper tissues are involved. The area is painless, white, and charred.

HISTORY/PE

- Patients may present with obvious skin wounds, but significant deep destruction may not be visible, especially with electrical burns.
- Determine whether inhalation of smoke occurred as in a closed-space fire (risk for CO poisoning) or burning carpets and textiles (risk for cyanide poisoning).
- Conduct a thorough airway and lung exam to assess for inhalation injury.

DIAGNOSIS

- **Best initial step:** Assess ABCs. If evidence of thermal or inhalation injury to the upper airway, intubate.
- **Next step:** Evaluate the percentage of body surface area (% BSA) involved (see Figure 2.17-13).
- In patients exposed to smoke, suspect inhalation injury, CO poisoning, and cyanide poisoning. Obtain a CXR, carboxyhemoglobin level, and lactate.
- Assess for circumferential eschar formation, which can obstruct venous and lymphatic drainage, leading to vascular compromise and compartment syndrome.

KEY FACT

Parkland formula: Fluids for the first 24 hours (in mL) = 4 × patient's weight in kg × % BSA. Give 50% of fluids over the first 8 hours and the remaining 50% over the following 16 hours.

KEY FACT

Endometritis is an additional cause of postoperative fever after C-section. Onset occurs anytime between POD 2–10.

KEY FACT

Immediate fever after administration of halothane or succinylcholine should raise concern for malignant hyperthermia. Assess for rigidity, metabolic acidosis, and electrolyte derangements. Treat with dantrolene and active cooling.

KEY FACT

Do not give nodal blockers if there is evidence of Wolff-Parkinson-White syndrome (δ waves) on ECG. Use procainamide instead.

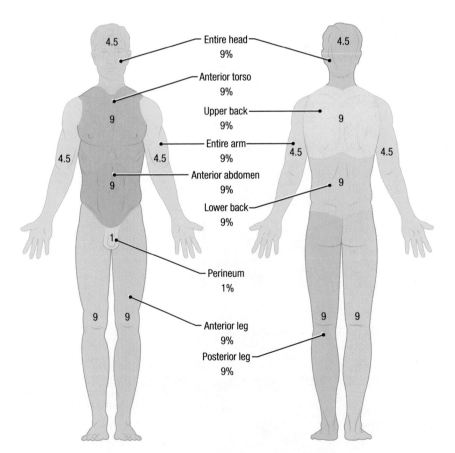

FIGURE 2.17-13. **The rule of 9's in the estimation of BSA.** Estimation of BSA is imperative in the evaluation of burn victims. (Reproduced with permission USMLE-Rx.com.)

TREATMENT

- **Best initial treatment:** Fluid repletion. For second- and third-degree burns, initiate fluids based on the Parkland formula. Titrate fluids to maintain at least 1 cc/kg/h urine output.
- Topical antimicrobials (eg, mafenide acetate [Sulfamylon] or silver sulfadiazine) can be used prophylactically when the epidermis is no longer intact. There is no proven benefit associated with the use of PO/IV antibiotics or corticosteroids.
- Perform escharotomy to relieve obstructed vascular flow in circumferential burns.
- Other management includes tetanus vaccination if appropriate, stress ulcer prophylaxis, and IV narcotic analgesia.

Postoperative Fever

Occurs in 40% of all postoperative patients. Timing after surgery determines the most likely cause. Fever before day 3 is rarely of infectious origin. Table 2.17-5 summarizes the most common etiologies based on postoperative day (POD) of onset.

Cardiac Life Support Basics

Table 2.17-6 summarizes the basic management of cardiac arrhythmias in an acute setting.

Shock

Defined as inadequate tissue-level oxygenation to maintain vital organ function. The multiple etiologies are differentiated by their cardiovascular effects and treatment options (see Table 2.17-7).

TABLE 2.17-5.   Postoperative Fever Timing

TIMING	ETIOLOGY	PREVENTION	MNEMONIC
Anytime	Drug reactions, malignant hyperthermia	N/A	Wonder drugs
POD 1–3	Atelectasis Pneumonia (day 3)	Incentive spirometry, early mobilization Antibiotics	Wind
POD 3–4	UTI	Short-term Foley use	Water
POD 4–5	Deep venous thrombosis/ pulmonary embolism	Early mobilization, heparin, sequential compression socks (SCDs)	Walking
POD 7+	Surgical site infection	Dressing changes, preoperative antibiotics	Wound

MNEMONIC

Possible causes of pulseless electrical activity—

5 H's and 5 T's

Hypovolemia
Hypoxia
Hydrogen ion: acidosis
Hyper/**H**ypo: K⁺, other metabolic
Hypothermia
Tablets: drug overdose, ingestion
Tamponade: cardiac
Tension pneumothorax
Thrombosis: coronary
Thrombosis: pulmonary embolism

KEY FACT

Avoid vasopressors in hypovolemic shock until adequate fluid resuscitation has been provided. Vasopressors ↑ total peripheral resistance and blood pressure but ↓ blood flow in tissues that undergo vasoconstriction (which can cause digital ischemia among other problems). Autoregulation reduces the effect of vasopressors on vital organs, ensuring they maintain perfusion.

KEY FACT

Heart rate is the first vital sign to change in hemorrhagic shock. BP falls only after ±1.5 L of blood loss.

Q

A 36-year-old woman is brought in by emergency medical services after suspected cocaine overdose. The patient is found to be in ventricular tachycardia and after cardioversion complains of abdominal pain. What study should be ordered?

TABLE 2.17-6. Management of Cardiac Arrhythmias[a,b]

Arrhythmia	Treatment
Asystole or pulseless electrical activity	Initiate CPR Give epinephrine or vasopressin; simultaneously search for the underlying cause (see the **5 H's and 5 T's** mnemonics) and provide empiric treatment
Ventricular fibrillation or pulseless ventricular tachycardia	Initiate CPR. Defibrillate with 120–200 J (biphasic) immediately → defibrillate again → epinephrine → defibrillate → amiodarone → defibrillate → epinephrine ("→" above represents 5 cycles of CPR followed by a pulse or rhythm check)
Supraventricular tachycardia	If unstable, perform synchronized electrical cardioversion If stable, attempt vagal maneuvers (Valsalva, carotid massage, or ALS) If resistant, give adenosine (If arrhythmia gets worse, think WPW) If resistant, give other AV-nodal blocking agents (CCBs or β-blockers) if rhythm fails to convert
Atrial fibrillation/ flutter	If unstable, perform synchronized electrical cardioversion at 120–200 J (biphasic) If stable, control rate with diltiazem or β-blockers and anticoagulate if duration is > 48 hours Elective cardioversion may be performed if duration is < 48 hours; otherwise, the clinician must r/o atrial thrombus with TEE before cardioversion (atrial synchronization can dislodge atrial thrombus after cardioversion)
Bradycardia	If symptomatic, give atropine If ineffective, use transcutaneous pacing, dopamine, or epinephrine Patient may require permanent pacemaker

[a]In all cases, disruptions of CPR should be minimized. After a shock or administration of a drug, CPR should be resumed immediately, and five cycles of CPR should be given before checking for a pulse or rhythm.

[b]Doses of electricity listed above assume a biphasic defibrillator.

Thermal Dysregulation

HYPOTHERMIA

Body temperature < 35°C (< 95°F) defines hypothermia. Shivering usually begins at < 35°C (< 95°F). Patients stop shivering at < 32°C (89.6°F) and develop confusion, lethargy, and possibly cardiac arrhythmias. Patients < 28°C (82.4°F) are usually comatose.

ETIOLOGY

- ↑ **Heat loss:** Cold environment (most common), burns, trauma.
- ↓ **Heat production:** Hypothyroidism, adrenal insufficiency, hypoglycemia.
- **Impaired regulation:** Spinal cord injury, cerebrovascular accident.

MANAGEMENT

- Directed at correcting body temperature regardless of etiology.
- Remove the patient from the cold or windy environment, and remove wet clothing. Direct warming method on severity of hypothermia:
  - **32–35°C:** Passive external rewarming. Remove wet clothing and cover with blankets or other insulation.

A

Cocaine use may lead to nonobstructive mesenteric ischemia because of perfusion deficits 2° to cardiac arrhythmias. Abdominal CT angiography should be ordered to screen for ischemia.

TABLE 2.17-7.   Types of Shock

Type	Major Causes	Cardiac Output	PCWP	PVR	Treatment
Hypovolemic	Trauma, blood loss, dehydration with inadequate fluid repletion, third spacing, burns	↓	↓	↑	Replete with isotonic solution (eg, LR or NS) or blood. Initiate blood transfusion in the setting of blood loss if blood pressure does not correct after 2 L isotonic crystalloid
Cardiogenic	CHF, arrhythmia, structural heart disease (severe mitral regurgitation, ventricular septal defect), MI (> 40% of left ventricular function)	↓	↑	↑	Identify the cause, and treat if possible. Give inotropic support with vasopressors such as dopamine (if hypotensive) or dobutamine (if not hypotensive). Intra-aortic balloon pump may help
Obstructive	Cardiac tamponade, tension pneumothorax, massive pulmonary embolism	↓ ↓	↑ ↓	↑ ↑	Treat the underlying cause: Pericardiocentesis, decompression of pneumothorax, thrombolysis. Equalization of pressures in all chambers distinguishes tamponade from other obstructive shock
Distributive		↑	↓	↓	
Septic	Bacteremia, especially gram ⊖ organisms				Administer broad-spectrum antibiotics. Measure central venous pressure (CVP), and give fluid until CVP = 8. Vasopressors (norepinephrine or dopamine) may be needed. Obtain cultures before administration of antibiotics
Anaphylactic	Bee sting, medications, food allergy				1:1000 epinephrine. Consider adjuncts H_1/H_2 antagonists and steroids
SIRS (systemic inflammatory response syndrome)	Pancreatitis, burns, trauma				Manage underlying cause
Neurogenic	Brain or spinal cord injury				Maintain pressures with fluid and pressor support

- **28–32°C:** Active external rewarming. Use warm blankets, warm water bath, or forced warm air (Bair Hugger).
- **< 28°C:** Active internal rewarming. Warm IV fluids, warm peritoneal/pleural lavage, or extracorporeal rewarming such as hemodialysis or ECMO.
- Use warm water bath to thaw frostbite. Patients will need narcotic analgesia for thawing.
- Monitor the ECG for arrhythmias such as bradycardia and slow atrial fibrillation, which can be common at < 30°C (< 86°F). The classic sign is the J wave (Osborn wave).
- Monitor and aggressively replace fluids. Monitor electrolytes and acid-base balance.
- Do not stop resuscitation efforts until the patient has been warmed.

KEY FACT

A patient is not dead until they are warm and dead. You cannot pronounce death until the body is rewarmed to 32°C.

Malignant hyperthermia and NMS should be ruled out in any suspected case of hyperthermia. Malignant hyperthermia would be seen after halothane exposure and NMS after a neuroleptic. Both conditions are treated with dantrolene, and bromocriptine is added for NMS.

Common microbiology of bites: *Pasteurella* species, *Capnocytophaga canimorsus, Bartonella,* and staphylococcus and streptococcus species.

Bites involving sharp teeth and resulting in deep puncture should not be sutured closed. Treat with amoxicillin/clavulanic acid, and monitor for developing deep tissue infections including osteomyelitis.

HYPERTHERMIA

Body temperature > 40°C (> 104°F) defines hyperthermia.

ETIOLOGY

- **Exposure:** Malignant hyperthermia, neuroleptic malignant syndrome (NMS), poisoning, overdose, withdrawal syndrome, environmental (heat, classically an athlete or military recruit).
- **Infectious:** Sepsis, meningitis/encephalitis, tetanus, typhoid, malaria.
- **Endocrine:** Thyroid storm, pheochromocytoma, diabetic ketoacidosis.
- **Neurologic:** Hypothalamic stroke, seizures, cerebrovascular accident.

MANAGEMENT

Directed at correcting body temperature regardless of etiology. Rapidly cool the patient with cold water, wet blankets, and ice. Give benzodiazepines to prevent shivering, which increases metabolic demand and heat generation. Rule out causes of fever such as infection or drug reaction.

Bites and Stings

Table 2.17-8 outlines the management of common bites and stings. Figures 2.17-14 and 2.17-15 summarize the recommended prophylaxis for rabies and tetanus.

Toxicology

HIGH-YIELD TOXICITIES

Carbon Monoxide Poisoning

A hypoxemic poisoning syndrome seen in patients who have been exposed to automobile exhaust, smoke inhalation, barbecues, or old appliances in poorly ventilated locations.

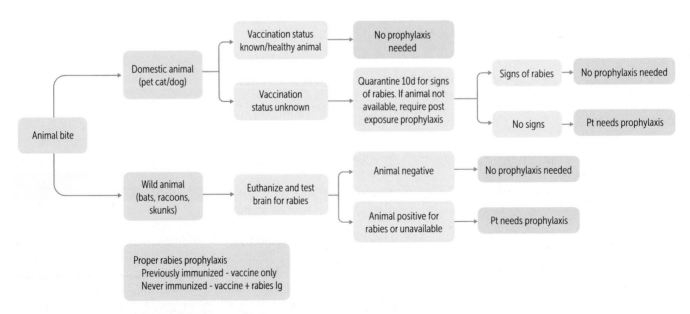

FIGURE 2.17-14. **Rabies postexposure prophylaxis algorithm.** (Reproduced with permission from USMLE-Rx.com.)

TABLE 2.17-8. Management of Bites and Stings

Source	Potential Complication	Management
Bees and wasps	Anaphylaxis	Antihistamines and steroids; IM epinephrine if anaphylaxis develops
Spiders	Black widow: Muscular spasms (can mimic rigid acute abdomen, but no rebound) Brown recluse: Necrosis, flulike symptoms, disseminated intravascular coagulation	Black widow: Antivenin. Classic treatment with Ca gluconate is largely proven ineffective Brown recluse: Cold compresses slow necrosis. Dapsone may help (contra in G6PD deficiency). Débridement should be limited to obviously necrotic tissue
Scorpions	In severe cases, neuromuscular toxicity manifests as cranial nerve dysfunction, excessive motor activity (can be mistaken for seizure), autonomic dysfunction (hypersalivation), and respiratory compromise	Antivenin if neuromuscular symptoms develop. If no antivenin, benzodiazepines and analgesics help pain and spasms
Snakes (Crotaline species: rattlesnake, copperhead)	Local necrosis, distributive shock, disseminated intravascular coagulation	Antivenin (CroFab) is the mainstay of treatment. Keep the affected limb below the heart Compression bands, tourniquets, prophylactic fasciotomy, and resection are ineffective or outdated treatments and probably the wrong answer
Dogs and cats	Infection, rabies/tetanus	Amoxicillin/clavulanate for puncture wounds, bites to hands/feet, and high-risk or immunocompromised patients Consider imaging cat bites for possible tooth fragments implanted in wound
Humans	Infection	Amoxicillin/clavulanate unless very minor
Rodents	Low risk for infection; not known to carry rabies Contact with wild rodents is a risk factor for leptospirosis	Local wound care only
Shellfish (*Vibrio vulnificus*)	Severe necrotizing fasciitis and hemorrhagic bullous lesions Increased risk in patients with preexisting liver disease (especially hemochromatosis)	IV doxycycline and ceftriaxone, emergent surgical débridement

History/PE

- Presents with headaches and confusion. Cherry red skin discoloration is rare. Coma or seizures occur in severe cases.
- Chronic low-level exposure may cause flulike symptoms with generalized myalgias, nausea, and headaches. Ask about symptoms in others living in the same house.
- Suspect smoke inhalation in the presence of singed nose hairs, facial burns, hoarseness, wheezing, or carbonaceous sputum.

Diagnosis

- Diagnose with serum carboxyhemoglobin level using co-oximetry (normal is < 5% in nonsmokers and < 10% in smokers).
- Check ABG, and perform an ECG in elderly patients and those with a history of cardiac disease.

A 44-year-old woman is brought to the ED following a motor vehicle collision. On arrival, her BP is 70/35 mm Hg and her heart rate 110 bpm. Physical exam reveals bruises over the chest and abdomen. A pulmonary artery catheter is placed and reveals a pulmonary capillary wedge pressure (PCWP) of 16 mm Hg. After resuscitation with 2 L of crystalloid, BP and heart rate measurements are 80/40 mm Hg and 125 bpm, respectively. PCWP is now 24 mm Hg. What is the most likely diagnosis?

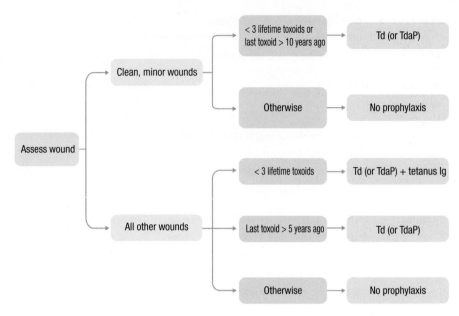

FIGURE 2.17-15. **Tetanus prophylaxis algorithm.** (Reproduced with permission from USMLE-Rx.com.)

Cardiogenic or obstructive shock probably caused by severe blunt trauma to the chest. The patient has signs of shock, and her ↑ PCWP suggests either a cardiogenic or an obstructive cause. Based on the mechanism of injury, she may have severe myocardial contusion or cardiac tamponade.

TREATMENT

- Treat with 100% O_2 facemask until the patient is asymptomatic and carboxyhemoglobin falls to normal.
- **Indications for hyperbaric O_2:** Pregnancy (↑ affinity of CO to fetal Hb); signs of CNS or cardiac ischemia; or severely ↑ carboxyhemoglobin (> 25%).
- Intubate early in patients with airway burns or smoke inhalation, as upper airway edema can rapidly lead to complete obstruction.

Methemoglobinemia

A syndrome of hypoxemia after exposure to an oxidizing agent (eg, local anesthetics, dapsone, nitrites) that oxidizes ferrous iron (Fe^{2+}) to ferric iron (Fe^{3+}), resulting in impaired oxygen transportation.

HISTORY/PE

- History of exposure to local anesthetic, nitrite, or dapsone.
- Cyanosis with "chocolate-colored blood" on blood draw.

DIAGNOSIS

- Do not rely on pulse oximetry and Pa_{O_2} (pulse oximetry will be low, and Pa_{O_2} will be falsely normal).
- Direct methemoglobin measurement using co-oximetry can confirm diagnosis.

TREATMENT

Methylene blue.

Arsenic Poisoning

- Exposure to pesticides, pressure-treated wood, and contaminated well water.
- **Acute:** Garlic breath, vomiting, watery diarrhea, prolonged QT interval on ECG.
- **Chronic:** Hypo or hyperpigmentation, peripheral neuropathy.
- Can be found in keratin (nails, hair).
- Treat with dimercaprol.

ANTIDOTES AND MANAGEMENT OF OTHER TOXIC INGESTIONS/OVERDOSES

Recent ingestions (< 2 h) should generally receive activated charcoal (exceptions are lithium, iron, lead, hydrocarbons, or toxic alcohols). Be careful in lethargic patients since aspiration can cause pneumonitis. Orogastric lavage is rarely indicated, but may help for lethal toxins ingested < 1 h prior. Ipecac syrup is an antiquated treatment for poisoning that is never used because of the risk for ↑ damage caused by emesis and the lack of demonstrated benefit.

Table 2.17-9 summarizes antidotes and treatments for substances commonly encountered in overdoses and intoxications.

KEY FACT

Serum cyanide concentration is a slow lab test that will not result in time to save the patient. Diagnose cyanide poisoning based on high clinical suspicion (inhalation of burning carpet/textiles and elevated lactate).

TABLE 2.17-9. **Antidotes and Management of Other Toxic Ingestions/Overdose**

Toxin	Antidote/Treatment	Notes
Acetaminophen	PO activated charcoal, IV *N*-acetylcysteine (repletes glutathione)	Charcoal is used if patient presents within 4 h of overdose along with NAC Always treat overdose > 7.5 g; otherwise get acetaminophen level
Acid/alkali ingestion	Assess ABCs, and remove affected clothing Upper endoscopy 6–24 h later Do not try to neutralize acid or base, and do not induce vomiting	Perform endoscopy too soon, and you may not see the full damage, too late and you may perforate Neutralization generates copious amounts of heat, and vomiting worsens esophageal injury, which is the worst part If the eyes are involved, the eyes should be irrigated with copious amounts of water for at least 15 minutes before traveling to the ED
Anticholinesterases, organophosphates	Atropine, pralidoxime (reactivates acetylcholinesterase)	
Antimuscarinic/anticholinergic agents	Physostigmine	
Arsenic, mercury, gold	Succimer, dimercaprol	
β-blockers	Glucagon	
Barbiturates (phenobarbital)	Urine alkalinization, dialysis, activated charcoal, supportive care	
Benzodiazepines	Supportive care (intubation), Flumazenil	Never use flumazenil in the setting of chronic use, even if acutely intoxicated. Can produce deadly withdrawal seizures
Copper, arsenic, lead, gold	Penicillamine	
Cyanide	Hydroxycobalamin, amyl nitrate, sodium nitrite, sodium thiosulfate	Nitrites induce methemoglobinemia, which binds cyanate
Digitalis	Anti-digitalis Fab in symptomatic patients (arrhythmia, AMS, AKI, hyperkalemia)	Do not treat hyperkalemia or hypocalcemia before giving antidote since these often correct once Na^+/K^+ pump is working
Heparin	Protamine sulfate	
Iron	Deferoxamine	Look for radiopaque tablets on x-ray in a child with hematemesis and metabolic acidosis

(continues)

TABLE 2.17-9. Antidotes and Management of Other Toxic Ingestions/Overdose *(continued)*

TOXIN	ANTIDOTE/TREATMENT	NOTES
Lead	Succimer, EDTA, dimercaprol	
Methanol, ethylene glycol (antifreeze)	Fomepizole > ethanol, dialysis, calcium gluconate for ethylene glycol	
Opioids	Naloxone	It is common to empirically treat patients found unconscious with naloxone
Salicylates	Urine alkalinization, dialysis, activated charcoal	
TCAs	Sodium bicarbonate, diazepam or lorazepam for seizures/agitation	Monitor closely and only give bicarb if QRS > 100 ms or ventricular arrhythmia
tPA, streptokinase	Aminocaproic acid	
Warfarin	FFP (immediate reversal in hemorrhaging pt), Vitamin K (long-term reversal)	

COMMON DRUG INTERACTIONS/REACTIONS

Table 2.17-10 outlines drug interactions and reactions that are commonly encountered.

TABLE 2.17-10. Drug Interactions and Reactions

INTERACTION/REACTION	DRUGS
Induction of P-450 enzymes	**Barb**iturates, **St**. John's wort, **P**henytoin, **R**ifampin, **G**riseofulvin, **C**arbamazepine (**Barb**ara **St**eals **P**hen-phen and **R**efuses **G**reasy **C**arbs)
Inhibition of P-450 enzymes	Quinidine, cimetidine, ketoconazole, INH, grapefruit, erythromycin, sulfonamides
Metabolism by P-450 enzymes	Sedatives: Benzodiazepines, barbiturates Cardiac drugs: Metoprolol, propranolol, nifedipine, warfarin, quinidine Anticonvulsants: Phenytoin, carbamazepine Other: Theophylline, amide anesthetics
↑ Risk for digoxin toxicity	Quinidine, cimetidine, amiodarone, CCBs
Competition for albumin-binding sites	Warfarin, ASA, phenytoin
Blood dyscrasias	Ibuprofen, quinidine, methyldopa, chemotherapeutic agents
Hemolysis in G6PD-deficient patients	Sulfonamides, INH, ASA, ibuprofen, nitrofurantoin, primaquine, pyrimethamine, chloramphenicol, dapsone
Gynecomastia	**S**pironolactone, **D**igitalis, **C**imetidine, chronic **A**lcohol use, **K**etoconazole (**S**ome **D**rugs **C**reate **A**wesome **K**nockers)
Stevens-Johnson syndrome	Lamotrigine, sulfonamides, penicillins
Photosensitivity	Tetracycline, amiodarone, sulfonamides
Drug-induced SLE	Procainamide, hydralazine, INH, penicillamine, chlorpromazine, methyldopa, quinidine

MAJOR DRUG SIDE EFFECTS

Table 2.17-11 outlines the major side effects of select drugs.

TABLE 2.17-11. Drug Side Effects

DRUG	SIDE EFFECTS
ACEIs	Cough, rash, proteinuria, angioedema, taste changes, teratogenesis (renal agenesis)
Acyclovir	Crystalluria → ATN 2/2 renal tubular obstruction (administer IV fluids with drug to lower risk for AKI)
Amantadine	Ataxia, livedo reticularis
Aminoglycosides (especially amikacin)	Ototoxicity, nephrotoxicity (acute tubular necrosis)
Amiodarone	Acute: AV block, hypotension, bradycardia Chronic: pulmonary fibrosis, peripheral deposition leading to bluish discoloration, arrhythmias, hypo-/ hyperthyroidism, corneal deposition
Amphotericin	Fever/rigors, nephrotoxicity, bone marrow suppression, anemia
Antihistamines (first-generation)	Potent anticholinergic effects (eye and oropharyngeal dryness, urinary retention)
Antipsychotics	Sedation, acute dystonic reaction, akathisia, parkinsonism, tardive dyskinesia, NMS
Azoles (eg, fluconazole)	Inhibition of P-450 enzymes
Azathioprine	Diarrhea, leukopenia, hepatotoxicity
AZT	Thrombocytopenia, megaloblastic anemia
β-blockers	Asthma exacerbation, masking of hypoglycemia, impotence, bradycardia, AV block, CHF
Benzodiazepines	Sedation, dependence, respiratory depression
Bile acid resins	GI upset, malabsorption of vitamins and medications
Carbamazepine	Autoinduction of P-450 enzymes (induces P-450 enzymes that break down carbamazepine—requires dose increase 2–3 weeks after initiation), agranulocytosis/aplastic anemia, liver toxicity
CCBs	Peripheral edema, constipation, cardiac depression
Chloramphenicol	Gray baby syndrome, aplastic anemia
Cisplatin	Nephrotoxicity, acoustic nerve damage
Clonidine	Dry mouth; severe rebound headache and hypertension
Clozapine	Agranulocytosis
Corticosteroids	Depression and other psychological conditions, hyperglycemia (acute), immunosuppression, bone mineral loss, osteonecrosis, thinning of skin, easy bruising, myopathy, cataracts (chronic)
Cyclophosphamide	Myelosuppression, hemorrhagic cystitis, bladder cancer

(continues)

TABLE 2.17-11. **Drug Side Effects** *(continued)*

DRUG	SIDE EFFECTS
Digoxin	GI disturbance, yellow visual changes, arrhythmias (eg, junctional tachycardia or SVT)
Diphenhydramine	Anticholinergic (tachycardia, hyperthermia, mydriasis, reduced bowel sounds) and antihistaminic (drowsiness, confusion)
Doxorubicin	Cardiotoxicity (cardiomyopathy), urine discoloration
Ethyl alcohol	Acidosis, renal dysfunction, CNS depression
Fluoroquinolones	Cartilage damage in children; Achilles tendon rupture in adults
Furosemide	Ototoxicity, hypokalemia, nephritis, gout
Gemfibrozil	Myositis, reversible ↑ in LFTs
Halothane	Hepatotoxicity, malignant hyperthermia
HCTZ	Hypokalemia, hyponatremia, hyperuricemia, hyperglycemia, hypercalcemia
HMG-CoA reductase inhibitors (statins)	Myositis, reversible ↑ in LFTs
Hydralazine	Drug-induced SLE
Hydroxychloroquine	Retinopathy (requires annual ophthalmologic exam for long-term use)
INH	Peripheral neuropathy (prevent with pyridoxine/vitamin B_6), hepatotoxicity, inhibition of P-450 enzymes, seizures with overdose, hemolysis in G6PD deficiency
MAOIs	Hypertensive tyramine reaction, serotonin syndrome (with meperidine)
Metformin	Lactic acidosis (acute kidney injury, dehydration, sepsis). Withhold metformin until condition improves
Methanol	Blindness, anion-gap metabolic acidosis
Methotrexate	Hepatic fibrosis, pneumonitis, anemia
Metoclopramide	Extrapyramidal symptoms: acute dystonia, akathisia, parkinsonism
Methyldopa	⊕ Coombs test, drug-induced SLE
Metronidazole	Disulfiram reaction, vestibular dysfunction, metallic taste
Mycophenolate mofetil	Bone marrow suppression

(continues)

TABLE 2.17-11. **Drug Side Effects** *(continued)*

Drug	Side Effects
Niacin	Cutaneous flushing
Nitroglycerin	Hypotension, tachycardia, headache, tolerance
Penicillamine	Drug-induced SLE
Penicillin/β-lactams	Hypersensitivity reactions
Phenytoin	Nystagmus, diplopia, ataxia, arrhythmia (in toxic doses), gingival hyperplasia, hirsutism, teratogenic effects
Prazosin	First-dose hypotension, priapism
Procainamide	Drug-induced SLE
Propylthiouracil	Agranulocytosis, aplastic anemia
Quinidine	Cinchonism (headache, tinnitus), thrombocytopenia, arrhythmias (eg, torsades de pointes)
Reserpine	Depression
Rifampin	Induction of P-450 enzymes; orange-red body secretions
Salicylates	Fever; hyperventilation with respiratory alkalosis and metabolic acidosis; dehydration, diaphoresis, hemorrhagic gastritis
SSRIs	Anxiety, sexual dysfunction, serotonin syndrome if taken with MAOIs
Succinylcholine	Malignant hyperthermia, hyperkalemia
TCAs	Coma, anticholinergic effects, seizures, QRS prolongation, arrhythmias
Tetracyclines	Tooth discoloration, photosensitivity, Fanconi syndrome, GI distress
Trazadone	Priapism ("Traza**done** = Traza**BONE**")
Trimethoprim	Megaloblastic anemia, leukopenia, granulocytopenia, hyperkalemia
Valproic acid	Teratogenicity leads to neural tube defects; rare fatal hepatotoxicity
Vancomycin	Nephrotoxicity, ototoxicity, "red man syndrome" (histamine release; not an allergy)
Vinblastine	Severe myelosuppression
Vincristine	Peripheral neuropathy, paralytic ileus

MANAGEMENT OF DRUG WITHDRAWAL

Table 2.17-12 summarizes common drug withdrawal symptoms and treatment.

RECOGNITION OF DRUG INTOXICATION

See the Psychiatry chapter for a summary of common drug intoxication symptoms.

TABLE 2.17-12. Symptoms and Treatment of Drug Withdrawal

DRUG	WITHDRAWAL SYMPTOMS	TREATMENT
Alcohol	Life-threatening (mortality up to 5%) Mild withdrawal: Tremor (first symptom), tachycardia, hypertension, agitation (within 48 hours) Alcoholic hallucinations: Visual hallucinations without delirium (12–48 hours) Delirium tremens: Visual hallucinations with severe autonomic instability, delirium, seizures, and possibly death (within 2–7 days)	Benzodiazepines (can require massive doses); thiamine, folate, and multivitamin replacement (banana bag—does not affect withdrawal, but most alcoholics are deficient)
Benzodiazepines and barbiturates	Life-threatening (mortality is rare) Tremor, rebound anxiety, insomnia, delirium/hallucinations, seizures May mimic alcohol withdrawal, but hypertension/tachycardia usually absent	Benzodiazepine taper
Cocaine/ amphetamines	Not life-threatening Depression, hyperphagia, hypersomnolence, constricted pupils	Intravenous benzodiazepines and supportive treatment Avoid pure β-blockers (lead to unopposed α activity, causing hypertensive crisis)
Opioids	Not life-threatening Anxiety, insomnia, flulike symptoms, piloerection, fever, rhinorrhea, lacrimation, yawning, nausea, stomach cramps, diarrhea, dilated pupils	Mild: Ondansetron, loperamide, benzodiazepines, and NSAIDs Severe: Clonidine for autonomic symptoms, buprenorphine or methadone for craving

Vitamin Deficiencies

Table 2.17-13 summarizes the signs and symptoms of key vitamin deficiencies.

TABLE 2.17-13. **Vitamin Deficiencies**

VITAMIN	SIGNS/SYMPTOMS OF DEFICIENCY
Vitamin A	Dry skin, night blindness, corneal degeneration, conjunctival keratinization
Vitamin B_1 (thiamine)	Beriberi (polyneuritis, dilated cardiomyopathy, high-output CHF, edema), Wernicke-Korsakoff syndrome (**COAT RACK**) Wernicke = **C**onfusion, **O**phthalmoplegia, **A**taxia, **T**hiamine **R**etrograde and **A**nterograde amnesia, **C**onfabulation = **K**orsakoff
Vitamin B_2 (riboflavin)	Angular stomatitis, cheilosis, corneal vascularization
Vitamin B_3 (niacin)	Pellagra (diarrhea, dermatitis, dementia). May be caused by carcinoid tumor ($\downarrow$ tryptophan, a precursor of niacin) and INH (vitamin B_6 is required for niacin synthesis)
Vitamin B_5 (pantothenate)	Dermatitis, enteritis, alopecia, adrenal insufficiency
Vitamin B_6 (pyridoxine)	Convulsions, irritability, peripheral neuropathy, and sideroblastic anemia Always supplement B_6 when administering INH
Vitamin B_{12} (cobalamin)	Megaloblastic anemia; glossitis; neurologic symptoms (eg, optic neuropathy, subacute combined degeneration, paresthesias)
Vitamin C	Scurvy: swollen gums, bruising, anemia, poor wound healing; immunosuppression
Vitamin D	Rickets in children (bending bones), osteomalacia in adults (soft bones), hypocalcemic tetany All breastfed babies should receive supplemental vitamin D
Vitamin E	$\uparrow$ Fragility of RBCs $\rightarrow$ hemolytic anemia, degeneration of posterior column May look like B_{12} deficiency with anemia and neurologic symptoms, but anemia is hemolytic rather than megaloblastic
Vitamin K	$\uparrow$ PT and aPTT, normal bleeding time. Neonatal hemorrhage Give all babies IM vitamin K (suspect neonatal hemorrhage in babies born at home)
Biotin	Dermatitis, enteritis Can be caused by ingestion of raw eggs or antibiotic use
Folic acid	Glossitis, megaloblastic anemia without neurologic symptoms More common than B_{12} deficiency since B_{12} stores in liver can last 3–5 years
Selenium	Cardiomyopathy (Keshan disease), impaired phagocytic function in macrophages
Zinc	Dysgeusia (impaired taste), impaired wound healing, alopecia, hypogonadism

NOTES

RAPID REVIEW

CARDIOVASCULAR

Classic ECG finding in atrial flutter	"Sawtooth" P waves
Definition of unstable angina	Angina that is new or worsening with no ↑ in troponin level
Antihypertensive for a diabetic patient with proteinuria	Angiotensin-converting enzyme inhibitor/angiotensin-receptor blocker
Beck triad for cardiac tamponade	Hypotension, distant heart sounds, and JVD
Drugs that slow heart rate	β-blockers, calcium channel blockers, digoxin, amiodarone
Hypercholesterolemia treatment that leads to flushing and pruritus	Niacin
Murmur—hypertrophic obstructive cardiomyopathy	Systolic ejection murmur heard along lateral sternal border that ↑ with ↓ preload (Valsalva maneuver)
Murmur—aortic insufficiency	Austin Flint murmur, a diastolic, decrescendo, low-pitched, blowing murmur that is best heard sitting up. ↑ With ↑ afterload (handgrip maneuver)
Murmur—aortic stenosis	Systolic crescendo/decrescendo murmur that radiates to neck. ↑ With ↑ preload (squatting maneuver)
Murmur—mitral regurgitation	Holosystolic murmur that radiates to axilla. ↑ With ↑ afterload (hand-grip maneuver)
Murmur—mitral stenosis	Diastolic, mid to late, low-pitched murmur preceded by an opening snap
Treatment for atrial fibrillation and atrial flutter	If unstable, cardiovert. If stable or chronic, rate control with CCBs or β-blockers
Treatment for ventricular fibrillation	Immediate defibrillation
Dressler syndrome	Autoimmune reaction with fever, pericarditis, and ↑ ESR occurring 2–4 weeks post-MI
IV drug use with JVD and a holosystolic murmur at the left sternal border. Treatment?	Treat existing heart failure, and replace the tricuspid valve
Diagnostic test for hypertrophic cardiomyopathy	Echocardiogram (showing a thickened left ventricular wall and outflow obstruction)
Pulsus paradoxus	↓ In systolic BP of > 10 mm Hg with inspiration. Seen in cardiac tamponade
Classic ECG findings in pericarditis	Low-voltage, diffuse ST-segment elevation
Eight surgically correctable causes of hypertension	Renal artery stenosis, coarctation of the aorta, pheochromocytoma, Conn syndrome, Cushing syndrome, unilateral renal parenchymal disease, hyperthyroidism, hyperparathyroidism

Evaluation of a pulsatile abdominal mass and bruit	Abdominal ultrasound and CT
Indications for surgical correction of abdominal aortic aneurysm	> 5.5 cm, rapidly enlarging, symptomatic, or ruptured
Treatment for acute coronary syndrome	ASA, heparin, clopidogrel, morphine, O_2, sublingual nitroglycerin, IV β-blockers
Metabolic syndrome	Abdominal obesity, high triglycerides, low HDL, hypertension, insulin resistance, prothrombotic or proinflammatory states
Appropriate diagnostic test? ◾ 50-year-old man with stable angina can exercise to 85% of maximum predicted heart rate ◾ 65-year-old woman with left bundle branch block and severe osteoarthritis has unstable angina	Exercise stress treadmill with ECG Pharmacologic stress test (eg, dobutamine echocardiogram)
Signs of active ischemia during stress testing	Angina, ST-segment changes on ECG, or ↓ BP
ECG findings suggesting MI	ST-segment elevation (depression means ischemia), flattened T waves, and Q waves
Coronary territories in MI	Anterior wall (LAD/diagonal), inferior (PDA), posterior (left circumflex/oblique, RCA/marginal), septum (LAD/diagonal)
Young patient with angina at rest and ST-segment elevation with normal cardiac enzymes	Prinzmetal angina
Common symptoms associated with silent MI	CHF, shock, altered mental status, unexplained fatigue, heartburn, shortness of breath, discomfort in the neck or jaw, and indigestion
Diagnostic test for pulmonary embolism	CT pulmonary angiogram
Protamine	Reverses the effects of heparin
Prothrombin time	The coagulation parameter affected by warfarin
Young patient with family history of sudden death collapses and dies while exercising	Hypertrophic cardiomyopathy
Endocarditis prophylaxis regimens	Oral surgery—amoxicillin for certain situations. GI or GU procedures—not recommended
Virchow triad	Stasis, hypercoagulability, endothelial damage
Most common cause of hypertension in young women	OCPs
Most common cause of hypertension in young men	Excessive EtOH
Figure 3 sign	Aortic coarctation
Water bottle–shaped heart	Pericardial effusion. Look for pulsus paradoxus

DERMATOLOGY

"Stuck-on" waxy appearance	Seborrheic keratosis
Red plaques with silvery-white scales and sharp margins	Psoriasis
Most common type of skin cancer. The lesion is a pearly-colored papule with a translucent surface and telangiectasias	Basal cell carcinoma
Honey-crusted lesions	Impetigo
Febrile patient with history of diabetes presents with a red, swollen, painful lower extremity	Cellulitis
⊕ Nikolsky sign, flaccid bullae	Pemphigus vulgaris
⊖ Nikolsky sign, tense bullae	Bullous pemphigoid
55-year-old obese patient presents with dirty, velvety patches on back of neck	Acanthosis nigricans. Check fasting blood glucose to rule out diabetes
Dermatomal distribution of crusted vesicles	Varicella zoster
Flat-topped, itchy, violet papules	Lichen planus
Irislike target lesions	Erythema multiforme
Lesion occurring in a geometric pattern in areas where skin comes into contact with clothing or jewelry	Contact dermatitis
Presents with one large patch and many smaller ones in a treelike distribution	Pityriasis rosea
Flat, often hypopigmented lesions on the chest and back. KOH prep has a "spaghetti-and-meatballs" appearance	Tinea (pityriasis) versicolor
Five characteristics of a nevus suggestive of melanoma	Asymmetry, border irregularity, color variation, large diameter, clinical evolution (ABCDE)
Premalignant lesion caused by sun exposure that can lead to SCC	Actinic keratosis
Crusting vesicles in all stages of evolution on entire body	Lesions of 1° varicella
"Cradle cap"	Seborrheic dermatitis Treat conservatively with bathing and moisturizing agents
Associated with *Propionibacterium acnes* and changes in androgen levels, and the treatment of last resort	Acne vulgaris Last-resort treatment is oral isotretinoin (requires monthly blood tests and two forms of contraception for women)
Painful, recurrent vesicular eruption of mucocutaneous surfaces	Herpes simplex
Inflammation and epithelial thinning of the anogenital area, predominantly in postmenopausal women	Lichen sclerosus
Exophytic nodules on the skin with scaling or ulceration. The second most common type of skin cancer	Squamous cell carcinoma

ENDOCRINOLOGY

Most common cause of hypothyroidism	Hashimoto thyroiditis
Lab findings in Hashimoto thyroiditis	High TSH, low T_4, antibodies to thyroid peroxidase (TPO)
Exophthalmos, pretibial myxedema, and ↓ TSH	Graves disease
Most common cause of Cushing syndrome	Iatrogenic corticosteroid administration. The second most common cause is Cushing disease
Post-thyroidectomy patient presents with signs of hypocalcemia and ↑ phosphorus	Hypoparathyroidism (iatrogenic)
"Stones, bones, groans, psychiatric overtones"	Signs and symptoms of hypercalcemia
Hypertension, hypokalemia, and metabolic alkalosis	1° Hyperaldosteronism (caused by Conn syndrome or bilateral adrenal hyperplasia)
Patient presents with tachycardia, wild swings in BP, headache, diaphoresis, altered mental status, and a sense of panic	Pheochromocytoma
Which should be used first in treating pheochromocytoma, α- or β-antagonists?	α-antagonists (phenoxybenzamine)
Patient with history of lithium use presents with copious amounts of dilute urine	Nephrogenic DI
Treatment of central DI	Administration of DDAVP
Postoperative patient with significant pain presents with hyponatremia and normal volume status	SIADH due to stress
Antidiabetic agent associated with lactic acidosis	Metformin
Patient presents with weakness, nausea, vomiting, weight loss, and new skin pigmentation. Lab results show hyponatremia and hyperkalemia. Treatment?	1° Adrenal insufficiency (Addison disease). Treat with glucocorticoids, mineralocorticoids, and IV fluids
Goal HbA_{1c} for a patient with DM	< 70%
Treatment of DKA	Fluids, insulin, and electrolyte repletion (eg, K+)
Bone pain, hearing loss, ↑ alkaline phosphatase	Paget disease
↑ IGF-1	Acromegaly
Galactorrhea, amenorrhea, bitemporal hemianopia	Prolactinoma
↑ Serum 17-hydroxyprogesterone	Congenital adrenal hyperplasia (21-hydroxylase deficiency)
Pancreas, pituitary, parathyroid tumors	MEN type 1

EPIDEMIOLOGY

How do you interpret the following 95% CI for an RR of 0.582: 95% CI 0.502, 0.673?	Data are consistent with RRs ranging from 0.502 to 0.673 with 95% confidence (ie, we are confident that, 95 out of 100 times, the true RR will be between 0.502 and 0.673)
Bias introduced into a study when a clinician is aware of the patient's treatment type	Observational bias
Bias introduced when screening detects a disease earlier and thus lengthens the time from diagnosis to death, but does not improve survival	Lead-time bias
If you want to know if geographic location affects infant mortality rate but most variation in infant mortality is predicted by socioeconomic status, then socioeconomic status is a _____	Confounding variable
The proportion of people who have the disease and test ⊕ is the _____	Sensitivity
Sensitive tests have few false ⊖s and are used to rule _____ a disease	Out
PPD reactivity is used as a screening test because most people with TB (except those who are anergic) will have a ⊕ PPD highly sensitive or specific?	Highly sensitive for TB Screening tests with high sensitivity are good for diseases with low prevalence
Chronic diseases such as systemic lupus erythematosus—higher prevalence or incidence?	Higher prevalence
Epidemics such as influenza—higher prevalence or incidence?	Higher incidence
What is the difference between incidence and prevalence?	Prevalence is the percentage of cases of disease in a population at one point in time. Incidence is the percentage of new cases of disease that develop over a given period among the total population at risk (prevalence = incidence × duration)
Cross-sectional survey—incidence or prevalence?	Prevalence
Cohort study—incidence or prevalence?	Incidence and prevalence
Case-control study—incidence or prevalence?	Neither
Describe a test that consistently gives identical results, but the results are wrong	High reliability (precision), low validity (accuracy)
Difference between a cohort and a case-control study	Cohort divides groups by an exposure and looks for development of disease Case-control divides groups by a disease and assigns controls, and then goes back and looks for exposures

Attributable risk?	The difference in risk in the exposed and unexposed groups (ie, the risk that is attributable to the exposure)
Relative risk?	Incidence in the exposed group divided by the incidence in the non-exposed group
Hypothetical study found an association between ASA intake and risk for heart disease. How do you interpret an RR of 15?	In patients who took ASA, the risk for heart disease was 15 times that of patients who did not take ASA
Odds ratio?	In cohort studies, the odds of developing the disease in the exposed group divided by the odds of developing the disease in the nonexposed group In case-control studies, the odds that the cases were exposed divided by the odds that the controls were exposed In cross-sectional studies, the odds that the exposed group has the disease divided by the odds that the nonexposed group has the disease
Most common cancer in men and most common cause of death from cancer in men	Prostate cancer is the most common cancer in men, but lung cancer causes more deaths
The percentage of cases within 1 SD of the mean? 2 SDs? 3 SDs?	68%, 95.4%, 99.7%
Birth rate?	Number of live births per 1000 population in 1 year
Mortality rate?	Number of deaths per 1000 population in 1 year
Neonatal mortality rate?	Number of deaths from birth to 28 days per 1000 live births in 1 year
Infant mortality rate?	Number of deaths from birth to 1 year of age per 1000 live births (neonatal + postnatal mortality) in 1 year
Maternal mortality rate?	Number of deaths during pregnancy to 90 days postpartum per 100,000 live births in 1 year

ETHICS

True or false: Once patients sign a statement giving consent, they must continue treatment	False. Patients may change their minds at any time Exceptions to the requirement of informed consent include emergency situations and patients without decision-making capacity
15-year-old pregnant girl requires hospitalization for preeclampsia. Is parental consent required?	No, parental consent is not necessary for the medical treatment of pregnant minors
Doctor refers patient for an MRI to a facility that doctor owns	Conflict of interest
Involuntary psychiatric hospitalization can be undertaken for which three reasons?	The patient is a danger to self, a danger to others, or gravely disabled (unable to provide for basic needs)

True or false: It is more difficult to justify the withdrawal of care than to have withheld the treatment in the first place	False. Withdrawing nonbeneficial treatment or treatment a patient no longer wants is ethically equivalent to withholding care
Mother refuses to allow her child to be vaccinated	Parent has the right to refuse treatment for his or her child as long as it does not pose a serious threat to child's well-being
When can a physician refuse to continue treating a patient on the grounds of futility?	When there is no rationale for treatment, maximal intervention is failing, a given intervention has already failed, and treatment will not achieve the goals of care
8-year-old child is in a serious accident and requires emergent transfusion, but her parents are not present	Treat immediately. Consent is implied in emergency situations
15-year-old girl seeking treatment for an STI asks that her parents not be told about her condition	Minors may consent to care for STIs without parental consent or knowledge
Conditions in which confidentiality must be overridden	Real threat of harm to third parties Suicidal intentions Certain contagious diseases Elder and child abuse
Involuntary commitment or isolation for medical treatment may be undertaken for what reason?	When treatment noncompliance represents a serious danger to public health (eg, active TB)
10-year-old child presents in status epilepticus, but her parents refuse treatment on religious grounds	Treat because the disease represents an immediate threat to the child's life
Son asks that his mother not be told about her recently discovered cancer	Physician can withhold information from the patient only in the rare case of therapeutic privilege or if patient requests not to be told

GASTROINTESTINAL

Patient presents with sudden onset of severe, diffuse abdominal pain. Exam reveals peritoneal signs, and x-ray of the abdomen reveals free air under the diaphragm. Management?	Emergent laparotomy to repair a perforated viscus
Most likely cause of acute lower GI bleeding in patients > 40 years of age	Diverticulosis
Diagnostic modality used when ultrasonography is equivocal for cholecystitis	HIDA scan
Risk factors for cholelithiasis	Fat, female, fertile, forty, flatulent
Inspiratory arrest during palpation of the RUQ	Murphy sign, seen in acute cholecystitis
Most common cause of SBO in patients with no history of abdominal surgery	Hernia
Most common cause of SBO in patients with a history of abdominal surgery	Adhesions

Identify key organisms causing diarrhea:

▪ Most common bacterial organism	*Campylobacter*
▪ Recent antibiotic use	*Clostridium difficile*
▪ Camping	*Giardia*
▪ Traveler's diarrhea	Enterotoxigenic *Escherichia*
▪ Church picnics/mayonnaise	*S aureus*
▪ Uncooked hamburgers	*E coli* O157:H7
▪ Fried rice	*Bacillus cereus*
▪ Poultry/eggs	*Salmonella*
▪ Raw seafood	*Vibrio*, HAV
▪ AIDS	*Isospora, Cryptosporidium, Mycobacterium avium* complex
▪ Pseudoappendicitis	*Yersinia, Campylobacter*

25-year-old Jewish man presents with pain and watery diarrhea after meals. Exam shows fistulas between the bowel and skin and nodular lesions on his tibias	Crohn disease
Inflammatory disease of the colon with ↑ risk for colon cancer	Ulcerative colitis (greater risk than Crohn)
Extraintestinal manifestations of IBD	Uveitis, ankylosing spondylitis, pyoderma gangrenosum, erythema nodosum, 1° sclerosing cholangitis
Medical treatment for IBD	5-ASA agents and steroids during acute exacerbations
30-year-old man with ulcerative colitis presents with fatigue, jaundice, and pruritus	Primary sclerosing cholangitis
Difference between Mallory-Weiss and Boerhaave tears	Mallory-Weiss: superficial tear in the esophageal mucosa. Boerhaave: full-thickness esophageal rupture
Charcot triad	RUQ pain, jaundice, and fever/chills
Reynolds pentad	Charcot triad plus shock and altered mental status
Medical treatment for hepatic encephalopathy	↓ Protein intake, lactulose, rifaximin
The first step in management of a patient with an acute GI bleeding episode	Manage ABCs
4-year-old child presents with oliguria, petechiae, and jaundice following an illness with bloody diarrhea. Most likely diagnosis and cause?	HUS caused by *E coli* O157:H7
Treatment after occupational exposure to HBV	If nonimmune, provide HBV immunoglobulin and initiate HBV vaccination series
Classic causes of drug-induced hepatitis	TB medications (isoniazid, rifampin, pyrazinamide), acetaminophen, and tetracycline
40-year-old obese woman with elevated alkaline phosphatase, elevated bilirubin, pruritus, dark urine, and clay-colored stools	Biliary tract obstruction

Hernia with highest risk for incarceration—indirect, direct, or femoral?	Femoral hernia
Severe abdominal pain out of proportion to the exam	Mesenteric ischemia
Diagnosis of ileus	Abdominal radiographs (could also perform CT scan)
50-year-old man with history of alcohol abuse presents with boring epigastric pain that radiates to the back and is relieved by sitting forward. Management?	Confirm diagnosis of acute pancreatitis with ↑ amylase and lipase Make the patient NPO, and give IV fluids, O_2, analgesia, and "tincture of time"

Colon cancer region based on symptoms:
    Anemia from chronic disease, occult blood loss, vague abdominal pain
    Obstructive symptoms, change in bowel movements
	Right sided: rare to have an obstruction
	
	Left-sided: "apple–core" lesion

Presents with watery diarrhea, dehydration, muscle weakness, and flushing	VIPoma (replace fluids and electrolytes, may need to surgically resect tumor, or use octreotide)
Presents with palpable, nontender gallbladder	Courvoisier sign (suggests pancreatic cancer)

HEMATOLOGY/ONCOLOGY

Four causes of microcytic anemia	**IRON LAST– IRON** deficiency**, L**ead poisoning, **A**nemia of chronic disease, **S**ideroblastic anemia, **T**halassemia
Elderly man with hypochromic, microcytic anemia is asymptomatic. Diagnostic tests?	Fecal occult blood test and sigmoidoscopy. Suspect colorectal cancer
Precipitants of hemolytic crisis in patients with G6PD deficiency	**Sell FAVA BEANS in INDIA** – Sulfa-drugs **FAVA Beans, I**nfections, **N**itrofurantoin, **D**apsone, **I**soniazid, **A**ntimalarials (quinines)
Most common inherited cause of hypercoagulability	Factor V Leiden mutation
Most common inherited bleeding disorder	von Willebrand disease
Most common inherited hemolytic anemia	Hereditary spherocytosis
Diagnostic test for hereditary spherocytosis	Osmotic fragility test
Pure RBC aplasia	Diamond-Blackfan anemia
Anemia associated with absent radii and thumbs, diffuse hyperpigmentation, café au lait spots, microcephaly, and pancytopenia	Fanconi anemia
Medications and viruses that lead to aplastic anemia	Chloramphenicol, sulfonamides, radiation, HIV, chemotherapeutic agents, hepatitis, parvovirus B19, EBV
How to distinguish polycythemia vera from 2° polycythemia	Both have ↑ hematocrit and RBC mass, but polycythemia vera should have normal O_2 saturation and low erythropoietin levels

TTP pentad?	**LMNOP – L**ow platelet count (thrombocytopenia), **M**icroangiopathic hemolytic anemia, **N**eurologic changes, "**O**bsolete" renal function, **P**yrexia
HUS triad?	Anemia (microangiopathic hemolytic anemia), thrombocytopenia, and acute renal failure
Treatment for TTP	Emergent large-volume plasmapheresis, corticosteroids, antiplatelet drugs Platelet transfusion is contraindicated!
Treatment for ITP in children	Usually resolves spontaneously. May require IVIG and/or corticosteroids
Which of the following are ↑ in DIC: fibrin split products, D-dimer, fibrinogen, platelets, and hematocrit?	Fibrin split products and D-dimer are ↑. Platelets, fibrinogen, and hematocrit are ↓
8-year-old boy presents with hemarthrosis and ↑ PTT with normal PT and bleeding time. Diagnosis? Treatment?	Hemophilia A or B. Consider desmopressin (for hemophilia A) or factor VIII or IX supplements
14-year-old girl presents with prolonged bleeding after dental surgery and with menses, normal PT, normal or ↑ PTT, and ↑ bleeding time. Diagnosis? Treatment?	von Willebrand disease. Treat with desmopressin, FFP, or cryoprecipitate
60-year-old African-American man presents with bone pain. What might a work-up for multiple myeloma reveal?	Monoclonal gammopathy, Bence Jones proteinuria, and "punched-out" lesions on radiographs of the skull and long bones
Reed-Sternberg cells	Hodgkin lymphoma
10-year-old boy presents with fever, weight loss, and night sweats. Exam shows an anterior mediastinal mass. Suspected diagnosis?	Non-Hodgkin lymphoma
Microcytic anemia with ↓ serum iron, ↓ TIBC, and normal or ↑ ferritin	Anemia of chronic disease
Microcytic anemia with ↓ serum iron, ↓ ferritin, and ↑ TIBC	Iron-deficiency anemia
80-year-old man presents with fatigue, lymphadenopathy, splenomegaly, and isolated lymphocytosis. What is the suspected diagnosis?	CLL
Patient with fatigue is found to have a ↓ hemoglobin and ↑ mean corpuscular volume. What are potential causes for this anemia?	↓ Vitamin B_{12} deficiency (pernicious anemia, vegetarian diet, Crohn/GI disorders) or folate deficiency (alcoholics)
Late, life-threatening complication of CML	Blast crisis (fever, bone pain, splenomegaly, pancytopenia)
Auer rods on blood smear	AML
AML subtype associated with DIC. Treatment?	M3 Retinoic acid
Electrolyte changes in tumor lysis syndrome	↓ Ca^{2+}, ↑ K^+, ↑ phosphate, ↑ uric acid

50-year-old man presents with early satiety, splenomegaly, and bleeding. Cytogenetics show t(9,22). Diagnosis?	CML
Patient on the chemotherapy service with ANC of 1000 is noted to have a fever of 38.8°C (102.1°F). Best next step?	Neutropenic fever is a medical emergency. Start broad-spectrum antibiotics
Virus associated with aplastic anemia in patients with sickle cell anemia	Parvovirus B19
25-year-old African-American man with sickle cell anemia has sudden onset of bone pain. Management of pain crisis?	O_2, analgesia, hydration, and, if severe, transfusion
Significant cause of morbidity in thalassemia patients. Treatment?	Iron overload. Use deferoxamine

INFECTIOUS DISEASE

The three most common causes of FUO	Infection, cancer, and autoimmune disease
Centor criteria for strep pharyngitis (1 point each)	Fever, tonsillar exudate, tender anterior cervical lymphadenopathy, lack of cough, 3–14 years of age
Causes of pneumonia in neonates?	GBS, *E coli*, *Listeria*
Causes of pneumonia in adults 40–65 years of age?	*S pneumoniae*, *H influenzae*, *Mycoplasma*
Treatment of tuberculosis by type	Active disease: INH + pyrazinamide + rifampin + ethambutol + vitamin B_6 Latent disease: INH for 9 months
Asplenic patients are particularly susceptible to these organisms	Encapsulated organisms—pneumococcus, meningococcus, *H influenzae*, *Klebsiella*
Causes of ring-enhancing brain lesions	Abscess, toxoplasmosis, metastasis, lymphoma, AIDS, neurocysticercosis
AIDS-defining illnesses	Esophageal candidiasis, CMV retinitis, Kaposi sarcoma, CNS lymphoma, PML, toxoplasmosis, PCP, invasive cervical/anal cancer, HIV encephalopathy
At what CD4 count should *Pneumocystis jiroveci* pneumonia prophylaxis be initiated in an HIV ⊕ patient? *Mycobacterium avium* complex (MAC) prophylaxis?	$\leq$ 200 cells/mm³ for *P jiroveci* (with TMP-SMX); $\leq$ 50–100 cells mm³ for MAC (with clarithromycin/azithromycin)
Causes of meningitis in neonates. Treatment?	GBS, *E coli*, *Listeria*. Treat with ampicillin + cefotaxime or gentamicin
Causes of meningitis in infants. Treatment?	*S pneumoniae*, *N meningitidis*, *H influenzae* type b. Treat with vancomycin + cefotaxime
What must always be done before LP?	Check for ↑ ICP. Look for papilledema
CSF findings: ■ Low glucose, PMN predominance ■ Normal glucose, lymphocytic predominance ■ Numerous RBCs in serial CSF samples ■ ↑ Gamma globulins	 Bacterial meningitis Aseptic (viral) meningitis SAH MS

Findings in 1° syphilis	Painless chancre and lymphadenopathy
Findings in 3° syphilis	Tabes dorsalis, gummas, Argyll Robertson pupils, aortitis, aortic root aneurysms
Characteristics of 1° Lyme disease	Erythema migrans
Characteristics of 2° Lyme disease	Arthralgias, migratory polyarthropathies, facial nerve palsy, myocarditis, third-degree heart block
SIRS criteria	Temp < 36°C (96.8°F) or > 38°C (100.4°F) Tachypnea > 20 bpm or Paco$_2$ < 32 mmHg Tachycardia > 90 bpm WBC < 4000, > 12,000, or > 10% bands
Risk factors for pyelonephritis	Pregnancy, vesicoureteral reflux, anatomic anomalies, indwelling catheters, kidney stones
Neutropenic nadir postchemotherapy	7–10 days
Classic physical findings for endocarditis	Fever, heart murmur, Osler nodes, splinter hemorrhages, Janeway lesions, Roth spots
Duke criteria for endocarditis	Major: Positive blood cultures, new murmur, positive echocardiogram Minor: Risk factors, > 38° C, vascular or immunologic phenomena, echocardiogram or culture evidence that does not meet major criteria
Aplastic crisis in sickle cell disease	Parvovirus B19

Name the organism:

▪ Branching rods in oral infection	*Actinomyces israelii*
▪ Weakly gram ⊕, partially acid-fast in lung infection	*Nocardia asteroides*
▪ Painful chancroid	*Haemophilus ducreyi*
▪ Dog or cat bite	*Pasteurella multocida*
▪ Gardener	*Sporothrix schenckii*
▪ Raw pork and skeletal muscle cysts	*Trichinella spiralis*
▪ Sheepherders with liver cysts	*Echinococcus granulosus*
▪ Perianal itching	*Enterobius vermicularis*
▪ Pregnant women with pets	*Toxoplasma gondii*
▪ Meningitis in adults	*Neisseria meningitidis*
▪ Meningitis in elderly	*Streptococcus pneumoniae*
▪ Meningoencephalitis in AIDS patients	*Cryptococcus neoformans*
▪ Alcoholic with pneumonia	*Klebsiella*
▪ "Currant jelly" sputum	*Klebsiella*
▪ Malignant external otitis	*Pseudomonas*
▪ Infection in burn victims	*Pseudomonas*
▪ Osteomyelitis from a foot wound puncture	*Pseudomonas*
▪ Osteomyelitis in a sickle cell patient	*Salmonella*

Patient presents with a pruritic papule with regional lymphadenopathy. Evolves into a black eschar after 7–10 days. Treatment?	Cutaneous anthrax. Treat with ciprofloxacin or doxycycline

55-year-old man who is a smoker and a heavy drinker presents with a new cough and flulike symptoms. Gram stain shows no organisms. Silver stain of sputum shows gram ⊖ rods. Diagnosis?	*Legionella* pneumonia
Patient from California or Arizona presents with fever, malaise, cough, and night sweats. Diagnosis? Treatment?	Coccidioidomycosis. Amphotericin B
Middle-aged man presents with acute-onset monoarticular joint pain and bilateral facial nerve palsy. What is the likely diagnosis, and how did he get it? Treatment?	Lyme disease, *Ixodes* tick bite, doxycycline
Patient develops endocarditis 3 weeks after receiving a prosthetic heart valve. What organism is suspected?	*S aureus* or *S epidermidis*
24-year-old man presents with soft white plaques on his tongue and the back of his throat. Diagnosis? Work-up? Treatment?	Candidal thrush. Work-up should include an HIV test. Treat with nystatin oral suspension
Patient develops endocarditis in a native valve after having a dental cleaning	*S viridans*

MUSCULOSKELETAL

Back pain that is exacerbated by standing and walking and relieved with sitting and hyperflexion of the hips	Spinal stenosis
Joints in the hand affected in rheumatoid arthritis	MCP and PIP joints. DIP joints are spared
Joint pain and stiffness that worsen over the course of the day and are relieved by rest	Osteoarthritis
Genetic disorder associated with multiple fractures and blue sclerae and commonly mistaken for child abuse	Osteogenesis imperfecta
Hip and back pain along with stiffness that improves with activity over the course of the day and worsens at rest. Diagnostic test?	Suspect ankylosing spondylitis. X-ray of sacroiliac joints
Arthritis, conjunctivitis, and urethritis in young men. Associated organisms?	Reactive arthritis. Most commonly associated with *Chlamydia,* also consider *Campylobacter, Shigella, Salmonella,* and *Ureaplasma*
55-year-old man has sudden, excruciating first MTP joint pain after a night of drinking red wine. Diagnosis, work-up, and chronic treatment?	Gout. Needle-shaped, negatively birefringent crystals are seen on joint fluid aspirate. Chronic treatment with allopurinol or probenecid
Rhomboid-shaped, positively birefringent crystals on joint fluid aspirate	Pseudogout
Elderly woman presents with pain and stiffness of the shoulders and hips. She cannot lift her arms above her head. Labs show anemia and ↑ ESR	Polymyalgia rheumatica
Bone is fractured in a fall on an outstretched hand	Distal radius (Colles fracture)
Complication of scaphoid fracture	Avascular necrosis

Signs suggesting radial nerve damage with humeral fracture	Wrist drop, loss of thumb abduction
Most common 1° malignant tumor of bone	Osteosarcoma
Headaches, soreness in jaw, pain on scalp, transient monocular blindness	Giant cell/temporal arteritis

NEUROLOGY

Unilateral, severe periorbital headache with tearing and conjunctival erythema	Cluster headache
Prophylactic treatment for migraine	Antihypertensives, antidepressants, anticonvulsants, dietary changes
Most common pituitary tumor. Treatment?	Prolactinoma. Dopamine agonists (eg, bromocriptine, cabergoline)
55-year-old patient presents with acute "broken speech." Type of aphasia? Lobe and vascular distribution?	Broca aphasia. Frontal lobe. Left MCA distribution
Most common cause of SAH	Trauma (second most common is berry aneurysm)
Crescent-shaped hyperdensity on CT that does not cross the midline	Subdural hematoma—bridging veins torn (seen in elderly and young children)
History significant for initial altered mental status with an intervening lucid interval. Diagnosis? Most likely source? Treatment?	Epidural hematoma. Middle meningeal artery. Neurosurgical evacuation
CSF findings with SAH	↑ ICP, RBCs, xanthochromia
Albuminocytologic dissociation	Guillain-Barré syndrome (↑ protein in CSF without a significant increase in cell count)
Cold water is flushed into a patient's ear, and the fast phase of the nystagmus is toward the opposite side. Normal or pathologic?	Normal
Most common 1° sources of metastases to the brain	Lung, breast, skin (melanoma), kidney, GI tract
May be seen in children who are accused of inattention in class and are often confused with ADHD. Treatment?	Absence seizures. Ethosuximide
Most frequent presentation of intracranial neoplasm	Headache. 1° Neoplasms are much less common than brain metastases
Most common cause of seizures in children (2–10 years of age)	Infection, febrile seizures, trauma, idiopathic
Most common cause of seizures in young adults (18–35 years of age)	Trauma, alcohol withdrawal, brain tumor
First-line medication for status epilepticus	IV benzodiazepine
Confusion, ophthalmoplegia, ataxia	Wernicke encephalopathy caused by a deficiency of thiamine
Most common causes of dementia	Alzheimer disease and vascular/multi-infarct
Combined UMN and LMN disorder	ALS

Rigidity and stiffness with unilateral resting tremor and masked facies	Parkinson disease
The mainstay of Parkinson therapy	Levodopa/carbidopa
Treatment for Guillain-Barré syndrome	IVIG or plasmapheresis. Avoid steroids
Rigidity and stiffness that progress to choreiform movements, accompanied by moodiness and altered behavior. Inheritance pattern?	Huntington disease. Autosomal dominant
6-year-old girl presents with a port-wine stain in the V$_1$ distribution as well as with intellectual disability, seizures, and ipsilateral leptomeningeal angioma	Sturge-Weber syndrome. Treat symptomatically. Possible focal cerebral resection of affected lobe
Multiple café-au-lait spots on skin	Neurofibromatosis type 1
Hyperphagia, hypersexuality, hyperorality, and hyperdocility	Klüver-Bucy syndrome (amygdala)
May be administered to a symptomatic patient to diagnose myasthenia gravis	Edrophonium

OBSTETRICS

Classic ultrasonography and gross appearance of complete hydatidiform mole	Snowstorm on ultrasonography. "Cluster-of-grapes" appearance on gross exam
Chromosomal pattern of a complete mole	46,XX
Molar pregnancy containing fetal tissue	Partial mole
Symptoms of placental abruption	Continuous, painful vaginal bleeding
Symptoms of placenta previa	Self-limited, painless vaginal bleeding
When should a vaginal exam be performed with suspected placenta previa?	Never
Antibiotics with teratogenic effects	Tetracycline, fluoroquinolones, aminoglycosides, sulfonamides
Medication given to accelerate fetal lung maturity	Betamethasone or dexamethasone for 48 hours
Most common cause of postpartum hemorrhage	Uterine atony
Treatment for postpartum hemorrhage	Uterine massage. If that fails, give oxytocin
Typical antibiotics for GBS prophylaxis	IV penicillin or ampicillin
Patient fails to lactate after delivery with marked blood loss	Sheehan syndrome (postpartum pituitary necrosis)
Uterine bleeding at 18 weeks' gestation. No products expelled. Cervical os open	Inevitable abortion
Uterine bleeding at 18 weeks' gestation. No products expelled. Cervical os closed	Threatened abortion

GYNECOLOGY

First test to perform when a woman presents with amenorrhea	Pregnancy test. Most common cause of amenorrhea is pregnancy
Term for heavy bleeding during and between menstrual periods	Menometrorrhagia
Cause of amenorrhea with normal prolactin, no response to estrogen-progesterone challenge, and a history of D&C	Asherman syndrome
Therapy for polycystic ovarian syndrome	Weight loss and OCPs. Consider metformin
Medication used to induce ovulation	Clomiphene citrate
Diagnostic step required in a postmenopausal woman who presents with vaginal bleeding	Endometrial biopsy
Indications for medical treatment of ectopic pregnancy	Patient stable. Unruptured ectopic pregnancy of < 35 cm at < 6 weeks' gestation
Medical options for endometriosis	OCPs, danazol, GnRH agonists
Laparoscopic findings in endometriosis	Powder burns, "chocolate cysts"
Most common location for an ectopic pregnancy	Ampulla of the oviduct
How to diagnose and follow a leiomyoma	Ultrasonography
Natural history of a leiomyoma	Regresses after menopause
Patient has ↑ vaginal discharge and petechial patches in the upper vagina and cervix	Trichomonal vaginitis
Treatment for bacterial vaginosis	Oral metronidazole
Most common cause of bloody nipple discharge	Intraductal papilloma
Contraceptive methods that protect against PID	OCPs and barrier contraception
Unopposed estrogen is contraindicated in which cancers?	Endometrial or estrogen receptor–⊕ breast cancer
Patient presents with recent PID with RUQ pain	Consider Fitz-Hugh–Curtis syndrome
Breast malignancy presenting as itching, burning, and erosion of the nipple	Paget disease
Annual screening for women with a strong family history of ovarian cancer	CA-125 and transvaginal ultrasonography
50-year-old woman leaks urine when laughing or coughing. Non-surgical options?	Kegel exercises, estrogen, pessaries for stress incontinence
30-year-old woman has unpredictable urine loss. Exam is normal. Medical options?	Anticholinergics (oxybutynin) or β-adrenergics (metaproterenol) for urge incontinence
Lab values suggestive of menopause	↑ Serum FSH

Most common cause of female infertility	Endometriosis
Two consecutive findings of ASCUS on Pap smear. Follow-up evaluation?	Colposcopy and endocervical curettage
Breast cancer type that ↑ future risk for invasive carcinoma in both breasts	Lobular carcinoma in situ

PEDIATRICS

Nontender abdominal mass associated with ↑ VMA and HVA	Neuroblastoma
Most common type of TEF? How does it present?	Esophageal atresia with distal TEF (85%). Inability to pass NG tube
Contraindications to vaccination	Life-threatening egg allergies (needs close observation for MMR and influenza). Encephalopathy within 7 days of pertussis vaccine. Personal history of intussusception (rotavirus vaccination), pregnant/immunocompromised patients (avoid live vaccinations). Weight < 2 kg for hepatitis B vaccine in newborn
Tests to rule out abusive head trauma	Ophthalmologic exam, CT, and MRI
Neonate has meconium ileus	Cystic fibrosis (Hirschsprung disease is associated with failure to pass meconium for 48 hours)
Bilious emesis within hours after the first feeding	Duodenal atresia
2-month-old baby presents with nonbilious projectile emesis. Diagnosis? Next steps in management?	Pyloric stenosis. Hydrate and correct metabolic abnormalities. Then correct pyloric stenosis with pyloromyotomy
Most common 1° immunodeficiency	Selective IgA deficiency
Infant has high fever and onset of rash as fever breaks. What is he at risk for?	Febrile seizures (caused by roseola infantum)
What is the immunodeficiency? ■ Boy has chronic respiratory infections. Nitroblue tetrazolium test is ⊖ ■ Child has eczema, thrombocytopenia, and high levels of IgA ■ 4-month-old boy has life-threatening *Pseudomonas* infection	Chronic granulomatous disease Wiskott-Aldrich syndrome Bruton's X-linked agammaglobulinemia
Acute-phase treatment for Kawasaki disease	High-dose ASA for inflammation and fever. IVIG to prevent coronary artery aneurysm
Treatment for mild and severe unconjugated hyperbilirubinemia	Phototherapy (mild) or exchange transfusion (severe). Do not use phototherapy for conjugated hyperbilirubinemia
Sudden onset of altered mental status, emesis, and liver dysfunction after ASA intake	Reye syndrome

Child has loss of red light reflex (white pupil). Diagnosis? Risk for which cancer is ↑?	Suspect retinoblastoma. Osteosarcoma
Vaccinations at a 6-month well-child visit	HBV, DTaP, Hib, IPV, PCV, rotavirus, influenza
Tanner stage 3 in a 6-year-old girl	Precocious puberty
Infection of small airways with epidemics in winter and spring	RSV bronchiolitis
Cause of neonatal RDS	Surfactant deficiency
Red "currant-jelly" stools, colicky abdominal pain, bilious vomiting, and a sausage-shaped mass in the RUQ	Intussusception
Congenital heart disease that causes 2° hypertension. Findings on physical exam?	Coarctation of the aorta. ↓ Femoral pulses
First-line treatment for otitis media	Amoxicillin
Most common pathogen causing croup	Parainfluenza virus type 1
Homeless child is small for his age and has peeling skin and a swollen belly	Kwashiorkor (protein malnutrition)
Defect in an X-linked syndrome with intellectual disability, gout, self-mutilation, and choreoathetosis	Lesch-Nyhan syndrome (purine salvage problem with HGPRTase deficiency)
Newborn girl has continuous "machinery murmur." What drug would you give?	PDA. Give indomethacin to close the PDA
Newborn girl with a posterior neck mass and swelling of the hands	Turner syndrome
Young child presents with proximal muscle weakness, waddling gait, and pronounced calf muscles	Duchenne muscular dystrophy
First-born female who was born in breech position is found to have asymmetric skin folds on newborn exam. Diagnosis? Treatment?	Developmental dysplasia of the hip. < 6 months Pavlik harness to maintain abduction
11-year-old obese African-American boy presents with sudden onset of limp. Diagnosis? Work-up?	Slipped capital femoral epiphysis. AP and frog-leg lateral x-rays
Active 13-year-old boy has anterior knee pain. Diagnosis?	Osgood-Schlatter disease

PSYCHIATRY

First-line pharmacotherapy for depression	SSRIs
Antidepressants associated with hypertensive crisis	MAOIs
Galactorrhea, impotence, menstrual dysfunction, and ↓ libido	Dopamine antagonists

17-year-old girl has left arm paralysis after her boyfriend dies in a car crash. No medical cause is found	Conversion disorder
Name the defense mechanism: - Mother who is angry at her husband yells at her child - Girl who is upset with her best friend acts overly kind - Hospitalized 10-year-old begins to wet his bed	 Displacement Reaction formation Regression
Life-threatening muscle rigidity, high fever, autonomic instability, confusion, and elevated creatine phosphokinase	Neuroleptic malignant syndrome
Amenorrhea, low body weight (< 85%), bradycardia, and abnormal body image in a young woman	Anorexia
35-year-old man has recurrent episodes of palpitations, diaphoresis, and fear of impending doom	Panic disorder
Most serious side effect of clozapine	Agranulocytosis
21-year-old man has 3 months of social withdrawal, worsening grades, flattened affect, and concrete thinking	Schizophreniform disorder (diagnosis of schizophrenia requires ≥ 6 months of symptoms)
Key side effects of atypical antipsychotics	Weight gain, type 2 DM, QT-segment prolongation
Young weight lifter receives IV haloperidol and complains that his eyes are deviated sideways. Diagnosis? Treatment?	Acute dystonia (oculogyric crisis). Treat with benztropine or diphenhydramine
Medication to avoid in patients with a history of alcohol withdrawal seizures	Neuroleptics, which can lower the seizure threshold
13-year-old boy has a history of theft, vandalism, and violence toward family pets	Conduct disorder. Associated with antisocial personality disorder in adults
Previously healthy 6-month-old girl has ↓ head growth, truncal discoordination, and ↓ social interaction	Rett disorder. Regression and loss of milestones is common. Stereotypical hand wringing
Patient has not slept for days, lost $20,000 gambling, is agitated, and has pressured speech. Diagnosis? Treatment?	Acute mania. Start an atypical antipsychotic and mood stabilizer (eg, lithium)
After a minor "fender bender," man wears a neck brace and requests permanent disability	Malingering
Health care worker presents with severe hypoglycemia. Blood analysis reveals no elevation in C-peptide	Factitious disorder
Patient spends most of his time acquiring cocaine despite losing his job and being threatened with legal charges	Substance use disorder
Medication to avoid in patients with PTSD	Benzodiazepines and opioids (have high addiction potential). Patients commonly have a history of substance abuse
Violent patient has vertical and horizontal nystagmus	PCP intoxication

Woman who was abused as a child frequently feels outside of or detached from her body	Depersonalization disorder
Schizophrenic patient takes haloperidol for 1 year and develops uncontrollable tongue movements. Diagnosis? Treatment?	Tardive dyskinesia. ↓ or discontinue haloperidol, and consider another antipsychotic (eg, risperidone, clozapine)
Man with major depressive disorder is counseled to avoid tyramine-rich foods with his new medication. What class of medications is he taking?	MAOIs

PULMONARY

Risk factors for DVT	Stasis, endothelial injury, and hypercoagulability (Virchow triad)
Criteria for exudative effusion	Pleural/serum protein > 0.5, OR pleural/serum LDH > 0.6
Causes of exudative effusion	Think of leaky capillaries ($2°$ to inflammation): malignancy, TB, bacterial or viral infection, PE with infarct, and pancreatitis
Causes of transudative effusion	Think of intact capillaries and ↑ hydrostatic pressure: HF, liver or kidney disease, and protein-losing enteropathy
Normalizing PCO_2 in a patient having an asthma exacerbation may indicate _____.	Fatigue and impending respiratory failure
Treatment for acute asthma exacerbation	β_2-agonists and corticosteroids
Treatment for acute COPD exacerbation	O_2, β_2-agonists (albuterol), muscarinic antagonist (ipratropium), corticosteroids, and $\pm$ antibiotics
Sarcoidosis	Dyspnea, bilateral hilar lymphadenopathy on chest x-ray (CXR), noncaseating granulomas, ↑ ACE, and hypercalcemia
PFTs of obstructive pulmonary disease	↓ FEV_1/FVC (< 0.7), ↑ TLC
PFTs of restrictive pulmonary disease	Normal or ↑ FEV_1/FVC, ↓ TLC
Honeycomb pattern on chest radiograph. Treatment?	Interstitial lung disease (AKA, diffuse parenchymal lung disease [DPLD]). Supportive care. Antifibrotic agents may help
Treatment for SVC syndrome	Radiation and endovascular stenting
Treatment for mild persistent asthma	Inhaled β_2-agonists and inhaled corticosteroids
Treatment for COPD exacerbation	O_2, bronchodilators, antibiotics, corticosteroids with taper, smoking cessation
Treatment for chronic COPD	Smoking cessation, home O_2, β_2-agonists (albuterol), anticholinergics (ipratropium), systemic or inhaled corticosteroids, flu and pneumococcal vaccines
Acid-base disorder in PE	Respiratory alkalosis with hypoxia and ↓ $PaCO_2$

NSCLC associated with hypercalcemia	SCC (ectopic PTHrP)
Lung cancer associated with SIADH	SCLC (ectopic ADH)
Lung cancer(s) associated with Lambert Eaton syndrome	SCLC
Lung cancer(s) highly related to cigarette exposure	SCLC, SCC
Tall white man presents with acute shortness of breath. Diagnosis? Treatment?	Spontaneous pneumothorax. Will regress spontaneously, but supplemental O_2 may be helpful
Treatment of tension pneumothorax	Immediate needle thoracostomy (over diagnostic) followed by chest tube placement
Characteristics favoring carcinoma in an isolated pulmonary nodule	Age > 45–50 years. Tobacco use. Lesions new or larger in comparison to old x-rays. Absence of calcification or irregular calcification. Size > 2 cm. Irregular margins
ARDS	Hypoxemia and pulmonary edema with normal PCWP
Sequelae of asbestos exposure	Pulmonary fibrosis, pleural plaques, bronchogenic carcinoma (mass in lung field), mesothelioma (pleural mass)
↑ Risk for what infection with silicosis?	*Mycobacterium tuberculosis*
Causes of hypoxemia	Right-to-left shunt, hypoventilation, low inspired O_2 tension, diffusion defect, V/Q mismatch
Classic chest radiographic findings for pulmonary edema	Cardiomegaly, prominent pulmonary vessels, Kerley B lines, "bat's-wing" appearance of hilar shadows, and perivascular and peribronchial cuffing
Chest radiography findings suggestive of PE	Westermark sign and Hampton hump (although most often normal)

RENAL/GENITOURINARY

Treatment of hypernatremia	NS if unstable vital signs. D_5W or 0.45% NS to replace free-water loss
Differential diagnosis of hypotonic hypervolemic hyponatremia	Cirrhosis, HF, nephrotic syndrome, AKI, CKD
Complication of overly rapid correction of hyponatremia (as may occur with 3% hypertonic saline therapy)	Central pontine myelinolysis (osmotic demyelination syndrome)
Peaked T waves and widened QRS	Hyperkalemia
Treatment of hyperkalemia	**C BIG K** (**C**alcium gluconate, **B**icarbonate, **I**nsulin + **G**lucose, **K**ayexalate)
T-wave flattening and U waves	Hypokalemia
Most common causes of hypercalcemia	Malignancy and hyperparathyroidism
First-line treatment for severe hypercalcemia (> 14 mg/dL)	IV hydration

Facial spasm elicited from tapping the facial nerve (Chvostek sign), carpal spasm after arterial occlusion by a BP cuff (Trousseau sign)	Hypocalcemia
Salicylate ingestion occurs in what type(s) of acid-base disorder?	Anion gap acidosis and 1° respiratory alkalosis caused by central respiratory stimulation
Acid-base disturbance commonly seen in pregnant women	Respiratory alkalosis
RTA associated with abnormal H+ secretion and nephrolithiasis	Type I (distal) RTA
RTA associated with abnormal HCO_3^- reabsorption and rickets	Type II (proximal) RTA
RTA associated with low aldosterone state	Type IV (distal) RTA
AKI in a patient with BUN/creatinine > 20:1 and/or Fe_{Na} < 1%	Prerenal (caused by ↓ renal perfusion)
Muddy brown casts	Acute tubular necrosis
Drowsiness, asterixis, nausea, and pericardial friction rub	Uremic syndrome seen in patients with renal failure
Hematuria, hypertension, oliguria, and RBC casts in the urine	Nephritic syndrome
Palpable purpura, arthralgias, abdominal pain	Henoch-Schönlein purpura
Glomerulonephritis with deafness	Alport syndrome
Glomerulonephritis with hemoptysis	Granulomatosis with polyangiitis (Wegener) and Goodpasture syndrome
Proteinuria (≥ 3.5 g/day), hypoalbuminemia, edema, hyperlipidemia, and thrombosis	Nephrotic syndrome
Waxy casts in urine sediment and Maltese crosses (seen with lipiduria)	Nephrotic syndrome
Most common form of nephrotic syndrome in adults	Focal segmental glomerulosclerosis
49-year-old man presents with acute-onset flank pain and hematuria	Nephrolithiasis
Most common type of nephrolithiasis	Calcium oxalate
Test of choice for nephrolithiasis	Noncontrast CT of abdomen
Ultrasonography shows bilateral enlarged kidneys with cysts. Associated brain anomaly?	ADPKD. Cerebral aneurysm
55-year-old man presents with irritative and obstructive urinary symptoms. Treatment options?	Probably BPH. Options include terazosin, finasteride, or surgical intervention (TURP)
55-year-old man is diagnosed with prostate cancer. Treatment options?	Watchful waiting, surgical resection, radiation therapy, and/or androgen suppression
50-year-old smoker with painless hematuria	Bladder cancer
Most common histology of bladder cancer	Transitional cell carcinoma

Hematuria, flank pain, and palpable flank mass	RCC
Most common type of testicular cancer	Seminoma, a type of germ cell tumor
Testicular cancer associated with ↑ β-hCG	Choriocarcinoma

SURGERY AND EMERGENCY MEDICINE

Class of drugs that may cause syndrome of muscle rigidity, hyperthermia, autonomic instability, and extrapyramidal symptoms	Antipsychotics (neuroleptic malignant syndrome)
Side effects of corticosteroids	Acute mania, immunosuppression, thin skin, osteoporosis, easy bruising, myopathies
Treatment for DTs	Benzodiazepines
Treatment for acetaminophen overdose	N-acetylcysteine
Treatment for opioid overdose	Naloxone
Treatment for benzodiazepine overdose	Flumazenil (monitor for withdrawal and seizures)
Treatment for neuroleptic malignant syndrome and malignant hyperthermia	Dantrolene
Treatment for malignant hypertension	Nitroprusside
Treatment of atrial fibrillation	Rate control, rhythm conversion, and anticoagulation
Treatment of SVT	If stable, rate control with carotid massage or other vagal stimulation. If unsuccessful, consider adenosine. If unstable, cardiovert (synchronized)
Causes of drug-induced SLE	INH, penicillamine, hydralazine, procainamide, chlorpromazine, methyldopa, quinidine
Macrocytic, megaloblastic anemia with neurologic symptoms	Vitamin B_{12} deficiency
Macrocytic, megaloblastic anemia without neurologic symptoms	Folate deficiency
Burn patient presents with cherry-red, flushed skin and coma. Sao_2 is normal, but carboxyhemoglobin is elevated. Treatment?	Treat CO poisoning with 100% O_2 or with hyperbaric O_2 if poisoning is severe or the patient is pregnant
Blood in urethral meatus or high-riding prostate	Bladder rupture or urethral injury
Test to rule out urethral injury	Retrograde cystourethrogram
Radiographic evidence of aortic disruption or dissection	Widened mediastinum (> 8 cm), loss of aortic knob, pleural cap, tracheal deviation to the right, depression of left main stem bronchus

Radiographic indications for surgery in patients with acute abdomen	Free air under the diaphragm, extravasation of contrast, severe bowel distention, space-occupying lesion (CT), mesenteric occlusion (angiography)
Most common organism in burn-related infections	*Pseudomonas*
Method of calculating fluid repletion in burn patients	Parkland formula: 24-hour fluids = 4 × kg × % BSA
Acceptable urine output in a trauma patient	50 cc/h
Acceptable urine output in a stable patient	30 cc/h
Signs of neurogenic shock	Hypotension and bradycardia
Signs of ↑ ICP (Cushing triad)	Hypertension, bradycardia, and abnormal respirations
↓ CO, ↓ PCWP, ↑ PVR	Hypovolemic shock
↓ CO, ↑ PCWP, ↑ PVR	Cardiogenic (or obstructive) shock
↑ CO, ↓ PCWP, ↓ PVR	Distributive (eg, septic or anaphylactic) shock
Treatment of septic shock	Fluids and antibiotics
Treatment of cardiogenic shock	Identify cause. Inotropes (eg, dobutamine)
Treatment of hypovolemic shock	Identify cause. Fluid and blood repletion
Treatment of anaphylactic shock	Epinephrine 1:1000 and diphenhydramine
Supportive treatment for ARDS	Low tidal volume ventilation
Signs of air embolism	Patient with chest trauma who was previously stable suddenly dies
Signs of cardiac tamponade	Distended neck veins, hypotension, diminished heart sounds (Beck triad). Pulsus paradoxus
Absent breath sounds, dullness to percussion, shock, flat neck veins	Massive hemothorax
Absent breath sounds, tracheal deviation, shock, distended neck veins	Tension pneumothorax
Treatment for blunt or penetrating abdominal trauma in a hemodynamically unstable patient	Exploratory laparotomy
↑ ICP in alcoholics or the elderly following head trauma. Can be acute or chronic. Crescent-shaped lesion on CT	Subdural hematoma
Head trauma with immediate loss of consciousness followed by a lucid interval and then rapid deterioration. Convex-shaped lesion on CT	Epidural hematoma
Best next step in patient with recent neck surgery, expanding neck mass/deviated trachea, and airway compromise (noisy breathing)	Wound exploration/evacuation of hematoma

TOP-RATED REVIEW RESOURCES

How to Use the Database

This section is a database of recommended clinical science review resources, question banks, and other test preparation tools marketed to medical students studying for the USMLE Step 2 CK. For each resource, we list the **Title**, the **First Author** (or editor), the **Current Publisher**, the **Copyright Year**, the **Edition**, the **Number of Pages**, the **ISBN**, the **Approximate List Price**, the **Format** of the resource, and the **Number of Test Questions**. Finally, each resource receives a **Rating**. The resources are sorted into a comprehensive section as well as into sections corresponding to the six clinical disciplines (internal medicine, neurology, OB/GYN, pediatrics, psychiatry, and surgery). Within each section, resources are arranged first by Rating, then by Author, and finally by Title.

For this edition of *First Aid for the USMLE Step 2 CK*, the database of review resources has been completely revised, with in-depth summary comments on more than 100 books and online and mobile applications. A letter rating scale with six different grades reflects the detailed student evaluations. Each resource receives a rating as follows:

A+	Excellent for boards review
A A–	Very good for boards review; choose among the group
B+ B	Good, but use only after exhausting better sources
B–	Fair, but there are many better books in the discipline; or low-yield subject material

The **Rating** is meant to reflect the overall usefulness of the resource in preparing for the USMLE Step 2 CK exam. This is based on a number of factors, including the following:

- Cost of the resource.
- Readability of the resource.
- Appropriateness and accuracy of the resource.
- Quality and number of sample questions.
- Quality of written answers to sample questions.
- Quality and appropriateness of the illustrations (eg, graphs, diagrams, photographs).
- Length of the text (longer is not necessarily better).
- Quality and number of other resources available in the same discipline.
- Importance of the discipline on the USMLE Step 2 CK exam.

Please note that **the rating does not reflect the quality of the resource for purposes other than reviewing for the USMLE Step 2 CK exam.** Many resources with low ratings are well written and informative but are not ideal for USMLE Step 2 CK preparation. We have also avoided listing or commenting on the wide variety of general textbooks available in the clinical sciences.

Evaluations are based on the cumulative results of formal and informal surveys of hundreds of medical students from medical schools across the country. The summary comments and overall ratings represent a consensus opinion, but there may have been a large range of opinions or limited student feedback on any particular resource. Please note that the data listed are subject to change.

We actively encourage medical students and faculty to submit their opinions and ratings of these clinical science review books so that we can update our database (see "How to Contribute," p. xiii). In addition, we ask that publishers and authors submit review copies of clinical science review books, including new editions, and books not included in our database, for evaluation. We also solicit reviews of new books or suggestions for alternate modes of study that may be useful in preparing for the exam, such as flash cards, computer-based tutorials, commercial review courses, and Internet Web sites.

DISCLAIMER/CONFLICT-OF-INTEREST STATEMENT

No material in this book, including the ratings, reflects the opinion or influence of the publisher. All errors and omissions will gladly be corrected if brought to the attention of the authors through our blog at www.firstaidteam.com. Please note that USMLE-Rx and the entire *First Aid for the USMLE* series are publications by the senior authors of this book; their ratings are based solely on recommendations from the student authors of this book as well as data from the student survey and feedback forms.

COMPREHENSIVE

		AUTHOR	PUBLISHER	TYPE	PRICE
A	*Master the Boards USMLE Step 2 CK*	Fischer	Kaplan Publishing, 2017, 4th ed., 752 pages, ISBN 9781506208534	Review	$54.99
A	*USMLE Step 2 Secrets*	O'Connell	Elsevier, 2017, 5th ed., 424 pages, ISBN 9780323496162	Review	$44.99
A⁻	*First Aid Cases for the USMLE Step 2 CK*	Le	McGraw-Hill Education, 2010, 2nd ed., 576 pages, ISBN 9780071625708	Review	$45.00
A⁻	*First Aid Q&A for the USMLE Step 2 CK*	Le	McGraw-Hill Education, 2010, 2nd ed., 768 pages, ISBN 9780071625715	Review/Test/1000 q	$52.00
A⁻	*Step-Up to USMLE Step 2*	Van Kleunen	Lippincott Williams & Wilkins, 2015, 3rd ed., 352 pages, ISBN 9781451189599	Review	$53.99
B⁺	*Boards & Wards for USMLE Steps 2 & 3*	Ayala	Lippincott Williams & Wilkins, 2012, 5th ed., 608 pages, ISBN 9781451144062	Review	$55.99
B⁺	*USMLE Step 2 Made Ridiculously Simple*	Carl	Medmaster Books, 2012, 5th ed., 381 pages, ISBN 9780940780996	Review	$29.95
B⁺	*Kaplan Medical USMLE Diagnostic Flashcards*	Fischer	Kaplan Publishing, 2012, 3rd ed., 408 cards, ISBN 9781609780371	Flashcards	$271.02
B⁺	*NMS Q&A Review for USMLE Step 2 CK*	Ibsen	Lippincott Williams & Wilkins, 2011, 4th ed., 384 pages, ISBN 9780781787390	Review/Test/1000 q	$53.99
B⁺	*Clinical Vignettes for the USMLE Step 2 CK: PreTest Self-Assessment & Review*	McGraw-Hill	McGraw-Hill Education, 2009, 5th ed., 292 pages, ISBN 9780071604635	Test/368 q	$41.00
B	*Physical Diagnosis: PreTest Self-Assessment & Review*	Bernstein	McGraw-Hill Education, 2010, 7th ed., 442 pages, ISBN 9780071633017	Test/500 q	$39.00
B	*USMLE Step 2 CK QBook*	Kaplan Medical	Kaplan Publishing, 2013, 6th ed., 540 pages, ISBN 9781419550485	Test/850 q	$49.99
B	*USMLE Steps 2 and 3: In Your Pocket*	McWilliams	Kaplan Publishing, 2014, 2nd ed., 480 pages, ISBN 9781609788988	Review	$34.99
B	*Déjà Review: USMLE Step 2 CK*	Naheedy	McGraw-Hill Education, 2010, 2nd ed., 348 pages, ISBN 9780071627160	Review	$25.00
B	*Brochert's Crush Step 2*	O'Connell	Elsevier Saunders, 2012, 4th ed., 352 pages, ISBN 9781455703111	Review	$41.95
B	*USMLE Step 2 Recall*	Ryan	Lippincott Williams & Wilkins, 2011, 2nd ed., 385 pages, ISBN 9781605479071	Review	$69.91

QUESTION BANKS

		AUTHOR	PUBLISHER	PRICE
A⁺	*UWorld Step 2 CK Qbank*	UWorld	www.uworld.com	$229–$649
A	*USMLE-Rx Step 2CK Qmax*	MedIQ Learning	www.usmle-rx.com	$78–$298
A⁻	*Kaplan QBank*	Kaplan	www.kaplanmedical.com	$80–$560
B	*USMLEasy*	McGraw-Hill Education	www.usmle-easy.com	$39–$169

INTERNAL MEDICINE, EMERGENCY MEDICINE, FAMILY MEDICINE

		AUTHOR	PUBLISHER	TYPE	PRICE
A	*Case Files: Emergency Medicine*	Toy	McGraw-Hill Education, 2017, 4th ed., 672 pages, ISBN 9781259640827	Review	$39.00
A⁻	*Step-Up to Medicine*	Agabegi	Wolters Kluwer Health, 2015, 4th ed., 560 pages, ISBN 9781496306142	Review	$61.99
A⁻	*First Aid for the Medicine Clerkship*	Kaufman	McGraw-Hill Education, 2010, 3rd ed., 432 pages, ISBN 9780071633826	Review	$50.00
A⁻	*Emergency Medicine: PreTest Self-Assessment & Review*	Rosh	McGraw-Hill Education, 2012, 3rd ed., 624 pages, ISBN 9780071773102	Test/500 q	$37.00
A⁻	*First Aid for the Emergency Medicine Clerkship*	Stead	McGraw-Hill Education, 2011, 3rd ed., 560 pages,, ISBN 9780071739061	Review	$50.00
A⁻	*Case Files: Family Medicine*	Toy	McGraw-Hill Education, 2016, 4th ed., 704 pages, ISBN 9781259587702	Review	$39.00
A⁻	*Case Files: Internal Medicine*	Toy	McGraw-Hill Education, 2016, 5th ed., 608 pages, ISBN 9780071843355	Review	$39.00
B⁺	*Medical Secrets*	Harward	Mosby, 2011, 5th ed., 640 pages, ISBN 9780323063982	Review	$46.99
B⁺	*Family Medicine: PreTest Self-Assessment & Review*	Knutson	McGraw-Hill Education, 2012, 3rd ed., 336 pages, ISBN 9780071760522	Test/500 q	$39.00
B	*Medicine Recall*	Bergin	Lippincott Williams & Wilkins, 2011, 4th ed., 848 pages, ISBN 9781605476759	Review	$55.99
B	*In A Page Emergency Medicine*	Caterino	Blackwell Publishing, 2003, 1st ed., 344 pages, ISBN 9781405103572	Review	$56.99
B	*Déjà Review: Family Medicine*	Perez	McGraw-Hill Education, 2011, 2nd ed., 402 pages, ISBN 9780071715157	Review	$25.00
B	*Déjà Review: Internal Medicine*	Saadat	McGraw-Hill Education, 2011, 2nd ed., 254 pages, ISBN 9780071715171	Review	$25.00
B	*Medicine: PreTest Self-Assessment & Review*	Smalligan	McGraw-Hill Education, 2012, 13th ed., 470 pages, ISBN 9780071761499	Test/500 q	$37.00
B	*Blueprints Medicine*	Young	Lippincott Williams & Wilkins, 2015, 6th ed., 416 pages, ISBN 9781469864150	Review/Test/100 q	$57.99
B⁻	*Déjà Review: Emergency Medicine*	Jang	McGraw-Hill Education, 2011, 2nd ed., 480 pages, ISBN 9780071715188	Review	$25.00

NEUROLOGY

		AUTHOR	PUBLISHER	TYPE	PRICE
A⁻	*Blueprints Neurology*	Drislane	Lippincott Williams & Wilkins, 2013, 4th ed., 256 pages, ISBN 9781451117684	Review/Test/100 q	$53.99
B⁺	*Neurology: PreTest Self-Assessment & Review*	Anschel	McGraw-Hill Education, 2012, 8th ed., 368 pages, ISBN 9781259009402	Test/500 q	$39.00
B	*Neurology Secrets*	Kass	Elsevier, 2016, 6th ed., 552 pages, ISBN 9780323359481	Review	$46.99
B	*Blueprints Clinical Cases in Neurology*	Sheth	Lippincott Williams & Wilkins, 2007, 2nd ed., 390 pages, ISBN 9781405104944	Test/200 q	$43.99

OB/GYN

		AUTHOR	PUBLISHER	TYPE	PRICE
A⁻	*Blueprints Obstetrics and Gynecology*	Callahan	Lippincott Williams & Wilkins, 2017, 7th ed., 529 pages, ISBN 9781496349507	Review/Test/150 q	$54.99
A⁻	*Case Files: Obstetrics and Gynecology*	Toy	McGraw-Hill Education, 2016, 5th ed., 624 pages, ISBN 9780071848725	Review	$39.00
B⁺	*First Aid for the Obstetrics & Gynecology Clerkship*	Kaufman	McGraw-Hill Education, 2017, 4th ed., 384 pages, ISBN 9781259644061	Review	$43.00
B⁺	*Obstetrics and Gynecology: PreTest Self-Assessment & Review*	Schneider	McGraw-Hill Education, 2012, 13th ed., 352 pages, ISBN 9780071761277	Test/500 q	$37.00
B	*Déjà Review: Obstetrics and Gynecology*	Miller	McGraw-Hill Education, 2011, 2nd ed., 462 pages, ISBN 9780071715133	Review	$25.00
B	*NMS Obstetrics and Gynecology*	Pfeifer	Lippincott Williams & Wilkins, 2011, 7th ed., 528 pages, ISBN 9781608315765	Review/Test/500 q	$56.99
B⁻	*Lange Q&A: Obstetrics and Gynecology*	Katz	McGraw-Hill Education, 2011, 9th ed., 404 pages, ISBN 9780071712132	Test/1300+ q	$53.00

PEDIATRICS

		AUTHOR	PUBLISHER	TYPE	PRICE
A⁻	*First Aid for the Pediatrics Clerkship*	Stead	McGraw-Hill Education, 2017, 4th ed., 576 pages, ISBN 9781259834318	Review	$55.00
A⁻	*Case Files: Pediatrics*	Toy	McGraw-Hill Education, 2015, 5th ed., 576 pages, ISBN 9780071839952	Review	$31.20
A⁻	*Pediatrics: PreTest Self-Assessment & Review*	Yetman	McGraw-Hill Education, 2016, 14th ed., 512 pages, ISBN 9780071838443	Test/500 q	$35.00
B⁺	*Déjà Review: Pediatrics*	Davey	McGraw-Hill Education, 2011, 2nd ed., 336 pages, ISBN 9780071715140	Review	$25.00
B	*Blueprints Pediatrics*	Marino	Lippincott Williams & Wilkins, 2013, 6th ed., 416 pages, ISBN 9781451116045	Review/Test/100 q	$52.99
B	*Pediatric Secrets*	Polin	Elsevier, 2015, 6th ed., 752 pages, ISBN 9780323310307	Review	$46.99
B⁻	*Lange Q&A: Pediatrics*	Jackson	McGraw-Hill Education, 2010, 7th ed., 326 pages, ISBN 9780071475686	Test/1000 q	$55.00
B⁻	*Pediatrics Recall*	McGahren	Lippincott Williams & Wilkins, 2011, 4th ed., 542 pages, ISBN 9781605476766	Review	$69.30

PSYCHIATRY

		AUTHOR	PUBLISHER	TYPE	PRICE
A	*First Aid for the Psychiatry Clerkship*	Stead	McGraw-Hill Education, 2018, 5th ed., 256 pages, ISBN 9781260143393	Review	$50.00
A⁻	*Psychiatry: PreTest Self-Assessment & Review*	Klamen	McGraw-Hill Education, 2015, 14th ed., 304 pages, ISBN 9789814670234	Test/500 q	$35.00
A⁻	*Case Files: Psychiatry*	Toy	McGraw-Hill Education, 2015, 5th ed., 544 pages, ISBN 9780071835329	Review	$35.00
B⁺	*Blueprints Psychiatry*	Murphy	Lippincott Williams & Wilkins, 2009, 5th ed., 176 pages, ISBN 9780781782531	Review/Test/100 q	$50.99
B⁺	*Lange Q&A: Psychiatry*	Blitzstein	McGraw-Hill Education, 2016, 11th ed., 304 pages, ISBN 9781259643941	Test/800+ q	$50.00
B	*NMS Psychiatry*	Thornhill	Lippincott Williams & Wilkins, 2011, 6th ed., 303 pages, ISBN 9781608315741	Review/Test/500 q	$50.44
B⁻	*Déjà Review: Psychiatry*	Gopal	McGraw-Hill Education, 2011, 2nd ed., 244 pages, ISBN 9780071715164	Review	$25.00

SURGERY

		AUTHOR	PUBLISHER	TYPE	PRICE
A	*Dr. Pestana's Surgical Notes: Top 180 Vignettes for the Surgical Wards*	Pestana	Kaplan Publishing, 2017, 3rd ed., 256 pages, ISBN 9781506208541	Review	$34.99
A⁻	*Case Files: Surgery*	Toy	McGraw-Hill Education, 2016, 5th ed., 736 pages, ISBN 978259585227	Review	$39.00
B⁺	*First Aid for the Surgery Clerkship*	Ganti	McGraw-Hill Education, 2016, 3rd ed., 512 pages, ISBN 9780071842099	Review	$50.00
B⁺	*Step-Up to Surgery*	Zaslau	Lippincott Williams & Wilkins, 2014, 2nd ed., 408 pages, ISBN 9781451187632	Review	$58.99
B	*Surgical Recall*	Blackbourne	Lippincott Williams & Wilkins, 2017; 8th ed., 640 pages, ISBN 9781496370815	Review	$49.99
B	*NMS Surgery*	Jarrell	Lippincott Williams & Wilkins, 2015, 6th ed., 575 pages, ISBN 9781608315840	Review/Test/350 q	$58.99
B	*Surgery: PreTest Self-Assessment & Review*	Kao	McGraw-Hill Education, 2012, 13th ed., 384 pages, ISBN 9780071761215	Test/500 q	$39.00
B	*Déjà Review: Surgery*	Tevar	McGraw-Hill Education, 2011, 2nd ed., 412 pages, ISBN 0071715126	Review	$25.00
B⁻	*Abernathy's Surgical Secrets*	Harken	Elsevier, 2017, 7th ed., 544 pages, ISBN 9780323478731	Review	$46.99
B⁻	*Blueprints in Surgery*	Karp	Lippincott Williams & Wilkins, 2009, 5th ed., 320 pages, ISBN 9780781788687	Review/Test/100 q	$33.05

COMMERCIAL REVIEW COURSES

Although commercial preparation courses can be helpful for some students, such courses are typically costly and require significant time commitment. They are usually most effective as an organizing tool for students who feel overwhelmed by the sheer volume of material involved in Step 2 CK preparation. Note, too, that multiweek courses may be quite intense and may thus leave limited time for independent study. Also note that some commercial courses are designed for first-time test takers, while others focus on students who are repeating the exam. In addition, some courses are geared toward IMGs who want to take all three Steps in a limited amount of time.

Student experience and satisfaction with review courses are highly variable. We suggest that you discuss options with recent graduates of the review courses you are considering. In addition, course content and structure can change rapidly. Some student opinions can be found in discussion groups on the World Wide Web. Contact information for some Step 2 CK commercial review courses is listed as follows:

Becker Professional Education
500 W Monroe
Chicago IL 60661
Phone: (800) 868-3900
http://www.becker.com

Kaplan Medical
6301 Kaplan University Avenue
Fort Lauderdale, FL 33309
Phone: (800) 527-8378
Email: customer.care@kaplan.com
www.kaplanmedical.com

Med School Tutors
641 Lexington Avenue
New York, NY 10022
Phone: (212) 327-0098
Fax: (347) 658-5978
Email: HQ@medschooltutors.com
https://www.medschooltutors.com

Northwestern Medical Review
4800 Collins Road, #22174
Lansing, MI 48909
Phone: (517) 347-6914
Fax: (517) 347-7005
Email: contactus@northwesternmedicalreview.com
http://www.northwesternmedicalreview.com

PASS Program
2302 Moreland Boulevard
Champaign, IL 61822
Phone: (217) 378-8018
Fax: (217) 378-7809
Email: info@passprogram.net
https://www.pass-program.com

ACRONYMS AND ABBREVIATIONS

Abbreviation	Meaning
A-a	alveolar-arterial (oxygen gradient)
AA	2° amyloidosis
AAA	abdominal aortic aneurysm
AAMC	Association of American Medical Colleges
ABG	arterial blood gas
ABI	ankle-brachial index
AC	abdominal circumference
ACA	anterior cerebral artery
ACD	anemia of chronic disease
ACE	angiotensin-converting enzyme
ACEI	angiotensin-converting enzyme inhibitor
ACh	acetylcholine
ACL	anterior cruciate ligament
ACLS	advanced cardiac life support (protocol)
ACTH	adrenocorticotropic hormone
AD	Alzheimer disease
ADA	American Diabetes Association, Americans with Disabilities Act
ADH	antidiuretic hormone
ADHD	attention-deficit hyperactivity disorder
ADP	autosomal-dominant polycystic kidney disease
AF	atrial fibrillation
AFI	amniotic fluid index
AFP	α-fetoprotein
Ag	antigen
AGC	atypical glandular cell
AHA	American Heart Association
AI	adrenal insufficiency
AICA	anterior inferior cerebellar artery
AIDS	acquired immunodeficiency syndrome
AIHA	autoimmune hemolytic anemia
AIN	acute interstitial nephritis
AKI	acute kidney injury
AL	1° amyloidosis
ALL	acute lymphocytic leukemia
ALP	alkaline phosphatase
ALS	amyotrophic lateral sclerosis
ALT	alanine aminotransferase
AMD	age-related macular degeneration
AML	acute myelogenous leukemia
ANA	antinuclear antibody
ANC	absolute neutrophil count

Abbreviation	Meaning
ANCA	antineutrophil cytoplasmic antibody
Anti-digitalis Fab	digitalis-specific antibody Fab fragments
AP	anteroposterior
APC	activated protein C; antigen-presenting cell
APL	acute promyelocytic leukemia
aPTT	activated partial thromboplastin time
ARB	angiotensin receptor blocker
ARDS	acute respiratory distress syndrome
ARF	acute renal failure
ARPKD	autosomal-recessive polycystic kidney disease
5-ASA	5-aminosalicylic acid
ASA	acetylsalicylic acid
ASC	atypical squamous cells
ASC-H	atypical squamous cells suspicious for high-grade dysplasia
ASC-US	atypical squamous cells of undetermined significance
ASD	atrial septal defect
ASO	antistreptolysin
AST	aspartate aminotransferase
ATN	acute tubular necrosis
ATRA	all-*trans* retinoic acid
AV	atrioventricular
AVM	arteriovenous malformation
AVN	avascular necrosis
AVNRT	atrioventricular nodal reentry tachycardia
AVRT	atrioventricular reciprocating tachycardia
AXR	x-ray of the abdominal
AZT	azidothymidine (zidovudine)
BAL	British anti-Lewisite (dimercaprol), bronchoalveolar lavage
BCC	basal cell carcinoma
BCG	bacille Calmette-Guérin
β-hCG	β-human chorionic gonadotropin
BID	twice a day
BMD	bone mineral density
BMI	body mass index
BMT	bone marrow transplantation
BP	blood pressure
BPAD	bipolar affective disorder
BPD	biparietal diameter, bipolar disorder

Abbreviation	Meaning
BPH	benign prostatic hyperplasia
bpm	beats per minute
BPP	biophysical profile
BPPV	benign paroxysmal positional vertigo
BSA	body surface area
BT	bleeding time
BUN	blood urea nitrogen
BW	birth weight
CABG	coronary artery bypass graft
CAD	coronary artery disease
CaEDTA	calcium disodium edetate
CAH	congenital adrenal hyperplasia
cAMP	cyclic adenosine monophosphate
c-ANCA	cytoplasmic antineutrophil cytoplasmic antibody
CBC	complete blood count
CBD	common bile duct
CBT	cognitive-behavioral therapy, computer-based testing
CCB	calcium channel blocker
CCP	cyclic citrullinated peptide
CCS	computer-based case simulation
CCSSA	Comprehensive Clinical Science Self-Assessment (test)
CD	cluster of differentiation
CEA	carcinoembryonic antigen
CF	cystic fibrosis
CFU	colony-forming unit
CGD	chronic granulomatous disease
cGMP	cyclic guanosine monophosphate
CHF	congestive heart failure
CHOP	cyclophosphamide, hydroxydaunorubicin, oncovin, prednisone
CI	confidence interval
CIN	candidate identification number, cervical intraepithelial neoplasia
CJD	Creutzfeldt-Jakob disease
CK	clinical knowledge, creatine kinase
CKD	chronic kidney disease
CK-MB	creatine kinase, MB fraction
CLL	chronic lymphocytic leukemia
CML	chronic myelogenous leukemia
CMP	comprehensive metabolic panel
CMV	cytomegalovirus
CN	cranial nerve
CNS	central nervous system
COMT	catechol-O-methyltransferase
COPD	chronic obstructive pulmonary disease
CPAP	continuous positive airway pressure
CPPD	calcium pyrophosphate deposition (disease)
CPR	cardiopulmonary resuscitation
Cr	creatinine

Abbreviation	Meaning
CREST	calcinosis, Raynaud phenomenon, esophageal dysmotility, sclerodactyly, and telangiectasia
CRL	crown-rump length
CRP	C-reactive protein
CS	clinical skills
CSA	central sleep apnea
CSD	combined system disease
CSF	cerebrospinal fluid
CST	contraction stress test
CT	computed tomography
CTS	carpal tunnel syndrome
CVA	cerebrovascular accident
CVID	common variable immunodeficiency
CVP	central venous pressure
CVS	chorionic villus sampling
CXR	chest x-ray
D&C	dilation and curettage
D&E	dilation and evacuation
DA	developmental age
DBP	diastolic blood pressure
DDAVP	desmopressin acetate
DES	diethylstilbestrol
DEXA	dual-energy x-ray absorptiometry
DFA	direct fluorescent antibody
DHEA	dehydroepiandrosterone
DHEAS	dehydroepiandrosterone sulfate
DI	diabetes insipidus
DIC	disseminated intravascular coagulation
DIP	distal interphalangeal (joint)
DIT	diiodotyrosine
DKA	diabetic ketoacidosis
DL_{CO}	diffusion capacity of carbon monoxide
DM	diabetes mellitus
DMARD	disease-modifying antirheumatic drug
DMD	Duchenne muscular dystrophy
DMSA	dimercaptosuccinic acid (succimer)
DNA	deoxyribonucleic acid
DNI	do not intubate
DNR	do not resuscitate
DPOAHC	durable power of attorney for health care
DPP-4	dipeptidyl peptidase-4
DRE	digital rectal exam
dsDNA	double-stranded deoxyribonucleic acid
DTaP	diphtheria, tetanus, acellular pertussis (vaccine)
DTRs	deep tendon reflexes
DTs	delirium tremens
DVT	deep venous thrombosis
EBV	Epstein-Barr virus
EC	emergency contraception
ECFMG	Educational Commission for Foreign Medical Graduates

Abbreviation	Meaning
ECG	electrocardiography
ECT	electroconvulsive therapy
ED	erectile dysfunction
EEG	electroencephalography
EF	ejection fraction
EFW	estimated fetal weight
EGD	esophagogastroduodenoscopy
ELISA	enzyme-linked immunosorbent assay
EM	electron microscopy, erythema multiforme
EMG	electromyography
EOM	extraocular movement
EPS	extrapyramidal symptoms
ER	emergency room, estrogen receptor
ERAS	Electronic Residency Application Service
ERCP	endoscopic retrograde cholangiopancreatography
ERV	expiratory reserve volume
ESR	erythrocyte sedimentation rate
ESRD	end-stage renal disease
ESWL	extracorporeal shock-wave lithotripsy
EtOH	ethanol
FAP	familial adenomatous polyposis
FAST	focused abdominal sonography for trauma (scan)
Fe_{Na}	fractional excretion of sodium
FEV_1	forced expiratory volume in 1 second
FFP	fresh frozen plasma
FHH	familial hypocalciuric hypercalcemia
FHR	fetal heart rate
Fio_2	fraction of inspired oxygen
FISH	fluorescence in situ hybridization
FL	femur length
FLAIR	fluid-attenuated inversion recovery (imaging)
FMG	foreign medical graduate
FNA	fine-needle aspiration
FOBT	fecal occult blood test
FRC	functional residual capacity
FSH	follicle-stimulating hormone
FSMB	Federation of State Medical Boards
FTA-ABS	fluorescent treponemal antibody absorption (test)
FTT	failure to thrive
5-FU	5-fluorouracil
FUO	fever of unknown origin
FVC	forced vital capacity
G6PD	glucose-6-phosphate dehydrogenase
GA	gestational age
GABA	gamma-aminobutyric acid
GAD	generalized anxiety disorder
GAF	global assessment of functioning
GAS	group A streptococcus
GBM	glioblastoma multiforme, glomerular basement membrane

Abbreviation	Meaning
GBS	group B streptococcus, Guillain-Barré syndrome
GCS	Glasgow Coma Scale
G-CSF	granulocyte colony-stimulating factor
GDMA2	gestational diabetes mellitus, insulin controlled
GERD	gastroesophageal reflux disease
GFAP	glial fibrillary acid protein
GFR	glomerular filtration rate
GGT	gamma-glutamyl transferase
GH	growth hormone
GI	gastrointestinal
GLP	glucagon-like peptide
GLP-1	glucagon-like peptide-1
GM-CSF	granulocyte-macrophage colony-stimulating factor
GNR	gram-negative rod
GnRH	gonadotropin-releasing hormone
GPA	granulomatosis with polyangiitis
GTD	gestational trophoblastic disease
GU	genitourinary
HAART	highly active antiretroviral therapy
HAV	hepatitis A virus
HbA_{1c}	hemoglobin A_{1c}
HbC	hemoglobin C
HBcAb	hepatitis B core antibody
HBcAg	hepatitis B core antigen
HBeAb	hepatitis E core antibody
HBeAg	hepatitis E core antigen
HBsAb	hepatitis B surface antibody
HBsAg	hepatitis B surface antigen
HBV	hepatitis B virus
hCG	human chorionic gonadotropin
HCL	hairy cell leukemia
HCTZ	hydrochlorothiazide
HCV	hepatitis C virus
HD	Huntington disease, Hodgkin disease
HDL	high-density lipoprotein
HDV	hepatitis D virus
HES	hypereosinophilic syndrome
HEV	hepatitis E virus
HGPRT	hypoxanthine-guanine phosphoribosyltransferase
HHS	hyperosmolar hyperglycemic state
HHV	human herpesvirus
5-HIAA	5-hydroxyindoleacetic acid
Hib	*Haemophilus influenza* type b
HIDA	hepato-iminodiacetic acid (scan)
HIT	heparin-induced thrombocytopenia
HIV	human immunodeficiency virus
HL	Hodgkin lymphoma
HLA	human leukocyte antigen
HMG-CoA	hydroxymethylglutaryl coenzyme A
HNPCC	hereditary nonpolyposis colorectal cancer

Abbreviation	Meaning
HOCM	hypertrophic obstructive cardiomyopathy
HPA	human placental antigen, hypothalamic-pituitary-adrenal (axis)
hpf	high-power field
HPV	human papillomavirus
HR	heart rate
HRT	hormone replacement therapy
HSIL	high-grade squamous intraepithelial lesion
HSV	herpesvirus
HTLV	human T-cell lymphotropic virus
HTN	hypertension
HUS	hemolytic-uremic syndrome
HVA	homovanillic acid
IBD	inflammatory bowel disease
IBS	irritable bowel syndrome
IC	inspiratory capacity
ICD	implantable cardiac defibrillator
ICP	intracranial pressure
ICU	intensive care unit
I/E	inspiratory to expiratory (ratio)
IFN-γ	Interferon-γ
Ig	immunoglobulin
IGF	insulin-like growth factor
ILD	interstitial lung disease
IM	intramuscular
IMED	International Medical Education Directory
IMG	international medical graduate
INH	isoniazid
INR	International Normalized Ratio
I/O	intake and output
IOP	intraocular pressure
IPF	idiopathic pulmonary fibrosis
ipsi	ipsilateral
IPV	inactivated polio vaccine
IRV	inspiratory reserve volume
ITP	idiopathic/immune thrombocytopenic purpura
IUD	intrauterine device
IUGR	intrauterine growth restriction
IUI	intrauterine insemination
IV	intravenous
IVC	inferior vena cava
IVDA	IV drug abuse
IVF	in vitro fertilization
IVIG	intravenous immunoglobulin
IVP	intravenous pyelography
JIA	juvenile idiopathic arthritis
JNC	Joint National Committee on Prevention, Detection, Evaluation, and Treatment of High Blood Pressure
JRA	juvenile rheumatoid arthritis
JVD	jugular venous distention
JVP	jugular venous pulse

Abbreviation	Meaning
KOH	potassium hydroxide
KS	Kaposi sarcoma
KSHV	Kaposi sarcoma–associated herpesvirus
KUB	kidney, ureter, bladder
LAD	left anterior descending (artery)
LAE	left atrial enlargement
LBBB	left bundle branch block
LBO	large bowel obstruction
LBP	low back pain
LCL	lateral collateral ligament
LDH	lactate dehydrogenase
LDL	low-density lipoprotein
LEEP	loop electrosurgical excision procedure
LES	lower esophageal sphincter
LFT	liver function test
LGV	lymphogranuloma venereum
LH	luteinizing hormone
LLQ	left lower quadrant
LLSB	lower left sternal border
LMN	lower motor neuron
LMP	last menstrual period
LMWH	low-molecular-weight heparin
LP	lumbar puncture
LR	lactated Ringer's, likelihood ratio
LSIL	low-grade squamous intraepithelial lesion
LTBI	latent tuberculosis infection
LUQ	left upper quadrant
LVH	left ventricular hypertrophy
LVOTO	left ventricular outflow tract obstructions
MAC	membrane attack complex, *Mycobacterium avium* complex
MALT	mucosa-associated lymphoid tissue
MAOI	monoamine oxidase inhibitor
mBPP	modified biophysical profile
MCA	middle cerebral artery
MCL	medial collateral ligament
MCP	metacarpophalangeal (joint)
MCV	mean corpuscular volume, meningococcal vaccine
MDD	major depressive disorder
MDE	major depressive episode
MDMA	3,4-methylenedioxymethamphetamine
MEN	multiple endocrine neoplasia
MGUS	monoclonal gammopathy of undetermined significance
MHA-TP	microhemagglutination assay–*Treponema pallidum*
MI	myocardial infarction
MIBG	metaiodobenzylguanidine (scan)
MIT	monoiodotyrosine
MM	multiple myeloma
MMA	methylmalonic acid
MMF	mycophenolate mofetil
MMR	measles, mumps, rubella (vaccine)

Abbreviation	Meaning
MoM	multiple of the median
MPTP	1-methyl-4-phenyl-1,2,3,6-tetrahydropyridine
MRA	magnetic resonance angiography
MRCP	magnetic resonance cholangiopancreatography
MRI	magnetic resonance imaging
MRSA	methicillin-resistant S aureus
MS	multiple sclerosis
MSAFP	maternal serum α-fetoprotein
MTP	metatarsophalangeal (joint)
MUA	manual uterine aspiration
MuSK	muscle-specific kinase
NBME	National Board of Medical Examiners
NEC	necrotizing enterocolitis
NF	neurofibromatosis
NG	nasogastric
NHL	non-Hodgkin lymphoma
NK	natural killer (cell)
Nl	normal
NMS	neuroleptic malignant syndrome
NNRTI	non-nucleoside reverse transcriptase inhibitor
NP	nasopharyngeal
NPH	normal pressure hydrocephalus; neutral protamine Hagedorn insulin
NPO	nil per os (nothing by mouth)
NPV	negative predictive value
NRTI	nucleoside/nucleotide reverse transcriptase inhibitor
NS	normal saline
NSAID	nonsteroidal anti-inflammatory drug
NSCLC	non–small cell lung cancer
NST	nonstress test
NSTEMI	non–ST-elevation myocardial infarction
NYHA	New York Heart Association
O&P	ova and parasites
OA	osteoarthritis
OCD	obsessive-compulsive disorder
OCP	oral contraceptive pill
OCPD	obsessive-compulsive personality disorder
OD	overdose
OP	oropharyngeal
OR	odds ratio, operating room
ORIF	open reduction and internal fixation
OSA	obstructive sleep apnea
OTC	over the counter
PA	posteroanterior
$Paco_2$	partial pressure of carbon dioxide in arterial blood
pANCA	perinuclear antineutrophil cytoplasmic antibody
Pao_2	partial pressure of oxygen in arterial blood
PAPP-A	pregnancy-associated plasma protein A

Abbreviation	Meaning
PAS	periodic acid–Schiff
PCA	posterior cerebral artery
PCI	percutaneous coronary intervention
PCL	posterior cruciate ligament
Pco_2	partial pressure of carbon dioxide
PCOS	polycystic ovarian syndrome
PCP	phencyclidine hydrochloride, *Pneumocystis carinii* (now *jiroveci*) pneumonia
PCR	polymerase chain reaction
PCV	polycythemia vera, pneumococcal vaccine
PCWP	pulmonary capillary wedge pressure
PDA	patent ductus arteriosus, posterior descending artery
PDD	pervasive developmental disorder
PDE	phosphodiesterase
PE	pulmonary embolism
PEA	pulseless electrical activity
PEEP	positive end-expiratory pressure
PET	positron emission tomography
PFT	pulmonary function test
PG	prostaglandin
$PGF_2\alpha$	prostaglandin $F_2\alpha$
PICA	posterior inferior cerebellar artery
PID	pelvic inflammatory disease
PIP	proximal interphalangeal (joint)
PKD	polycystic kidney disease
PKU	phenylketonuria
PMI	point of maximal impulse
PML	promyelocytic leukemia
PMN	polymorphonuclear (leukocyte)
PND	paroxysmal nocturnal dyspnea
PNH	paroxysmal nocturnal hemoglobinuria
PO	per os (by mouth)
Po_2	partial pressure of oxygen
Po_4	phosphate
POC	product of conception
PPD	purified protein derivative (of tuberculin)
PPI	proton pump inhibitor
PPROM	preterm premature rupture of membranes
PPV	pneumococcal polysaccharide vaccine, positive predictive value
PR	per rectum, progesterone receptor
PRN	pro re nata (as needed)
PROM	premature rupture of membranes
PSA	prostate-specific antigen
PT	prothrombin time
PTH	parathyroid hormone
PTHrP	parathyroid hormone–related protein
PTSD	post-traumatic stress disorder
PTT	partial thromboplastin time
PUD	peptic ulcer disease
PUVA	psoralen plus ultraviolet A
PVC	premature ventricular contraction

Abbreviation	Meaning
PVR	peripheral vascular resistance
PVS	persistent vegetative state
RA	rheumatoid arthritis
RAI	radioactive iodine
RBBB	right bundle branch block
RBC	red blood cell
RCA	right coronary artery
RCC	renal cell carcinoma
RCT	randomized controlled trial
RDS	respiratory distress syndrome
RDW	red cell distribution width
REM	rapid eye movement
RF	rheumatoid factor
RLQ	right lower quadrant
ROM	range of motion, rupture of membranes
RPR	rapid plasma reagin
RR	relative risk
RS	Reed-Sternberg (cell)
RSV	respiratory syncytial virus
RTA	renal tubular acidosis
RTI	reverse transcriptase inhibitor
RUQ	right upper quadrant
RV	residual volume
RVH	right ventricular hypertrophy
SAAG	serum-ascites albumin gradient
SAB	spontaneous abortion
SAH	subarachnoid hemorrhage
Sao_2	oxygen saturation in arterial blood
SARS	severe acute respiratory syndrome
SBO	small bowel obstruction
SBP	systolic blood pressure
SBS	shaken baby syndrome
SCC	squamous cell carcinoma
SCD	sickle cell disease
SCFE	slipped capital femoral epiphysis
SCID	severe combined immunodeficiency
SCLC	small cell lung cancer
SD	standard deviation
SE	status epilepticus
SES	socioeconomic status
SGLT	sodium-glucose transporter
SIADH	syndrome of inappropriate secretion of antidiuretic hormone
SIDS	sudden infant death syndrome
SIRS	systemic inflammatory response syndrome
SJS	Stevens-Johnson syndrome
SLE	systemic lupus erythematosus
SMA	superior mesenteric artery
SNRI	serotonin-norepinephrine reuptake inhibitor
SQ	subcutaneous
SRP	sponsoring residency program
SSRI	selective serotonin reuptake inhibitor

Abbreviation	Meaning
SSSS	staphylococcal scalded-skin syndrome
STD	sexually transmitted disease
STEMI	ST-elevation myocardial infarction
SVC	superior vena cava
SVT	supraventricular tachycardia
T_3	triiodothyronine
T_4	thyroxine
TAB	therapeutic abortion
TAH/BSO	total abdominal hysterectomy/bilateral salpingo-oophorectomy
TB	tuberculosis
TBG	thyroxine-binding globulin
TCA	tricyclic antidepressant
TEE	transesophageal echocardiography
TEF	tracheoesophageal fistula
TEN	toxic epidermal necrolysis
Th	T-helper
TFT	thyroid function test
TIA	transient ischemic attack
TIBC	total iron-binding capacity
TID	three times a day
TIMI	Thrombosis in Myocardial Infarction (study)
TLC	total lung capacity
TM	tympanic membrane
TMA	transcortical motor aphasia
TMJ	temporomandibular joint
TMP-SMX	trimethoprim-sulfamethoxazole
TMS	transcranial magnetic stimulation
TNF	tumor necrosis factor
TNM	tumor, node, metastasis (staging)
TOEFL	Test of English as a Foreign Language
ToRCHeS	toxoplasmosis, other agents, rubella, cytomegalovirus, herpes simplex
tPA	tissue plasminogen activator
TP-EIA	*Treponema pallidum* enzyme immunoassay
TPN	total parenteral nutrition
TPO	thyroid peroxidase
TP-PA	*Treponema pallidum* particle agglutination (test)
TRAP	tartrate-resistant acid phosphatase
TSA	transcortical sensory aphasia
TSH	thyroid-stimulating hormone
TSS	toxic shock syndrome
TSST	toxic shock syndrome toxin (S aureus toxin)
TTP	thrombotic thrombocytopenic purpura
TURP	transurethral resection of the prostate
TV	tidal volume
UA	urinalysis
UMN	upper motor neuron
URI	upper respiratory infection

Abbreviation	Meaning
USB	upper sternal border
USMLE	United States Medical Licensing Exam
USPSTF	United States Preventive Services Task Force
UTI	urinary tract infection
UV	ultraviolet
VA	Department of Veterans Affairs
VC	vital capacity
VCUG	voiding cystourethrography
VDRL	Venereal Disease Research Laboratory
VF	ventricular fibrillation
VIN	vulvar intraepithelial neoplasia
VIP	vasoactive intestinal peptide
VLDL	very low density lipoprotein

Abbreviation	Meaning
VMA	vanillylmandelic acid
VOC	vaso-occlusive crisis
VOR	vestibulo-ocular reflex
VP	ventriculoperitoneal
V/Q	ventilation/perfusion (scan)
VRSA	vancomycin-resistant *S aureus*
VSD	ventricular septal defect
VT	ventricular tachycardia
VUR	vesicoureteral reflux
vWD	von Willebrand disease
vWF	von Willebrand factor
VZV	varicella-zoster virus
WBC	white blood cell
WPW	Wolff-Parkinson-White

NOTES

COMMON LABORATORY VALUES

* = Included in the Biochemical Profile (SMA-12)

Blood, Plasma, Serum	Reference Range	SI Reference Intervals
* Alanine aminotransferase (ALT, GPT at 30°C)	8–20 U/L	8–20 U/L
Amylase, serum	25–125 U/L	25–125 U/L
* Aspartate aminotransferase (AST, GOT at 30°C)	8–20 U/L	8–20 U/L
Bilirubin, serum (adult)		
Total // Direct	0.1–1.0 mg/dL // 0.0–0.3 mg/dL	2–17 μmol/L // 0–5 μmol/L
* Calcium, serum (Total)	8.4–10.2 mg/dL	2.1–2.8 mmol/L
* Cholesterol, serum	140–250 mg/dL	3.6–6.5 mmol/L
* Creatinine, serum (Total)	0.6–1.2 mg/dL	53–106 μmol/L
* Electrolytes, serum		
Sodium	135–147 mEq/L	135–147 mmol/L
Chloride	95–105 mEq/L	95–105 mmol/L
Potassium	3.5–5.0 mEq/L	3.5–5.0 mmol/L
Bicarbonate	22–28 mEq/L	22–28 mmol/L
Gases, arterial blood (room air)		
P_{O_2}	75–105 mm Hg	10.0–14.0 kPa
P_{CO_2}	33–44 mm Hg	4.4–5.9 kPa
pH	7.35–7.45	[H+] 36–44 nmol/L
* Glucose, serum	Fasting: 70–110 mg/dL	3.8–6.1 mmol/L
	2-h postprandial: < 120 mg/dL	< 6.6 mmol/L
Growth hormone - arginine stimulation	Fasting: < 5 ng/mL	< 5 μg/L
	provocative stimuli: > 7 ng/mL	> 7 μg/L
Osmolality, serum	275–295 mOsm/kg	275–295 mOsm/kg
* Phosphatase (alkaline), serum (p-NPP at 30°C)	20–70 U/L	20–70 U/L
* Phosphorus (inorganic), serum	3.0–4.5 mg/dL	1.0–1.5 mmol/L
* Proteins, serum		
Total (recumbent)	6.0–7.8 g/dL	60–78 g/L
Albumin	3.5–5.5 g/dL	35–55 g/L
Globulins	2.3–3.5 g/dL	23–35 g/L
* Urea nitrogen, serum (BUN)	7–18 mg/dL	1.2–3.0 mmol urea/L
* Uric acid, serum	3.0–8.2 mg/dL	0.18–0.48 mmol/L
Cerebrospinal Fluid		
Glucose	40–70 mg/dL	2.2–3.9 mmol/L
Hematologic		
Erythrocyte count	Male: 4.3–5.9 million/mm³	$4.3\text{–}5.9 \times 10^{12}$/L
	Female: 3.5–5.5 million/mm³	$3.5\text{–}5.5 \times 10^{12}$/L
Hematocrit	Male: 41–53%	0.41–0.53
	Female: 36–46%	0.36–0.46
Hemoglobin, blood	Male: 13.5–17.5 g/dL	2.09–2.71 mmol/L
	Female: 12.0–16.0 g/dL	1.86–2.48 mmol/L

(continues)

Hematologic (continued)

Hemoglobin, plasma	1–4 mg/dL	0.16–0.62 µmol/L
Leukocyte count and differential		
Leukocyte count	4500–11,000/mm³	4.5–11.0 × 10⁹/L
Segmented neutrophils	54–62%	0.54–0.62
Band forms	3–5%	0.03–0.05
Eosinophils	1–3%	0.01–0.03
Basophils	0–0.75%	0–0.0075
Lymphocytes	25–33%	0.25–0.33
Monocytes	3–7%	0.03–0.07
Mean corpuscular hemoglobin	25.4–34.6 pg/cell	0.39–0.54 fmol/cell
Platelet count	150,000–400,000/mm³	150–400 × 10⁹/L
Prothrombin time	11–15 seconds	11–15 seconds
Reticulocyte count	0.5–1.5% of red cells	0.005–0.015
Sedimentation rate, erythrocyte	Male: 0–15 mm/h	0–15 mm/h
(Westergren)	Female: 0–20 mm/h	0–20 mm/h
Proteins, total	< 150 mg/24 h	< 0.15 g/24 h

Index